Intrapartum Management Modules

FOURTH EDITION

A Perinatal

Education

Program

Intrapartum Management Modules

FOURTH EDITION

A Perinatal Education Program

EDITORS

BETSY B. KENNEDY, RN, MSN

Assistant Professor
Vanderbilt University School of Nursing
Nashville, Tennessee

DONNA JEAN RUTH, RN, MSN

Clinical Learning Consultant
Nursing Education and Development
Vanderbilt University Medical Center
Nashville, Tennessee

E. JEAN MARTIN, RN, MS, MSN, CNM

Professor Emeritus
College of Nursing, Graduate Nurse-Midwifery
Medical University of South Carolina
Charleston, South Carolina

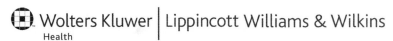
Wolters Kluwer | Lippincott Williams & Wilkins
Health

Philadelphia • Baltimore • New York • London
Buenos Aires • Hong Kong • Sydney • Tokyo

Senior Acquisitions Editor: Margaret Zuccarini
Managing Editor: Annette Ferran
Editorial Assistant: Brandi Spade
Production Project Manager: Cynthia Rudy
Director of Nursing Production: Helen Ewan
Senior Managing Editor / Production: Erika Kors
Design Coordinator: Holly Reid McLaughlin
Cover Designer: Bess Kiethas
Interior Designer: Lisa Delgado
Manufacturing Coordinator: Karin Duffield
Production Services / Compositor: Aptara, Inc.

4th edition

9 8 7 6 5 4 3 2 1

Printed in the United States of America

Library of Congress Cataloging-in-Publication Data

Intrapartum management modules : a perinatal education program / editors, Betsy B. Kennedy, Donna Jean Ruth, and E. Jean Martin. — 4th ed.
    p. ; cm.
  Includes bibliographical references and index.
  ISBN-13: 978-0-7817-8168-8 (alk. paper)
  ISBN-10: 0-7817-8168-X (alk. paper)
 1. Maternity nursing—Programmed instruction. 2. Labor (Obstetrics)—Programmed instruction. 3. Delivery (Obstetrics)—Programmed instruction. I. Kennedy, Betsy B. II. Ruth, Donna Jean. III. Martin, E. Jean (Elizabeth Jean)
  [DNLM: 1. Labor, Obstetric—Programmed Instruction. 2. Delivery, Obstetric—nursing—Programmed Instruction. 3. Maternal-Child Nursing—methods—Programmed Instruction. 4. Prenatal Care—methods—Programmed Instruction. WY 18.2 I61 2009]
  RG951.I57 2009
  618.407—dc22

                                                        2008004767

LWW.com

This edition continues to be dedicated to you, the reader, who in rendering care touches not only the body, but perhaps the soul. On behalf of the mothers and babies you care for in a knowledgeable, safe, and sensitive manner—"thank you."

CONTRIBUTORS

Julie M. Arafeh, RNC, MSN
Perinatal Outreach Coordinator
Assistant Director of the Center for Advanced Pediatric
    and Perinatal Education
Stanford University
Palo Alto, California

Suzanne McMurtry Baird
Assistant Professor
Vanderbilt University School of Nursing
Nashville, Tennessee

Sarah Branan, MSN, RN
Registered Nurse
Greenville Hospital System University Medical Center
Greenville, South Carolina

Angel Carter, MSN, APRN, NNP
Coordinator Neonatal Follow-Up Clinic
Monroe Carell, Jr. Children's Hospital at Vanderbilt
Nashville, Tennessee

Susan Drummond, RN, MSN
Assistant in Obstetrics
Vanderbilt University Medical Center
Nashville, Tennessee

Elizabeth Fritz, RN, MSN
Nurse Educator, Labor and Delivery
Vanderbilt University Medical Center
Nashville, Tennessee

Kelly Gee, MSN, RNC, WHNP
Clinical Nurse Practitioner
Morgan Stanley Children's Hospital of New York
Presbyterian Columbia University Medical Center
New York, New York

Mary Jo Gilmer, PhD, MBA, RN
Professor and Director, Clinical Management Program
Co-Director, Pediatric Advanced Comfort Team
Vanderbilt University School of Nursing
Nashville, Tennessee

Marcella T. Hickey, RN, MSN, CNM
Professor Emeritus
Graduate Nurse–Midwifery, College of Nursing
Medical University of South Carolina
Charleston, South Carolina

Elizabeth Howard, CNM, PhD
Clinical Teaching Associate
Brown Medical School
Providence, Rhode Island

Anne Moore, MSN, RNC, FAANP
Professor of Nursing/Women's Health Nurse Practitioner
Vanderbilt University School of Nursing
Nashville, Tennessee

Mary Copeland Myers, CNM, MSN, CDE
Instructor
University of South Carolina, Upstate
Spartanburg, South Carolina

Judith H. Poole, PhD, RNC
Nurse Manager, Birthing Care/Special Maternity Care
Presbyterian Hospital
Charlotte, North Carolina

Erin Rodgers, RN, BSN, MSN
Instructor
Vanderbilt University School of Nursing
Nashville, Tennessee

Nancy Webster Smith, RN, MSN, CNM
Nurse-Midwife
Mt. Pleasant, South Carolina

Francilla Thomas, RNC, MSN, EFMC
Clinical Nurse III
Morgan Stanley Children's Hospital of New York
Presbyterian Columbia University Medical Center
New York, New York

Penny Spencer Waugh, MSN, RNC
Clinical Instructor, Clinical Liaison
Vanderbilt University School of Nursing
Nashville, Tennessee

Ann Mogabgab Weathersby, RN, MSN, CNM
Assistant Manager of Obstetrics and Gynecology
Piedmont Practice Service Director
Kaiser Permanente
Atlanta, Georgia

Kimberly Yeager, RN, BSN
Director of Training and Research
Center for Advanced Pediatric and Perinatal Education
Stanford University
Palo Alto, California

REVIEWERS

Carol Abrahams, RN, MS
Perinatal Clinical Nurse Specialist
California Pacific Medical Center
San Francisco, California

Joanne E. Foresman, RNC, MSN
Nurse Clinician
St. John's Mercy Medical Center
St. Louis, Missouri

Ann C. Holden, RN, BScN, MSc, PNC
Manager, Family Birthing Center and Childbirth
and Parenting Services
St. Joseph's Health Center
Toronto, Ontario

Mary Lou Moore, PhD, RNC, FACCE, FAAN
Associate Professor, Department of Obstetrics
and Gynecology
Wake Forest University School of Medicine
Winston-Salem, North Carolina

Virginia Bradford Pearson, RN, MSN
Maternal–Child Nursing Instructor
Ellisville, Mississippi

Kathleen Simpson, PhD, RNC, FAAN
Perinatal Clinical Nurse Specialist
St. John's Mercy Medical Center
St. Louis, Missouri

FOREWORD

This book would not exist without the foresight and leadership of Henry C. Heins, Jr., MD, MPH. Dr. Heins initiated the original perinatal outreach program for South Carolina, and writing for that program began. Members of the Department of Pediatrics, University Health Sciences Center, Charlottesville, Virginia, pioneered one of the first self-instructional perinatal outreach programs in the United States. They generously granted permission for the use of their highly successful text format, style, and program plan on which this book, in its several editions, is based. Their program on maternal, fetal, and newborn evaluation and care continues to be updated and available. Components of the program and a web address constitute a "resource of note" that is highly recommended for all users of this book: Kattwinkel, J., Cook, L. J., Hurt, H., Nowacek, G. A., Short, S. G., & Crosby, W. M. (2007), *Perinatal Continuing Education Program.* The Maternal and Fetal set (2 books) and related products were developed by the University of Virginia and leading perinatal medicine experts. To obtain information or to order, visit the AAP Bookstore at www.aap.org.

Dr. Faith J. Hohloch, BSN, MA, EdD, Professor of Nursing, Ret., has. . . "read the book". . . as she proofed every word! I am so grateful for these insightful eyes!

The research, theory, and practice base of perinatal care is ever-evolving. Betsy Kennedy and Donna Ruth have graciously, with extraordinary efficiency and competency, undertaken revisions to the third edition to bring you this fourth edition. I acknowledge my gratitude and confidence in the "new team."

E. Jean Martin, RN, MS, MSN, CNM

PREFACE

While the phenomenon of birth has not changed, our knowledge base continues to expand. The clinical issues facing those who provide intrapartum care are becoming increasingly complex. Providing "best" care for women and their families during childbearing involves being clinically safe, accurate, therapeutic, and sensitive to individual needs. Earning and maintaining this kind of competency is not easy. You must be educated, updated, and motivated. It is our hope that this text helps you with all three.

In this fourth edition of *Intrapartum Management Modules*, each module has been updated with great care to reflect "best practices" and current evidence. Trends and issues in care have been presented. An introduction to cultural competence in caring for women during the intrapartum period is now included in the Overview of Labor module. The Intrapartum Fetal Monitoring module has been extensively revised to reflect the NICHD nomenclature. The discussion of liability issues in the intrapartum period has been expanded to address the most commonly litigated areas and strategies to avoid malpractice claims. New modules, including Intimate Partner Violence, Operative and Assisted Births, and Intrapartum Emergencies, have been added to better address the challenges caregivers may face in the intrapartum period. The appendices have also undergone extensive revision.

Great care has been taken to ensure that the drugs and treatments presented in the text are accurate at the time of publication. However, technology and knowledge expand exponentially with every passing day. With each revision we will continue to update content so that it best reflects current practice.

The focus of this book has always been on perinatal care in the intrapartum period and will continue to be so. The topics covered should be pertinent for anyone working in an intrapartum setting, primarily staff nurses, but also nurse midwives, nurse practitioners, family practice physicians, physician assistants, and nursing and medical students. This book is not intended to replace standard texts, but rather used as a self-paced, self-instructional manual. The material is presented along with pertinent skills and practice/review questions. Posttests with answers are included for validation of your comprehension of the material. If you are using this text as an adjunct to unit orientation, the modules should be completed within the orientation period, usually 12 weeks.

Remember that your care during the intrapartum period has profound effects upon the woman and her family. You will be remembered for your interactions, and perhaps preserved on film or in digital images for the family to look at again and again. But as Jean has stated, "the dynamics of such interactions work both ways . . . the gratitude is ours for being allowed to participate in one of life's most incredible events!"

Betsy B. Kennedy, RN, MSN
Donna Jean Ruth, RN, MSN

ACKNOWLEDGMENTS

We have often commented during the revision of this text that the process is akin to giving birth. To undertake such a project is exciting, daunting, a little frightening, and more work than you ever thought possible, but ultimately richly rewarding.

We are incredibly blessed and grateful to have inherited such a fine work from Jean Martin. She has created a text and an informational "voice" that is well loved by those caring for women during this unique time. We have heard from many that they relied on the text during their training and education, as evidenced by the worn appearance, dog-eared pages, and markings in the margins. Jean has seen the text through three editions and was an integral part of this one as well, sharing her wisdom, experience, and editorial skills! We know how much of herself she has shared in her dedication to this work and thank her for the opportunity to continue the tradition.

We gratefully acknowledge all past contributors to the text and thank all the new contributors for sharing their expertise and time. They are valued friends, colleagues, and experts from across the country.

The beautiful image on the cover was created by Lana Feole. Thank you for taking a very inarticulate expression of our vision and turning it into a perfect representation of our feelings and the content of this text. Many thanks to Will Gustafson for being the technical mastermind who assisted in transmission of the image.

The editorial staff at Wolters Kluwer Health | Lippincott Williams & Wilkins extended to us great patience, kindness, and support throughout this process. Their guidance and reassurance were helpful beyond measure. We thank everyone who worked on the text, for without them it would not be in your hands.

We would also like to thank the Vanderbilt University Medical Center Labor and Delivery Unit and the Vanderbilt University School of Nursing. Again, their support for our work on this project was essential in its completion.

Last, but most important, a heartfelt thank you to our families and friends for their love and support as we were away from them, working to meet deadlines and maintain the standard of excellence set by the previous editions.

Betsy B. Kennedy, RN, MSN
Donna Jean Ruth, RN, MSN

CONTENTS

MODULE

1

Overview of Labor

E. JEAN MARTIN ■ BETSY B. KENNEDY

Objectives

As you complete this module, you will learn:

1. Current theories and concepts on labor physiology and initiation
2. The stages of labor
3. The anatomic divisions of the uterus undergoing labor
4. Characteristics and terms used to describe uterine contractions
5. Characteristics of normal uterine contractions
6. Appropriate timing of vaginal examination to evaluate cervical dilatation
7. Techniques for evaluating uterine contractions
8. Effective ways to support the laboring woman
9. A definition of cultural competence and characteristics of a culturally competent practitioner
10. Questions to be used for a cultural assessment tool

Key Terms

When you have completed this module, you should be able to recall the meaning of the following terms. You should also be able to use the terms when consulting with other health professionals. The terms are defined in this module or in the glossary at the end of this book.

cervix
contraction
corticotropin-releasing factor (CRF)
cultural competence
cytokines
decidua
endogenous

gap junctions
macrophages
parturition
placenta
progesterone
prostaglandins

Labor and Birth: A Medical View

Identifying Features of Labor

▶ **What is labor?**

Labor can be defined medically as regular, progressively intense uterine contractions that, over time, produce cervical effacement and dilatation, leading to the development of expulsive forces adequate to move the fetus through the birth canal against the resistance of soft tissue, muscle, and the bony structure of the pelvis.

NOTE: *Uterine contractions in the absence of cervical change is not labor.*

A number of biochemical, physiologic, and pharmacologic pathways are thought to exist; it is through these pathways that term labor is initiated and maintained. The exact mechanism for the onset and maintenance of labor has not yet been fully revealed. Improved experimental laboratory techniques and increasingly sophisticated research approaches *in humans* are leading to better understanding of the numerous hormonal interactions in human labor and birth; however, these are processes that are not able to be directly investigated.

> Ancient civilizations believed that the fetus was delivered head first so that it could kick its legs against the top of the uterus and propel itself through the birth canal![1]

There is no doubt that, under hormonal influences, the uterus is maintained in a quiescent state throughout most of pregnancy. Certainly, a dramatic physiologic change is involved in taking a pregnancy from the state of relatively low-level antepartum uterine contractility to the coordinated, intense uterine contractility of labor. However, rather than an active process initiated by uterine stimulants, labor may be promoted as a result of the removal of the inhibitory effects of pregnancy on the myometrium.[1] In addition, there is substantial evidence from the research that indicates the fetus plays an important role in the timing of labor. In fact, there may be a "parturition cascade" that involves the fetus, the mother, and the placenta.[1]

Labor Initiation and Maintenance

- During quiescence, the uterus is maintained by inhibitors such as progesterone, prostacyclin, relaxin, nitric oxide, adrenomedullin, and other substances.
- In the weeks and days before term, all parts of the uterus undergo preparation for labor and delivery (*parturition*).[2]
- Hormonal mediators from the placenta and maternal and fetal endocrine glands are believed to effect the regulation of the uterine musculature (myometrium).
- In pregnancy the lining of the uterus (the endometrium) is referred to as the *decidua*. Experiencing marked change in thickness and vascularity, the decidua has the capacity to alter hormonal proportions (e.g., estrogen increases over progesterone content) and enzymes and to nourish the embryo. Special decidual cells called macrophages synthesize prostaglandins and another group of compounds called cytokines.[3]
- Direct tissue-to-tissue communication occurs among uterine musculature, the decidua, and fetal membranes.[3]
- The uterine myometrium consists of thick and thin contractile fibers grouped in bundles. Few intracellular contacts between them exist until late in pregnancy. At that time, areas between muscle fiber cells develop pathways for communication (cell to cell). These pathways are called gap junctions. They are clearly present in great numbers as parturition nears. These efficient cell-to-cell gap junctions serve as channels for the transfer of chemical and electrical signals from one muscle fiber cell to another. Simultaneous contractions of a majority of cells are needed to make an effective contraction. This synchronization of the uterine muscle fibers leads to efficient, coordinated *contractions,* which soften, thin, and dilate the cervix.[2]
- A placental hormone called *corticotropin-releasing factor (CRF)* is released into maternal circulation early in the second trimester, with concentrations rising significantly as pregnancy advances. CRF production increases the strength of contractions and stimulates production of oxytocin and prostaglandins.[4]
- *Prostaglandins* are chemicals derived from the fetus, amniotic membranes, decidua, and other sources. These prostaglandins, particularly PGF and PGE_2, cause smooth muscle contraction and vasoconstriction, soften ("ripen") cervical tissue, and modulate hormonal activity.[3,5]
- *Cytokines* are an important group of compounds. These compounds have numerous functions in labor physiology, which act either synergistically or antagonistically.
- Calcium (the calcium ion) is vital for the contractile process in myometrial cells, which depends on the influx of extracellular free calcium. The calcium ion also plays a critical role in transmitting signals of excitation from the myometrial cell membranes to the contractile complex inside the cell.[2]

NOTE: *Agents that block this movement of calcium, called calcium channel blockers (e.g., nifedipine), are in fact used as tocolytic agents for the purpose of suppressing uterine contractility.*

- Once the uterus has been prepared, myometrial activity may be initiated by the fetoplacental unit and the mother, through the secretion of hormones and mechanical stretch of the uterus.[1]
- The nonpregnant or very early gravid uterus is not sensitive to oxytocin. However, oxytocin is secreted in pulses of low frequency throughout pregnancy.[2]
- As the uterus gradually approaches term, it is thought that the myometrium becomes increasingly responsive to oxytocic hormones, mainly PGE and PGF. Toward the end of pregnancy, the number of oxytocin receptors increases, peaking in the myometrium and decidua in early labor.
- Secretion of oxytocin seems to be in a pulsatile fashion, even in labor[2] (Figures 1.1 and 1.2.
- Maternal plasma concentrations of endogenous oxytocin are equivalent to a range of 4 to 6 mU/min during the first stage of labor.[6]

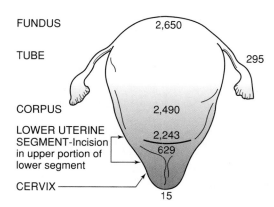

FIGURE 1.1 Distribution of oxytocin receptors in a pregnant human uterus, removed in preterm labor at 34 weeks. Numbers denote oxytocin receptors (OTRs) per unit measurement (fmol/mg DNA). (Reprinted with permission from Fuchs, A. R., & Fuchs, R. [1996]. Physiology and endocrinology of parturition. In S. G. Gabbe, J. R. Niebyl, & J. L. Simpson [Eds.]. *Obstetrics: Normal and problem pregnancies* [3rd ed., p. 123]. New York: Churchill Livingstone.)

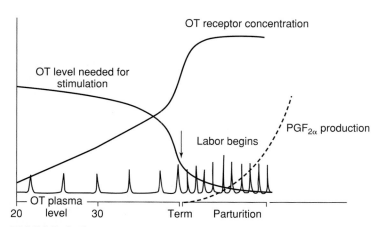

FIGURE 1.2 Diagrammatic representation of the concentration of myometrial oxytocin, the level of oxytocin needed to elicit contractions, and maternal plasma oxytocin levels at the end of gestation and during labor. Oxytocin is secreted in pulses of low frequency. During labor, pulse frequency increases. Fetal secretion of oxytocin can be considerable and may contribute to the oxytocin level reaching the myometrium. PGF production does not increase significantly until labor is in progress and then increases progressively throughout the third stage of labor. OT, oxytocin. (Reprinted with permission from Fuchs, A. R., & Fuchs, R. [1996]. Physiology and endocrinology of parturition. In S. G. Gabbe, J. R. Niebyl, & J. L. Simpson [Eds.]. *Obstetrics: Normal and problem pregnancies* [3rd ed., p. 124]. New York: Churchill Livingstone.)

Identifying Stages and Phases of Labor

▶ **How are the parts of the labor process described?[1-4]**

For the sake of description, labor is divided into the following four stages:

Stage I   Stage I begins with the onset of regular uterine contractions and lasts until full dilatation of the cervix is achieved. Dilatation is the *gradual opening of the cervical entrance* to the uterus. Stage I can be divided further into *two phases,* which are predictable in normal labor.

Latent phase—begins with fairly regular contractions until rapid cervical dilatation begins. It usually lasts several hours, but duration is variable.

Active phase—begins with rapid cervical dilatation and lasts until full dilatation of the cervix occurs. It usually begins around 2 to 4 cm dilatation.

Stage II   Stage II begins with full cervical dilatation (10 cm) and lasts until the baby is born. During this phase, the presenting part of the fetus descends through the maternal pelvis. Stage II may be accompanied by an increase in bloody show, feelings of pressure in the rectum, nausea and vomiting, and desire to push or bear down.

Stage III   Stage III is that part of the process after the birth of the baby during which the placenta is delivered.

Stage IV   Stage IV is that part of the process after the delivery of the placenta in which the uterus effectively contracts, preventing excessive bleeding. This is a period of adjustment as the mother's body functions begin to stabilize.

> Careful assessment of the laboring woman's progress through this predictable pattern can be helpful in early detection of problems.

Evaluating Contractions

▶ **How is the uterus suited to accomplish labor and birth?**

The uterus is composed of *three* layers of tissue. These layers are arranged as shown in Figure 1.3.

1. **Perimetrium**—a thick outer membrane covering the uterus.
2. **Myometrium**—the middle layer that contains special muscle cells called myometrial cells.
3. **Endometrium**—the innermost layer containing glands and nutrient tissue.

Figure 1.4 illustrates the changes in the uterus and cervix as normal labor progresses.

Under the influence of myometrial contractions, labor progresses with the uterus becoming separated into *two distinct parts.* The upper portion becomes *thicker* and more powerful because of shortening and thickening of the myometrial fibers. This prepares the uterus to exert the effort necessary to push the baby out at birth. The lower portion of the uterus becomes *thinner, softer, and more relaxed* as the myometrial fibers relax and become longer. As a result, the baby can more easily be pushed out at birth.

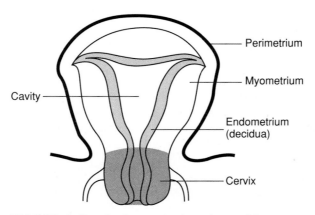

NOTE: The endometrium is altered through hormonal influences during pregnancy to become what is called the decidua, which functions to maintain the pregnancy.

FIGURE 1.3   The three major tissue layers of the uterus.

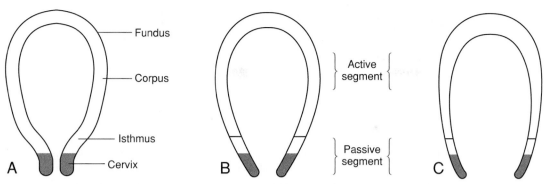

FIGURE 1.4 Changes in the uterus and cervix as normal labor progresses. **A.** Uterus and cervix at term. **B.** Uterus and cervix early in stage I. **C.** Uterus and cervix in stage II.

Downward pressure caused by the contraction of the fundal segment is gradually transmitted to the passive lower segment or cervical portion, causing effacement (thinning of the cervix) and dilatation. The cervix is drawn upward and over the baby, allowing the baby to descend into the passageway. The cervix is made up of an inner part called the internal os and an outer part called the external os. Figure 1.5 demonstrates how the internal and external os change position as effacement occurs.

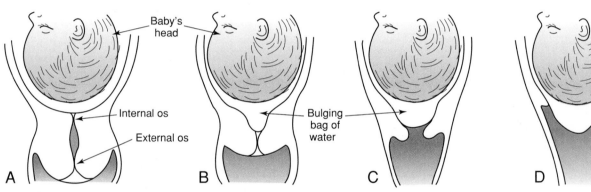

FIGURE 1.5 **A.** Cervix before effacement begins. **B.** Effacement in its early phase. **C.** Effacement with some dilatation. **D.** Complete effacement and dilatation.

▶ How are uterine contractions described?

Contractions have a wavelike pattern that can be divided into segments (Fig. 1.6).

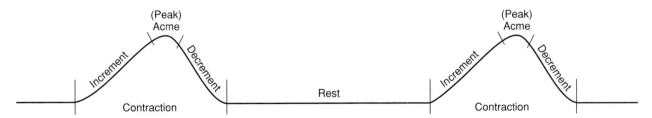

FIGURE 1.6 The segments of a contraction.

- Increment—usually makes up the *longest* part of the contraction.
- Acme—the *shortest,* but most intense, part of the contraction.
- Decrement—a fairly rapid diminishing of the contraction.

Four characteristics of a contraction have been identified:
1. **Frequency**—This is how often the contractions are occurring. Contractions can begin 10 to 15 minutes apart, but get closer together as labor progresses. They can occur as frequently as 2 to 3 minutes apart late in the labor process. It is important to remember that the frequency of contractions does not reflect the intensity.

2. **Regularity**—As labor becomes well established, contractions occur with a rhythmic pattern.
3. **Duration**—The length of contractions increases as labor progresses. Contractions in early labor can be as short as 30 seconds and gradually increase to as long as 90 seconds.
4. **Intensity**—This characteristic can be assessed as mild, moderate, or strong. The strength of contractions increases as labor intensifies. Other variables that affect the intensity (strength) of contractions include parity, the condition of the cervix, pain medication, and the use of exogenous oxytocin. To obtain an estimate of the intensity, you can palpate the mother's abdomen with your hand. A true assessment of the contraction's intensity can be obtained only by using an internal uterine monitor, which is described in detail in Module 6.

NOTE: In normal labor, *the intensity (or amplitude) of the contraction varies from 30 to 55 mmHg and the frequency is two to five contractions every 10 minutes. During the second stage of labor, peak intensity of contractions may reach 65 mmHg. In prolonged labor, the intensity of the contractions is less than 25 mmHg and the frequency is fewer than two contractions every 10 minutes.* No labor is occurring if the intensity is less than 15 mmHg.

Montevideo units may be measured with the use of an internal pressure monitor to determine "adequate" labor. This is discussed further in Module 6.

The duration and frequency of a contraction can be diagrammed as in Figure 1.7.

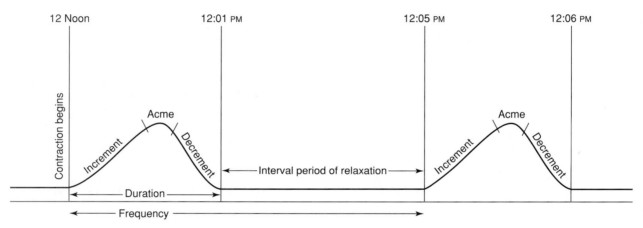

FIGURE 1.7   Frequency and duration of contractions.

Notice that the duration of a contraction is timed from the beginning of the increment to the end of the decrement. The frequency of a contraction is timed from the beginning of one contraction to the beginning of the next.

Although the interval between contractions is referred to as a period of relaxation, in fact, the uterus never entirely relaxes between contractions. It maintains what is called a resting tone, a result of increased tension and thickening of muscle fibers in the upper portion of the uterus. Contractions are assessed in three basic ways:

1. **Subjectively**—This is a description given by the patient. She will respond to questions such as "When did they start?" "How often are they coming?" "How long do they last?" and "Are they getting stronger?"
2. **Palpation**—This is an efficient method of assessment using the palmar surface of the fingertips. Fingertips should be kept moving throughout the contraction to continually palpate the changing uterus through the abdominal wall (Figure 1.8).

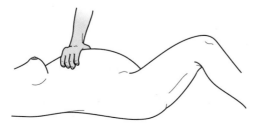

FIGURE 1.8   Palm or surface of the fingers palpates for intensity and duration of a contraction.

The intensity of the uterine contraction can be described as follows:
- Mild—The uterus can be indented with gentle pressure.
- Moderate—The uterus indents only with firm pressure at the peak of a contraction.
- Strong—The uterus feels firm or hard and cannot be indented at the peak of a contraction.

Your moving fingertips pick up the changes within a contraction as it gains in intensity and then recedes. Do this carefully so that you do not cause discomfort to the laboring woman.

3. **Electronic fetal monitoring**—This type of fetal monitoring can be either external or internal. The external method involves the use of electronic equipment that measures and records the frequency and duration of contractions. The intensity of contractions can be truly measured only with the internal method. True representation of heart rate variability is obtained only with the internal method (fetal spiral electrode).

If you are assessing contractions, it is suggested that you sit at the bedside for 20 to 40 minutes (depending on the general frequency of contractions), with your fingertips lightly placed over the fundal portion of the mother's abdomen. This enables you to detect accurately the beginning and end of the contraction. You cannot depend on signals from the mother—such as restlessness or a statement that the contraction is beginning—because she is often unaware of the initial changes in the uterine muscle.

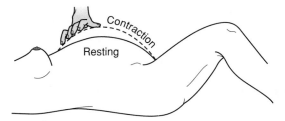

When feeling for the general intensity and duration of a contraction, the best area of the mother's abdomen on which to place your fingertips is near the top of the uterus (Figure 1.9).

FIGURE 1.9 The palpating fingers are placed near the top of the uterus.

The reason for placing your fingertips near the top of the uterus is that the uterus has pacemakers located there. These pacemakers are a group of highly excitable myometrial cells that are responsible for starting contractions (Figure 1.10). They are located on either side of the uterus near the oviducts or fallopian tubes: *The contraction begins at the top of the uterus and sweeps down over the main body of the uterus.*

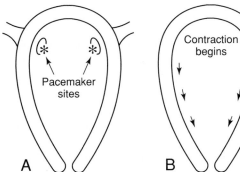
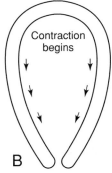

FIGURE 1.10 **A.** Sites where the uterine contraction begins (pacemaker sites). **B.** Contraction pathway.

Each contraction wave has three components:

1. **Propagation** of the wave starts at the pacemaker site. The wave starts above and moves downward toward the lower part of the uterus.
2. **Duration** of the contraction lessens progressively as the wave moves away from the pacemaker. Throughout any contraction the upper portion of the uterus is in action for a longer period than the lower portion.
3. **Intensity** of the contraction decreases from the top to the bottom of the uterus; that is, the upper segment of the uterus contracts more strongly than the lower.

NOTE: Analysis of wave properties of the uterine contraction indicates that the full impact of the contraction is not felt at the cervix until the last half of the contraction.

Vaginal examination to determine cervical dilatation should be performed throughout a contraction and not between contractions. The woman should be prepared for this and helped to understand why the examination is done during a contraction. It is imperative that the examiner also understand the rationale. Vaginal examinations between contractions in actively laboring women do not always provide a true picture of what is happening to the cervix. Vaginal examinations during labor are discussed in Module 5.

To obtain a true assessment of contraction length and frequency, carefully palpate the abdomen for at least 30 minutes.

NOTE: When using electronic uterine and fetal monitoring, always palpate uterine contractions and auscultate maternal and fetal heart rates in the first few minutes of using the equipment and periodically throughout labor. This validates that the equipment is working properly.

Labor and Birth: Reflections From a Different View

"Birth is not only about making babies. Birth is also about making mothers—strong, competent, capable mothers who trust themselves and know their inner strength."[7]

The experience of pregnancy and childbirth, although shared with husbands or partners, is uniquely female. It is life altering, one of nature's most powerful events. The manner in which a woman experiences birth has profound implications, possibly affecting the quality of her immediate infant interaction and subsequent parenting. Research shows that childbirth affects a woman's self-esteem and can also affect her emotional availability to her infant.[8]

McKay[9] maintains that the birth setting and its participants powerfully influence the childbirth experience, shaping roles and the amount of control held by the woman herself, those who support her, and her caregivers. McKay goes on to state, "The outcome can be an environment of support, enabling the woman to experience her power and control or, at the opposite end of the spectrum, [the result is] managed birth where the principal actors are the caregivers, their procedures, and technology" (p. 283). Supporting the woman and her family in any birth setting, through any type of birth, and providing sensitive care is the nurse's privilege and honor.

Supporting the Laboring Woman

Effective labor support involves the following:
- A thorough understanding of the physiologic and anatomic adaptations involved in labor and birth.
- Compassion for the enormous but individualized adaptive responses required on the part of the woman and her family in the birth process.

- Knowledge of the woman's (and her support person's) preparation, understanding, and goals for the birth experience.
- Commitment to provide continuous support for the woman and her family and to work at facilitating this philosophy of care on the birth unit.

> The continuous presence of a support person reduces the likelihood of medication for pain relief, operative vaginal delivery, cesarean delivery, and a 5-minute Apgar score of less than 7.[10]

It is important to remember that families today are diverse in nature. The mother's primary support person may be her husband, a male partner, a female relative, a female partner, or even a male partner who is not the father of the baby.[11] The mother is the only one who can determine who is important to her, and who she wants to support her during this experience.[11] Respect the mother's preferences and needs in support of the family.

Ongoing efforts are directed at making birthing units in hospitals more family centered, homelike, and baby friendly. The World Health Organization has promoted the Baby-Friendly Hospital Initiative, urging hospitals worldwide to be baby friendly by giving support to breast-feeding. However, much more current research and understanding of babies, their intimate relationship with their mothers, and their developmental life in the womb (i.e., in cognitive, sensory, and emotional dimensions) need to be embraced and applied to 21st century obstetric practices.[12]

> "Babies are not what we thought they were in the 19th century or even what we thought they were twenty-five years ago.... The finding's of psychology are so revolutionary that virtually everything we believed a quarter of a century ago has been discredited and a new encyclopedia of knowledge has been written" (p. 127).[13]

Chamberlain has conducted extensive research and written about prenatal and newborn clinical findings for years.[13,14] He believes that a new paradigm for a new view of babies, both the newborn and unborn, is in order, stating that "babies of whatever age are aware, expressive, and affected by their interactions with us." (p. 130)[13] This is important information for everyone who has a role in birthing and caring for babies: nurses, physicians, midwives, practitioners, childbirth educators, and parents.

The Coalition for Improving Maternity Services has outlined steps for mother-friendly care and examined evidence based support for each of the steps. The Coalition is part of a global effort to promote normal childbirth and promote care that is "mother friendly." Foundations for this initiative include the following[15]:

- Birth is a normal, healthy, natural process that may take place in a variety of settings, including homes, birth centers and hospitals.
- Women should be empowered and confident in their ability to give birth and care for their new baby. The encounters and experiences that occur during this time may have profound and long-lasting effects.
- Every woman should have the opportunity to have a positive birth experience in her choice of setting. Her personal preferences, well-being, right to information and autonomy, and privacy should be respected.
- Interventions should not be routinely applied. Any necessary interventions should be based on the most up-to-date, quality evidence.
- Caregivers are responsible for the quality of care provided. Individuals (mothers and their families) are responsible for making informed choices about their health care.

It may be a challenge for caregivers, and even women, to trust birth; however, it should be the goal of all who provide care to protect, promote and support the process.[15]

> It is something to be able to paint a particular picture, or to carve a statue, and so to make a few objects beautiful; but it is far more glorious to carve and paint the very atmosphere and medium through which we look, which morally we can do. To affect the quality of the day, that is the highest of the arts.
>
> —Henry David Thoreau, *Walden*

9

Specific practices that provide support for the laboring woman, her unborn baby, and her coach include the following:

1. Assist women in the transition from home to the hospital.
   - Recognize that this is a vulnerable time and the mother may not know the "right" time to arrive at the birth setting, hospital, or birthing center.[16]
   - Welcome the mother into the new environment.
2. *Make the mother and her unborn baby the central focus in the situation* and include her coach through all phases of labor and birth.
   - Introduce yourself and others who might be providing care.
   - Inform the mother and her coach of her progress.
   - Include the mother and her coach in conversations with others.
   - Offer choices when possible.
   - Actively support the coach in his or her efforts to help the mother.
   - Think of the unborn baby as a sensing, responsive, and social being as you give care. Use touch, sound, and light as soothing, even therapeutic, elements.
3. Ensure the mother's privacy.
   - Try to provide a private labor room.
   - Orient the mother to her surroundings.
   - Keep the mother draped adequately.
   - Request the mother's permission for procedures and examinations and keep her coach updated and involved.
   - Control the environment according to the mother's wishes (e.g., a darkened or bright room, open or closed door, quiet atmosphere).
4. Promote preparedness.
   - Assess the mother's knowledge level and preparedness. Give information about labor and birth that addresses where she is in labor. Use simple, direct terminology appropriate to her level of understanding and ability to take it in at the time. Orient the mother and coach to the expected time frame for labor. Update this as necessary.
   - Instruct the mother and coach in relaxation, breathing, and pushing techniques. For mothers who have attended classes, these techniques might need to be reviewed. Give brief, practical instructions to the unprepared mother.
5. Instill confidence.
   - Praise the efforts of the mother and her coach.
   - Speak positively about labor and delivery events. For example, when giving a sedative, tell the mother that the medication will help her to relax.
   - Stay with the mother if she is without a coach. If you must leave her for a brief time, tell her why and when you will return.
   - Provide a call light or buzzer when you are out of the room.
   - Inform the mother and coach in advance of special procedures or examinations.
   - Use vocabulary that is suited to the needs of the mother and coach and ensure that they understand.
   - Encourage a family member to remain with the mother throughout labor and include this person in your explanations and care. Remember, coaches need reassurance too.
6. Apply culturally competent care to each woman and family.

▶ What is culturally competent care?

Perinatal care is often directed to women and families from diverse cultures; 1 in every 10 people in the United States is an immigrant.[17] Major cultural groups in the United States include African Americans/blacks, American Indians/Alaska Natives, Asian Americans/Pacific Islanders, Hispanics/Latinos, and whites/Caucasians. The majority of these immigrants are women and for many of them the first exposure to health care may be maternity care.[18] These women and their families approach childbirth within their cultural context, that is, a set of core values, cultural beliefs, and practices. It is essential to provide care that is sensitive, responsive, and individualized.[18] Without cultural knowledge, delivery of appropriate, respectful care is difficult.[19]

Cultural competence is generally considered a process of developing cultural awareness, cultural knowledge, cultural skill, cultural encounters, and cultural desire.[20] It is the motivation of the care provider that initiates the process. Providing care in a culturally competent manner is a progressive and developmental, but conscious, process that should be a focus for the clinically competent care provider.

Cultural competence is further described by Rorie, Paine, and Barger[21] as a set of behaviors, attitudes, and policies that enable a system, agency, and/or individual to function effectively with culturally diverse patients and communities. Groups might also include the homeless, migrants, refugees, or same sex couples. These authors go on to outline traits that identify the culturally competent practitioner (Display 1.1).

| **DISPLAY 1.1** | CHARACTERISTICS OF THE CULTURALLY COMPETENT PRACTITIONER |

Moves from cultural unawareness to an awareness of and sensitivity to own cultural heritage.
Recognizes own values and biases and is aware of how he or she may effect patients from other cultures.
Demonstrates comfort with cultural differences that exist between self and patients.
Knows specifics about the particular cultural group(s) with which he or she works.
Understands the historical events that may have caused harm to particular cultural groups.
Respects and is aware of the unique needs of patients from diverse communities.
Understands the importance of diversity within as well as between cultures.
Endeavors to learn more about cultural communities through patient interactions, participation in cultural diversity workshops and community events, readings on cultural dynamics, and consultations with community experts.
Makes a continuous effort to understand the other's point of view.
Demonstrates flexibility and tolerance of ambiguity; is nonjudgmental.
Maintains a sense of humor and an open mind.
Demonstrates a willingness to relinquish control in clinical encounters; to risk failure; and to look within for the source of frustration, anger, and resistance.
Acknowledges that the process is as important as the product.

Adapted with permission from Rorie, J. L., Paine, L. L., & Barger, M. K. (1996). Cultural competence in primary care services. *Journal of Nurse Midwifery, 41*(2), 99.

Many birth units are developing cultural assessment tools focusing on cultural practices unique to childbirth to be used for bedside assessment. The use of a tool ensures consistency in that all patients are asked the same questions. Questions to consider for a cultural assessment tool[17]:

- Where were you born?
- How long have you lived in the United States?
- Who are your major support people?
- What languages do you speak and read?
- What are your religious practices?
- What are your food preferences?
- What is your economic situation?
- What does childbearing represent to you?
- How do you view childbearing?
- Are there any maternal precautions or restrictions?
- Is birth a private or social experience?
- How would you like to manage labor pain?
- Who will provide labor support?
- Who will care for the baby?
- Do you use contraception?

It is important to ask these questions in a conversational, nonjudgmental tone.[17] Open-ended questions should be used. If the mother does not speak English, then an interpreter should be used if available. The use of a female interpreter is best; remember too that a member of the mother's family, especially another child, should not be used as an interpreter. Address questions to the mother, not the interpreter, in short, but clear sentences.

The care of the laboring woman is addressed further in Module 5.

PRACTICE/REVIEW QUESTIONS

After reviewing this module, answer the following questions.

1. Define *labor* in your own words. Compare your definition with that presented in the text.

   _____

   _____

2. There is probably one predominant factor that results in rhythmic contractions leading to labor initiation and birth.

   a. True

   b. False

3. Current evidence shows that the functions of the uterus during labor are controlled by hormonal mediators from the placenta and the maternal and fetal glands.

   a. True

   b. False

4. Match the actions listed in Column B with the description of probable hormones, chemicals, or functions in labor listed in Column A.

   Column A

   1. _____ Calcium ions

   2. _____ Decidua

   3. _____ Increased number of oxytocin receptor sites in the myometrium

   4. _____ Prostaglandins

   5. _____ Oxytocin

   6. _____ Both maternal and fetal signals

   Column B

   a. Part of the endometrium; in pregnancy plays an important role in increasing estrogen content and synthesizing prostaglandins

   b. Secretion is pulsatile even during labor

   c. Results in increasing uterine sensitivity to oxytocin

   d. Derived from the fetus, decidua, and amniotic membranes

   e. Initiation of labor

   f. Vital for the contractile process in myometrial cells

5. When does Stage I begin and end? _____

6. Describe each of the two phases of Stage I.

   Latent phase: _____

   Active phase: _____

7. When does Stage II begin and end? _____

8. Describe what occurs in Stage III. _____

9. Describe what occurs in Stage IV. _____

10. Briefly describe why it is important to assess what stage of labor a woman is in.

    _____

    _____

11. What are the three layers of tissue that make up the uterus?

    a. _____

    b. _____

    c. _____

12. Which layer of the uterus contains special muscle cells that aid in expulsion of the baby at birth?

    _____

13. What does *effacement* mean when referring to the labor process?

    _____

    _____

14. Describe the changes that take place in the uterus as labor progresses.

    Upper portion: _____

    Lower portion: _____

15. Label the following diagram of the uterus.

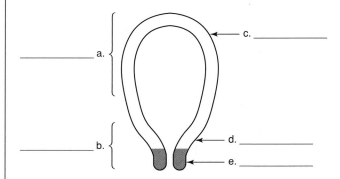

16. Which group of women is likely to experience effacement before labor actually begins?

    _____

17. The longest part of a contraction is the _____ segment.

18. The shortest and most intense part of a contraction is the _____ segment.

19. The contraction diminishes in the _____ segment.

20. List the four characteristics of a contraction.

    a. _____

    b. _____

    c. _____

    d. _____

21. For each of the following statements, identify the characteristics of a contraction that is described.

    a. Contractions last for 15 seconds: _____

    b. An internal electronic monitor is needed to assess this characteristic: _____

    c. Contractions are 6 minutes apart: _____

    d. There is an established, predictable pattern:

       _____

22. Match the appropriate labor description in Column A with the contraction intensity described in Column B.

    Column A

    1. _____ Normal labor

    2. _____ No labor

    3. _____ Prolonged labor

    Column B

    a. The intensity of the contraction is less than 15mm Hg.

    b. The intensity of the contraction is less than 25 mmHg (and the frequency is fewer than 2 contractions every 10 minutes).

    c. The intensity of contractions varies from 30 to 55 mmHg (and the frequency is 2 to 5 contractions every 10 minutes).

23. Refer to the following diagram below to answer questions a through d.

    a. What is the duration of the contractions? _____

       _____

    b. What is the frequency? _____

       _____

    c. How long can the woman relax? _____

       _____

    d. At what time will the next contraction begin? _____

       _____

24. List three ways to assess contractions.

    a. _____

    b. _____

    c. _____

25. What is the most efficient method of assessing contraction intensity?

    _____

26. What part of the hand is used to assess contractions?

    _____

27. Approximately how long would you need to remain at the bedside to assess contractions?

    _____

28. Where should you palpate the mother's abdomen and why? _____

    _____

29. a. To obtain a true assessment of cervical dilatation, when is the best time to perform a vaginal examination? _____

    b. Why? _____

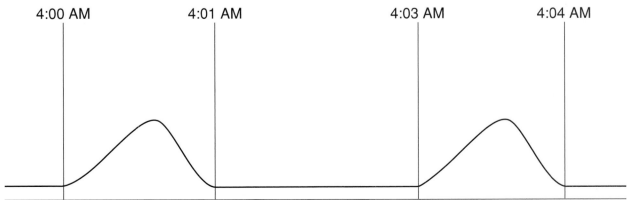

4:00 AM   4:01 AM   4:03 AM   4:04 AM

30. State three evidence-based outcomes when a laboring woman has a continuous supportive person with her.

    a. _____

    b. _____

    c. _____

31. Which is *not necessarily* effective in providing support for the laboring woman?

    a. Telling her in advance about special procedures, even though the procedure might be uncomfortable for her

    b. Protecting her privacy

    c. Keeping the visit of family members limited

    d. Including her in conversations when speaking with others in the room about her progress

32. In general, effective support during labor depends on which of the following?

    a. The health professional's interest and compassion

    b. The health professional's understanding of the physiologic and anatomic aspects of the birth process

    c. The health professional's appreciation of the psychological aspects of the birth process

    d. Knowledge of the level of preparation and the goals of the couple

    e. All of these

33. One of the first steps in becoming culturally competent is to increase awareness and sensitivity to one's own cultural heritage.

    a. True

    b. False

34. Relinquishing control in clinical situations does not play any role in culturally competent care.

    a. True

    b. False

35. When working with a non–English-speaking client, the nurse should address all questions directly to an interpreter.

    a. True

    b. False

36. The use of a cultural assessment tool increases consistency of care.

    a. True

    b. False

PRACTICE/REVIEW ANSWER KEY

1. *Labor* is a process involving a series of integrated uterine contractions occurring over time, leading to the development of expulsive forces adequate to propel the fetus through the birth canal against the resistance of soft tissue, muscle, and the bony structure of the pelvis.

2. b, False

3. a, True

4. 1. f
   2. a
   3. c
   4. d
   5. b
   6. e

5. Stage I begins with true labor and ends with full dilatation of the cervix.

6. The *latent phase* begins with regular contractions and *lasts until* rapid cervical *dilatation begins.*
   The *active phase* begins with rapid cervical dilatation and lasts until *full dilatation* of the cervix occurs.

7. Stage II begins with full dilatation of the cervix and lasts until the baby is born.

8. In Stage III, the placenta is delivered.

9. In Stage IV, the uterus contracts and the mother's body functions begin to stabilize.

10. Assessment of a woman's progress through the stages of labor is helpful in detecting problems.

11. a. Perimetrium
    b. Myometrium
    c. Endometrium

12. Myometrium

13. In labor, *effacement* refers to the thinning of the cervix.

14. The upper portion of uterus becomes thicker because of shortening and thickening of the myometrial fibers.
    The lower portion of uterus becomes thinner, softer, and more relaxed as myometrial fibers become longer.

15. a. Active fundal segment
    b. Passive segment
    c. Fundus
    d. Isthmus
    e. Cervix

16. Mothers experiencing their first labor

17. Increment

18. Acme

19. Decrement

20. a. Frequency
    b. Regularity
    c. Duration
    d. Intensity

21. a. Duration
    b. Intensity
    c. Frequency
    d. Regularity

22. 1. c
    2. a
    3. b

23. a. 1 minute
    b. every 3 minutes
    c. 2 minutes
    d. 4:06 AM

24. a. Subjectively
    b. By palpation
    c. With use of electronic fetal monitoring

25. Internal electronic monitoring

26. Palmar surface of fingertips

27. At least 30 minutes

28. Fingertips should be placed lightly over the fundal portion of the abdomen, which is near the top of the uterus. This is an appropriate area because this is where contractions begin and end.

29. a. Throughout the entire contraction
    b. Because of the nature of the contraction wave, the full effects of the contraction forces on cervical dilatation will be appreciated only at the peak and toward the end of the contraction.

30. Any three of the following:
    a. Less likelihood of medication need for pain relief
    b. Less likelihood of need for vaginal operative delivery
    c. Less likelihood of need for cesarean delivery
    d. Less likelihood of Apgar score of less than 7 at 5 minutes

31. c, Keeping the visit of family members limited

32. e, All of these

33. a, True

34. b, False

35. b, False

36. a, True

REFERENCES

1. Liao, J. B., Buhimschi, C. S., & Norwitz, E. R. (2005). *Normal labor: Mechanism and duration. Obstetrics and Gynecology Clinics of North America, 32,* 145–164.
2. Kilpatrick, S. & Garrison, E. (2007). Normal labor and delivery. In S. G. Gabbe, J. R. Simpson, J. R. Niebyl, H. Galan, L. Goetzl, E.R.M. Jauniax & M. Landon (Eds.), *Obstetrics: Normal and problem pregnancies* (5th ed.). New York: Churchill Livingstone.
3. Cunningham, F. G., Leveno, K. J., Bloom, S. L., Hauth, J. C., Gilstrap, L. C., III, & Wenstrom, K. D. (Eds.) (2005). *Williams obstetrics* (22nd ed.). New York: McGraw-Hill.
4. Farrington, P. F. & Ward, K. (2003). Normal labor, delivery and puerperium. In J. R. Scott, P. J. DiSaia, C. Hammond, & W. N. Spellacy (Eds.), *Danforth's obstetrics & gynecology* (8th ed.). Philadelphia: Lippincott Williams & Wilkins.
5. Pozaic, S. (1999). Induction and augmentation of labor. In L. K. Mandeville, & N. H. Troiano (Eds.), *AWHONN's high-risk and critical care intrapartum nursing* (2nd ed., pp. 142–145). Philadelphia: Lippincott Williams & Wilkins.
6. Simpson, K. R. (2002). *Cervical ripening and induction and augmentation of labor.* (Practice Monograph). Washington, DC: Association of Women's Health, Obstetric and Neonatal Nurses.
7. Rothman, B. K. (1996). Women providers and control. *Journal of Obstetric, Gynecologic, and Neonatal Nursing, 25*(3), 254.
8. Peterson, G. (1996). Childbirth: the ordinary miracle—Effects of childbirth on women's self-esteem and family relationships. *Pre- and Perinatal Psychology Journal, 11*(2), 101–109.
9. McKay, S. (1991). Shared power: The essence of humanized childbirth. *Pre- and Perinatal Psychology, 54*(4), 283–296.
10. Taylor, J. S. (2002) Caregiver support for women during childbirth: Does the presence of a labor support person affect maternal-child outcomes? *American Family Physician, 66*(7), 1205–1206.
11. Tillett, J. (2006). Are open visitation policies beneficial for women? *Journal of Perinatal and Neonatal Nursing, 20*(3), 193–194.
12. Chamberlain, D. B., & Arms, S. (1999). Obstetrics and the prenatal psyche. *Journal of Prenatal and Perinatal Psychology and Health, 14*(1–2), 97–118.
13. Chamberlain, D. B. (1999). Babies are not what we thought: Call for a new paradigm. *Journal of Prenatal and Perinatal Psychology and Health, 14*(1–2), 127–144.
14. Chamberlain, D. B. (1994). The sentient prenate: What every parent should know. *Pre- and Perinatal Psychology Journal, 9*(1), 9–31.
15. Lothian, J. A. (2001). Back to the future: Trusting birth. *Journal of Perinatal and Neonatal Nursing, 15*(3), 13–22.
16. Low, L. K., & Moffat, A. (2006). Every labor is unique, but "call when your contractions are 3 minutes apart." *Maternal Child Nursing, 31*(5), 307–312.

17. Moore, M. L., & Moos, M. (2003). *Cultural competence in care of childbearing families.* White Plains, NY: March of Dimes Birth Defects Foundation Education Services.

18. Cooper, M., Grywalski, M., Lamp, J., Newhouse, L., & Studlien, R. (2007). Enhancing cultural competence: A model for nurses. *Nursing for Women's Health, 11*(2), 148–159.

19. Kim-Godwin, Y. S. (2003). Postpartum beliefs and practices among non-western cultures. *Maternal Child Nursing, 28*(2), 75–78.

20. Camphina-Bacote, J. (2003). *The process of cultural competence in the delivery of healthcare services.* Cincinnati, OH: Transcultural C.A.R.E. Associates.

21. Rorie, J. L., Paine, L. L., & Barger, M. K. (1996). Cultural competence in primary care service. *Journal of Nurse Midwifery, 4*(2), 99.

SUGGESTED READINGS

Brach, C., & Fraser, I. (2000). *Can cultural competency reduce racial and ethnic health disparities? A review and conceptual model.* Agency for Healthcare Research and Quality. Rockville, MD: U.S. Department of Health and Human Services.

Enkin, M., Keirse, M. J. N. C., Neilson, J., Crowther, C., Duley, L., Hodnett, E., & Hofmeyer, J. (2000). *A guide to effective care in pregnancy and childbirth* (3rd ed.). New York: Oxford University Press.

Goer, H. (1999). *The thinking woman's guide to a better birth.* New York: Berkley Publishing Group.

Lowdermilk, D. L., Perry, S. E., & Bobak, I. M. (Eds.). (2007). *Maternity & women's health care* (9th ed.). St. Louis: Mosby.

Mandeville, L. K., & Troiano, N. H. (1999). *High-risk & critical care intrapartum nursing* (2nd ed.). Philadelphia: Lippincott Williams & Wilkins.

Pillitteri, A. (1999). *Maternal & child health nursing* (3rd ed.). Philadelphia: Lippincott.

Simkin, P., & Ancheta, R. (2000). *The labor progress handbook.* Malden, MA: Blackwell Scientific.

Simpson, K. R., & Creehan, P. A. (2007). AWHONN's *Perinatal nursing* (3rd ed.). Philadelphia: Lippincott Williams & Wilkins.

Willis, W. O. (1999). Culturally competent nursing care during the perinatal period. *Journal of Perinatal Nursing, 13*(3), 45–59.

MODULE

2 Maternal and Fetal Response to Labor

E. JEAN MARTIN ■ BETSY B. KENNEDY

Identifying Features of the Pelvis That Make It Adequate for Labor

As you complete Part 1 of this module, you will learn:

1. Critical factors involved in labor
2. The significance of each type of pelvis to the birth process
3. Features of the pelvis that affect labor
4. Limitations of pelvic evaluation methods

When you have completed Part 1 of this module, you should be able to recall the meaning of the following terms. You should also be able to use the terms when consulting with other health professionals. The terms are defined in this module or in the glossary at the end of this book.

fetal attitude	fetal presentation
fetal lie	molding
fetal position	pelvic planes

Features of the Pelvis That Make It Adequate for Labor

There are four factors, often referred to as the "four Ps," that affect the progress of labor.

1. *Passage* involves
   - the size of the pelvis
   - the shape of the pelvis
   - the ability of the cervix to dilate and the vagina to stretch
2. *Passenger* involves
   - fetal *size,* particularly the fetal head
   - fetal *attitude,* which describes the relation of the fetal head, shoulder, and legs to one another
   - fetal *lie,* which refers to the relationship of the long axis ($\updownarrow$) of the fetus to the long axis ($\updownarrow$) of the mother
   - fetal *presentation,* which describes that part of the fetus entering the pelvis first
   - fetal *position,* which refers to the direction toward which the presenting part is pointing—front, side, or back of the maternal pelvis
3. *Powers* involves
   - the frequency, duration, and intensity of uterine contractions
   - abdominal pressures resulting from pushing, which occur in stage II of labor
4. *Psyche* involves
   - the mother's physical, emotional, and intellectual preparation
   - her previous childbirth experiences
   - her cultural attitude
   - support from significant people in the mother's life

For labor to progress smoothly, there must be adaptations of both fetal and maternal factors. Abnormalities of any of these critical factors can mean risk for baby, mother, or both.

▶ **What makes a pelvis adequate for labor?**

The size and the shape of the pelvis make it adequate for labor. The female pelvis is uniquely suited to the demands of childbearing. However, not all women possess the same type of pelvis. The following four classic types of pelves are based on differences in shapes, diameters, and angles[1,2] (Display 2.1). In clinical practice, consistent prediction of a successful vaginal delivery cannot be done based on pelvis shape classification.[3]

DISPLAY 2.1	CLASSIC TYPES OF PELVES

TYPE	FEATURES
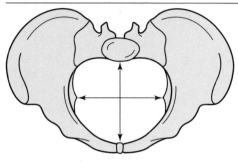 **A.** Gynecoid pelvis	• Typical female pelvis • Adequate for labor and birth • Found in 50% of women
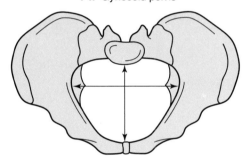 **B.** Android pelvis	• Typical male pelvis • Narrow dimensions • Slow descent of fetal head • Associated with the halting of labor • Forceps delivery often required • Found in 20% of women
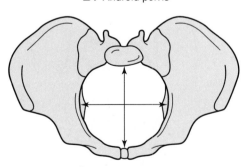 **C.** Arthropoid pelvis	• Apelike pelvis • Adequate for labor and birth • Found in 25% of women
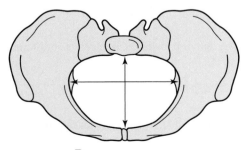 **D.** Platypelloid pelvis	• Unfavorable for labor • Frequent delay in descent • Found in 5% of women

A woman can have a pelvis that has a combination of characteristics from these classic types. Mixed architectural features are encountered frequently in clinical practice.[4]

In obstetrics, the pelvis is divided into the following parts (Fig. 2.1):
1. *False pelvis*—where there is ample room
2. *True pelvis*—which contains important narrow dimensions through which the fetus must pass

There is a ridge that provides an imaginary dividing line between the two areas. This ridge is the boundary for the inlet to the true pelvis.

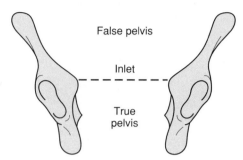

FIGURE 2.1 False pelvis and true pelvis.

NOTE: The false pelvis has no obstetric significance, whereas the true pelvis has great significance.

The *true pelvis* can be divided into three key areas (Fig. 2.2):
1. Inlet
2. Pelvic cavity, which extends from the inlet to the outlet
3. Outlet

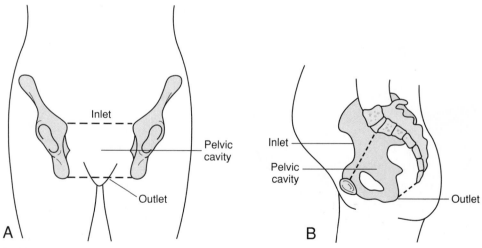

FIGURE 2.2 **A.** Front view of pelvis. **B.** Side view of pelvis.

The *pelvic planes* are imaginary flat surfaces passing across parts of the true pelvis at different levels. Three important planes are shown in Figure 2.3.

▶ How is the adequacy of the pelvis evaluated?

The relationship of the fetal size to the pelvis must be evaluated. This relationship probably changes depending on the forces and stages of labor. Positioning of the mother can bring about subtle changes in one or two pelvic dimensions (e.g., the McRoberts maneuver; see Modules 13 and 18). Dynamic changes in the fetal head, thorax, and abdomen are believed to occur as the

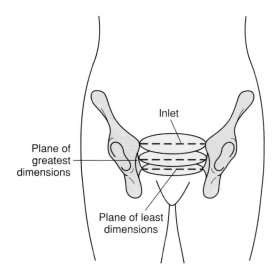

Inlet

Plane of greatest dimensions

Plane of least dimensions

The plane of least dimensions is the narrowest section of the pelvis. Occasionally, labor stops because the fetus cannot descend past this area.

FIGURE 2.3 Pelvic planes.

pelvic passageway is negotiated during descent. Efforts to predict fetal–pelvic disproportion have included the following[1]:

1. Clinical pelvimetry
   - Estimation of pelvic shapes and dimensions by the examiner
   - Wide margin of error depending on the examiner's skill
2. X-ray pelvimetry
   - Potential fetal exposure to low-dose radiation
   - Can provide critical pelvic diameters not otherwise obtainable
   - Sometimes used in breech presentations
   - Has been replaced by other pelvic imaging methods
3. Ultrasonography
   - Uses sound waves, not ionizing energy
   - Not useful for evaluating maternal pelvic measurement
   - Useful for precisely measuring fetal biparietal diameters and fetal head circumference
4. Computed tomographic (CT) pelvimetry (CT scanning)
   - Has replaced x-ray pelvimetry at many institutions
   - Accuracy is improved over conventional x-ray pelvimetry
   - Involves a lower fetal radiation exposure than x-ray
   - Maternal movement during procedure needs to be minimal to prevent distortion
   - Expense is comparable to that of conventional x-ray
5. Magnetic resonance imaging
   - Offers accurate pelvic measurements and complete fetal imaging
   - Has the potential to aid in diagnosing soft tissue dystocia and obstructed labor
   - Use is limited by expense, length of time needed to obtain the study, and availability of equipment

Imaging studies, although readily defining values for the parameters of the true bony pelvis, have not been shown to consistently predict women at risk for cephalopelvic disproportion.[4] Radiographic studies are generally avoided during pregnancy because of the theoretical risk of radiation exposure to the fetus. Clinical pelvimetry is a skill that must be mastered, yet still may not allow prediction of the adequacy of a woman's pelvis to deliver the baby. Currently, a "trial of labor" is used to determine if the woman's pelvis is adequate for delivery of the baby.

Additional considerations include the following:
- Except for some relaxation of the pelvic joints because of hormonal influences, the bones of the pelvis cannot expand.
- The soft tissues of the birth canal (the cervix and pelvic floor musculature) provide resistance during labor. The cervix undergoes biochemical changes that increase its elasticity. The musculature of the pelvic floor facilitates rotation and flexion for the fetal head.
- The relationship of the fetal head size to the pelvis is important.
- The fetal head has the ability to change shape to fit through the pelvis. This ability of the head to change shape is called *molding.*

- Because of the tilt of the pelvis, the fetus descends through this pathway during labor and birth, as shown in Figure 2.4.

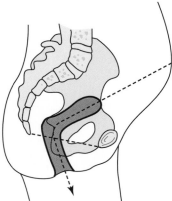

FIGURE 2.4 Pathway of fetal descent.

PRACTICE/REVIEW QUESTIONS

After reviewing Part 1, answer the following questions.

1. List four critical factors involved in the labor process.

   a. _____

   b. _____

   c. _____

   d. _____

2. Match the definition in Column B with the correct term in Column A.

   Column A

   1. _____ Lie
   2. _____ Attitude
   3. _____ Position
   4. _____ Presentation

   Column B

   a. Relationship of the long axis of the fetus to the long axis of the mother
   b. That part of the fetal body that is entering the pelvis
   c. The relationship of fetal parts to one another
   d. The direction toward which the presenting part is pointing with respect to the front, side, or back of the mother's pelvis

3. List the four main types of pelves.

   a. _____

   b. _____

   c. _____

   d. _____

4. The pelvis best suited for labor and birth is the _____ pelvis. This type of pelvis is found in _____ % of women.

5. The pelvis that has narrow dimensions and is likely to result in labor stopping or a forceps delivery is the _____ pelvis. This type of pelvis is found in _____ % of women.

6. Match the areas of the pelvis with the correct numbers in the diagram.

   _____ a. Inlet

   _____ b. False pelvis

   _____ c. True pelvis

   _____ d. Outlet

   _____ e. Plane of least dimensions

7. The true pelvis is made up of three key planes called:

   a. _____

   b. _____

   c. _____

8. The planes of the true pelvis are critical because

   _____

   _____

9. Name two ways in which the female pelvis is evaluated for adequacy.

   a. _____

   b. _____

10. Explain how it is possible for the fetal head to fit through the rigid, bony pelvis.

    _____

    _____

PRACTICE/REVIEW ANSWER KEY

1. a. Passage
   b. Passenger
   c. Power
   d. Psyche

2. 1. a
   2. c
   3. d
   4. b

3. a. Gynecoid
   b. Android
   c. Platypelloid
   d. Anthropoid

4. Gynecoid; 50

5. Android; 20

6. a. 1
   b. 2
   c. 5
   d. 3
   e. 4

7. a. Least dimensions
   b. Greatest dimensions
   c. Pelvic inlet

8. The fetus must pass through these areas, some of which are narrow.

9. a. X-ray
   b. Pelvic examination

10. The head flexes and the bones of the scalp mold somewhat.

PART 2

Identifying Relationships Between the Fetus and Pelvis

As you complete Part 2 of this module, you will learn:

1. Relationships of the fetal position and presenting part to the outcome of labor
2. Landmarks used to identify the position of the fetus
3. Features of the pelvis that affect labor
4. How to determine and describe fetal lie, presentation, attitude, and position

When you have completed Part 2 of this module, you should be able to recall the meaning of the following terms. You should also be able to use the terms when consulting with other health professionals. The terms are defined in this module or in the glossary at the end of this book.

biparietal diameter	mentum
denominator	occiput
fetal anencephaly	placenta previa
fetal hydrocephaly	prematurity
fontanelle	sinciput
grand multiparity	suture
hydramnios	vertex

Relationships Between the Fetus and Pelvis

▶ **How does the fetal passenger accommodate to the pelvis during labor?**

The position of the fetus as the mother is ready to go into labor largely determines how smoothly the labor and delivery will progress. The fetal head is the largest part of the baby and is composed of both fixed and flexible parts. You must become familiar with the parts of the fetal skull because the identification of certain landmarks will assist you when performing vaginal examinations to determine the mother's labor progress. The skull consists of three major divisions (Fig. 2.5):

1. Face
2. Back of the skull
3. Cranium, or top of the skull

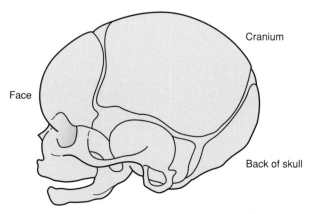

FIGURE 2.5 Major divisions of the fetal skull.

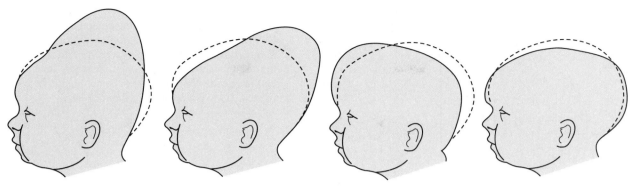

FIGURE 2.6 Molding of the fetal head in different cephalic presentations.

The bones of the face and the back of the skull are fused and fixed, but the cranium consists of several large bones that are not fused together at the time of birth. This permits the shape of the head to change somewhat as the fetus passes through the narrow, rigid pelvis (Fig. 2.6).

> The force of uterine contractions on the fetal head can cause overlapping of the cranial bones; this is called *molding* and can be felt during a vaginal examination.

▶ **What other landmarks of the fetal skull are used in describing the fetal head?**

There are four landmarks that are important in describing the general areas of the fetal head (Fig. 2.7):
1. *Sinciput*—brow area
2. *Vertex*—area between the anterior and posterior fontanelles
3. *Occiput*—area beneath the posterior fontanelle where the occipital bone is located
4. *Mentum*—fetal chin

NOTE: *Learn these terms now; later in this module they are used to denote which part of the fetal head is leading as the fetus descends.*

If looking down at the fetal cranium, you would see the divisions between the bones of the head, as depicted in Figure 2.8.

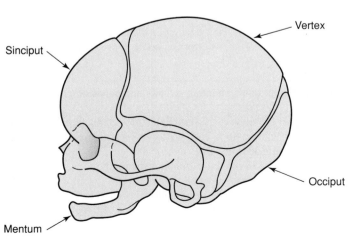

FIGURE 2.7 Bony landmarks used in describing areas of the fetal head.

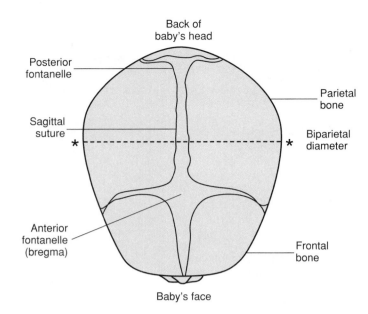

A *suture* is a space between the cranial bones that is covered by a membrane. A *fontanelle*, or *fontanel*, is a space covered by a membrane where the cranial sutures meet. Feeling the suture lines and fontanelles during a vaginal examination helps in identifying the position of the fetal head.

FIGURE 2.8 Suture, fontanelle, and bony landmarks used in describing the position of the fetal head.

There are two important *landmarks* formed by the sutures that are useful in identifying the position of the fetal head in the pelvis.

1. *Anterior fontanelle* (Fig. 2.9)—is *diamond-shaped* and measures 2 × 3 cm. This is sometimes referred to as the *bregma*. When the head is *moderately* flexed or hyperextended, this fontanelle can be palpated. It remains open approximately 18 months after birth to allow for brain growth.

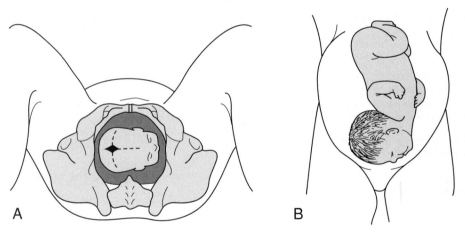

FIGURE 2.9 **A.** Vaginal view (hyperextended head). **B.** Abdominal view (hyperextended head).

2. *Posterior fontanelle* (Fig. 2.10)—is *smaller* and *triangular* in shape. When the head is well flexed, this fontanelle can be felt. The posterior fontanelle closes approximately 12 weeks after birth.

▶ **How is the position of the fetus in the mother's abdominal cavity and pelvis described?**

You must understand the relationship of the fetus to the mother's abdominal and pelvic cavities because careful observation of these relationships can alert you to potential problems. To review, four aspects of this relationship are as follows:

1. *Lie*—the relationship of the long axis of the fetus to that of the mother
2. *Presentation*—that part of the fetus entering the pelvic inlet first
3. *Attitude*—the relationship of the fetal parts (e.g., chest, chin, arms) to each other
4. *Position*—the relationship of the presenting part to a specific area of the mother's pelvis

NOTE: *Station also describes a relationship between the presenting part of the fetus and the maternal pelvis. This is discussed in Part 3.*

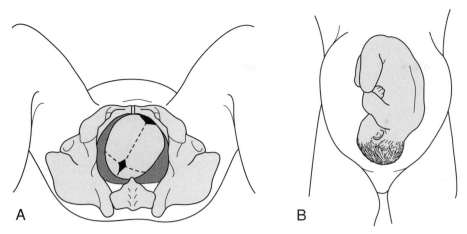

FIGURE 2.10 **A.** Vaginal view (normal flexed head). **B.** Abdominal view (normal flexed head).

Types of Fetal Lie

Figure 2.11 illustrates types of fetal lie. Display 2.2 illustrates longitudinal and transverse lies.

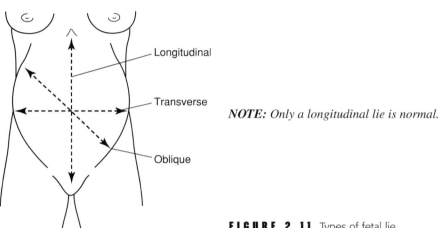

NOTE: Only a longitudinal lie is normal.

FIGURE 2.11 Types of fetal lie.

DISPLAY 2.2 ILLUSTRATIONS OF FETAL LIE

A longitudinal lie, occurring in 99.5% of pregnancies, is when the long axis of the fetal body is parallel to the mother's spine.
A longitudinal lie can be either *cephalic* or *breech.*

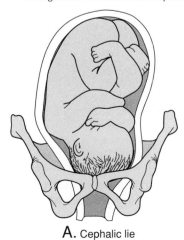

When the head is leading, it is called a *cephalic lie.*

A. Cephalic lie

display continues on page 28

27

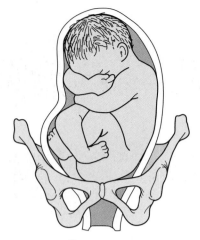

B. Breech lie

If the buttocks are coming first, it is called a *breech lie.*

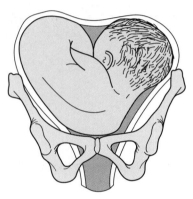

C. Transverse lie

The fetus can assume a *transverse lie,* in which the long axis of the fetus lies directly across the mother's spine. It occurs in approximately 0.3% of pregnancies.

Transverse lie is often associated with the following[5]:
1. *Grand multiparity* (having five or more pregnancies)
2. A small (contracted) pelvis
3. Placenta previa
4. Polyhydramnios
5. Fetal prematurity
6. Uterine anomalies

*Most women at 37 weeks gestation with a transverse lie convert to a longitudinal lie, but the risk of morbidity from cord prolapse and uterine rupture is great. Therefore, **vaginal delivery is not possible with a transverse lie**. External version may be attempted; if it fails, a cesarean delivery is planned.*

Types of Fetal Attitude

Attitude refers to the relationship of the fetal parts to each other. Normally, the attitude is one of *flexion* or *extension* in relation to the fetal spine. Adequate flexion creates the smallest cephalic diameter to facilitate delivery (Display 2.3).

DISPLAY 2.3 ILLUSTRATIONS OF FETAL ATTITUDE

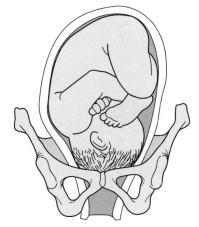

Flexion is when the chin is near the chest, the arms and legs are folded in front of the body, and the back is curved.

> This position of the fetus presents the smallest possible fetal head measurements in relation to the pelvic passageway and is the only normal attitude.

A. Attitude of flexion

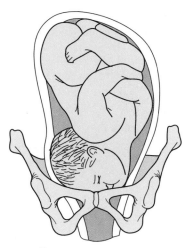

Extension occurs when the head is bent back and the chest and abdomen are slightly curved.

> In the extreme of this position, the fetal face is the leading part as it descends through the pelvis. It is traumatic for the baby, who is often not deliverable vaginally because a larger diameter of the fetal head presents, unlike when the head is well flexed.

B. Attitude of extension

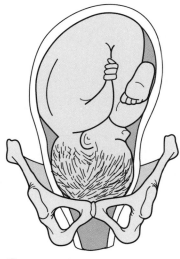

Military attitude occurs when the fetal position is not one of flexion or extension.

C. Military attitude (neither flexed nor extended)

display continues on page 30

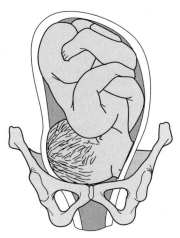

Partial extension occurs when there is moderate extension of the head.

D. Attitude of partial extension.

The *cephalic prominence* describes that part of the fetal head that can be felt by placing both hands on the sides of the uterus and feeling down toward the pelvis. When the head is in normal flexion, the cephalic prominence is felt on the opposite side of the fetal back; in Figure 2.12, it is found in the lower left of the mother's abdomen.

Hyperextension of the head results in the face presenting for birth. The cephalic prominence is felt on the same side as the fetal back; in Figure 2.13 it is found in the lower right of the mother's abdomen.

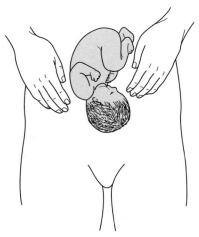

FIGURE 2.12 Position of the cephalic prominence in normal flexion.

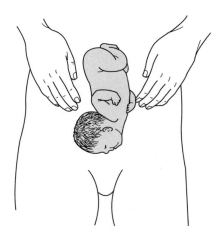

FIGURE 2.13 Position of the cephalic prominence in hyperextension.

The location of the cephalic prominence can aid in diagnosing the attitude of the fetus and any malpositions (discussed further in Module 4, Skill Unit 2).

Types of Fetal Presentation

Presentation refers to that part of the fetus entering the pelvic inlet first. The main presentations are as follows (Table 2.1):
- Shoulder
- Breech
- Cephalic

TABLE 2.1	TYPES OF FETAL PRESENTATION	
Shoulder	Either shoulder leads	Fortunately, shoulder presentation rarely occurs.
Breech	Buttocks lead	Breech presentation occurs in 3%–4% of pregnancies and is more common in preterm pregnancies.[1]
Cephalic	Head leads	Cephalic presentation occurs in 96%–97% of term pregnancies.[1]

NOTE: The term "compound presentation" is used when there is more than one fetal part presenting at the pelvic inlet. If the umbilical cord is present at the inlet, it is known as a funic presentation.

Shoulder Presentation

The shoulder is entering the pelvis first (Fig. 2.14). This presentation occurs infrequently.

Breech Presentation

The buttocks or breech enters the pelvis first (Figs. 2.15, 2.16, and 2.17). Breech presentation can be complete, frank, or footling. The prevalence of breech presentation depends on gestational age, occurring more frequently in earlier gestations.

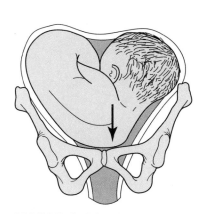

FIGURE 2.14 Shoulder presentation.

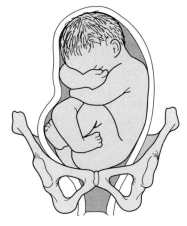

FIGURE 2.15 Complete breech presentation.

> Risk factors for breech presentation include:
> Placenta previa
> Hydramnios
> Twin pregnancies
> Preterm labor/birth
> Previous breech delivery
> Grand multiparity
> Fetal hydrocephaly
> Fetal anencephaly
> Uterine anomalies

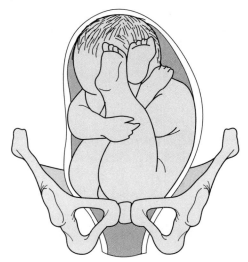

FIGURE 2.16 Frank breech presentation.

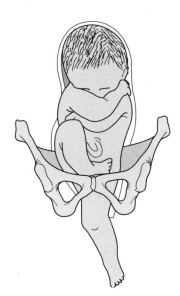

FIGURE 2.17 Footling breech presentation.

Cephalic Presentation

Cephalic presentation (96% to 97% of term pregnancies) can occur[1]:

When the head is *well flexed* and the vertex presents first, as in Figure 2.18.
When the head is *poorly flexed* and the brow presents first, as in Figure 2.19.
When the head is *poorly flexed* and the face presents first, as in Figure 2.20.

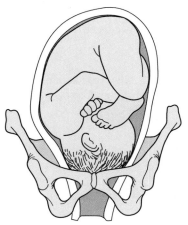

> This is the only normal presentation.

FIGURE 2.18 Vertex presents in cephalic presentation.

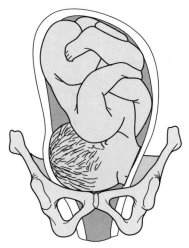

FIGURE 2.19 Brow presents in cephalic presentation.

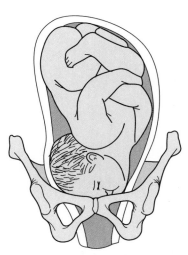

FIGURE 2.20 Face presents in cephalic presentation.

Types of Fetal Position

▶ **How are the fetal positions described?**

"Position" refers to the relationship of the presenting part to a specific area on the woman's pelvis. In describing fetal position, certain landmarks on the fetus, called *denominators,* are used.

In *vertex* presentations, the *occiput* is the denominator (Fig. 2.21).

In *face* presentations, the *mentum* (chin) is the denominator (Fig. 2.22).

In *breech* presentations, the *sacrum* is the denominator (Fig. 2.23).

In *shoulder* presentations, the *scapula,* or the *acromial process,* is the denominator (Fig. 2.24).

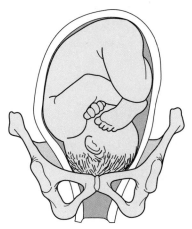

FIGURE 2.21 Vertex presentation with occiput as the denominator.

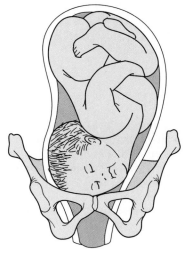

FIGURE 2.22 Face presentation with chin as the denominator.

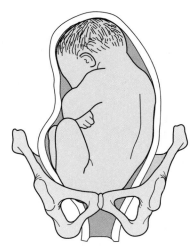

FIGURE 2.23 Breech presentation with sacrum as the denominator.

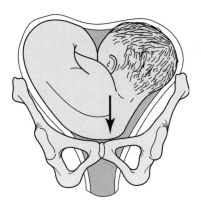

FIGURE 2.24 Shoulder presentation with the scapula (acromial process) as the denominator.

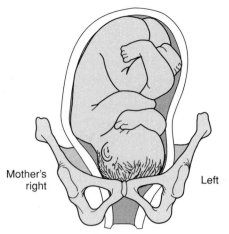

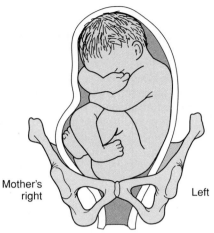

FIGURE 2.25 Occiput leading and pointing to mother's right.

FIGURE 2.26 Sacrum leading and pointing to mother's left.

Having determined which denominator is the leading part of the fetus, its *position* can be described further. Note whether the denominator is pointing to the left (**L**) or right (**R**) side of the mother's pelvis. For example:

The *occiput* of the fetus leads and points to the mother's *right* (Fig. 2.25).

The *sacrum* of the fetus leads and points to the mother's *left* (Fig. 2.26).

Finally, in describing position, note whether the denominator is in the front (anterior), directly to the side (transverse), or in the back (posterior) of the *mother's* pelvis (Display 2.4).

DISPLAY 2.4 EXAMPLES OF DENOMINATOR POSITIONS IN CEPHALIC PRESENTATION

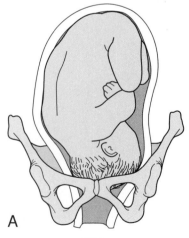

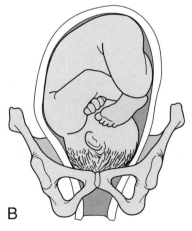

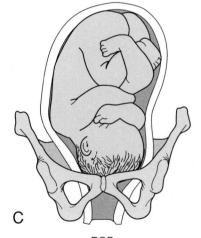

A

ROA

Occiput is in the **A**nterior (front) of the pelvis.

R	Right
O	Occiput
A	Anterior

B

ROT

Occiput is **T**ransverse (to the side) of the pelvis.

R	Right
O	Occiput
T	Transverse

C

ROP

Occiput is in the **P**osterior (back) of the pelvis.

R	Right
O	Occiput
P	Posterior

Display 2.5 shows breech positions.
Display 2.6 shows a face presentation with the *mentum* (chin) leading.

DISPLAY 2.5 EXAMPLES OF DENOMINATOR POSITIONS IN BREECH PRESENTATION

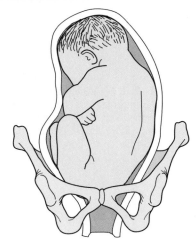

A

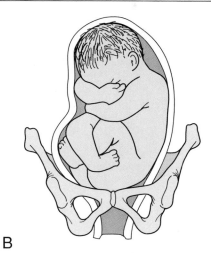

B

LSA

Sacrum is in the **A**nterior (front) of the pelvis.

L   Left
S   Sacrum
A   Anterior

LSP

Sacrum is in the **P**osterior (back) of the pelvis.

L   Left
S   Sacrum
P   Posterior

DISPLAY 2.6 EXAMPLE OF DENOMINATOR POSITION IN CEPHALIC PRESENTATION WITH FACE PRESENTING

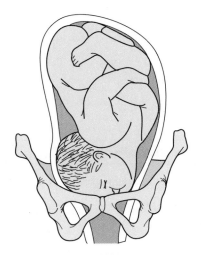

LMA

The **M**entum (chin) is in the **L**eft **A**nterior of the pelvis.

L   Left
M   Mentum
A   Anterior

Vertex Positions

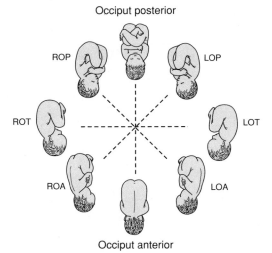

Occiput posterior

ROP

LOP

ROT

LOT

ROA

LOA

Occiput anterior

NOTE: The occiput is the denominator.

FIGURE 2.27 Variety of fetal positions with vertex presentations. (Adapted with permission from Oxorn, H. [1986]. *Oxorn-Foote human labor & birth* [5th ed., p. 59]. New York: Appleton-Century-Crofts.)

Breech Positions

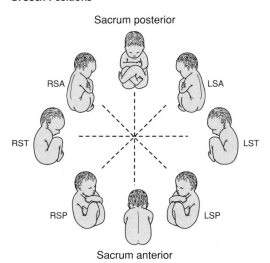

Sacrum posterior

RSA

LSA

RST

LST

RSP

LSP

Sacrum anterior

NOTE: The sacrum is the denominator.

FIGURE 2.28 Variety of fetal positions with breech presentations. (Adapted with permission from Oxorn, H. [1986]. *Oxorn-Foote human labor & birth* [5th ed., p. 59]. New York: Appleton-Century-Crofts.)

Figures 2.27 and 2.28 illustrate how various positions for vertex and breech presentations can be described.

► How can fetal position and presentation be determined?

It is important to determine fetal position and presentation to predict the course of labor. Several methods are available:
- Combined abdominal inspection and palpation (Leopold's maneuvers)
- Vaginal examination
- Ultrasonography
- CT scanning
- X-ray examination

Because x-rays are known to be harmful to the fetus if used frequently or in early pregnancy, they are used only when fetal position cannot be determined in any other way.

PRACTICE/REVIEW QUESTIONS

After reviewing Part 2, answer the following questions.

1. Label the following diagrams.

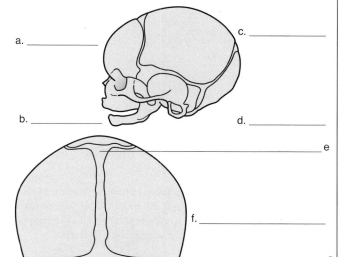

a. _____

b. _____

c. _____

d. _____

e _____

f. _____

g _____

2. The posterior fontanelle closes approximately _____ months after birth. It is _____ shaped and can be felt when the head is _____ flexed.

3. The anterior fontanelle closes approximately _____ months after birth. It is _____ shaped and can be felt when the head is _____ flexed.

4. The only normal lie is _____.

5. A longitudinal lie can be_____, when the head leads, or _____, when the buttocks come first.

6. Why is vaginal delivery impossible with a transverse lie?
   _____
   _____

7. The only normal attitude is one of _____
   _____

8. Why is a fetus positioned in extreme extension often not deliverable vaginally?
   _____
   _____

9. Locating the cephalic prominence is helpful in diagnosing fetal _____ and malpositions.

10. The three primary types of presentations are:
    a. _____ (approximately 96%)
    b. _____ (3% to 4% of pregnancies)
    c. _____ (infrequent)

11. The only normal presentation is _____, when the _____ presents first.

12. Prematurity, placenta previa, and/or grand multiparity can be associated with a _____ presentation.

13. State the denominator used to describe the fetal position in each of the following presentations.

Fetal Position	Denominator
a. Vertex	_____
b. Face	_____
c. Breech	_____
d. Shoulder	_____

14. Fully describe each of the following according to fetal lie, presentation, and position.

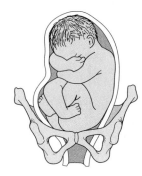
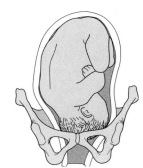

a. _____
   _____
   _____

b. _____
   _____
   _____

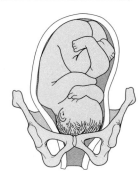
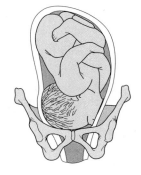

c. _____
   _____
   _____

d. _____
   _____
   _____

15. State five ways in which fetal position and presentation can be determined.

    a. _____

    b. _____

    c. _____

    d. _____

    e. _____

16. The term *position* refers to which of the following?

    a. The relationship of the long axis of the fetus to that of the mother

    b. The part of the fetus that first enters the inlet of the pelvis

    c. The degree of descent of the fetus through the maternal pelvis

    d. The relationship of a specific point of the fetus to one of the four quadrants of the mother's pelvis

17. Which statement accurately describes the fetal attitude, lie, presentation, and position in the following illustration?

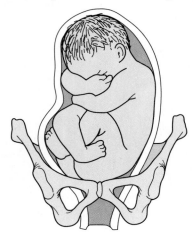

    a. Attitude is one of extension, longitudinal lie, breech presentation, and position is LSP.

    b. Attitude is one of flexion, longitudinal lie, breech presentation, and position is LSA.

    c. Attitude is one of flexion, longitudinal lie, breech presentation, and position is LSP.

    d. Attitude is one of extension, longitudinal lie, cephalic presentation, and position is RSP.

PRACTICE/REVIEW ANSWER KEY

1. a. Sinciput
   b. Mentum
   c. Vertex
   d. Occiput
   e. Posterior fontanelle
   f. Sagittal suture
   g. Anterior fontanelle (bregma)

2. 3; triangular; well

3. 18; diamond; moderately

4. longitudinal

5. cephalic; breech

6. Vaginal delivery is not possible with a transverse lie because the long axis of the fetus lies across the mother's spine.

7. Flexion

8. In extreme extension, the face is often the leading part as the fetus descends through the pelvis. This is traumatic for the baby. A larger diameter is presented to the vaginal passageway than when the head is well flexed.

9. Attitude

10. a. Cephalic
    b. Breech
    c. Shoulder

11. Cephalic; vertex

12. Breech

13. a. Occiput
    b. Mentum
    c. Sacrum
    d. Scapula or acromial process

14. a. Longitudinal (breech) lie
       Breech presentation
       LSP
    b. Longitudinal (cephalic) lie
       Cephalic presentation
       ROA
    c. Longitudinal (cephalic) lie
       Cephalic presentation
       ROP
    d. Longitudinal (cephalic) lie
       Cephalic presentation
       LMT (you may interpret the diagram to be LMA)

15. a. Abdominal inspection and palpation
    b. Vaginal examination
    c. Ultrasonography
    d. CT scanning
    e. X-ray examination

16. d. The relationship of a specific point of the fetus to one of the four quadrants of the mother's pelvis.

17. c. Attitude is one of flexion, longitudinal lie, breech presentation, and position is LSP.

PART 3

Describing Fetal Descent During Labor

Objectives

As you complete Part 3 of this module, you will learn:
1. How to describe the descent of the fetus
2. The significance of engagement and pelvic adequacy
3. How fetal descent through the pelvis is evaluated
4. How molding of the fetal head can affect the evaluation of descent

Key Terms

When you have completed Part 3 of this module, you should be able to recall the meaning of the following terms. You should also be able to use the terms when consulting with other health professionals. The terms are defined in this module or in the glossary at the end of this book.

caput succedaneum	multipara
dipping	primigravida
engagement	station
floating	

Fetal Descent During Labor

▶ **How is the descent of the fetus described and assessed?**

The degree of descent of the fetus through the pelvis is assessed by abdominal, vaginal, and rectal examination. The relationship of the presenting part of the fetus to an imaginary line drawn between the ischial spines of the pelvis is called *station.*

To measure station, a scale of −3 to +5 is used. The numbers represent the distance in centimeters of the presenting part to the ischial spines (Fig. 2.29). The ischial spines are approximately halfway between the pelvic inlet and the pelvic outlet. When the presenting fetal part (e.g., the head) is at the level of the ischial spines, it is said to be at *station 0.*

An older, less objective measurement of station uses a scale of −3 to +3 to describe the relationship of the presenting fetal part to the ischial spines. The long axis of the birth canal is divided into thirds. If the presenting part is above the spines and at the level of the pelvic inlet, it is said to be at −3 station. If it has descended one third the distance past the inlet, it is at −1 station. A similar division is assigned to the distances between the ischial spines and the pelvic outlet. If the level of the presenting part is one third or two thirds the distance between the spines and the outlet, it is said to be +1 or +2 station, respectively. When the presenting fetal part descends to the bony outlet, it is resting on the muscles of the vaginal opening and is at +3 station (Fig. 2.30).

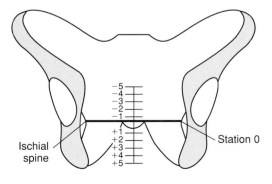

Ischial spine

Station 0

FIGURE 2.29 Levels of progress through the pelvis using a scale of −3 to +5.

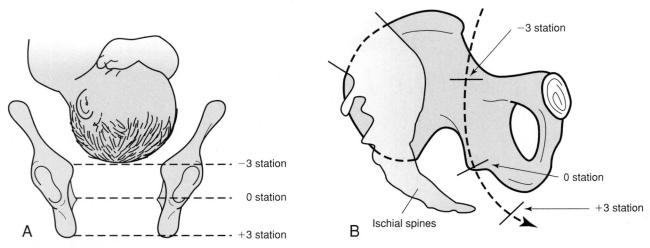

FIGURE 2.30 **A.** Descent of the presenting fetal part to station −3. Front view using a scale of −3 to +3. **B.** Descent pathway, side view.

It is important that the same scale be understood and used consistently by all staff within the labor and delivery unit.

▶ When is the pelvis considered adequate?

When the presenting part of the fetal head is at station 0, the widest part of the head usually has passed through the inlet and the pelvis is then thought to be adequate. This is called *engagement* (Fig. 2.31).

Vaginal examination will assist you in determining the amount of descent.

Caution:
- In women with deep pelves, this relationship might not be exact, and even though engagement has occurred, the presenting part can be slightly above the spines.
- Sometimes the fetal scalp becomes edematous with the pressure of labor exerted on it. This can be felt as a soft, swollen layer over the hard bony surface of the skull and is called *caput succedaneum.* Also, it is possible for molding of the fetal skull to occur, which can distort the examiner's evaluation of the fetal head descent.

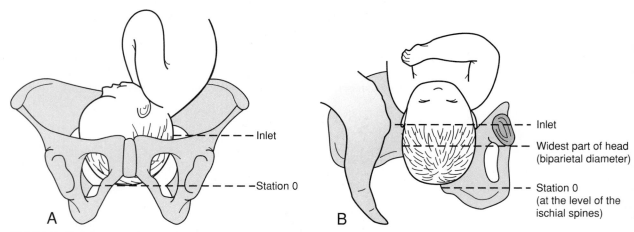

FIGURE 2.31 Engaged presenting fetal head. **A.** Front view. **B.** Side view.

If the fetal head is severely molded, there is considerable caput succedaneum, or both, engagement might not have taken place *even though the tip of the presenting part is at station 0.*

Progressive cervical dilatation without fetal descent can suggest fetal–pelvic disproportion.

For women pregnant for the first time (*primigravidas*), engagement occurs approximately 2 to 3 weeks before labor begins.

For women who have had more than one pregnancy (*multiparas*), engagement occurs any time before or during labor.

Other terms used to describe the relationship of the fetal presenting part to the pelvic passageway are as follows:

Floating—when the presenting part is entirely out of the pelvis and can be moved by the examiner abdominally just above the symphysis pubis bone (Fig. 2.32) This may also be referred to as "ballottment."

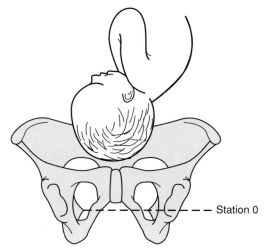

FIGURE 2.32   Floating. Fetal head is entirely out of the pelvis.

Dipping—when the presenting part has descended into the false pelvis but is not through the inlet. The examiner has to feel more deeply abdominally, and the presenting part is not easily moved (Fig. 2.33).

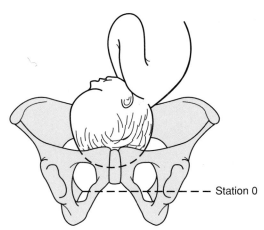

FIGURE 2.33   Dipping. Fetal head is approaching but not through the pelvic inlet.

▶ **What else can station tell you?**

You should recognize some situations that can predict problems[2]:
- An unengaged presenting part in a primigravida can indicate fetal–pelvic disproportion and bears careful watching. However, this actually happens frequently, and women often make good progress in labor.
- The occurrence of disproportion is more likely when the presenting part is high (e.g., station −3, as labor begins).
- Women who begin labor with high presenting parts tend to have achieved less cervical dilatation during early labor. Women with presenting parts at lower stations (station 0 or +2) tend to have cervices that are more effaced and dilated at the beginning of labor.
- The higher the station, the longer labor tends to be.
- Dysfunctional (nonprogressive) labor is more common when the presenting part is at a high station.
- The high presenting part that descends rapidly is usually not related to abnormal labor.

PRACTICE/REVIEW QUESTIONS

After reviewing Part 3, answer the following questions.

1. When the presenting fetal part is at the pelvic inlet, it is said to be at _____ station.

2. When the presenting fetal part is at the level of the ischial spines, it is said to be at _____ station.

3. When the presenting fetal part is halfway between the ischial spines and the pelvic outlet, it is at _____ station.

4. When the widest part of the fetal head has passed through the pelvic inlet, _____ has occurred.

5. When engagement has taken place, the pelvis is thought to be _____.

6. What effect does molding have on assessment for the amount of descent? _____

_____

7. Why is it important to assess the degree of descent?

_____

PRACTICE/REVIEW ANSWER KEY

1. −3

2. 0

3. Close to +2 station using the −3 to +3 scale; at +3 station using the −3 to +5 station

4. Engagement

5. Adequate

6. Sometimes, if severe molding of the fetal head has occurred, the examiner's assessment of the amount of descent can be distorted. That is, engagement might not have occurred even though the leading edge of the presenting part is at 0 station.

7. Assessment of the degree of descent is necessary to determine normal/abnormal progress in labor over time.

Evaluating for Fetal Malpresentation

Objectives

As you complete Part 4 of this module, you will learn:

1. What is meant by *fetal malpresentation*
2. To identify maternal and fetal conditions that can lead to fetal malpresentation
3. What to do if you suspect a fetal malpresentation

Key Terms

When you have completed Part 4 of this module, you should be able to recall the meaning of the following terms. You should also be able to use the terms when consulting with other health professionals. The terms are defined in this module or in the glossary at the end of this book.

anoxia   prolapsed cord

dystocia

Fetal Malpresentation

▶ **What is fetal malpresentation?**

Malpresentation means that some other part of the fetus, such as buttocks, shoulder, or face, is presenting at or near the pelvic inlet.

Maternal and Fetal Conditions That Can Lead to Fetal Malpresentation

Maternal factors leading to malpresentation include the following:
- Contracted (small) pelvis (the most commonly occurring factor)
- Lax abdominal muscles so that the uterus and fetus fall forward, preventing good fetal descent
- Uterine tumors (fibroids), which can block the entry to the pelvic passageway
- Uterine malformations, which can prevent efficient labor
- Abnormalities of placental size or location that lead to the fetus assuming a position unfavorable to labor and/or descent

Fetal factors leading to malpresentation include the following:
- Breech presentation or transverse lie
- Abnormal fetal attitude (e.g., hyperextension)
- Multiple pregnancy
- Fetal abnormalities (e.g., hydrocephalus)
- *Hydramnios* (excessive amounts of fluid permit greater freedom for fetal movement and, therefore, abnormal positions)

Effects of Malpresentation on Labor

- Weak and irregular contractions that are inefficient
- Prolonged labor
- Slow and incomplete cervical dilatation
- Failure of presenting part to descend
- Increased need for operative delivery
- Increased risk of uterine rupture

Effects of Malpresentation on the Mother

- Maternal exhaustion because of prolonged labor
- Greater chance of lacerations along the birth canal because of wider presenting parts
- Heavier bleeding because of lacerations and/or an exhausted uterus, which fails to contract after delivery
- Increased risk of infection caused by the following:
  - Early rupture of membranes
  - Increased blood loss
  - Tissue damage because of lacerations and bruising
  - Prolonged labor
- Decreased peristalsis of the bowel and bladder

Effects of Malpresentation on the Fetus

- Difficult fit through the pelvis, which leads to edema of the presenting part and excessive molding
- Long labor, which can be hard on the fetus, increasing the possibility of anoxia and intrauterine death
- Increased incidence of forceps and cesarean birth
- More frequently occurring prolapsed cord

▶ What should you do if you suspect fetal malpresentation?

The nurse is often the first person to recognize a malpresentation such as breech presentation. Fetal malpresentation is detected through careful abdominal palpation and vaginal examination. If you suspect malpresentation during your nursing assessment, take the following steps:

1. Alert the primary care provider immediately.
2. Monitor the baby closely until the primary care provider arrives.
3. Closely assess the mother's status and progress in labor. Do not leave her alone.

For all patients who have a breech presentation or any presentation that does not fit the pelvis well or is not settled well into the pelvis, it is essential to inspect the perineum, listen to fetal heart tones, and conduct a vaginal examination as soon as the membranes rupture.

> When the presenting part fails to fit the pelvic inlet closely, the danger of a prolapsed cord exists.

A vaginal examination should be performed in the following situations:

- There is unexplained fetal distress (this is especially true when the presenting part is high).
- The membranes rupture with a high presenting part.
- The membranes rupture in a woman presenting with a malpresentation.
- The baby is premature.
- There is a twin gestation.

▶ Why is it necessary to be able to recognize a breech presentation?

A prolapsed cord can occur in a breech presentation because the pelvic cavity is not well filled when the feet or buttocks are coming first. Once the cord is out of the uterus or vagina, the fetal blood and oxygen supply can be blocked because of (a) a drop in temperature, (b) spasm of the blood vessels, or (c) compression between the pelvic brim and the presenting part. When a prolapsed cord occurs, a delay of more than 30 minutes in delivering the baby increases fetal mortality fourfold.[2] (Prolapsed cords are discussed further in Module 18.)

PRACTICE/REVIEW QUESTIONS

After reviewing Part 4, answer the following questions.

1. Define *malpresentation.* _____

   _____

2. State at least four maternal or fetal factors that can lead to malpresentation.

   a. _____

   b. _____

   c. _____

   d. _____

3. Why is it critical that you be able to recognize a breech

   presentation? _____

   _____

PRACTICE/REVIEW ANSWER KEY

1. *Malpresentation* means that a part other than the vertex, such as buttocks, shoulder, or face, is presenting at or near the pelvic inlet.

2. Maternal factors are a contracted pelvis, lax abdominal muscles, uterine tumors blocking entry to the pelvic passageway, uterine malformations preventing efficient labor, and abnormalities of placental size or locations. Fetal factors are breech or transverse lie, abnormal fetal attitude, multiple pregnancy, fetal abnormalities, and hydramnios.

3. A prolapsed cord can occur in a breech presentation. The prolapsed cord can result in blockage of blood supply to the fetus, which could result in fetal death.

REFERENCES

1. Cunningham, F. G., Leveno, K. J., Bloom, S. L., Hauth, J. C., Gilstrap, L. C., III, & Wenstrom, K. D. (Eds.) (2005). *Williams Obstetrics* (22nd ed.). New York: McGraw-Hill.
2. Oxorn, H. (1986). *Oxorn-Foote human labor & birth* (5th ed.). New York: Appleton-Century-Crofts.
3. Yeomans, E. R. (2006). Clinical pelvimetry. *Clinical Obstetrics and Gynecology, 49*(1), 140–146.
4. Liao, J. B., Buhimschi, C. S., & Norwitz, E. R. (2005). Normal labor: Mechanism and duration. *Obstetrics and Gynecology Clinics of North America, 32*, 145–164.
5. Stitely, M. L., & Gherman, R. B. (2005). Labor with abnormal presentation and position. *Obstetrics and Gynecology Clinics of North America, 32*, 165–179.

MODULE

3

Admission Assessment of the Laboring Woman

E. JEAN MARTIN ■ DONNA JEAN RUTH

Skill Unit 1

Physical Examination of the Laboring Woman

Skill Unit 2

Testing for Ruptured Membranes
- Sterile Speculum Examination
- Nitrazine Paper Test

Skill Unit 3

Fern Testing for Ruptured Membranes

Skill Unit 4

Vaginal Examination

Objectives

As you complete this module, you will learn:

1. Key questions to ask the woman being admitted to the labor unit
2. To identify factors that makes the laboring woman a high-risk patient
3. To recognize those characteristics that help to distinguish between true labor and false labor
4. Physical assessment skills used in admitting the laboring woman
5. How to use the fern test, the Nitrazine paper test, and a sterile speculum examination to determine whether membranes have ruptured
6. To evaluate cervical effacement, dilatation, fetal presentation, and station during labor
7. The importance of preparing for and informing the expectant mother of examination and test procedures

Key Terms

When you have completed Part 1 of this module, you should be able to recall the meaning of the following terms. You should also be able to use the terms when consulting with other health professionals. The terms are defined in this module or in the glossary at the end of this book.

ABO incompatibility	meconium
abruptio placentae	meconium aspiration syndrome (MAS)
amniotic fluid index (AFI)	microcephaly
arborization	multipara
bradycardia	nullipara
chancroid	oligohydramnios
chorioamnionitis	perinatal
cleft palate	perinatal morbidity
clonus	perinatal mortality
Down's syndrome	postterm infant
eclampsia	pyloric stenosis
esophageal atresia	Rh incompatibility
group B streptococcus (GBS)	spina bifida
herpes simplex virus (HSV) type 1, type 2	tachycardia
	term infant
hydramnios (polyhydramnios)	thrombophlebitis
macrosomia	vertical transmission

Identifying Critical Information

> ▶ **What critical information must be identified for the woman being admitted to the labor unit?**

Certain information is needed immediately to evaluate the following:

- The extent of the woman's labor
- Her general physical condition
- Her risk status
- Her preparation for labor and delivery

This assessment must be carried out quickly to determine how active the labor is and to become alert to women with a history of rapid deliveries or those with problems denoting risk.

Questions	*Information Needed*
1. What made you come to the hospital?	1. Presenting complaint
2. When were you told the baby was due?	2. Expected date of delivery/confinement (EDD/EDC) and how it was determined: • by dates • by size • by ultrasound and during which trimester the ultrasound was performed
3. How many babies have you had?	3. Projection about possible rapid labor due to multiparity
4. When did your labor begin? How far apart are the contractions? Have they changed in intensity? Have you had any bleeding?	4. Stage of labor she is in: • Frequency, duration, and intensity of contractions • Amount and character of bloody show • Identification of abnormal bleeding versus bloody show
5. Has the bag of water (membranes) broken, and when did it occur? What color was the fluid?	5. Whether or not membranes have ruptured Risk of chorioamnionitis owing to prolonged rupture of membranes Presence or absence of meconium-stained or bloody amniotic fluid
6. How has your pregnancy been? Did you have any problems that required special treatment? Have you had any bleeding?	6. Any abnormalities in her pregnancy—specifically ask about problems with blood pressure (BP), bleeding, or infections
7. When did you last have anything to eat or drink? What were these foods?	7. Extent of gastric fullness
8. Are you allergic to any foods or drugs that you know of?	8. Any known allergies to drugs
9. Who has come with you? Will they be staying with you during labor?	9. Presence of a support system
10. Have you had any preparation for this labor and delivery?	10. Knowledge level regarding the birth experience
11. Is there anything special about your pregnancy that I should know?	11. To elicit information that could affect her labor/delivery or the newborn Opportunity for woman to share specific concerns regarding her care

Guidelines for History Taking

- Maintain eye contact.
- **Introduce yourself** and confirm the name by which the woman wishes to be called.
- Inform the woman that you need to ask several questions and that you will stop whenever a contraction begins. Explain that you will be writing down notes to enter into her chart.
- Ask open-ended questions when possible. For example, "Can you tell me about any infections (or problems) you have had during this pregnancy?" instead of "Have you had an infection (or problem) during this pregnancy?" and "What preparation have you had for your labor and delivery?" instead of "Have you attended childbirth preparation classes?"

You might need to ask specific questions to follow-up on her answers to your open-ended questions.

Identifying the High-Risk Mother and Fetus

▶ How can you identify a mother and fetus who are at risk?

Mothers with high-risk pregnancies tend to have high-risk babies. These patients need to be identified as early as possible on admittance to the labor unit. Women who begin pregnancy as a low-risk patient may develop complications that make them high risk during the labor and delivery process. Assessment on admission and throughout the labor process will help to identify these women in a timely manner.

Taking a good history and reviewing the prenatal record of the woman when she is admitted to the labor unit is necessary for identifying the high-risk intrapartal patient. Risk status may have changed in the period between her last prenatal visit and admission for delivery.

Every year, American women die of pregnancy-related complications during their pregnancies or within 1 year of delivery. Leading causes include hemorrhage, preeclampsia, eclampsia, emboli, and infection. The risk of pregnancy-related death is four times higher for African-American women and two times greater for Hispanic women than that for Caucasian women.[1]

Risk Factors for Laboring Women

Age 16 years or younger
Nulliparous at age 35 or older
Multiparous at age 40 or older
Fifth or more pregnancy
Height 60 inches or less
Prepregnant weight of 20% less than or 20% more than standard for height and age
Little or no weight gain during pregnancy
Heavy cigarette smoking
Rh incompatibility or ABO incompatibility problems
Previous premature deliveries
Previous birth to a large infant (>4,000 g/ 9 lb—*macrosomia*)
Previous perinatal loss
Less than a high school education or in the poverty-level income group
Single marital status
Unplanned pregnancy
Little or no antenatal care
History of a congenital anomaly or medical disorder, such as anemia, diabetes, renal disease, cardiac problems, malignant tumors, or psychiatric disorders
Symptoms of oral (type 1) or genital (type 2) *herpes simplex virus* (HSV) or a current positive herpes culture; current symptoms, especially significant if the genital herpes infection present is the woman's first infection (primary infection) experienced during pregnancy
Lesions appear as blister-like vesicles, which progress to a crusted or ulcer-type appearance. HSV of either type 1 or 2 can be shed at the cervix in symptomatic and asymptomatic women. Women with prior HSV type 2

> Maternal smoking is associated with preterm labor and delivery, neonatal and fetal death, birth defects, and other pregnancy complications.[2]

> Maternal poverty and low levels of education are factors associated with the low birth weight infants.[3]

> **NOTE:** *Ulcerative genital complaints are symptomatic of many kinds of infections (e.g., chancroid, secondary infected syphilis, contact dermatitis).*

Primary HSV is a first infection with the virus. It has a 33% to 50% neonatal transmission rate in women who deliver vaginally.[4]
Nonprimary first episode HSV is a recurrent infection but is first clinically recognized. It has a 2% to

infections who are asymptomatic have a low risk of shedding the virus during delivery.

5% transmission rate. *Recurrent HSV and genital lesions at the time of delivery* have a 0% to 3% transmission rate.

Universal viral culturing is not recommended at the time of delivery for asymptomatic women with a history of recurrent infection or whose partner has had a herpetic lesion.

Viral cultures are costly and imprecise. A negative culture does not rule out the possibility of neonatal infection because the culture sensitivity is well below 100%.[5]

Partner currently has or has a history of herpes

Active herpes in a partner can expose the sexually active mother and can unwittingly infect a newborn after birth. Parents should be educated on the possible risk that HSV imposes on the newborn. Sources of risk include children, grandparents, and so on, who have oral lesions as well. Contact with the newborn should be avoided by anyone with a current infection.

At risk for hepatitis B carrier status and no documentation of a negative screen

Newborns born vaginally or by cesarean delivery to a mother with active HSV lesions should be physically separated from other babies and managed with contact precautions while in the nursery. An isolation room is not necessary. The neonate may stay with the mother in a private room after she has been instructed on proper preventive care to reduce postpartum transmission.

See Appendix A for further discussion.

The hepatitis B virus can be transmitted to the fetus during delivery and, perhaps, in rare cases, transplacentally. See Module 11 for a complete discussion.

At risk for HIV infection

History of previous obstetric complications, such as preeclampsia, multiple pregnancy, or hydramnios

Abnormal presentation (breech presentation or transverse lie)

Prenatal and intrapartum administration of zidovudine to HIV-infected pregnant women has been shown to decrease transmission to newborns by 68%.[4] See Module 10 for a complete discussion of HIV in pregnancy.

Fetus has failed to grow normally or fetus does not reach the expected size for dates

A preterm birth is one that occurs before 37 completed weeks of gestation. *Gestational age is more important than weight in determining perinatal morbidity or mortality.* (See Module 8.)

► **Can women who are clearly at risk for problems during labor be identified ahead of time?**

The following factors are associated with the development of complications for either the mother or the baby both during and after labor and delivery.

Factors Identified From the Mother's History

- Diabetes
- Preeclampsia or eclampsia
- Rh sensitization
- Sickle cell disease
- Heart disease
- Sexually transmitted infections
- Chronic hypertension
- Previous perinatal loss
- Anemia
- Renal disease
- Carrier state for blood-borne infectious disease (e.g., hepatitis B, syphilis, or HIV)
- Group B streptococcus (GBS) carrier status

> Women who are partners of intravenous drug abusers, bisexual males, or those who have multiple partners exhibit high-risk behavior for sexually transmitted diseases, some of which could be life threatening to both the mother and the fetus. Screening for syphilis, hepatitis B, and HIV infection is strongly recommended.

> Between 10% and 30% of pregnant women are colonized with GBS. Vertical transmission of GBS during labor and delivery may result in infection in the newborn during the first week of life.[6] See Appendix A for a complete discussion of GBS.

Factors That Develop During Pregnancy

- Preeclampsia
- Postterm pregnancy (more than 42 weeks' gestation)
- Hydramnios or oligohydramnios
- Third trimester bleeding of undetermined origin
- Abruptio placentae or placenta previa

Factors Related to the Fetus

- Irregularity in fetal heart rate (FHR) or nonreassuring FHR patterns
- Intrauterine growth restriction
- Prematurity
- Malpresentation, such as breech
- Significant increase or decrease in current fetal activity
- Meconium-stained amniotic fluid

Factors Developing During Early Labor

- Amnionitis
- Premature labor
- Premature rupture of membranes (PROM)
- Fresh meconium-stained fluid
- Abnormal fetal heart tones or nonreassuring FHR patterns
- Suspected cephalopelvic disproportion

> The presence of any one of these factors requires that the mother and fetus be continually evaluated throughout labor. Electronic fetal monitoring is recommended.

Determining True Labor

▶ Is the woman in true labor?

The uterus undergoes intermittent contractions once pregnancy is established. These contractions are called Braxton-Hicks contractions, and they are often associated with false labor. After the 28th week of pregnancy, these contractions become definite and more noticeable by the woman.

As the 37th week of pregnancy approaches, contractions can be strong and are sometimes perceived by the expectant mother as a sign of true labor. Braxton-Hicks contractions usually stop or become highly irregular with a change of activity.

True Labor

Show—is often present. Show is blood-tinged mucus released from the cervical canal as labor nears or begins. It is pink, red, or brownish.

NOTE: *Bloody show without contractions indicates that the body is preparing for labor but labor is not present without regular contractions lasting approximately 1 minute.*

Contractions—tend to occur at regular intervals. They start at the back and sweep around to the abdomen, increasing in intensity and duration over several hours. They often intensify with walking.

NOTE: *Regular and intensifying contractions are the single most important indication that labor might have begun.*

Fetal movement—no significant change is noted.
Cervix—becomes effaced and dilated.

NOTE: *Progressive cervical dilatation is the hallmark of progress in labor.*

Walking—increases the intensity of contractions.
Sedation—does not stop true labor.

In addition, for some women:
Bowel status—can have loose stools 1 or 2 days before the onset of labor.
Nesting—women tend to experience a flurry of activity in housecleaning 1 or 2 days before the onset of labor.

False Labor

Show—is absent or can be related to intercourse or to a recent vaginal examination. It is brownish when the bleeding occurs hours before discovery.

Contractions—are irregular. They can be felt only in the back or in the lower abdomen. They do not intensify with walking and gradually diminish over several hours.

Fetal movement—can increase for a short time or remain the same.
Cervix—no change is noted or very small changes in thinning out (effacement) occur. Contractions help to bring about effacement.

Walking—does not change the intensity of contractions.
Sedation—tends to stop false labor or prodromal labor.

Bowel status—is usually unchanged.

Nesting—none is present.

If uncertainty exists regarding the status of labor, the mother might need to walk for 2 to 3 hours, taking frequent rests. Walking often assists in establishing a good contraction pattern.

When the mother is asked to walk, tell her to return if any of the following occur:
- Bag of water breaks
- Contractions become more frequent than 3 to 4 minutes apart
- Bloody show increases
- Nausea and vomiting occur
- Urge to push occurs
- Contractions become so strong that she is having difficulty coping

Evaluating the Status of Membranes

▶ What is meant by "membranes"?

While developing inside the uterus, the fetus lives in a sac. The sac has two layers: the inner layer, called the *amnion,* and the outer covering, called the *chorion.* This sac is filled with fluid that is made up of water, various chemicals (e.g., salts), and particles that come from the fetus itself (e.g., body cells and hair).

▶ What is normal amniotic fluid like?

By the end of pregnancy, the uterus contains approximately 1 L of amniotic fluid. The fluid is clear or straw colored and has a characteristic (not foul) odor. When tested for its acid–base content, it ranges from neutral to slightly alkaline. A close relationship exists between the status of the fluid and the health of the fetus. By studying various components of amniotic fluid, one can learn much about the gender, health, and maturity of the baby.

▶ Does the fluid serve a special purpose?

The fetus derives many benefits from amniotic fluid, which does the following:
- **Protects** the fetus from a direct blow. Pressure from a blow spreads in all directions within the fluid-filled sac, so the fetus does not receive the full impact of the blow.
- **Provides** a fluid environment in which the fetus moves. This fluid continually changes in amount and consistency, promoting the growth and development of the fetus.
- **Prevents** loss of heat and permits the fetus to maintain a constant body temperature.
- **Provide**s a source of oral intake. The fetus swallows amniotic fluid from approximately the fourth month until delivery.
- **Acts** as a collection system for the waste products of the fetus. The fetus urinates into the amniotic fluid from the fourth month until delivery.

▶ What can happen to the amniotic fluid and membranes that indicates a problem?

A. Premature Rupture of Membranes (PROM) Before Labor Begins With a Term Fetus at 37 Completed Weeks or More Gestational Age

Membranes ("bag of waters") can rupture before labor begins. The break in the membranes can be complete, with a large gushing of fluid from the birth canal, or a small tear with a slow leak.

> Most women go into labor spontaneously within a few hours after membranes rupture.

B. Preterm Premature Rupture of Membranes (pPROM) Before Labor Begins With a Preterm Fetus 36 Weeks or Less Gestational Age

When rupture occurs before the fetus has reached the 37th completed week of gestation, perinatal morbidity and mortality increase. These women should be monitored for signs and symptoms of infection

> BE PREPARED FOR THE BIRTH OF A HIGH-RISK INFANT.

C. Meconium-Stained Amniotic Fluid

Fetal stool is referred to as *meconium.* It is largely made up of water, but also contains proteins, cholesterol, lipids, vernix, and other substances. Large concentrations of bile pigments give meconium its green color. Meconium present for more than 24 hours begins to turn yellow-green. Bacteria are not present in fresh meconium.

Meconium at delivery in a term fetus is present between 12% and 20% of the time. It is seldom present in the preterm fetus, yet approaches an incidence of 25% to 30% in the postterm infant.[7]

Fetal physiologic mechanisms that result in relaxation of the sphincter required for meconium passage are not well understood. Three theories have been suggested to explain fetal passage of meconium. The theories are listed below.

- May be in response to a hypoxic event and therefore may signal fetal compromise[8]
- May be the result of vagal stimulation from transient umbilical cord entrapment and resultant peristalsis[9]
- May represent normal gastrointestinal tract maturation under neural control and is a normal physiologic process[10]

The significance of meconium-stained amniotic fluid as a predictor of fetal compromise may depend on the following:

- Concentration and type of meconium (e.g., thick or thin; color; amount)
- Gestational age
- Stage of labor when the meconium is passed (often not known)
- The presence of other fetal compromise markers such as FHR abnormalities or oligohydramnios

Meconium aspiration syndrome (MAS) is thought to be caused by an initial hypoxic event resulting in the release of meconium into the amniotic fluid. The normal fetal response to hypoxemia is to gasp, and thus in this instance, the meconium is aspirated and can be seen below the vocal cords on examination.

> The pathophysiologic process set up in MAS often leads to a poor perinatal outcome.

> *NOTE: MAS is significantly associated with fetal acidemia at birth; there is increasing evidence that infants with MAS have suffered chronic hypoxia before birth.*[11,12]

Related Facts

Meconium is rarely passed before the 34th gestational week.

Clinical studies indicate an association between the passage of meconium and high-risk clinical situations, including the following:

- Acute chorioamnionitis
- PROM
- Abruptio placentae
- Cocaine use
- Postterm pregnancy

Meconium alone is not an indicator of fetal hypoxia. Look at other fetal assessment parameters.

MECONIUM STAINING, ACCOMPANIED BY A NONREASSURING FETAL HEART RATE PATTERN **MAY** INDICATE NONREASSURING FETAL STATUS.

Electronic fetal monitoring is recommended when meconium-stained amniotic fluid is present.

> Be prepared for the birth of a highrisk infant.

Postterm pregnancies are defined at those lasting beyond 42 weeks gestation.

In postterm laboring women, you should look for the following:

- The presence of meconium-stained fluid
- The absence of any amniotic fluid—This should alert you to the almost certain presence of meconium even though you cannot see it!
- Placental dysfunction—Watch for late decelerations
- Umbilical cord compression—Watch for variable decelerations
- Macrosomia

> Primigravidas are more likely to have prolonged pregnancies.

Suctioning should be anticipated and the neonatal specialist alerted (Display 3.1).

DISPLAY 3.1 | SELECTIVE SUCTIONING IN INFANTS WITH MECONIUM-STAINED AMNIOTIC FLUID

1. If meconium is present, the mouth and hypopharynx should be suctioned with a mechanical device before delivery of the shoulders in a cephalic presentation. In a breech presentation, suctioning should be done after delivery of the head.
2. If meconium is present and the newborn is depressed, the infant should be intubated. The trachea should be suctioned to removed meconium and other aspirated material.
3. If meconium is present and the newborn is vigorous, there is no evidence that tracheal suctioning is necessary and the attempt to intubate a vigorous newborn may cause injury to the vocal cords. Use a bulb syringe or large-bore catheter to clear secretions from the nose and mouth.
4. Vigorous is defined as strong respiratory efforts, good muscle tone and a heart rate greater than 100 bpm.

> When suctioning with a mechanical apparatus, set the suction pressure so that when the suction tubing is occluded, the negative pressure is approximately 100 mmHg.

> The presence of meconium-stained amniotic fluid, no matter what the color, should alert you to the potential for fetal aspiration of meconium. Prompt suctioning of the mouth and nose of the infant with suction apparatus before delivery of the baby's shoulders and trunk is important to reduce the occurrence of MAS (a form of aspiration pneumonia that occurs most often in term or postterm infants who have passed meconium in utero). Even when suctioning is done, meconium aspiration can be present because aspiration can occur in utero.

D. Infection

Amniotic membranes and fluid can become infected, especially after 24 hours of ruptured membranes. Infection can be detected by the presence of a foul odor, fundal tenderness, and an elevated temperature in the mother.

> In all instances of *premature rupture of membranes*, the woman's temperature should be taken and recorded every 2 hours. An elevated temperature (99.6°F) can indicate the presence of an infection and should be reported immediately to the primary care provider.

E. Port Wine–Colored Amniotic Fluid–
AN EMERGENCY

Port wine–colored amniotic fluid is an indicator of a premature separation of the placenta from the uterine wall, called *abruptio placentae* (Display 3.2). (See Module 18.)

DISPLAY 3.2 | SIGNS OF ABRUPTIO PLACENTAE

The following signs indicate that the placenta has partially or totally separated from the uterine wall:
- Tender abdomen
- Hard or rigid tone to abdomen
- Absence of fetal heart tones
- Mother has had a few sharp piercing pains in her abdomen in the past 1 or 2 hours
- Mother may or may not have vaginal bleeding

Abruptio placentae occurs in approximately 1 in 200 pregnancies. Factors that may predispose a woman to developing abruptio placentae include the following:

- Hypertension
- Hydramnios
- Multiple pregnancies
- Trauma
- History of heavy smoking
- Cocaine use (especially intravenous use or smoking "crack")

F. Hydramnios/Oligohydramnios

There can be too much or too little fluid within the amniotic sac. Normally, the fluid volume is about 1 L toward the end of pregnancy. The presence of 2 L or more of amniotic fluid is considered excessive and called *polyhydramnios* or *hydramnios.* The mother's abdomen may look unusually large, tight, and glistening.

When there is less than 500 mL of fluid, the condition is called *oligohydramnios.*

Ultrasonic techniques are used to measure amounts of amniotic volume. One method of calculation involves adding the depth in centimeters of the largest vertical pocket of fluid in each of four equal uterine quadrants. The numerical value is called the *amniotic fluid index* (AFI).[14]

Reference ranges have been established from 16 weeks onward and the measurement is reported as a number (e.g., 24 cm).

Clinical studies indicate that the AFI tends to be reliable in determining normal and increased fluid, but may not be accurate in diagnosing oligohydramnios.[15] Factors such as maternal hydration/dehydration and altitude may affect the AFI.

Hydramnios, an AFI of greater than 20 to 25 cm, is commonly associated with fetal malformations and chromosomal abnormalities including:

- hydrocephaly, microcephaly and anencephaly
- spina bifida
- cleft palate
- esophageal atresia
- pyloric stenosis
- Down's syndrome
- congenital heart disease

Oligohydramnios, an AFI of 5 cm or less, while not common early in pregnancy, is associated with poor fetal outcomes. When pregnancies continue beyond term, diminished fluid volume is often found. Oligohydramnios may be associated with the following conditions:

- chromosomal abnormalities
- congenital anomalies

> Amniotic fluid increases to about 1 L by 36 weeks and then begins to decrease. In postterm pregnancies, the amniotic fluid volume may be only 100 to 200 mL.[13]

> Common maternal antepartal conditions associated with hydramnios include:
> - Diabetes
> - Multifetal pregnancies
>
> Be alert for maternal intrapartal complications such as the following:
> - Placental abruption
> - Dysfunctional labor patterns
> - Postpartum hemorrhage

> Cord compression during labor is common with oligohydramnios. Whenever women are diagnosed as having oligohydramnios or when there is no amniotic fluid on rupture of membranes, electronic fetal monitoring is recommended.

- postterm pregnancies
- ruptured membranes
- maternal hypertension
- preeclampsia
- intrauterine growth restriction
- defects of the fetal urinary tract

Oligohydramnios is primarily associated with the following:
- Congenital defects of the fetal urinary tract
- Intrauterine growth restriction
- Postterm pregnancies

PRACTICE/REVIEW QUESTIONS
After reviewing this part, answer the following questions.

1. List at least five types of information you need to elicit from a woman being admitted to the labor unit.

   a. _____

   b. _____

   c. _____

   d. _____

   e. _____

2. Which of the following are considered high-risk categories for a laboring woman? Select all that apply.

   a. Age of 37 years

   b. Unmarried

   c. High school graduate

   d. Fourth pregnancy

   e. Previous perinatal loss

   f. First pregnancy

   g. Current history of an active herpes lesion

3. Which of the following factors predict a strong possibility of problems developing for the mother or baby during or after labor and delivery? Select all that apply.

   a. Maternal history of heavy smoking

   b. Fresh, meconium-stained fluid

   c. Induction of labor

   d. Fetal tachycardia

   e. Multiple pregnancies

   f. Mild anemia

   g. Prematurity

4. A birth occurring before _____ completed weeks' gestation is identified as preterm birth.

5. A fetus of more than _____ completed weeks' gestation (postterm) is considered high risk.

6. Which of the following is (are) an indication of *true* labor? Select all that apply.

   a. Pinkish mucus present

   b. Regular and intensifying contractions

   c. Loose stools 1 to 2 days before labor

   d. Effaced cervix

   e. Increase in fetal movement

7. Define *primary HSV infection.*

   _____

   _____

8. Define *nonprimary first episode HSV.*

   _____

   _____

9. Amniotic fluid generally peaks in volume by the _____ gestational week and then slowly _____ until the _____ week. It can _____ quickly after 40 weeks.

10. Which of the following descriptions are characteristic of normal amniotic fluid? Select all that apply.

    a. Clear or straw colored

    b. Neutral to slightly acid

    c. Composed of water, salts, and other particles from the fetus

    d. Alkaline

11. Which of the following situations indicates that you should prepare for the birth of a high-risk infant? Select all that apply.

    a. Rupture of membranes before labor begins with a 38-week gestational age fetus

    b. Rupture of membranes before labor begins with a fetus less than 37 weeks' gestational age

    c. A laboring woman at a documented 43 weeks' gestation

    d. Rupture of membranes with little fluid at 41 weeks' gestation

12. Which of the following can indicate that the fetus is in distress? Select all that apply.

   a. Greenish-brown meconium staining with a cephalic presentation

   b. Mother's temperature of 99°F

   c. Tender abdomen

   d. Excessive amniotic fluid

   e. Port wine–colored amniotic fluid

   f. Absence of amniotic fluid

13. State the difference between PROM (premature rupture of membranes) and pPROM (preterm premature rupture of membranes). _____

_____

14. Meconium passage at delivery in a term fetus is present in approximately _____% of women. Two situations that increase the chances of this happening are

_____ and _____.

15. Thick, meconium-stained amniotic fluid does not seem to increase the risk of a low Apgar score.

   a. True

   b. False

16. The American Academy of Pediatrics recommends that, in a vigorous and spontaneously breathing infant who may have aspirated meconium, aggressive suctioning may not be warranted.

   a. True

   b. False

17. When pregnancy is prolonged beyond 42 completed weeks of gestation, one should be prepared for a high-risk baby that is _____.

18. In prolonged pregnancies, one should watch for placental dysfunction that can be reflected in an electronic fetal monitoring strip depicting _____.

19. Suctioning done on infants with moderate or thick meconium-stained amniotic fluid ensures that meconium aspiration will not occur.

   a. True

   b. False

20. The amniotic fluid index (AFI) is defined as

_____

_____.

21. The AFI tends to be less reliable in diagnosing

_____.

22. If a woman is diagnosed as having oligohydramnios, electronic fetal monitoring is recommended.

   a. True

   b. False

PRACTICE/REVIEW ANSWER KEY

1. Presenting complaint and symptoms, EDD/EDC, stage of labor, abnormalities in pregnancy, time of last snack or meal, known allergies to drugs, support system, review of patient's history (family and past history, current laboratory data, present obstetric status).

2. a, b, e, g

3. b, d, e, g

4. 37

5. 42

6. a, b, d, e, g

7. *Primary HSV* is a first infection with the virus; it can be symptomatic or asymptomatic.

8. *Nonprimary first episode HSV* is actually a recurrent infection but at the time is first clinically diagnosed as such.

9. 36th, decreases, 40th, decreases

10. a, c, d

11. b, c, d

12. a, c, e, f

13. PROM pertains to rupture of membranes after the 37th completed gestational week, whereas pPROM signifies rupture of membranes before the 37th completed gestational week.

14. Seven percent to 22% (some say 30%); any two of the following: acute chorioamnionitis, premature rupture of membranes, abruptio placentae, cocaine use, postterm pregnancy

15. b. False

16. a. True

17. Postmature/dysmature (see glossary)

18. Late decelerations

19. b. False

20. A numerical value expressing calculations of amniotic fluid volume found during ultrasonography as compared with standardized values for normal pregnancies at expressed gestational weeks.

21. Oligohydramnios

22. a. True

SKILL UNIT 1 | PHYSICAL EXAMINATION OF THE LABORING WOMAN

This section details how to perform a modified physical examination to screen for problems in the woman being admitted to labor and delivery. Study this section and then attend a skill practice and demonstration session scheduled with your preceptor. You will need to demonstrate the examination and correctly interpret the results. The steps of the examination are summarized at the end of this unit.

ACTIONS	REMARKS

What Are the Techniques to Be Used in Performing the Physical Examination?

1. *Inspection*—observing the general health and outstanding characteristics of the patient in a thorough, unhurried manner
2. *Palpation*—feeling or touching parts to be evaluated
3. *Auscultation*—listening, usually with a stethoscope, for the sounds produced by the body

The physical examination of the laboring woman is not as extensive as that given at her first prenatal visit.

What Steps Should You Take to Prepare for the Examination?

1. Ask the woman to empty her bladder.

A full bladder can make examination of the abdomen or bladder uncomfortable.

2. Follow a logical order of assessment. Use all of your senses as the assessment is carried out.

In general, it is suggested that you begin at the head of the patient and work toward the toes. You are not likely to miss anything this way.

3. Explain to the woman what you are doing.
4. Warm your hands by rubbing them together or holding them under warm water.
5. Chart your findings in a logical order.

Unless you have a checklist, chart your findings in the same order in which you conduct the examination.

When Is the Best Time to Perform the Physical Examination?

The initial assessment is carried out immediately to evaluate the labor and any signs of problems.

The examination is conducted as quickly as possible. The woman can then assume a side-lying or upright sitting position. Cardiac output is better for the mother, and uteroplacental circulation for the fetus is optimized in these positions.

Assess the following:
General appearance
• Look for edema in face, hands, and feet
Vital signs
Abdominal
• Determine the frequency, duration, and intensity of contractions
Fetal position
Fetal heart tones
Height of the fundus (top of uterus)
Perform a vaginal examination to determine the following:
Cervical effacement
Cervical dilatation and station
Amount of bloody show
Whether membranes have ruptured
Amount of amniotic fluid

Early and careful assessment of the patient's physical status will provide clues to problems.

For example, if the BP is elevated, evaluate for the following:
• Edema in hands and feet
• Protein in the urine
• Presence of headache and blurred vision
• Elevated preeclampsia laboratory indices
• Epigastric pain
In the presence of vaginal bleeding, the digital examination may be deferred until the location of the placenta can be verified and placenta previa ruled out.

NOTE: Women with preterm or term pregnancies who are not in labor and who present with ruptured membranes and no signs of fetal distress should not

Vaginal examination should not be performed on a nonlaboring woman who presents with ruptured membranes. A sterile speculum examination using strict aseptic techniques will tell you whether she is

undergo a digital vaginal examination on arrival. Wait for the primary care provider to arrive.

dilated. A single vaginal examination can compromise both mother and fetus by leading to chorioamnionitis. Management of the expectant woman depends on whether membranes have ruptured, not on dilatation.

> If the fetus is in a transverse or breech position and labor is active, you need to alert the primary care provider immediately. If the membranes are ruptured and there are signs of fetal distress, you need to perform a digital vaginal examination to assess the progress of the labor and to check for a prolapsed cord.

What Position Is Best for the Examination?

Ask the patient to lie on her back as you begin the examination.
Elevate the head of the bed or the examining table enough to make the patient comfortable.

You need to ensure that the patient is not flat on her back to avoid supine hypotension syndrome.

Completing a General Assessment

Give *thoughtful attention* to the general appearance of the patient.
Note the following:
    Signs of distress
    Skin color
    Movements
    Personal hygiene
    Odor
    Facial expression
    Speech
    Manner
    Mood
    State of awareness

The woman who comes to the labor unit in active labor might appear stressed because contractions are strong and frequent. Note how she is coping with them—whether she is using a breathing technique or tensing up. You can reinforce her technique or teach her an effective one.
If she has come with a support person, find out whether she wishes the support person to remain with her during as much of the admission as possible. If she has no partner, you may need to assume a supporting role.

Vital Signs

1. Blood pressure: Be sure to assess BP between contractions.
    a. The cuff must fit snugly on the arm and be of appropriate size. The cuff should be approximately 20% wider than the width of the arm.
    b. Take BP measurements with the woman in a sitting position or left lateral (side-lying) position.
    c. Taking BP measurements using the Korotkoff IV (muffled) sound or the V (disappearing) sound has been an issue. A recent consensus states that the Korotkoff V sound should be used for reading the diastolic pressure.[16]

A cuff too small or too large can result in BP readings that are inaccurately high or low, respectively.

BP in the arteries is affected by position. When sitting, the pressure in the brachial artery is highest; when lying on the right or left side, it is lowest.
The method for taking BP readings (e.g., patient position and which Korotkoff sound to use) should be consistently used by all caretakers on the unit.

> An elevated systolic but normal diastolic BP can indicate anxiety.

*Compare the reading you obtain
with the mother's prenatal BP readings.*

The patient may have a hypertensive disorder
if the BP is:

- 140/90 mm Hg or higher (mild hypertension)
- 160/110 mm Hg or higher (severe hypertension)

You also need to do the following:

- Determine whether the mother's urine has protein in it
- Check for facial, fingertip, and pretibial edema
- Test for hyperreflexia
- Ask the mother if she is having headaches or blurred vision or is seeing spots before her eyes
- Notify the primary care provider immediately of proteinuria (other than trace), BP elevations approaching 140/90 mm Hg, hyperreflexia, marked edema (>2+), and complaints of headaches or blurred vision or spots before the eyes.

To assess for the presence of hypertension in the mother, *her baseline BP must be known.*

A woman with either of these BP changes can have pregnancy-induced hypertension, chronic hypertension, or gestational hypertension.

Women presenting before term (less than 37 weeks) with flu-like symptoms, nausea, vomiting, or gastrointestinal upset should be assessed for HELLP syndrome. This assessment should include laboratory studies of the platelet count and liver functions. Elevated BP *may not* be present. These women are very ill and need immediate evaluation and intervention (see Module 9).

2. Pulse (normal range, 60 to 90 bpm)

Increased pulse rate can result from excitement, anxiety, dehydration, pain, and, in rare cases, cardiac problems.

3. Respirations

Avoid counting respirations during a uterine contraction because they can be abnormally high or low as a result of stress or because of the use of a breathing technique.

4. Temperature (normal range, 97.6°F to 99.6°F [36.2°C to 37.6°C])

Look for signs of infection or dehydration if the temperature is above 99.6°F.

NOTE: *In the past, an increase of 30 mmHg systole or 15 mmHg diastole above a baseline BP on at least two occasions 6 hours apart was diagnostic for pregnancy-induced hypertension. This is no longer considered a reliable diagnostic marker. However, rising systolic and/or diastolic BP readings are always cause for increased surveillance of the pregnant woman. See Module 9 for a detailed discussion of this topic.*

Abdomen

1. Inspect for scars, striae (stretch marks), rashes, and symmetry of the abdomen.

Striae are shiny, reddish lines that appear on the breasts, abdomen, thighs, and buttocks of approximately half of pregnant women as a result of stretching of the skin and underlying tissue.

2. If you detect a scar that the woman tells you is the result of surgery done on the uterus and the woman is in active labor, notify the primary care provider immediately.

Vertical scars from previous classic cesarean births are much more likely to rupture than horizontal scars down low on the abdomen.

3. Assess the following:
   - Fundal height
   - Fetal position
   - Fetal heart tones

An abnormal shape of the abdomen should alert you to fetal malposition (such as a transverse lie)

See Skill Unit 1, Measuring Fundal Height, in Module 4.

Bladder

Gently palpate the lower abdominal area just above the symphysis pubis bone to determine bladder fullness or tenderness.

Suprapubic tenderness might suggest a bladder infection. Signs and symptoms of elevated temperature, burning on urination, and frequency of urination should be discussed.

Lower Extremities

1. Inspect for the presence of *varicosities.* If present, feel for warmth.

Warmth over a varicosity can indicate a *thrombophlebitis* (inflammation of a vein associated with a blood clot). The primary care provider should be alerted.

Using both hands, palpate for *tenderness,* beginning behind the knee and working your way down the leg to the ankle (Fig. 3.1)

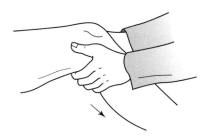

FIGURE 3.1

If the woman experiences tenderness to your touch, dorsiflex the foot (i.e., bend it back toward the knee) and ask her whether this causes any calf pain (Fig. 3.2). Calf pain with dorsiflexion of the foot indicates possible thrombophlebitis. This is called Homans' sign.

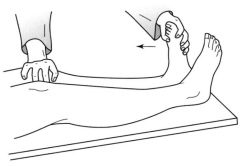

FIGURE 3.2

2. Press firmly with the thumb approximately 5 seconds over the pretibial (shin) area to test for *edema* in both legs (Fig. 3.3).

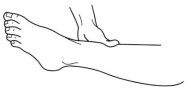

FIGURE 3.3

Edema of the legs measuring 3+ and 4+ is often accompanied by facial and hand edema. When 3+ to 4+ edema is present, the woman should be assessed for preeclampsia. Evaluate for the following:
- BP
- Proteinuria
- Headaches or visual disturbances

Pretibial edema is assessed as follows:
  1+ = small suggestion of fullness felt
  2+ = sense of fullness
  3+ = blanching of the skin and depression seen as finger presses down
  4+ = indentation made by finger pressure (pitting), which remains for several seconds and gradually declines
Edema is not considered a reliable diagnostic criterion for preeclampsia.

3. To elicit a deep tendon reflex, the patient must be relaxed. Position the leg by supporting the knee with one hand or arm in a partially flexed position while asking the patient to relax that leg completely (Fig. 3.4). Briskly tap the patellar tendon just below the kneecap. This can also be done with the patient in a sitting position (Fig. 3.5). Watch for some degree of a brisk jerk.

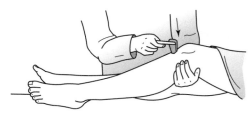

FIGURE 3.4

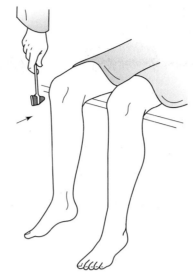

FIGURE 3.5

NOTE: Many women, including adolescents, have brisk reflexes. Do not consider this a major indication of a pathologic condition.

Test for clonus if reflexes are 4+ (hyperactive). Support the knee in a partially flexed position. With your other hand, sharply dorsiflex the foot and maintain it in dorsiflexion (see Fig. 3.2). If clonus is present, you will see the foot moving back and forth in small rhythmic movements.

Reflexes are graded on a 0 to 4+ scale.

4+ = extremely brisk (called hyperactive); often indicates a disease state of the central nervous system

3+ = brisker than average

2+ = average, normal

1+ = somewhat diminished, low normal

0 = flat, no response

The presence of clonus indicates that the central nervous system is highly irritated, although in some patients it can simply be the result of anxiety. Clonus may be associated with moderate to severe preeclampsia.

You will need to attend a skill session(s) to practice these skills with the help of your preceptor. Mastery of the skill is achieved when you can demonstrate techniques of physical assessment, including the following:

- Preparatory steps
- Logical order
- Appropriate positions for examining various areas of the body
- Accurate assessment of vital signs
- Abdomen (fundal height, fetal position, and fetal heart tones are demonstrated in Module 4)
- Bladder
- Lower extremities, including checking for edema, reflexes, tenderness, and clonus

SKILL UNIT 2 | TESTING FOR RUPTURED MEMBRANES

- *Sterile Speculum Examination*
- *Nitrazine Paper Test*

This section details accurate ways to test for the rupture of amniotic membranes. Study this section and then attend a skill practice and demonstration scheduled with your preceptor. You will need to demonstrate that you can perform and interpret the steps of this procedure. These steps are summarized at the end of this unit.

ACTIONS	REMARKS

Selecting the Speculum

1. The speculum is composed of two blades and a handle. A thumb piece attaches to the top blade; the bottom blade is fixed (Fig. 3.6).

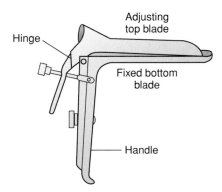

Hinge · Adjusting top blade · Fixed bottom blade · Handle

FIGURE 3.6

The top blade is hinged, and the thumb piece controls its motions (Fig. 3.7).

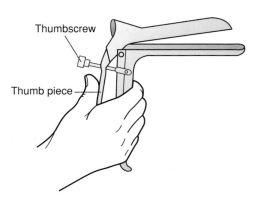

Thumbscrew · Thumb piece

FIGURE 3.7

The thumbscrew, when turned, tightens and fixes the top blade in position (Fig. 3.8).

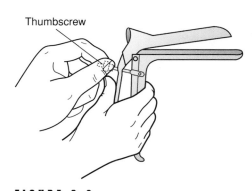

Thumbscrew

FIGURE 3.8

When the speculum is opened by using the thumb piece, a space is created between the blades, which, if placed in the vagina, permit a clear view of the vaginal walls and cervix (Fig. 3.9).

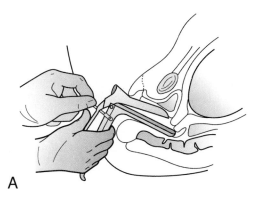

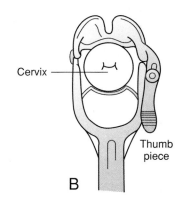

Cervix

Thumb piece

A

B

FIGURE 3.9

2. Two basic types of specula are as follows:
   a. The Graves speculum (Fig. 3.10 a & b)
   - Is the most common
   - Is used in the examination of the adult female
   - Comes in two sizes, standard and large, which vary in length from 3.5 to 5.0 inches and in width from 0.75 to 1.50 inches

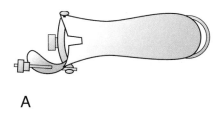

A

FIGURE 3.10 Graves speculum.

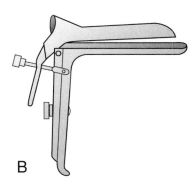

B

   b. The Pedersen speculum (Fig. 3.11 a & b)
   - Is as long as the Graves speculum but narrower and flatter
   - Is used more in women who have not had intercourse, women who have never had a baby, or women who are so tense that insertion of the Graves speculum is difficult

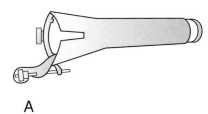

A

FIGURE 3.11 Pedersen speculum.

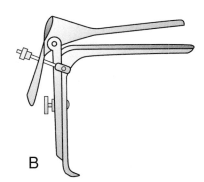

B

Preparing the Woman

3. Tell the woman what you are going to be doing in terms she can understand.

An informed woman is more relaxed. She is more likely to cooperate with you throughout the examination.

4. Ask the woman to empty her bladder.

A full bladder can make the examination uncomfortable for the woman and more difficult to perform.

5. Have the woman remove her underclothing and lie on the examining table. Assist her to relax with her legs bent, feet resting flat on the table or in the stirrups. Place a pillow under her head and ask that she rest her hands across her abdomen or at her sides.

This increases her comfort and relaxation. Sometimes women put their hands above their heads during a vaginal examination, which tightens abdominal muscles and makes the examination more difficult and uncomfortable.

What Should You Do Before Beginning the Examination?

6. Drape the mother's legs so that you cover her up to her knees. Make sure that you can see her face when you are sitting down.

7. Position a gooseneck lamp so that the perineum is well lit.

If the perineum appears wet and glistening, there is a good chance that the membranes have ruptured.

8. Position the stool on which you will sit for the examination so that you will not need to move it again.

9. Select the appropriate speculum. The speculum must be *sterile.*

10. Wash your hands.

11. Put on sterile gloves.

12. If you are alone, open the package containing the sterile speculum in such a way that you can grasp the handle for removal after you have put on a sterile glove.

The appropriate speculum is the one that will cause the least amount of discomfort to the woman while providing a good view of the vagina and cervix.

It is a good idea to have someone assist you and support the woman throughout the examination.

Take care! Maintaining strict aseptic technique throughout the sterile speculum examination can reduce the risk of chorioamnionitis if membranes are ruptured.

What Is the Best Way to Begin the Examination?

13. Sit down on the stool and ask the woman to separate or spread her legs. *Do not try to use force, or even to gently separate her legs.*

Because this examination is an intrusive procedure, it should be carried out when the woman is ready for it.

14. Tell the woman *how to relax.* If she knows a relaxation and breathing technique learned previously, have her use it. If not, have her do slow, deep, relaxed breathing. Ask her to let herself go limp, to think of herself as a rag doll.

15. If the woman becomes upset or tense during the examination, *stop whatever you are doing.* Do not remove your fingers; simply hold your hand still. Find out what is bothering her. Try to distinguish among discomfort as a result of pressure, fear, and actual pain. Wait until she has regained control, helping her to relax.

16. Hold the speculum near the gooseneck lamp to warm it. Often, additional lubricant is not needed because the vagina is moist from bloody show when the mother goes into labor. If a lubricant is needed, only *sterile* water should be used.

If you use running tap water or a lubricant, you will lose the sterility of the speculum. This could introduce an infectious organism to the mother and to the fetus if membranes are ruptured.

17. Tell the woman what you are doing as you touch her inner thigh with the back of the gloved hand that is not holding the speculum.

This accustoms her to your touch and prepares her for the more intrusive part of the examination.

18. Using this same hand, place two fingers just inside the introitus and gently press down on the base of the vagina.
19. With your other hand, introduce the *closed* speculum past your fingers at approximately a 45-degree angle downward (Fig. 3.12). Keep a moderate downward pressure on the blades to avoid upward pressure on the sensitive bladder and top vaginal wall.

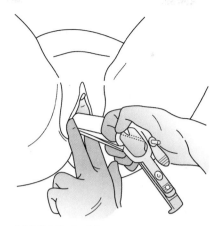

FIGURE 3.12

20. After the speculum is in the vagina, remove your fingers from the base of the vaginal opening. Turn the blades of the speculum into a horizontal position, all the while keeping a moderate downward pressure (Fig. 3.13).

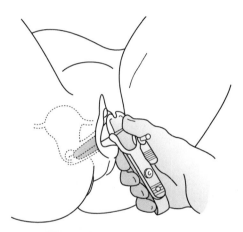

FIGURE 3.13

21. Tell the woman she might feel pressure. Move your thumb to the thumb piece and press to open the blades so that the cervix is in view (Fig. 3.14).
22. Sweep the blades slowly upward by gently pressing on the handle. If this does not bring the cervix into view, close the blades and withdraw the speculum a little. Warn the mother of the extra pressure she might feel. Then, while pressing down firmly, move the blades toward the back of the vagina again. Sometimes the tip of the blades needs to be directed more anteriorly or posteriorly, depending on the position of the cervix.
23. When the cervix is in view, tighten the thumbscrew to keep the blades open.

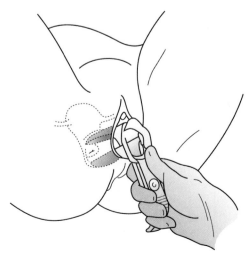

FIGURE 3.14

What Will You See If the Membranes Are Ruptured?

24. Fluid will be seen leaking from the cervical opening.

> Viewing leaking fluid from the cervical opening is the best method for determining that the membranes have ruptured.

Note the color and odor.

- *Deep yellow color* indicates the release of meconium approximately 1 to 2 days previously.
- *Greenish-brown color* indicates a more recent passage of meconium.

Use this opportunity to screen for any signs of abnormalities, such as bleeding. Heavy bloody show can alert you to an advanced state of labor.

25. Obtain a specimen of the suspected leaking fluid by placing a *sterile* cotton-tipped applicator into the pool of fluid accumulating in the lower blade (Fig. 3.15).

Amniotic fluid is clear or straw colored. It does not have an unpleasant odor.

The presence of meconium may be an indication of a potentially poor outcome for the fetus and requires further evaluation. It is not necessarily a predictor of poor fetal outcome, but it must be evaluated in light of other assessment and findings (e.g., FHR tracings). The release of meconium during labor may indicate that the fetus is stressed. (This might not be true if the fetus is in a breech position.)

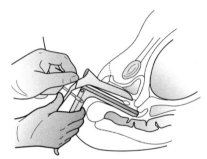

FIGURE 3.15

Nitrazine paper contains a dye that changes color when alkaline substances such as amniotic fluid moisten it.

26. Touch the cotton-tipped applicator or cotton ball on a fresh strip of Nitrazine paper, moistening it well.

How Do You Interpret the Color Change?

27. Compare the color that appears on the moistened paper against the standard color chart.

Findings on Nitrazine Paper		
Color	**pH**	**Interpretation**
Yellow	5.0	
Olive	5.5	Probably membranes are *not* ruptured
Olive-green	6.0	
Blue-green	6.5	Probably membranes are ruptured
Blue-gray	7.0	
Deep blue	7.5	May be caused by blood or cervical mucus

Be aware of the possibility of false-positive readings.

A standard color chart can be found on the box of Nitrazine paper, with a range of colors used to interpret the alkaline nature of substances. Because amniotic fluid is neutral (pH 7.0) or slightly alkaline (pH 7.25), it changes the yellow color of Nitrazine paper.

The pH values of blood, vaginal mucus, and certain secretions from vaginal infections are also alkaline. If the amount of amniotic fluid is small or absent but the above substances are present in large amounts, a false-positive test could result.

The Nitrazine test is not considered a definitive test for diagnosing ruptured membranes. See the fern test for this.

How Do You Remove the Speculum?

28. Release the thumbscrew on the thumb piece. Hold the blades apart by pressing on the thumb piece and begin withdrawing the speculum until the cervix is released from between the blades.

29. Release your pressure on the thumb piece and allow the blades to close. Avoid pinching the vaginal tissue or pubic hair when the blades close. Rotate the blades to a sideways position and exert downward pressure. As the blades are eased out, hook your index finger over the top blade to control it.

   This avoids pressure to the sensitive urethra and top vaginal wall.

30. Note the odor of any vaginal discharge pooled in the bottom blade.

   Foul-smelling discharge might indicate amniotic fluid infection.

31. Deposit the speculum in the proper container.

32. Wipe any moisture or discharge from the perineal area.

You will need to attend a skill session(s) to practice this skill with the help of your preceptor. Mastery of the skill is achieved when you can demonstrate the following:
- Selection and operation of an appropriately sized speculum for a variety of women
- Positioning and preparation of the woman for speculum examination
- The procedure for a sterile speculum examination
- How to obtain a specimen for Nitrazine paper testing
- Interpretation of color changes indicating that membranes have ruptured

SKILL UNIT 3 | FERN TESTING FOR RUPTURED MEMBRANES

This section details how to do the fern test to determine whether membranes have ruptured. Study this section and then attend a skill practice and demonstration section scheduled with your preceptor. You will need to demonstrate that you can perform the procedure and correctly interpret the results. These steps are summarized at the end of this unit.

ACTIONS	REMARKS
Preparing to Conduct the Test	
1. Who might need this test? • Any pregnant woman suspected of having ruptured membranes	Amniotic fluid contains a high amount of a salt called sodium chloride. If drops of the fluid are spread on a glass slide, allowed to dry, and examined through a microscope, a characteristic palm leaf pattern can be seen. This is why it is called *arborization* or the fern test.
2. What equipment is needed? • Sterile gloves • Sterile speculum • Two clean microscope slides • Two small, sterile cotton-tipped applicators	No bacteria or other foreign material should be introduced into the vagina if ruptured membranes are suspected.
Performing the Test	
1. Assemble all the necessary equipment.	
2. Explain to the woman exactly what you will be doing.	Many people use no lubricant. If a lubricant is needed for the speculum examination, use only sterile water. There is some concern that water dilutes the amniotic fluid specimen and interferes with the arborization process.

3. Help her assume the position for a speculum examination.
4. Put on sterile gloves.
5. Insert the sterile speculum.
6. Locate the cervix.
7. Insert a sterile cotton-tipped applicator and place it in the fluid accumulating in the lower blade. Be certain to use pooled fluid in the lower blade. Avoid touching the cervical opening.
8. Roll the cotton-tipped applicator on the first slide, spreading the specimen *thinly* over at least two thirds of the slide (Fig. 3.16).
9. Repeat the procedure but place the second cotton-tipped applicator in the back of the vagina below the cervix.

If the membranes are ruptured, fluid can leak from the cervix if the woman is asked to cough or bear down.

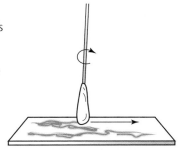

FIGURE 3.16

10. Roll the cotton-tipped applicator on the second slide.

Testing from two different areas offers a better chance of obtaining leaking fluid, which might otherwise be overlooked.

11. Allow the slide to dry for 5 to 7 minutes.

Some people remove the speculum and dip the cotton-tipped applicator in the fluid that has pooled in the lower blade.

Drying permits the sodium chloride in the amniotic fluid to "arborize," or develop the typical "ferning" pattern (Fig. 3.17).

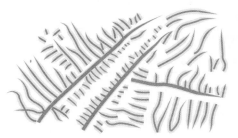

FIGURE 3.17

12. Put the microscope on *low* power and examine all areas of each slide for the ferning pattern. If you have any doubt about the ferning pattern you see under low power, check again under high power.

The presence of the ferning pattern is a positive test result for ruptured membranes. Cervical and vaginal fluids per se do not fern. If you see ferning on the first slide, it is not necessary to check the second slide. However, you should always check the second slide if you do not see ferning on the first slide.

You will need to attend a skill session(s) to practice this skill with the help of your preceptor. Mastery of the skill is achieved when you can demonstrate the following:
- Collection of a specimen for testing
- Preparation of the slides for microscope viewing
- Use of low and high power on the microscope
- Interpretation of the ferning pattern seen under the microscope

SKILL UNIT 4 | VAGINAL EXAMINATION

This section details how to perform a vaginal examination to determine cervical effacement, dilatation, the status of membranes, and fetal presenting part and station. Study this section and then attend a skill practice and demonstration session scheduled with your preceptor. You will need to demonstrate that you can perform the procedure and correctly interpret the results. These steps are summarized at the end of this unit.

ACTIONS	REMARKS

Preparing the Woman for a Vaginal Examination

Information you need before performing a vaginal examination:
- Gravidity
- Parity
- Gestational age
- History of any bleeding/spotting
- History of possible ruptured membranes

Caution: *If membranes are ruptured and the mother is not in active labor, do not perform a digital vaginal examination. Perform a speculum examination to obtain fluid for fern test and to visually assess cervical status*

1. Ask the woman to empty her bladder before the examination.

   A full bladder makes the abdomen difficult to palpate thoroughly and is uncomfortable for the woman.

2. Tell the woman, in terms she can understand, what you will be doing and share your findings with her throughout the examination using her name.

   An informed woman is more relaxed. She is more likely to cooperate with you throughout the examination. The woman has a right to know what is being done in regard to her body.

3. Warn the woman in advance if you are going to be exerting extra pressure or doing something that might be particularly uncomfortable.

4. Help her to lie down on the examining table with legs bent so that her feet are resting on the table or in the stirrups. Place a pillow under her head and ask that she rest her hands across her abdomen or at her sides.

   This increases her comfort and relaxation. Sometimes women put their hands over their heads during a vaginal examination, which tightens abdominal muscles and makes the examination more difficult or uncomfortable.

5. Drape the woman's legs to avoid unnecessary exposure. Make sure that you can see her face whether you are sitting or standing for any part of the examination.

   The message given to the woman is that you respect her modesty and privacy. This will help her to relax. Making sure that you can see her face at all times might reassure her and enables you to note expressions of fear, discomfort, or embarrassment.

6. *Has the mother had any bleeding during the last part of her pregnancy?*

   Do you see signs of bleeding that might be more than just bloody show? Blood running down her legs or bright red bleeding is abnormal.

   If you note any bleeding, do not proceed with the examination.

   Vaginal examinations are never done by the nurse if the woman has a history of bleeding. Sometimes the placenta grows partially or completely over the cervix. This condition is called *placenta previa* and is rare (Fig. 3.18). A digital vaginal examination might cause severe bleeding and place both mother and fetus in danger.

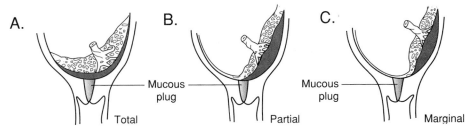

FIGURE 3.18 Types of placenta previa.

Getting Ready to Do a Vaginal Examination

7. Wash your hands and put on gloves.
   - If ruptured membranes are suspected, always use sterile gloves.
   - If membranes are intact, clean or sterile gloves can be used.
8. Ask the woman to separate or spread her legs. Do not try to use force or even gently separate her legs.
9. Tell the woman how to relax. If she knows a relaxation and breathing technique learned previously, have her use it. If not, have her do slow, deep, relaxed breathing. Ask her to let herself go limp, to think of herself as a rag doll.
10. Ask the woman if you may proceed now. Watch your facial expression. Remain focused on the woman. Share your findings with her to the extent possible for the situation. Acknowledge the discomfort the examination may be causing her—even offer an apology.

This procedure describes a two-gloved approach. One gloved hand is used to separate the labia (step 13) and the other gloved hand conducts the vaginal/cervical examination.

This examination is an intrusive procedure. It should be carried out when the woman is ready for it.

This appropriately gives the woman some control, is empowering, and is humanizing in a difficult situation.

Performing the Examination

If the woman becomes upset or tense during the examination, *stop whatever you are doing.* Do not remove your fingers; simply hold your hand still. Find out what is bothering her. Try to distinguish between discomfort as a result of pressure, or fear, and actual pain. Wait until she has regained control, helping her to relax.

11. Generously lubricate the index and middle fingers of your examining hand with lubricating gel. As you squeeze the tube, let the lubricant drop onto your outstretched fingers. Do not wipe your fingers against the mouth of the tube to obtain the lubricant. The lubricant should be considered clean only—not sterile.
12. Be sure that you have good lighting. A lamp is usually necessary.
13. Separate the labia with your gloved fingers (Fig. 3.19). Inspect the general area of the introitus (vaginal opening).

If it is uncertain whether the membranes have ruptured and a compelling reason exists for performing the examination, use only sterile water because some substances interfere with the Nitrazine paper color change.

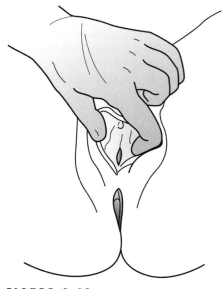

FIGURE 3.19

Look for the following:
- Amount of bloody show
- Wet, glistening perineum
- Malodorous discharge

Which might indicate the following:
Labor is advanced.
Membranes have ruptured.
Infection of the amniotic fluid and membranes is present.

- Deep yellow or greenish-brown discharge

- Ulceration of the labia
- Blisters or raised vesicles on the labia

Elicit signs and symptoms of current infection.

> **STOP THE EXAMINATION. NOTIFY THE PRIMARY CARE PROVIDER IMMEDIATELY.**

> Newborns delivered through an infected birth canal should be isolated to protect other newborns in the nursery. The mucous membranes (e.g., eyes, nasopharynx) of the newborn should be cultured at 24 to 48 hours after birth to avoid positive cultures resulting from contamination from the mother.[5]

14. Insert the first finger of the other sterile gloved hand and then the second finger gently into the vagina. The hand should be turned sideways in this initial step. Continue to apply downward pressure as you insert the fingers to avoid pressing on the anterior vaginal wall or urethra. The thumb and forefinger on one hand separate the labia widely to expose the vaginal opening and prevent the examining fingers from touching the labia (Fig. 3.20).

Presence of greenish-brown fluid indicates fresh meconium. In cephalic presentations, it can indicate that the fetus is in distress.
Syphilis (chancre) or an HSV infection might be present.
HSV infection might be present.

The appearance of a raised vesicle or a blistered area can mean that the mother has an active HSV infection. Mothers with herpes virus blisters on the cervix or genitalia can pass the disease on to a newborn delivered vaginally. In primary genital herpes infections, these babies experience high morbidity and mortality.

NOTE: Herpetic lesions of either type 1 or type 2 can appear anywhere on the body. Sometimes cervical shedding of the virus occurs in a woman who has a herpetic lesion elsewhere on the body. Cervical shedding of the herpes virus can also occur in asymptomatic patients. Current research shows some correlation between HSV infection during pregnancy and cervical shedding at the time of delivery. Fortunately, the incidence of neonatal HSV infection is low when compared with the incidence of known HSV infection in pregnant women.[5]

Current delivery recommendations for pregnant women with genital herpes infection include the following considerations:
- If there are no active lesions at term in a woman with intact membranes who has had active HSV lesions during pregnancy, vaginal delivery is acceptable.[5]
- If there are active lesions near or at term in a woman who is in labor or who has ruptured membranes, cesarean delivery is recommended.[5]

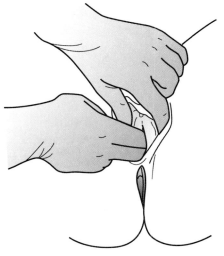

FIGURE 3.20

If you are doing a vaginal examination with one hand, avoid sweeping contaminants into the vagina by separating the labia with the thumb and little finger as you introduce the examining fingers.

The length of the vagina varies in women, but is usually 3 to 4 cm.

15. Move your fingers the full length of the woman's vagina. During the examination, the fourth and fifth fingers should not touch the rectal area. Keep the thumb straight up and stretched out. Keep the fourth and fifth fingers bent inward and touching the palm of your hand (Fig. 3.21).

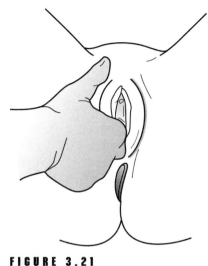

FIGURE 3.21

Assessing Progress in Labor

16. Are the membranes ruptured?
    Palpate for a soft, movable, bulging sac through the cervix (Fig. 3.22). Watch for running fluid during the examination.

    If the membranes are not ruptured, they tend to bulge. If they are ruptured, amniotic fluid is likely to leak during the examination.

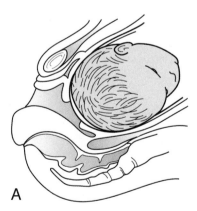

A   B

FIGURE 3.22   Membranes. **A.** Watchglass shape. **B.** Bulging into the cervix.

17. What is the degree of cervical dilatation?

    Dilatation is measured in centimeters. One finger represents approximately 1.5 to 2.0 cm dilatation. Measurement of dilatation can be from 0 to 10 cm in diameter.

18. What is the degree of cervical effacement?
    Palpate the thickness of the cervix. Estimate the degree of thinness in percentages.

    Effacement is measured in percentage. The uneffaced cervix by digital examination is approximately 2.0 to 2.5 cm (1 inch) thick and would be described as 0% effaced. A cervix measuring approximately 1 cm (0.5 inch) is 50% effaced. Transvaginal ultrasound is often used to measure cervical length in women suspected of cervical incompetency or at risk for preterm labor. The normal cervical length as measured by transvaginal ultrasound at midpregnancy is approximately 4 cm (1.6 inches).

19. What is the presenting part of the fetus?
    Palpate for the presenting part. If you feel:
    • The hard skull with the sagittal suture and follow it to the posterior or anterior fontanelle, it is a *cephalic presentation.*
    • The softer buttocks, it is a *breech presentation.*
    • Irregular, knobby parts like facial features, it is a *face presentation.*

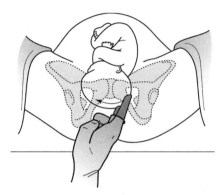

FIGURE 3.23 Identification of the posterior fontanelle.

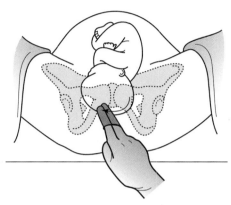

FIGURE 3.24 Identification of the anterior fontanelle.

20. What is the station? Has engagement occurred?
    Locate the lowest portion of the presenting part and then sweep the fingers deeply to one side of the pelvis to feel for the ischial spines (Fig. 3.25). Imagine a straight line from one spine to the other. To determine station, estimate how far (in centimeters) the tip of the presenting part is above or below the ischial spine (see Part III in Module 2). For example, if the fetal head is approximately 1 to 2 cm below the ischial spines, it is at +1 station.
    Engagement occurs when the widest part of the fetal head has entered the inlet of the pelvis. Commonly, this occurs when the tip of the presenting part has reached the level of the ischial spines (i.e., station 0).

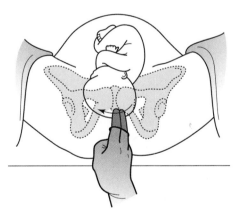

FIGURE 3.25

Station provides some information about the descent of the fetus through the pelvis. If the station is judged to be beyond 0, the pelvis is probably adequate for labor.

Examination between contractions tells you about the degree of dilatation and effacement when the presenting part is not under the pressure of contraction. Examination during a contraction tells you the full extent of dilatation, effacement, and descent. It provides you with a clearer picture of how the laboring woman is doing.

> A vaginal examination can *begin* between contractions but should be *continued* throughout a contraction in the laboring woman.

21. Remove your fingers and discard the glove.

Informing the Mother

22. Tell the woman your findings and relate them to her progress in labor. Praise the woman for whatever you can at that point (e.g., working with you during the examination, achieving progress in labor to whatever degree, and recognizing the need to come in and be evaluated).	Information can be reassuring and supportive for the woman and for her support system. Find some words of empowerment from the examination!

You will need to attend a skill session(s) to practice this skill with the help of your preceptor. Mastery of the skill is achieved when you can demonstrate the following:

- Preparation and positioning of the woman for a vaginal examination
- Techniques used in a vaginal examination
- Accurate assessment of the status of membranes, cervical dilatation and effacement, fetal presentation, and station

REFERENCES

1. U.S. Department of Health and Human Services, Center for Disease Control. (2007). Maternal Mortality and Related Concepts. *Vital and Health Statistics* Series 3, Number 33. February 2007. Hyattsville, Maryland. DHHS Publication No. (PHS) 2007-1417.

2. Yu, S. M., Parth, C. H., & Schwalberg, R. H. (2002). Factors associated with smoking cessation among pregnant versus non-pregnant women. *Maternal Child Health Journal, 6*(2), 89–97.

3. U.S. Department of Health and Human Services, Health Resources and Services Administration, Maternal and Child Health Bureau. (2005). *Child Health USA* 2005. Rockville, MD: U.S. Department of Health and Human Service.

4. American Academy of Pediatrics and American College of Obstetricians and Gynecologists. (2002). *Guidelines for perinatal care* (5th ed.). Washington, D.C.: Author.

5. American College of Obstetricians and Gynecologists. (1999). *Management of herpes in pregnancy* [ACOG Practice Bulletin No. 8.] Washington, D.C.: Author.

6. American College of Obstetricians and Gynecologists. (2002). *Prevention of early-onset group B streptococcal disease in newborns* [ACOG Committee Opinion No. 279]. Washington, D.C.: Author.

7. Cunningham, F. G., Leveno, L., Bloom, S. L., Hauth, J. C., Gilstrap, L. C., & Wenstrom, K. D. (2005). Abnormalities of the placenta, umbilical cord and membranes. In *Williams Obstetrics* (22nd ed. pp. 619–630). New York: McGraw-Hill.

8. Walker, J. (1953). Fetal anoxia. *Journal of Obstetrics and Gynecology, British Commonwealth, 61*(4), 162.

9. Hon, E. H., Bradfield, A. M., & Hess, O. W. (1961). The electronic evaluation of the fetal heart rate. *American Journal of Obstetrics and Gynecology, 82*(1), 291.

10. Mathews, T. G., & Warshaw, J. B. (1979). Relevance of the gestational age distribution of meconium passage in utero. *Pediatrics, 64*(3), 30.

11. Ramin, K. D., Levono, K. J., & Kelly, M. S. (1996). Amniotic fluid meconium: A fetal environmental hazard. *Obstetrics and Gynecology, 87*(4), 181.

12. Ghidini, A., & Spong, C. Y. (2001). Severe meconium aspiration syndrome is not caused by aspiration of meconium. *American Journal of Obstetrics and Gynecology, 185*(2), 931.

13. Cunningham, F. G., Leveno, L., Bloom, S. L., Hauth, J. C., Gilstrap, L. C., & Wenstrom, K. D. (2005). Disorders of amniotic fluid volume. In *Williams Obstetrics* (22nd ed. pp. 525–534). New York: McGraw-Hill.

14. Phelan, J. P., Smith, C. V., & Broussard, P. (1987). Amniotic fluid volume assessment with the four-quadrant technique at 36–42 weeks' gestation. *Journal of Reproductive Health, 32*(3), 540.

15. Magann, E. F., Doherty, D. A., & Chauhan, S, P. (2003). Effect of maternal hydration on amniotic fluid volume. *Obstetrics and Gynecology, 101*, 1261.

16. National Institutes of Health, National Heart, Lung and Blood Institute, National High Blood Pressure Education Program. (2000). *Working Group report on high blood pressure in pregnancy* [NIH publication number 00-3029]. Bethesda, MD: National Institutes of Health.

MODULE

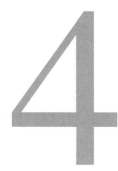

Admission Assessment of the Fetus

E. JEAN MARTIN ■ DONNA JEAN RUTH

As you complete this module, you will learn:

1. Methods of determining fetal health
2. How to calculate the date of delivery and gestational age
3. Methods used to obtain an accurate estimated date of confinement (EDC)
4. The relationship of fetal activity to fetal physiology and development
5. What fetal movement tells us about fetal health
6. What to teach expectant mothers about fetal movement counting (maternal assessment measures for fetal activity)
7. The significance of the fetal alarm signal
8. Nursing implications for telephone triage when the expectant mother reports decreased fetal movement
9. Newer appreciations of the true capacities of the developing fetus and how to use this in humanizing the fetus for the mother and father during fetal assessment
10. An organized approach to evaluating fundal height and fetal lie, presentation, and position (Leopold's maneuvers), as well as how to estimate fetal weight and amniotic fluid in its extremes of low and high volumes
11. Clinical issues when findings for fundal height and fetal lie, presentation, and position vary from expected norms
12. What can and cannot be assessed with the auscultation method
13. How to apply an organized approach in locating and counting fetal heart rate (FHR) in intermittent auscultation (IA)
14. Definitions for and the significance of variations in FHR
15. Differentiation of sounds and rates when listening for fetal heart tones (FHTs)
16. Terminology to use when interpreting and charting FHRs heard by the auscultation method
17. Guidelines for fetal surveillance while caring for low- and high-risk laboring women

When you have completed this module, you should be able to recall the meaning of the following terms. You should also be able to use the terms when consulting with other health professionals. The terms are defined in this module or in the glossary at the end of this book.

acidosis	hypoxia
ballottement	oligohydramnios
fetal bradycardia	postterm
fetal tachycardia	semi-Fowler's position

Assessing Fetal Health

► **How can you assess fetal health at the time of admission?**

As the laboring woman is admitted to the hospital, it is important to keep in mind that two patients are being admitted: the mother and the fetus.

There are several things that you can do to gather important information about fetal health:

- Estimate the gestational age of the fetus using the EDC or estimated date of delivery (EDD).
- Measure the fundal height of the uterus.
- Evaluate fetal position.
- Ask about fetal movement.
- Listen to FHTs.

Gestational Age

▶ How is gestational age estimated?

Evaluating fetal size, development, and maturity to identify gestational age depends on the initial determination of when the pregnancy began. Predicting the EDC is another way of looking at gestational age. One can use the following equation, known as Naegels's rule, to determine an EDC. Follow these two simple steps.

1. Determine the date of the mother's last normal menstrual period (LNMP).
2. Count back 3 months from the date of the LNMP and add 7 days, adjusting the year if appropriate.
   EXAMPLE: If the LNMP began August 18, 2007, the EDC is May 25, 2008.
   Less than 5% of women deliver on the date predicted, which demonstrates that it is truly an estimate.

▶ What can go wrong in estimating the EDC and gestational age?

Many women cannot remember the date of their LNMP. Many also do not realize that an unusually short "period" can occur while they are pregnant. Implantation of the fertilized egg with a small amount of bleeding typically occurs about the same time in the menstrual cycle when a period is expected. Occasionally, a pregnancy is achieved during an amenorrheic period, when there is no menstruation. Amenorrhea may occur in women experiencing conditions such as diabetes, thyroid problems, obesity, eating disorders, and breastfeeding. Precise knowledge of the gestational age of the fetus is essential to providing ideal prenatal care.

Obtaining an Accurate EDC

An EDD or EDC represents a calculation for an average length of gestation in an average woman and appears to be 283 to 284 days, with a standard deviation in humans of 8 to 15 days, rather than the 280 days calculated by Naegele's rule. Often, the diagnosis of pregnancy begins when a woman presents with a positive home pregnancy test and cessation of menstrual periods. It is incumbent upon the provider to establish an accurate EDD or EDC. The following are methods the provider may use to establish the EDD or EDC.

1. Use of the woman's LNMP. Use the following steps to help establish the LNMP:
   - Explore with the woman whether her last menstrual period was normal in length, amount, color, and expected onset.
   - If the last menstrual period was abnormal but the previous one was normal, use the first day of the last *normal* period.
   - Jog the woman's memory with special dates like holidays, birthdays, and so forth, to help her recall the date of her LNMP.
2. If the pregnancy occurred during a period of amenorrhea, the provider may use the following techniques to help establish the EDC/EDD by doing the following:
   - Asking the woman about her history of sexual intercourse.
   - Questioning the woman about her use of birth control.
   - Identifying the date the woman felt quickening, which is when the mother first feels the fetus moving. (This is generally at 16–18 gestational weeks for multigravidas and 18–20 gestational weeks for primigravidas.)
   - Noting when FHTs are first heard (using a Doptone, FHTs can be heard between 10 and 12 weeks. Using a fetoscope, FHTs can be heard between 18 and 20 weeks).
3. Use ultrasound to establish the EDD/EDC, remembering that the earlier ultrasound examination is done, the more accurate the information.
   - In the first trimester, the crown–rump length of the fetus is accurate to within 3 to 5 days.
   - In the second trimester, the biparietal diameter (BPD) and femur length (FL) are accurate to within 7 to 11 days. The head circumference (HC) and abdominal circumference (AC) may also be measured.
   - In the third trimester, all individual measurements become less accurate. Estimates are improved by taking an average of the various parameters (BPD, FL, HC, and AC).[1]

A simple way to remember degrees of accuracy when reviewing EDDs by ultrasound follows:

- First trimester—accuracy ±1 week
- Second trimester—accuracy ±2 weeks
- Third trimester—accuracy ±3 weeks

NOTE: *Using an accurate LNMP for calculating the EDD is as reliable as using ultrasound in the second trimester.*

Fetal Physiology and Movement

▶ What does fetal movement tell us about fetal health?

Much of the literature agrees that the five primary situations that place the fetus at risk for intrauterine fetal death are as follows:

- *Postterm* (beyond 42 weeks' gestation)
- Hypertension
- Diabetes
- Intrauterine growth restriction (IUGR)
- Previous stillbirth

The widespread use of real-time ultrasound allows for direct measurement of fetal movements. Fetal breathing and body movements are important functions in utero and are necessary for appropriate growth and development.

Fetal activity requires oxygen consumption. When subjected to a hypoxic occurrence, one of the first fetal physiologic adjustments made is to economize movement. Compromise of fetal oxygenation elicits an adaptive response to decrease activity, thereby decreasing oxygen need. This adaptive response can result from a physiologic or a pathophysiologic event. Fetal movements serve as an indirect measure of central nervous system function.

> Healthy fetuses have recognizable patterns of movement in utero.

Adequate functioning of the uteroplacental unit is necessary for the fetus to accomplish and maintain patterns of healthy behavior.

Biologic factors affecting fetal breathing and body movements include the following:

- The maturity level of fetal status in awake/sleep states
- Gestational age
- Time of day
- Relationship to maternal meals (research shows a positive correlation with maternal eating/drinking and breathing movements *but not with body movements*)

> A decrease in fetal activity may be a marker for fetal hypoxia and/or acidosis.

- Maternal drug ingestion

Some clinical situations in pregnancy that put the fetus at risk include:

- Diabetes mellitus and gestational diabetes
- Intrauterine growth restriction or suspected IUGR
- History of previous IUGR
- Chronic hypertension
- Pregnancy-induced hypertension
- Systemic lupus erythematosus
- Multiple pregnancy
- Oligohydramnios
- Postterm pregnancy
- Rh disease (which is much less prevalent today)

NOTE:
- *Meconium aspiration and cord accidents are among the most common causes of stillbirth in women having antepartal testing, such as nonstress tests and biophysical profiles.*
- *Studies show that cessation of fetal movement is highly correlated with impending fetal death. However, there is no general consensus as to what constitutes decreased fetal movement.*[2]

> Unfortunately, at this time, evidence-based data are inconsistent in demonstrating that fetal movement assessment results in a reduction in fetal deaths.[3]

Assessing Fetal Movement/Activity

Make time during each prenatal visit to discuss fetal movement and activity. The mother's perception of fetal movement has been shown to correlate with ultrasound detection of movement 80% to 90%.[4] Yet, although fetal movement and activity are considered a positive sign of fetal health, decreased fetal movement may not always be an ominous sign. Many factors can impact fetal movement and activity. These factors include:

Time of day—near term fetal movements in the late evening are increased, which may be due to increased periods of fetal wakefulness. Maternal perception of these movements is also increased.

Gestational age—preterm fetuses, particularly those less than 28 weeks' gestation, are more active and their movements are more sporadic. As the fetus matures, the sleep/wake cycle stabilizes, leading to more predictable patterns of movement.

Placental location—may dull the maternal perception of movement.

Maternal smoking—increases fetal activity.

Maternal alcohol ingestion—decreases fetal activity.

Maternal medications—may cause either an increase or decrease depending on the type and effect of the medication.

Decreased uterine space—as the fetus grows it has less room to move.

NOTE: Women often report "less fetal movement" as term approaches. This change always requires careful evaluation, although what the mother perceives as "less movement" is often a result of less room in utero for the fetus to put "momentum" behind movements. The mother's perception of a significant change always requires further exploration.

The normal fetus may move as many as 100 times per hour or as few as 4 times per hour. It is important to discuss with the woman the normal pattern of movement for her fetus. Attention should be given to any complaint of a decrease in the normal pattern of movement in the fetus. A period of decreased fetal movement commonly precedes fetal death, but the absence of perceived fetal movements does not necessarily indicate fetal death or compromise.

Any time an expectant woman calls reporting decreased fetal activity, it requires follow-up. (See Module 15 for discussion of telephone triage.)

Far too many expectant mothers avoid seeking care because they do not trust what they feel. Many have no prior frame of reference for what they are experiencing, but they also fear being seen as bothersome or a worrier. Anyone who might be a first-line contact for the expectant woman must be sensitized to demonstrate a caring concern.

If a mother calls reporting decreased fetal movement, explore her background for normalcy. Ask how today's fetal movements compare with those of the previous day and the days preceding. When movement is present but perceived as lessening, you might instruct the mother as follows:

- Drink two to three glasses of water or juice and then lie down and count fetal movement for 1 to 2 hours. Either the mother calls to report the results to the nurse (not the office staff or secretary) or the nurse calls the mother back. An outcome should be known and a record kept of all calls to and from the unit, practice, or clinic. Four movements in an hour are considered reassuring.

  OR

- Come to the appropriate site for further evaluation. Practice on the far side of caution. You will never regret it! The mother will sleep better, so will you, and the baby has a better chance for a good outcome.

Most of the time, ultrasound and/or EFM reveal a normal FHR and activity pattern. Praise the mother for her vigilance, and as she leaves, offer professional assurance that you or the staff are there to help her in the weeks ahead.

Fetal Movement Counts (a.k.a "Kick Counts")

Fetal movement counts have been utilized in the past as a simple, inexpensive, and noninvasive means of fetal surveillance for pregnant women. It is very popular because it can be done at home and has no contraindications. The rationale for fetal movement counting is the hope that fetal death can be prevented by acting immediately when there is a decrease in fetal movement. However, limitations of the test include the fact that the ideal number of movements or kicks has not been established, nor has the ideal duration for movement counting been clearly defined.[5] Additionally, the period between decreased fetal movement and fetal death may be too short for timely intervention in some clinical situations such as placental abruption or cord accidents.

Despite the fact that there is not enough evidence to recommend formal fetal movement counts for all expectant women, they are widely prescribed in both low- and high-risk women.[3] Fetal movement counts in high-risk women may begin as early as 28 weeks' gestation and in low-risk women at 32 to 36 weeks' gestation.

Many different methods have been devised to assess fetal movement. The intent of all methods is to have the expectant woman achieve a daily awareness of the patterns and level of activity exhibited by her baby in utero. One of the most popular is the "count to 10" method. This method requires that the mother dedicate 1 hour or less every day to tracking her baby's movements. The short time commitment seems to enhance compliance.[6]

The steps in the "Count to 10" method are described below.

1. Ask the woman to select a specific time each day to count movements. Mothers often select the time of day when the baby is most active.
2. Have her assume a comfortable position that allows her to rest on her side.
3. Count each movement until 10 movements are felt. It can take from a few minutes to 1 hour to complete the test. Most women feel 10 movements in 2 hours.
4. After 10 movements have been perceived, the count is discontinued.
5. If, after 2 hours the woman has not felt 10 movements, she should notify her provider immediately. **Do not wait until the next day to notify the provider.**

Humanizing the Fetus for Parents

The three Skill Units presented in this module not only offer methods to assess fetal health but involve a unique opportunity to help the mother and father or support person perceive the fetus as a developing human. While conducting any of the skills outlined, you can interact with the fetus through abdominal massaging, speaking to, and commenting about the fetus to the mother.

Research is revealing amazing true capacities of prenates—(the unborn): "their precocious sensory development, their exquisite sensitivity and responsiveness, and their ability to learn from what is happening in the world of their mother and father."[7]

Modern technologies allow observation of the unborn's behavior throughout the entire period of gestation. Chamberlain, in "Prenatal body language: A new perspective on ourselves,"[8] describes (1) early and self-initiated spontaneous movement that expresses interest and personality; (2) prenatal pain perception, preferences, learning, memory, and emotional states of fear, anger, and smiling; and (3) interactive movements between twins in utero and between the fetus and parents with play periods.

Reactive movements or behaviors of the fetus are cited by Chamberlain with the following examples:

- Coughing or laughing in the mother brings about movement in nearly all fetuses between 10 and 15 weeks' gestation.
- Fetuses sometimes react to the needle during an amniocentesis by moving away from the needle or even attacking it.
- A bright light shining through the abdominal wall and fixed on the fetal head (vertex) increases the fetus' heartbeat.
- Some fetuses react to high-volume rock music and violent movies with vigorous movements that can even be painful to the mother.
- Lullabies, children's songs, and melodious classical music sometimes are seen to have a calming effect.

So, as you measure the fundus and palpate the maternal abdomen, talk to the baby and comment to the mother about any response you get. Educate and encourage the mother about fetal hearing and sensory perceptions. Babies will thrive on nurturing attention after birth but what has become clear in the cited studies is that babies thrive with attention *before* birth.

PRACTICE/REVIEW QUESTIONS

After reviewing this module, answer the following questions.

1. State four ways to gather information about fetal health when the mother is admitted to the labor unit.

   a. _____

   b. _____

   c. _____

   d. _____

2. If the LNMP is June 6, 2007, when is the EDC?

   _____

3. Pregnancy can be achieved during an amenorrheic period if the woman has diabetes or thyroid problems.

   a. True

   b. False

4. An estimated date of delivery (EDD or EDC) represents a calculation for the average woman and appears to be

   _____ days rather than _____ days.

5. State three top predictors with reliable criteria for accuracy in dating a pregnancy.

   a. _____

   b. _____

   c. _____

6. The mother can identify quickening around the 12th to 14th week of pregnancy.

   a. True

   b. False

7. A small amount of bleeding can occur with implantation.

   a. True

   b. False

8. Five primary clinical situations that put the fetus at risk for intrauterine fetal death are:

   a. _____

   b. _____

   c. _____

   d. _____

   e. _____

9. When the fetus is deprived of sufficient oxygen, a physiologic adaptive response is _____

   _____.

10. A *postdate pregnancy* is defined as one that has gone beyond which gestational week?

    a. 40

    b. 41

    c. 42

11. A significant overall decrease in fetal activity:

    a. Can be related to the awake/sleep state of the fetus

    b. Can signal a sign of maturity

    c. Can be a marker for fetal hypoxia

    d. Should be expected before the onset of labor

12. Name 10 clinical situations in which the fetus is at risk.

    a. _____

    b. _____

    c. _____

    d. _____

    e. _____

    f. _____

    g. _____

    h. _____

    i. _____

    j. _____

13. At what gestational age is it recommended that fetal movement counting begin for the situations you have

    listed in question 12? _____

14. Maternal intake of alcohol has a profound effect on fetal gross body movements.

    a. True

    b. False

15. Select *two* statements that reflect what is known about fetal body movement.

    a. The more immature the fetus, the more sporadic the movements.

    b. Between 30 and 40 weeks' gestation, fetal body movement is present 10% of the time.

    c. Movements significantly increase during active labor.

    d. The expectant woman perceives movements more in the afternoons.

16. Maternal perceptions of fetal activity (select two):

    a. Are not reliable

    b. Are influenced by the time of day

    c. Are reliable

    d. Correlate poorly with actual fetal movement

17. A low-risk expectant woman who has been doing fetal movement counting since 36 weeks' gestation is now at 38 weeks' gestation. She phones you with her concern that on doing fetal movement counting this evening, she counted only six movements in 1 hour. She usually has no trouble getting 10 movements in 1 hour. A reasonable response to her would be:

    a. "Come right in and let us evaluate what is going on."

    b. "Drink 1 or 2 glasses of fluids, go to bed this evening, but call your primary care provider in the morning."

    c. "Take a walk and relax. Call tomorrow if you continue to have fewer than 10 movements in 1 hour."

    d. "Drink 1 or 2 glasses of fluids, continue your counting for 1 more hour, and call me back with your results. I'll want to talk with you then."

18. Select your response for question 17 if the mother had a history of stillbirth at 38 weeks' gestation with her last pregnancy and currently has gestational diabetes. You would choose response:

    a. "Come right in and let us evaluate what is going on."

    b. "Drink 1 or 2 glasses of fluids, go to bed this evening, but call your primary care provider in the morning."

    c. "Take a walk and relax. Call tomorrow if you continue to have fewer than 10 movements in 1 hour."

    d. "Drink 1 or 2 glasses of fluids, continue your counting for 1 more hour, and call me back with your results. I'll want to talk with you then."

19. An insulin-dependent mother at 35 weeks' gestation calls to state that the baby has been moving a lot less over the past 2 days. When she is placed on the electronic fetal monitor, fetal activity with FHR accelerations is seen over 25 minutes. Subsequent to being reassured and sent home, she calls again 4 days later worried because, again, fetal movement appears significantly different. What will you recommend to her?

_____

_____

PRACTICE/REVIEW ANSWER KEY

1. Any four of the following:
   a. Estimate gestational age of fetus and EDC.
   b. Measure the fundal height of the uterus.
   c. Evaluate fetal position.
   d. Listen to FHTs.
   e. Ask about fetal movement.

2. March 13, 2008

3. a. True

4. 283 to 284; 280

5. a. Basal body temperature with a coital record demonstrating ovulation and sustained temperature elevation

   b. Transvaginal ultrasound 4 to 5 weeks from the LNMP to identify the gestational sac and/or ultrasound between 7 and 13 weeks (first trimester) using fetal crown–rump length (accurate within 3–5 days)

   c. hCG levels in urine or blood serum by 8 to 9 days after ovulation

6. b. False

7. a. True

8. a. Postterm
   b. Hypertension
   c. Diabetes
   d. Intrauterine growth restriction
   e. Decreased fetal movement

9. To decrease fetal movement

10. c. 42

11. c. Can be a marker for fetal hypoxia

12. Any 10 of the following:
    a. Pregestational diabetes mellitus
    b. Suspected IUGR
    c. History of previous IUGR
    d. Chronic hypertension
    e. Pregnancy-induced hypertension
    f. Systemic lupus erythematosus
    g. Multiple pregnancy
    h. Oligohydramnios
    i. Previous stillbirth
    j. Postterm
    k. Rh disease (less prevalent today)

13. 28 weeks' gestation

14. a. True

15. a. The more immature the fetus, the more sporadic the movements; and
    b. Between 30 and 40 weeks' gestation, fetal body movement is present 10% of the time.

16. b. Are influenced by the time of day; and
    c. Are reliable

17. d. "Drink 1 or 2 glasses of fluids, continue your counting for 1 more hour, and call me back with your results. I'll want to talk with you then."

NOTE: *Some may select A, which is always a safe response. The majority of expectant women, however, will get 10 movements with one additional hour of counting. That is reassuring.*

18. a. "Come right in and let us evaluate what is going on."

19. Tell her to come in for evaluation.

SKILL UNIT 1 | MEASURING FUNDAL HEIGHT

This section details how to measure the height of the uterine fundus to obtain information about fetal growth and body size. Study this section and then attend a skill practice and demonstration session scheduled with your preceptor. You will need to demonstrate the examination and correctly interpret the results. The steps of the examination are summarized at the end of this unit.

Physical examination techniques used in fetal assessment are structured in the sequence given here, that is, first measuring fundal height, then determining presentation and position, and finally auscultating for FHTs. There is a good reason for this. Measuring fundal height before any abdominal palpation is carried out reduces the likelihood of stimulating contractions or fetal activity, both of which could alter the height of the fundus. Occasionally, when the woman assumes a supine position on the examination table, a contraction is stimulated. This is especially true in the late second trimester and third trimester. Wait until the contraction has subsided before taking the measurement. Moving on to determining fetal lie, presentation, and position will then prepare you to know where to look for FHTs, the final assessment technique.

ACTIONS	REMARKS

Measure the Fundal Height

1. Ask the woman to empty her bladder. Assist the woman to a supine position on the examination table. Avoid elevating the woman's trunk or flexing her knees, if possible. This may not be a comfortable position for her, so be prepared to move through the assessment without delay. When finished, elevate the examination table to her comfort.	A full bladder gives a falsely high fundal height of as much as 2 to 3 cm.
	Maternal position does influence fundal height measurement as seen in the Engstrom et al. study.[9]
	No research data exist to support the use of a position other than supine for obtaining fundal height measurements.
2. Always inspect the maternal abdomen before beginning fundal height measurements. Look at the abdominal shape. An elongated shape probably denotes a vertical lie; a triangular shape may indicate a transverse lie.	
Facing the woman's head, place your hands on each side of the uterus approximately halfway between the symphysis and the fundus (Fig. 4.1). Feel along the sides of the uterus upward toward the fundus. As you near the top, your hands will begin to come together. They will meet at the top of the fundus.	This assists in identifying exactly where the fundus is located.

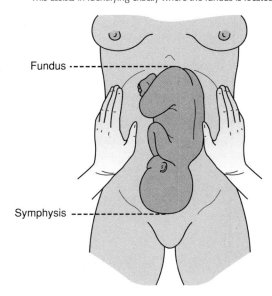

Fundus

Symphysis

FIGURE 4.1

The fundal height is measured in centimeters.

3. Place the zero line of the tape measure on the anterior border of the symphysis pubis and stretch the tape over the midline of the abdomen to the top of the fundus (Fig. 4.2).

NOTE: The tape should be brought over the curve of the fundus. The measurement is read at the lowermost edge of the curved fundus.

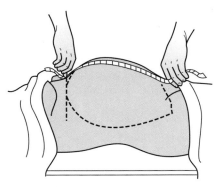

Slight variations in the way people measure the curve of the fundus result in discrepancies between examiners. **It is essential for clinicians to standardize their fundal height measurement technique so that all measurements are obtained in the same position and use the same anatomic landmarks.**[9]

FIGURE 4.2

Interpret the Movement

4. Estimating gestational age from fundal height is based on a simple rule: After the 20th week of pregnancy, the height of the fundus in centimeters equals the number of weeks of gestation, ±2 cm. This is a general rule and best applied between the 20th and 32nd weeks (Fig. 4.3).

Generally, the height of the uterus increases by approximately 1 cm per week after the 20th week. It is a way of assessing the growth of the fetus within the uterus when measured regularly.

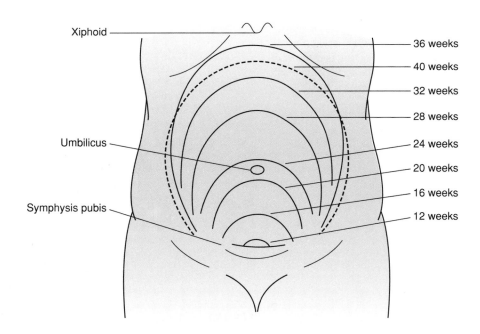

Xiphoid

Umbilicus

Symphysis pubis

36 weeks
40 weeks
32 weeks
28 weeks
24 weeks
20 weeks
16 weeks
12 weeks

FIGURE 4.3

APPROXIMATE HEIGHT OF THE FUNDUS DURING PREGNANCY

Week	Location of the Uterus
1 to 2	The uterus is a pelvic organ for the first 3 months of pregnancy, palpable on vaginal examination.
12	The uterus fills the pelvic cavity. The fundus is felt level with or just above the upper margin of the symphysis pubis. The uterus is the size of a small grapefruit and feels globular and firm.
16	The fundus is halfway between the symphysis pubis and the umbilicus and is ovoid in shape.
20	The fundus is approximately 1 to 2 fingerbreadths below the umbilicus.
24	The fundus is 1 to 2 fingerbreadths above the umbilicus and can rotate to the right; it feels less firm.
28	The fundus is halfway between the umbilicus and the xiphoid, approximately 3 fingerbreadths above the umbilicus.
32	The fundus is three fourths the distance between the umbilicus and the xiphoid, or approximately 3 fingerbreadths below the xiphoid.
36	The fundus is at or just below the xiphoid.
40	The fundus drops several fingerbreadths, particularly in primigravidas.

(Adapted from Carr, K. C. [1976]. *Perinatal nurse clinician program. Maternal-fetal pathway syllabus.* Seattle: University of Washington; as appears in Blackburn, S., & Loper, D. [1992]. *Maternal, fetal and neonatal physiology: A clinical perspective.* Philadelphia: WB Saunders.)

> **NOTE:** *If the fetus is growing abnormally slowly or quickly, the fundal height will be too low or too high to give an accurate gestational age.*

Finding an Abnormal Fundal Height

5. What if you find a *low fundal height* for gestational age? When you measure the mother's abdomen and find it is more than 2 cm less than what would be expected for her due date, it can indicate growth restriction in the fetus.

> A lack of increase in fundal height over 3 consecutive weeks often indicates fetal growth restriction. *Poor prenatal weight gain in a mother who is average size or smaller adds to the probability of this diagnosis.*

Consistently low fundal heights can mean that the fetus has a slow growing rate. This is called *intrauterine growth restriction* and can be a cause of serious problems in newborns. Fetuses with IUGR require vigilant assessment and follow-up.

Low fundal height can occur with a transverse lie. Careful abdominal palpation should be done.

There are multiple causes for IUGR. When IUGR is identified, the provider should be vigilant in trying to establish the cause when possible. See Display 4.1.

DISPLAY 4.1	MATERNAL, FETAL, AND PLACENTAL FACTORS AFFECTING IUGR

MATERNAL FACTORS	FETAL FACTORS	PLACENTAL FACTORS
Nutritional status	Chromosomal abnormalities	Impaired umbilical blood exchange
Extremes in maternal age	Structural anomalies	Inadequate development or maintenance
Smoking	Multifetal gestation	of the placental vascular beds
Alcohol consumption	Premature infants	Elevated maternal serum α-fetoprotein levels
Illicit drug use	Intrauterine infections	
Medications		
Poor obstetric history		
Maternal disease states		

You need to do the following:
• Review the woman's medical and prenatal history for the following:
  • Heart disease
  • Elevated blood pressure
  • Exposure to communicable diseases

The longer a pregnancy goes beyond the due date, the more likely it is that the fetus will not only fail to gain weight, but may lose weight.

- An incidence of fever, chills, vomiting, or diarrhea
- Smoking and drinking habits
- Drug use
- Note the fundal height measurements throughout pregnancy.
- Assess the mother for signs of preeclampsia (hypertension, edema, and proteinuria).
- Consult/notify the care provider.

> Nonreassuring FHR tracings often occur during labor and delivery in a seriously growth-restricted fetus. If the mother is in a level I hospital, transferring her to a level II or level III hospital for labor and delivery may be necessary. Resuscitation equipment and personnel skilled in its use must be available throughout the labor and birth of this high-risk infant.

> Intense antepartum surveillance is recommended for the fetus with IUGR. Delivery before term may be necessary if testing indicates fetal compromise.

6. What if a *high fundal height for gestational age* is found?

A high fundal height of more than 2 cm above the norm for gestational age can mean that the fetus is large but healthy. However, you need to do the following:

- Palpate the mother's abdomen for the presence of an excessive amount of fluid (hydramnios).
- Palpate for the presence of twins.
- Review the mother's prenatal and medical history. Look for the following:
  - The presence of a consistently high fundal height
  - History of diabetes mellitus
  - Schedule an ultrasound examination for measurement of the amniotic fluid index.

Excessive amounts of fluid may be present in the following clinical conditions:

- Twin gestations.
- Fetuses with congenital anomalies.
- Women who have diabetes mellitus or syphilis.
- Women who have blood incompatibility–Rh isoimmunization.

Diabetic mothers have large babies who often look mature but are not. Immature lungs often lead to serious problems for the baby. (See Module 12.)

> Diabetic screening is recommended for all pregnant patients whether by patient's history, clinical risk factors, or laboratory screening tests that measure blood glucose levels.[10]

You will need to attend a skill lesson(s) to practice this skill with the help of your preceptor. Mastery of the skill is achieved when you can do the following:
- Identify the anterior border of the symphysis pubis bone as your starting point for measuring fundal height.
- Attain the same fundal height measurements as your coordinator or preceptor.
- Accurately interpret your measurements as normal, high, or low.
- Describe the implications for management of mothers with low and high fundal height measurements.

SKILL UNIT 2 | EVALUATING FETAL LIE, PRESENTATION, AND POSITION USING LEOPOLD'S MANEUVERS

This skill unit details how to use a systematic approach in abdominal palpation to determine fetal presentation and position. Study the section and then attend a skill practice and demonstration session scheduled by your preceptor. You will need to demonstrate that you can perform Leopold's maneuvers and correctly identify a variety of fetal lies, positions, and presentations. These steps are summarized at the end of this skill unit.

ACTIONS	REMARKS

Prepare the Mother

1. Ask the mother to empty her bladder.
2. Assist the mother onto the examining table. She should lie on her back.
3. Slightly elevate her head and shoulders. Ask her to bend her knees so that the soles of her feet rest flat on the table (Fig. 4.4).

Abdominal muscles are relaxed, and palpating for the fetal parts is generally easier.

Moderately flexed knees decreases abdominal muscle tightening.

A towel or small pillow may be placed on one side of the mother's hips and back to induce a lateral tilt. This is especially important if the woman is experiencing supine hypotension (faintness from diminished circulation to heart or brain while supine).

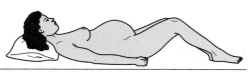

FIGURE 4.4

4. Carry out the examination between contractions if labor has begun.

Determine the Presenting Part and Lie

5. Warm your hands by washing them under warm water or rubbing them together.
   Always inspect the maternal abdomen before beginning any palpation. Look for an elongated abdomen denoting a probable vertical lie or a triangular-shaped abdomen indicating a possible transverse lie. Use gentle but firm motions.

Cold hands cause abdominal muscles to contract and tighten.

> Leopold's maneuvers should be done systematically to obtain the best results.

6. **First maneuver:** Grasp the lower portion of the abdomen just above the symphysis pubis between the thumb and fingers of one hand (Fig. 4.5). Use your other hand to steady the uterus by placing it on the fundus.

NOTE: Many authors/diagrams exchange the third maneuver depicted in this skill unit for the first maneuver. Either approach is fine.

Beginning the maneuvers by attempting to determine what is in the lower aspect of the uterus seems efficient; after 26 weeks' gestation, the hard head is more easily palpated than the softer breech. In 90% of fetal positions, the head can be identified near or in the pelvis.

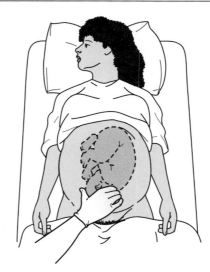

FIGURE 4.5

7. Attempt to move the head from side to side to see whether it is:
   - Floating—out of the pelvis
   - Dipping—partially into the pelvis
   - Approaching engagement—fixed in the pelvis and unmovable

If the head is identified here, you know that the:
   - Lie is *longitudinal.*
   - Presentation is *cephalic.*

Locate the Back and Small Parts

8. **Second maneuver:** Move your hands to the sides of the abdomen. Use one hand to steady the uterus and palpate with the other hand for the fetal back or small parts, such as hands and feet (Fig. 4.6). Keeping the fingers together, apply firm circular motions with the palmar surface of the hands.
   Avoid any poking motion with the ends of the fingers because this can cause discomfort and will not elicit the information being sought.

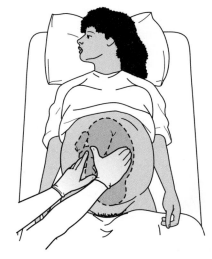

FIGURE 4.6

The side where the fetal back is located will feel firmer and smoother. The side where the fetal hands, elbows, knees, and feet are will feel softer and knobby and have more "give" as you palpate.

Examine the Fundus

9. **Third maneuver:** Move your hands up the sides of the abdomen to the fundus (Fig. 4.7). Palpate for the breech or head, depending on what you felt in the lower abdomen on the first maneuver. The breech is usually found in the fundus.
   If you think you feel the head in the fundal area, tap it sharply with your fingers to see if it will bounce back.
   Ask yourself if what you are feeling confirms what you felt in the lower abdomen on the first maneuver.

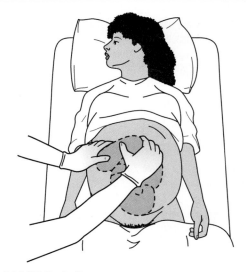

FIGURE 4.7

The breech will feel firm and broad compared with the hard and smaller head. The breech is also less movable.
The head is small and mobile and will bounce or rise up in the amniotic fluid against your fingers. This is called *ballottement.* It might help to confirm your palpation. The breech is not as mobile and does not tap well.

Locate the Cephalic Prominence

10. **Fourth maneuver:** Turn and face the mother's feet. Attempt to locate the cephalic prominence by moving your hands down the sides of the abdomen toward the symphysis pubis (Fig. 4.8).

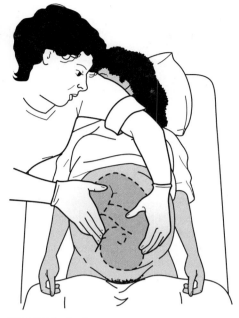

FIGURE 4.8

Note whether the head is:
- Free and floating

OR
- Flexed and approaching engagement

11. As you carry out the entire procedure, ask yourself the following:
- Is there fetal movement?
- How large is the fetus?
- Is there one fetus or more than one?
- Is the height of the fundus appropriate for the gestational age of the fetus?

The cephalic prominence, or brow, is located on the side where there is greatest resistance to the downward movement of the fingers. When the head is well flexed, it is found on the opposite side from the fetal back (Fig. 4.9). When the fetal head is not well flexed or is hyperextended, the cephalic prominence is found on the same side as the back.

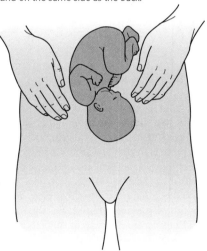

FIGURE 4.9

NOTE: Throughout the maneuvers, be sensitive to the feel of fluid "fullness." Amniotic fluid volume normally increases to about 1 L (1 quart) or a little more by 36 weeks' gestation but begins to decrease thereafter. With experience, one can sense whether the uterus is very full and tense, possibly as a result of excessive amniotic fluid (hydramnios). On the other hand, if the fundal height has been below normal, the palpation "sense" may be that there is greatly diminished fluid (oligohydramnios).

<table>
<tr>
<td>

Hydramnios (polyhydramnios) is generally defined as more than 2,000 mL (2 L). It occurs in about 1% of all pregnancies and is often associated with fetal malformations, especially of the central nervous system or gastrointestinal tract.

</td>
<td>

In the ACOG Practice Bulletin on Antepartum Fetal Surveillance, oligohydramnios is defined as a nonultrasonographically measurable vertical pocket of amniotic fluid greater than 2 cm or an amniotic fluid volume of 5 cm or less.[5]

</td>
</tr>
</table>

NOTE: *In postterm pregnancy, oligohydramnios is common and associated with increased risk of meconium-stained amniotic fluid and cesarean birth for nonreassuring heart rates. Oligohydramnios has been considered an indication for delivery of a postterm pregnancy, although the effectiveness of this approach has not been established by randomized investigation.*[5]

You will need to attend a skill session(s) to practice this skill with the help of your preceptor. Mastery of the skill is achieved when you can do the following:
- Prepare the woman and yourself for the examination.
- Systematically approach abdominal palpation using the first through fourth Leopold's maneuvers.
- Correctly identify fetal lie, presentation, and position on three different patients.

SKILL UNIT 3 | AUSCULTATION OF FETAL HEART TONES

This skill unit will teach you how to find and count the FHR and what to do if you hear a FHR that is not reassuring. Study this section and then attend a skill practice and demonstration session scheduled by your preceptor. You will need to demonstrate that you can perform the procedure and correctly interpret the findings. These steps are summarized at the end of this skill unit.

Introduction

The goal of FHR assessment is to detect any signs of fetal compromise. Early intervention may result in healthier neonatal outcomes. To date, neither IA nor electronic FHR monitoring (EFM) has been effective in predicting the extent of fetal compromise in utero. When reassuring signs are present during auscultation or electronic fetal monitoring, fetal well-being is a reliable interpretation. The information presented in this unit is limited to a discussion of auscultation of the FHR during admission assessment.

Auscultation of the fetal heart is the practice of using a device to listen to the fetal heart sounds (sometime referred to as the FHT). Intermittent auscultation refers to the assessment of the FHT at selected intervals during labor. Overall IA has been reported as equivalent to EFM in terms of neonatal morbidity and mortality outcomes based on randomized controlled trials (RTC).

Decisions regarding the use of IA or EFM should, in the best practice approach, be a mutual one between each woman and her provider and should be shaped by patient history and risk status, hospital policies and procedures, and the availability of personnel trained in IA. The RTC comparing outcomes between IA and EFM were based on a 1:1 nurse to patient ratio, so staffing patterns may be a consideration when selecting IA or EFM as the primary method of fetal surveillance in labor.

ACTIONS	REMARKS

Assemble the Equipment

1. The basic types of auscultation devices are as follows:
   a. A modified stethoscope worn on the head of the listener so that bone conduction from the skull increases hearing ability. Sounds associated with the actual opening and closing of fetal ventricular valves can be heard.

a. DeLee–Hillis fetoscope with headpiece (Fig. 4.10).

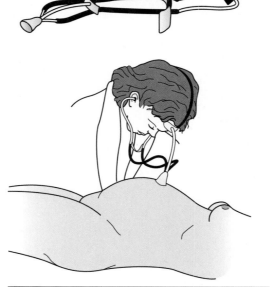

FIGURE 4.10

b. A large, heavy bell that magnifies fetal heart sounds.

b. Leff stethoscope (Fig. 4.11).

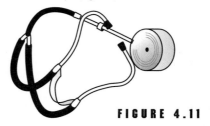

FIGURE 4.11

c. An electronic device that uses ultrasound technology to detect fetal heart motion such as the moving heart walls or valves and converts the ultrasound information into a sound that represents the cardiac activity. Some Doppler devices have been developed that can be submerged under water for use in women laboring in tubs.[11]

NOTE: If the EFM ultrasound transducer (Doppler) is used for FHR auscultation, the paper recorder should not be running. If a tracing of the FHR is produced, it cannot be considered auscultation alone and the tracing produced requires interpretation.[11]

c. Doptone (ultrasound; Fig. 4.12).

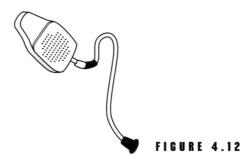

FIGURE 4.12

Determine Fetal Position and Presentation

2. Raise the head of the bed so that the woman is in a semi-Fowler's position or place a small pillow or rolled towel under the woman's hip to avoid the supine position.

   Explain the procedure to the woman and the father or support person.

3. Determine fetal position and presentation through Leopold's maneuvers. Determine where the *fetal back* is.

If the woman is not flat on her back, there is less chance of poor circulation back to the heart and head and, therefore, less risk of her becoming faint (supine hypotensive syndrome).

Begin preparing the woman to attend to the explanation of your examination findings and to turn inward to the unborn.

The FHTs are transmitted through the convex portion of the fetus because that is the part in close contact with the uterine wall. In most breech (Fig. 4.13) and cephalic presentations (Fig. 4.14), FHTs are best heard through the fetal back (*).

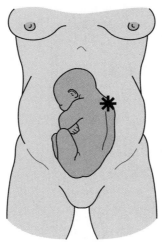

FIGURE 4.13 Breech presentation.

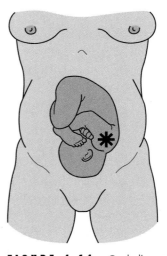

FIGURE 4.14 Cephalic presentation.

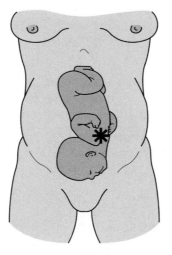

FIGURE 4.15 Face presentation.

In a face presentation (Fig. 4.15), the fetal back becomes concave, and the best place to listen for heart sounds is over the more convex chest.

Position the Fetoscope

4. Position the fetoscope or Doptone on the appropriate quadrant of the mother's abdomen. Use firm pressure. In **ROA** (Fig. 4.16), sounds are best heard in the right lower quadrant.

   In posterior positions, such as **LOP** (Fig. 4.17) or **ROP** (Fig. 4.18), sounds are best heard at the mother's side. In the breech position (Fig. 4.19), sounds are best heard above the mother's umbilicus on her left side.

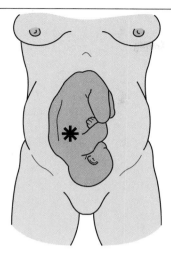

FIGURE 4.16   ROA.

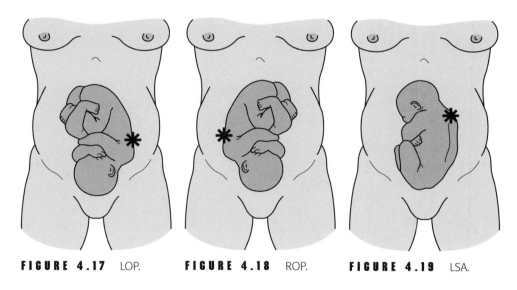

FIGURE 4.17   LOP.   **FIGURE 4.18**   ROP.   **FIGURE 4.19**   LSA.

Review common fetal positions discussed in Module 2, Part 2.

Guidelines for Listening and Interpretation

5. Guidelines that can aid you in locating the fetal heart beat are as follows:

   a. *Between the 10th and 16th weeks of pregnancy, use a Doptone.* Apply a small amount of conduction gel to the contact portion of the Doptone. Begin listening at the upper border of the pubic hair. If you are unable to hear fetal tones, slowly move the instrument up toward the mother's umbilicus. Generally only light pressure is needed. You will need to apply more gel if the search is extensive.

   The ultrasound instrument is more sensitive than the fetoscope. It picks up FHTs about the 10th week of gestation. Conduction gel aids in the transmission of ultrasound waves.

   b. *Between the 16th and 24th weeks of pregnancy,* measure off two fingerbreadths above the pubic hairline and listen along the midline of the abdomen.

   A regular fetoscope can pick up FHTs by the 18th or 20th week of pregnancy.

c. *After the 24th week of pregnancy,* search the abdomen in a methodical manner. Place the feto-scope or Doptone at position 1, as shown in Figure 4.20. If nothing is heard, move to position 2 in the lower left quadrant. Continue following the numbered positions.

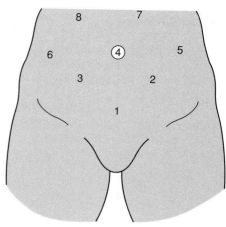

FIGURE 4.20 Methodical search pattern for FHTs. (Adapted with permission from Wheeler, L. A. [1979]. *Fetal assessment. Series 2: Prenatal Care, Module 3* [p. 19]. White Plains, NY: The National Foundation—March of Dimes.)

If you do not detect FHTs at these eight positions, begin a systematic search of the abdomen. Place the feto-scope or Doptone at the umbilicus and move it cen-timeter by centimeter outward along a spoke-like pat-tern. Follow the sequence of numbers in Figure 4.21.

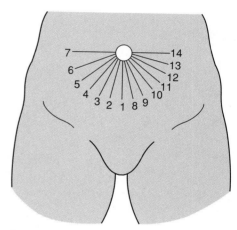

FIGURE 4.21 Systematic search pattern for FHTs. (Adapted with permission from Wheeler, L. A. [1979]. *Fetal assessment. Series 2: Prenatal Care, Module 3* [p. 19]. White Plains, NY: The National Foundation—March of Dimes.)

Differentiating Sounds and Rates

6. Listening
   You may hear a soft "blowing" sound of maternal blood coursing through the uterine arteries; this is referred to as *the uterine soufflé.*

   This is synonymous with the *maternal heart rate.*

   A distinct "swishing" sound may be heard; this is synonymous with blood coursing through the umbilical artery and is referred to as the *funic soufflé.*

   This reflects the *FHR.*

Fetal heart valve opening and closing have very distinct cardiac sounds—not muffled or swishing sounds as in the uter-ine or funic soufflé. Check the woman's radial pulse while counting FHR.

The goal in assessing FHR is to search for and count the fetal cardiac sound.

This distinguishes the maternal heart rate from the FHR, which is usually about double the maternal pulse.

Auscultation: What can be assessed?

Fetal heart rate baseline rate: This is obtained by auscultation between palpated contractions when the fetus is not moving. Baseline FHR is between 110 and 160 beats per minute (bpm) in the normal term infant.

Fetal bradycardia is defined as a baseline rate below 110 bpm.

Fetal tachycardia is defined as a baseline over 160 bpm.

Rhythm is assessed for regularity and is described as regular or irregular.

Increases and decreases from the FHR baseline: may be heard and should be charted.

For example, FHR 144 bpm by auscultation, regular rhythm, audible acceleration.

Abrupt or gradual decreases from the baseline may also be heard but the decelerations that can be visually assessed with EFM cannot be identified based on auditory assessment.[12]

7. Charting: Document each period of auscultation with a description of baseline rate, rhythm, and the presence of gradual or abrupt decreases or increases from the baseline.

The FHR must be counted long enough to pick up changes in rate and rhythm. To determine a baseline, the FHR should be listened to for a full 60 seconds. If tachycardia or bradycardia is detected, more frequent auscultation must be done. It is important to distinguish if the change is a brief, isolated increase or decrease from the baseline or a change in the baseline rate. [11]

Irregular rhythms should be further assessed by ultrasound or cardiography to rule out artifact or to determine the type of dysrhythmia present. Fortunately, most dysrhythmias are benign and convert to normal rhythm after birth.

Dysrhythmias should be reported to the provider.

NOTE: Although auscultation allows the listener to hear gradual or abrupt changes from the baseline, baseline variability and the types of deceleration (late, variable, or early) cannot be identified with IA. There is no research to support that the expert listener can make these distinctions.[11]

A clear, organized record of FHR assessments is a professional and legal obligation.

Intrapartum Guidelines

8. Assessment during labor:
   Intermittent auscultation requires a 1:1 nurse-to-patient ratio.

   Support of the laboring woman and her partner should be a significant goal of care regardless of the type of fetal surveillance chosen.

   During labor, the Association of Women's Health, Obstetric and Neonatal Nurses (AWHONN) recommends that FHR be counted **after** uterine contractions for at least 30 to 60 seconds.[11]

   In the low-risk laboring woman: The American College of Obstetricians and Gynecologists (ACOG) and AWHONN advise assessing the FHR every 30 minutes during active labor. Frequency of assessments increases to every 15 minutes once 10 cm dilatation is achieved and the second stage of labor has begun.[11]

   In the high-risk laboring woman: Assess the FHR a minimum of every 15 minutes during active labor and every 5 minutes during the second stage of labor.

   Evaluate FHR characteristics before and after special events during labor (e.g., spontaneous and artificial rupture of membranes, administration of medication, ambulation, or a labor-initiating event).

There is a potential need to increase or realign staffing patterns to meet the 1:1 nurse-to-patient ratio that is recommended based on RCT comparing auscultation and EFM.

Fetal well-being during labor is assessed by the response of the FHR to uterine contractions.

When the mother is pushing during Stage II of labor, assessing the FHR after every contraction enables you to detect abrupt or gradual changes from baseline.

Continuous EFR and uterine contractions in the high-risk mother may give a more precise measurement of fetal response to the stress of uterine contractions.

Each institution should have a written policy that describes FHR assessment and auscultation guidelines during first and second stages of labor. **Readers are urged to study AWHONN's monograph *Fetal Heart Rate Auscultation* (2000), by Feinstein, Sprague, and Trepanier, which provides an excellent overview on the topic.**

REFERENCES

1. Cunningham F. G., Leveno K. J., Bloom S. L., Hauth, J. C., Gilstrap L. C., & Wenstrom K. D. (2005). Ultrasonography and Doppler. In *Williams Obstetrics* (22nd ed.). New York: McGraw-Hill.

2. Sinha, D., Sharma, A., Nallaswamy, V., Jayagopal N., & Bhatti, N. (2007). Obstetric outcome in women complaining of reduced fetal movements. *Journal of Obstetrics and Gynaecology, 27*(1), 41–43.

3. Mangesi, L., & Hofmeyr, G. Y. (2007). Fetal movement counting for assessment of fetal wellbeing. *Cochrane Database of Systemic Reviews, 1,* 1–16.

4. Moore, T. R., & Pinquadok, K. (1989). A prospective evaluation of fetal movement screening to reduce the incidence of antepartum fetal death. *American Journal of Obstetrics and Gynecology, 160*(5, Pt 1), 1075–1080.

5. American College of Obstetricians and Gynecologists. (1999). *Antepartum fetal surveillance.* [Practice bulletin no. 9]. Washington DC: Author.

6. Rayburn, W. R. (1990). Fetal body movement monitoring. *Obstetrics and Gynecology Clinics of North America, 17*(1), 85–110.

7. Chamberlain, D. B. (1999, Fall/Winter). Life in the womb: Dangers and opportunities. *Journal of Prenatal and Perinatal Psychology and Health, 14*(1–2), 31.

8. Chamberlain, D. B. (1999, Fall/Winter). Prenatal body language: A new perspective on ourselves. *Journal of Prenatal and Perinatal Psychology and Health, 14*(1–2) 173–176, 179–180.

9. Engstrom, J. L., McFarlin, B. L., & Sampson, M. B. (1993). Fundal height measurement. *Journal of Nurse-Midwifery, 38*(6), 318.

10. American Academy of Pediatrics and American College of Obstetricians and Gynecologists. (2002). *Guidelines for perinatal care* (5th ed.). Washington DC: Author.

11. Feinstein, N. F., Sprague, A., & Trepanier, M. J. (2000). *Fetal heart rate auscultation* (AWHONN Symposium). Washington DC: Association of Women's Health, Obstetric and Neonatal Nurses.

12. Moffatt, F. W., & Feinstein, N. (2003). Techniques for fetal heart assessment. In Feinstein, N., Torgersen, K. L., & Atterbuty, J. (Eds.), *AWHONN fetal heart rate monitoring principles and practices* (pp. 77–106). Washington DC: Association of Women's Health, Obstetric and Neonatal Nurses.

MODULE

5 Caring for the Laboring Woman

E. JEAN MARTIN ■ DONNA JEAN RUTH

Skill Unit 1

Friedman Graph: Plotting and Analysis

Skill Unit 2

Techniques for Breathing and Effleurage

Skill Unit 3

Techniques for Second Stage and Birth

Key Terms

When you have completed this module, you should be able to recall the meaning of the following terms. You should also be able to use the terms when consulting with other health professionals. The terms are defined in this module or in the glossary at the end of this book.

conduction anesthesia
doula
epinephrine
hyperventilation
lithotomy

spaces used in conduction anesthesia:
    arachnoid space
    extradural space
    subdural space

The Purpose of Intrapartum Care

Intrapartal care is essential to the goals of promoting a safe passage for both mother and baby, to minimize risks to both mother and baby, and to promote a healthy outcome and positive experience. Labor and delivery are natural process and if this basic and reasonable tenet can be accepted, most woman do well with supportive care and limited interventions.

Knowledgeable, clinically competent, caring, and skillful individuals are needed in labor and delivery units. Every laboring woman deserves kindness, compassion, and support as she navigates the process of giving birth. Think of this aspect of your caregiving as an art. Every art form asks from the artist something of himself or herself and this is no different. On your busy day, your tired day, the day when sad things happen on the unit, when difficulties occur at home, or when assignments are not to your liking, you must still enter a room and provide care.[1] Nurses today have limited time to spend providing supportive care.[2] This requires efficient use of therapeutic support for women and their support person(s) and leads to confidence of the mother in her providers.[3]

Studies indicate that the satisfaction a woman experiences during childbirth is related to either her ability to remain in control or to influence what happens to her.[4] Maternal perception of control is closely related to satisfaction, and the issue of control can be seen in terms of power. Both the birth setting and its participants powerfully influence the process of childbirth, shaping the role and amount of control held by a laboring woman, those who support her, and her caregivers. The birth experience belongs to the laboring woman and all efforts should be made to support, accommodate, and encourage her and her support persons. Care providers should be committed to meeting the needs of the laboring women and their support persons and not committed to arbitrary and restrictive rules.

The goals of intrapartum care are to do the following:
- Promote maternal coping behaviors
- Provide a safe environment for mother and fetus
- Support the mother and her family throughout the labor and birth experience
- Follow through on the mother's desires and choices throughout labor, whenever possible
- Provide comfort measures and pain relief as needed
- Offer reassurance and information, doing so with attention to the mother's and family's cultural needs

The caregiver should do the following:
- Create an environment sensitive to the psychological, spiritual, and cultural needs of the mother and her family
- Monitor maternal and fetal well-being
- Listen actively
- Recognize that language can have a powerful influence over maternal perceptions of the birth experience[5]
- Use language that is culturally appropriate, provides positive reinforcement, and empowers women and their families
- Touch so as to be therapeutic
- Use knowledge of both nonpharmacologic and pharmacologic therapies for pain relief
- Integrate the mother's support person(s) in all of these responsibilities so that he, she, or they become an essential and valued part of the profound experience of birth.

Cultural Sensitivity

Diversity is the norm in our society, requiring health care providers to be aware of beliefs and cultural practices of the families for which they care. Quality of care can be measured by cultural competency or the ability of a provider to incorporate knowledge of beliefs and cultural norms as they relate to the birth experience.[6] Women give birth within the context of their cultural background and traditional norms, including factors such as dietary practices and birth rituals. Language represents one example of cultural influences that significantly affect health care needs. Other cultural norms surrounding birth need to be addressed by the caregiver. Food intake, positioning, support behaviors, and early infant caretaking all may be influenced by culture. A cultural assessment should be done to ensure the caregiver has adequate knowledge of beliefs about labor support, drug therapies, and taboos.[6,7]

Maternal and Fetal Assessment During Labor: Auscultation and Electronic Fetal Monitoring

Both observation and technical skill are used to identify changes in maternal status, fetal position, presentation, and descent. These, combined with experience in fetal heart rate (FHR) monitoring techniques, provide the caregiver with the ability to monitor maternal and fetal well-being.

Guidelines for Documentation of Maternal and Fetal Status

The Association of Women's Health, Obstetric and Neonatal Nurses (AWHONN) has established guidelines for documentation during labor and birth. Documentation of care is essential because liability issues are a concern. "Documentation through the stages of labor includes maternal and fetal physiologic status, labor progression, risk status, and the meeting of educational needs."[8] The caregiver should maintain a flow sheet or written narrative of maternal and fetal status throughout labor. The documentation may be done in either electronic or written forms. This allows for a permanent record and creates a visual perspective of what transpired during labor.

Selecting a Fetal Heart Rate Assessment Technique

The goals of FHR monitoring during labor are to assess fetal well-being and detect signs of potential fetal compromise so that appropriate interventions may be initiated. Once you have studied Module 6, you will recognize that monitoring techniques involve the ability to differentiate reassuring from nonreassuring FHR changes. Assessment of the FHR may be accomplished by one of the following methods:

1. Auscultation with a stethoscope or a Doppler ultrasound device
2. Continuous electronic monitoring

Whichever method is used, nurses must be proficient, knowledgeable, and able to interpret the findings. FHR auscultation requires the nurse to be actively involved during labor, which may result in more supportive behavior; however, it does take more time. Circumstances such as staffing, provider and patient preference, and risk status often dictate the appropriate use of monitoring techniques.

Guidelines for the Auscultation of Fetal Heart Rate[9]

- When auscultation of the FHR is required every 15 minutes, the nurse-to-patient ratio must be 1:1 (one nurse to one patient).
- Clinical skills for auscultation, contraction palpation, and recognition of significant heart rate changes are essential (see Module 4, Skill Unit 3).
- Perform Leopold's maneuvers to identify the location of the fetal vertex, buttocks, and back. Fetal heart tones are best heard over the fetal back (in normal fetal flexed positions).
- Palpate for uterine contraction frequency, duration, intensity, and resting tone.
- Take the maternal radial pulse while listening to fetal heart tones to differentiate maternal and FHRs. This helps to prevent false conclusions about fetal status.
- *Count the FHR **after** uterine contractions for at least 30 to 60 seconds. This is helpful in evaluating fetal response to a contraction.*
- When differences are noted between counts, longer periods for recounting should be used to clarify the changes (i.e., type of periodic change and abrupt versus gradual change).

Recommended Frequency of Fetal Heart Rate Assessments During Labor

Low-risk women	Every hour in latent phase
	Every 30 minutes in active labor
	Every 15 minutes in stage II of labor
High-risk women	Every 30 minutes in latent phase
	Every 15 minutes in active labor
	Every 5 minutes in stage II of labor

NOTE: Evaluate fetal heart tones:
- *Before artificial rupture of membranes*
- *After artificial and spontaneous rupture of membranes*
- *Before and after ambulation*
- *Before administering medication*
- *At peak times of medication effect*
- *After procedures such as catheterizations and vaginal examinations*

Electronic Fetal Heart Rate Monitoring

Electronic FHR monitoring offers both visual and auditory monitoring on a continuous basis. External monitoring provides data on uterine contraction patterns and timing, as well as the FHR. Continuous electronic monitoring should be considered for the high-risk expectant woman. Meeting the high-risk criteria for auscultation can be disruptive to the woman; external or internal monitoring, if called for, can furnish critical information in a less distracting manner. The decision to use electronic fetal monitoring depends on maternal desires, provider decision by the physician or midwife, unit staffing patterns, and status of labor progress. *All women with nonreassuring FHR patterns should have continuous monitoring. Other clinical situations that call for consideration of continuous electronic fetal monitoring are discussed in this text.*

Evaluating Patterns of Labor

► What is the normal pattern of labor for nulliparous women?

Although each woman's labor and birth experience is unique, the pattern of normal labor is fairly predictable for both the nulliparous and the multiparous woman. In the early 1960s, an obstetrician named Emanuel Friedman published a study showing that *cervical dilatation and descent of the fetus occur within certain time frames, which can be plotted on a graph.* This has been used to measure normal limits for different phases of labor in the nulliparous and the multiparous woman. Using the graph, caregivers can objectively document labor progress. In general, primiparous women progress an average of 1.2 cm per hour during the first stage of labor; multiparas progress an average of 1.5 cm per hour. However, Friedman's work was based on 100 "normal labors" that included women with multiple gestations and fetal malpresentations.[10]

More recent information shows that labor progress may vary by race and ethnicity, timing and dosing of epidurals, use of oxytocin and misoprostol, fetal size and position, maternal psyche, labor positions, and pelvic structure, all of which should be considered when determining appropriate lengths of labor.[11–14] In addition, women who receive regional anesthesia experience a longer second stage.[15] This information allows a better understanding of the variation of length of normal labor. Experienced clinicians commonly can predict the length of labor based on maternal characteristics and FHR changes. However, vaginal examinations are necessary to confirm the status and progress of labor, and the Friedman graph can be used to identify potential problems with the progress of labor. *This allows consideration of a variety of factors, including medical and psychological issues that may inhibit labor progress.*

► What are the elements of a sensitive vaginal examination?

A vaginal examination provides important information but requires a skillful approach. The technical aspects of vaginal examination are well known and are addressed in Module 3. The manner in which the caregiver approaches and conducts the examination must be sensitive, thoughtful, and woman focused. A vaginal examination is an extremely invasive procedure. Without a thoughtful and sensitive approach, women may feel violated and demeaned. Women who have a history of sexual abuse may find that examinations are difficult and provide a trigger for memories of previous experiences.[16,17]

Before the examination, the caregiver should **review the maternal history** for the following information before conducting the examination:
- Gravidity
- Parity
- Gestational age
- History of ruptured membranes
- History of bleeding/spotting
- History of the present labor
  - When contractions began
  - When they became regular
  - Frequency and duration

- **Fetal history**
  - Recent movement pattern
  - Lie
  - Presentation
  - Heart rate

- **History of sexual abuse**—be sensitive to emotional reactions to the examination in women with a history of sexual abuse. Reactions may include
  - Inability to relax during the examination
  - Tightening of vaginal muscles
  - Body language that suggests fear and/or anxiety such as covering the eyes or crying

> **NOTE:** *Before performing an initial vaginal examination*
> - *Palpate the abdomen for fetal lie and presentation.*
> - *Listen to fetal heart tones.*
> - *Ask about bleeding history.*
> - *Ask about possible ruptured membranes.*

During the physical evaluation, the examiner should look for the following findings.

External
- Fluid
- Bloody show

Cervical
- Effacement
- Dilatation
- Position (i.e., anterior, midline, posterior)

Membranes
- Intact
- Ruptured

Presentation
- Leading part
- Degree of flexion
- Molding
- Caput
- Degree of descent

Take care to do the following:
- Introduce yourself.
- Keep vaginal examinations to a minimum. A good reason must exist for doing one. You must make your decision based on the information that needs to be obtained.
- Ensure privacy and draping.
- **Ask the woman's permission to do the examination.** This might require negotiating with her about the examination. Wait for explicit consent; tell her what you want to do and why. If she says "no," wait a while. Give her time to prepare herself. Most women give consent after a few minutes.
- Consider the optimal position for you and the mother. Experience in performing examinations while mothers are in alternative positions such as squatting or side-lying may optimize her tolerance of the examination.
- Have an organized approach to conducting the examination. If possible, perform the examination between contractions. If an examination is necessary during a contraction, start before the contraction so that the mother does not have to react to both at once; minimize finger/hand movement as much as possible.
- Use solution or lubricant sparingly. Too much lubrication makes the area around the perineum wet and cold. Obtain all cultures and check Nitrazine paper before using lubricants that may interfere with results.
- ***Take care that you put on gloves discreetly while standing at the bedside; do it as quietly and unobtrusively as possible. Avoid postures such as holding the gloved hand up in a fist as you wait to begin the examination.*** [15a]
- Keep the mother in focus throughout the examination.
- Watch your facial expressions—you are conveying a message.
- Forewarn the mother that the examination might be uncomfortable.
- Pay attention to what the mother says about the pain; acknowledge the discomfort and apologize for it.
- Share your findings with the mother. Use positive language whenever possible ("You are still 5 cm dilated but are now 100% effaced, so some progress has been made.").
- Clean and dry the mother's perineum and change bed pads if needed.

Care of the Mother During Active Labor

▶ **What are the major needs of the woman in active labor?**

Assessment of Maternal and Fetal Vital Signs

If, on admission of a mother in early labor, a normal baseline FHR pattern has been obtained by auscultation or electronic monitoring, FHR evaluation can be carried out less frequently than every 30 minutes, but should be done at least hourly. When active labor begins, evaluation intervals

TABLE 5.1	ASSESSMENT OF LABOR PROGRESS		
	LATENT PHASE	**ACTIVE LABOR**	**STAGE II**
Vital signs	Every 4 hr	Every 4 hr	
Blood pressure	Every 60 min	Every 30 min	
Contractions	Every 30 min to 1 hr	Every 30 min	
Fetal heart rate	Low risk: every hr	Low risk: every 30 min	Low risk: every 15 min
	High risk: every 30 min	High risk: every 15 min	High risk: every 5 min
Show	Every hr	Every 30 min	Every 10 to 15 min

Data from Sleutel, M. R. (2000). Intrapartum nursing care: A case study of supportive interventions and ethical conflicts. *Birth, 27,* 38–45.

of 15 to 30 minutes are appropriate, depending on risk status as outlined previously. Many providers prefer a "baseline strip" with electronic FHR monitoring; however, there is no research to suggest a difference in outcome when this strategy is used. See Table 5.1 for a summary of assessment recommendations.

Maternal vital signs should be assessed on admission. Be alert to any abnormal findings and consider possible explanations. An increased pulse rate often precedes a rise in temperature. Keep this in mind, especially in women who have ruptured membranes. Increases in heart rate and blood pressure (BP) may be due to pain or anxiety, but do not assume this. Repeat your assessments and if the findings remain abnormal alert the provider.

Support

Women tend to cope better, relax more readily, cooperate with treatment, describe their babies more positively, have a more positive recall of the experience, and adjust more easily to parenthood when they receive kind and sensitive care during their labor. Women who are provided support in labor have shorter labors; use less medication; have less incidence of forceps-assisted, vacuum-assisted, or cesarean births; and have babies with fewer low Apgar scores.[18] Our understanding of physiology shows us that undue fetal stress may occur if the laboring woman is anxious or frightened, as a result of increased catecholamine levels and vasoconstriction. This may contribute to a compromised fetal state in some cases.

Knowledge is empowering. Keeping women informed during labor about what to expect, interpreting the sensations they are experiencing and explaining their progress in labor are important elements of care.
The following elements are essential to cover when providing supportive care:
- Helping the woman to feel that she can handle the sensations, intensity, and effort required of labor by giving constant feedback, explaining everything, being positive, and validating her efforts
- Reviewing with her how to breathe and how to position herself, placing her hands on the fundus to feel the oncoming contraction, and showing her the baby's progress in a mirror, if desired
- Recognizing that the woman might have an unrealistic view of labor and what it involves, and following through by anticipating information needs
- Discussing potential barriers to labor progress such as fear, anxiety, or a history of sexual abuse or domestic violence
- Being concrete and specific, with an understanding that information might need to be repeated and skills reinforced and validated

In addition, a significant family member or friend should be encouraged to stay to support the mother. The support person needs nursing care too. Show him or her how to offer support and praise his or her efforts. Provide snacks and fluids for the support person if available in the labor area. Be sure to determine whether a support person has any special needs that may require attention.

Ambulation and Positioning

Healthy laboring women should be encouraged to change positions based on their comfort needs and position of the baby. Women who ambulate while in labor have shorter labors, less use of anesthesia, and report greater satisfaction with the birth process.[19] Positions that women find helpful in labor include positions listed in Table 5.2 and shown in Figure 5.1.

TABLE 5.2	MATERNAL POSITIONS FOR LABOR
IN BED	**OUT OF BED**
Upright	Standing/walking/dancing
Semisitting	Sitting on a birth ball
	Sitting on a side chair or rocking chair
	Sitting on the toilet
	Sitting in a tub
Hands and knees	Hands and knees in the shower or tub
Lateral	Side-lying in a tub
Exaggerated lateral	
Squatting	Squatting in the shower or on the floor

From Simkin, P. (1995). Reducing pain and enhancing progress in labor: A guide to nonpharmacologic methods for maternity caregivers. *Birth, 22*(3), 161–170.

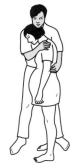 Standing

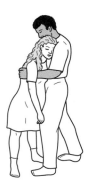 Standing, leaning forward

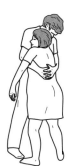 Slow dancing

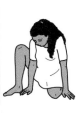 The lunge (standing)

The lunge (kneeling)

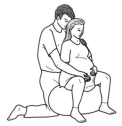 Sitting upright

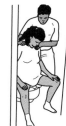 Sitting on commode

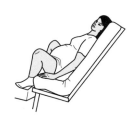 Semisitting

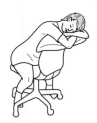 Sitting, leaning forward with support

 Hands and knees

 Kneeling over chair seat

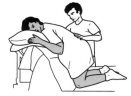 Kneeling, leaning on raised head of bed

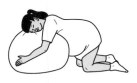 Kneeling over birth ball

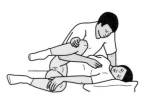 Side-lying

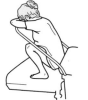 Squatting

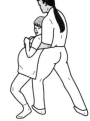 Supported squat

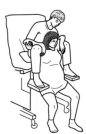 The dangle

FIGURE 5.1 Maternal positions for labor and birth. *Top row.* Upright positions. *Second row.* Sitting positions. *Third row.* Kneeling positions. *Fourth row.* Second-stage positions. (Adapted with permission from Simkin, P. [1995]. Reducing pain and enhancing progress in labor: A guide to nonpharmacologic methods for maternity caregivers. *Birth* 22[3], 161–170.)

Positions that may provide comfort and help rotate a fetus from a posterior position include the following[20]:
- Knee press
- Lunge
- Pelvic rocks on hands and knees
- Exaggerated lateral position

Nurses should be advocates for promoting optimal positioning in labor and for birth. Encourage the laboring woman to select her positions within the bounds of safety and with consideration of fetal monitoring and special procedures. When she is in bed, promote right or left side-lying or sitting.

> Supine positions result in the heavy uterus resting on the major veins leading back to the heart, diminishing cardiac input. This may result in supine hypotension and fetal bradycardia. The risk is greatest when a lithotomy position is assumed.

> Laboring women should be encouraged to avoid remaining on their backs and to change position frequently.

It is not likely that a supine position must be maintained during labor for any reason. However, during a cesarean birth, the supine position cannot be avoided. To prevent supine hypotension, raise the woman's right hip with a pillow or wedge so that the uterus can be shifted to the left. Raising the right hip relieves pressure on the vena cava and may improve circulation to the maternal heart, lungs, uterus, and placenta, resulting in fewer low Apgar scores.[20]

Fluids and Food

The policy of NPO (nothing by mouth) during labor is, unfortunately, a well-established routine in many hospitals. This practice dates back to 1946 when it was suggested that aspiration of acidic gastric contents was a significant cause of maternal morbidity and mortality.[21] Although the risk of aspiration has decreased significantly since the 1940s, mandatory fasting for laboring women is a practice that continues in many hospitals today. Consider the following:
- Aspiration during general anesthesia in operative deliveries is directly related to difficult intubation, regardless of the patient's oral intake.
- Experts in anesthesiology agree that substandard management of anesthesia is a primary cause of pulmonary aspiration.
- The NPO status results in increased gastric acidity.
- Regional blocks have little effect on gastric emptying time and greatly reduce the risk of aspiration pneumonia.
- A regional block is appropriate for most emergency cesarean deliveries.
- Routine intravenous (IV) fluid administration can induce fluid overload, hyperglycemia in the fetus, and hypoglycemia in the newborn, and can alter plasma sodium levels.[22]
- Hydration and the energy needs of the laboring woman are akin to the needs of a competitive athlete. Deprivation of food and fluid can directly affect labor progress and outcome.[22]
- In 1999, the American Society of Anesthesiologists revised their recommendations regarding oral intake in labor. Clear liquids recommended include water, fruit juices without pulp, carbonated beverages, clear teas and coffee, flavored gelatin, fruit ices, popsicles, and broth. They recommend restrictions on a case-by-case basis only for those women who may be at increased risk for aspiration.[23]

Women should be informed about the small but serious risk of aspiration related to oral intake during labor. It should be clear that the risk is from anesthesia and that if the labor deviates from normal, she may be asked to refrain from further oral intake.[22]

Intravenous Hydration

Intravenous fluids are indicated when the mother must be NPO. Those IV solutions that contain glucose are controversial and may result in fetal hyperglycemia and subsequent reactive hypoglycemia, hyperinsulinemia, acidosis, jaundice, and transient tachypnea of the new-born.[24,25] When IV solutions are indicated, solutions that do not contain glucose are a better choice. Another question is the amount of IV solution required to hydrate laboring women. Results of a study indicated that 125 mL/hr (which is the usual amount ordered) may be insufficient to meet the needs of laboring women and that the resulting dehydration may cause complications of labor.[26] This study indicated that 250 mL/hr was a more appropriate rate to maintain hydration. At present, most practice related to IV solution selection and rate is based mostly on tradition, and additional studies are needed to guide best practice.

Bladder Status

Provide the woman with the opportunity to empty her bladder every 2 hours. A full bladder can halt progress in labor, especially descent of the presenting part. If the woman is ambulating, urination is much more likely to be addressed by the mother because of increased pressure from the presenting part that is evident with upright positions.

Assessing Progress in Labor

Analysis of labor by plotting progress on a labor graph in the nulliparous and multiparous woman has provided a norm for evaluating progress in labor for many years. Although Friedman's norms are cited here, it is important to refrain from using these norms as rigid criteria for judging the adequacy of progress in every woman. Many factors, including maternal positions affecting gravity during labor, race, ethnicity, and the use of regional anesthesia, need to be considered when assessing progress in labor.[11]

▶ **If plotted on a graph, what does the normal labor pattern look like?**

Two major physiologic and anatomic events occur during labor:
1. Cervical dilatation
2. Fetal descent

Cervical Dilatation

Friedman found that most women in labor for the first time (nulliparas) experienced a cervical dilatation rate that, when plotted on a graph, looks like Figure 5.2.

Notice that during the fourth hour of labor, exactly 2 cm of dilatation has been achieved; at 10 hours, 3 cm of dilatation has occurred. Dilatation then progresses rapidly. The graph shows that the nulliparous woman achieves full dilatation after *14 hours* of labor.

For the multiparous woman, cervical dilatation occurs more quickly. See the graph in Figure 5.3.

The multiparous woman reaches full dilatation after an average of *8 hours* of labor.

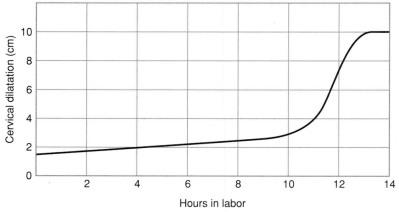

FIGURE 5.2 Labor progress of nulliparas. (Adapted from Friedman, E. A. [1967]. *Labor: Clinical evaluation and management* [p. 40]. New York: Appleton-Century-Crofts.)

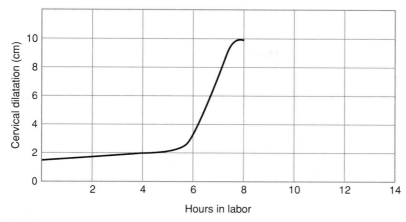

FIGURE 5.3 Labor progress of multiparas. (Adapted from Friedman, E. A. [1967]. *Labor: Clinical evaluation and management* [p. 38]. New York: Appleton-Century-Crofts.)

The normal labor patterns of cervical dilatation have an S-shaped curve. Friedman found that this curve could be divided into two major phases: *latent* and *active*. The S curve is marked to show the occurrence of these phases, in Figure 5.4.

The *latent phase* (preparatory phase) extends from the onset of regular contractions to the beginning of the active phase, when dilatation occurs more rapidly. It usually extends over several hours and appears as a nearly flat line on the graph. At the end of the latent phase, the cervix is soft, well effaced, and dilated approximately 3 cm. The latent phase can be prolonged if the laboring woman is given heavy sedation.

The *active phase* (dilatational phase) begins at the end of the latent phase, with a sharp upswing in the curve as the rate of dilatation increases rapidly. This phase ends at complete dilatation. Effective labor begins with the active phase.

The active phase is subdivided into three parts:

1. *Acceleration phase*—when the cervix begins to dilate rapidly
2. *Phase of maximum slope*—when the incline on the graph is very steep because most of the cervical dilatation happens at this time
3. *Deceleration phase*—when the rate of cervical dilatation slows (this happens just before complete dilatation; sometimes it is short or not present at all)

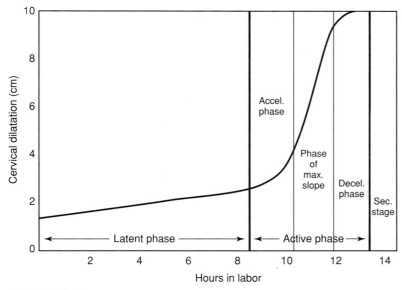

FIGURE 5.4 Phases of the cervical dilatation pattern in nulliparas. (Adapted from Friedman, E. A. [1967]. *Labor: Clinical evaluation and management* [p. 30]. New York: Appleton-Century-Crofts.)

The *rate of cervical dilatation* during the active phase is as follows:
- 1.2 cm or more per hour in *nulliparas*
- 1.5 cm or more per hour in *multiparas*

Overall, the *length of the first stage of labor* is shown in Table 5.3.

TABLE 5.3	LENGTH OF THE FIRST STAGE OF LABOR	
	AVERAGE (HR)	**UPPER NORMAL (HR)**
Nulliparas	13.3	28.5
Multiparas	7.5	20

► **What can go wrong with the progress of cervical dilatation in labor?**[10]

Certain factors can affect cervical dilatation. Some women have a dilatation pattern that, when graphed, differs from the normal S-shaped curve. Four major abnormal labor dilatation patterns have been identified. They are referred to as patterns of *dysfunctional labor*. Each pattern can be easily distinguished when plotted (Fig. 5.5).

Dysfunctional Labor Patterns for Nulliparas

Dysfunctional labor patterns occur in both the latent phase (prolonged latent phase) and the active phase. Active phase disorders fall into two categories:
1. Progressing too slowly (protraction)
2. Failing to progress (arrest)

Both dilatation and/or descent can be involved. Protraction and arrest disorders must be separated because treatment differs for each. Both are associated with increased perinatal morbidity.

A **prolonged latent phase** is longer than 20 hours in the nullipara and 14 hours in the multipara. It is associated with the following:
- An unripe cervix
- Too-early use of analgesics or sedatives
- Too-early use of conduction anesthesia

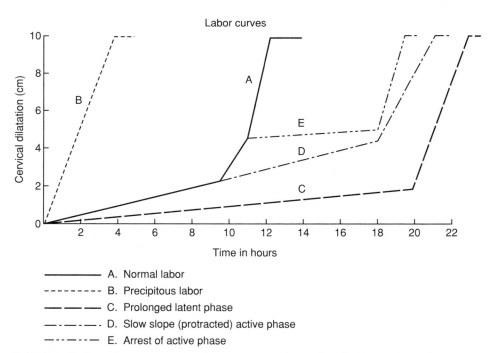

FIGURE 5.5 Labor patterns of nulliparous women. (Reproduced with permission from Malinowski, J. S. [1983]. *Nursing care of the labor patient* [2nd ed., p. 109]. Philadelphia: FA Davis.)

Prolonged latent phase accounts for nearly one third of abnormal labors in nulliparas and more than half in multiparas.

Treatment Consists of the Following:
- Support and therapeutic rest with sedation
- Oxytocin stimulation

NOTE: *Artificial rupture of membranes as a treatment method usually is not effective.*

A **protracted active phase** occurs when dilatation is less than 1.2 cm per hour in the nullipara and less than 1.5 cm per hour in the multipara. It is associated with the following:
- Cephalopelvic disproportion
- Minor malpresentations, such as posterior or transverse occiput
- Amniotomy before or at onset of labor
- Administration of conduction anesthesia before active labor is well established

Treatment Consists of the Following:
- Cesarean section for women with confirmed cephalopelvic disproportion
- Support
  - Explain the situation of slow progress to the woman and her family.
  - Ensure adequate fluid and electrolyte intake.
  - Anticipate with the woman and her family the course that labor is likely to take, explaining that progress will likely be slow but steady; cooperation is given more readily when full explanations are offered.

NOTE: *Friedman did not find oxytocin augmentation to be of value in women with protraction disorders. Others have found oxytocin augmentation to be useful in correcting protraction disorders. Therefore, in nulliparous women with suboptimal progress of labor, it is reasonable and safe to use oxytocin to determine if labor will progress.*[27]

Secondary arrest of the active phase occurs when cervical dilatation stops in the active phase. This is diagnosed when the arrest has lasted for 2 hours or more, as assessed by two vaginal examinations done 2 hours apart. Arrest is also seen when the deceleration phase lasts longer than 3 hours in the nullipara or longer than 1 hour in the multipara. It is associated with the following:
- Use of excessive sedation or conduction anesthesia
- Malpositions
- Cephalopelvic disproportion
- Artificial rupture of membranes

Secondary arrest of active phase occurs in 1 of 20 nulliparas in labor and in slightly fewer multiparas.

> Current studies show a good outcome for babies born after secondary arrest occurs *if delivered by a spontaneous vaginal birth.* A good outcome is less likely when a forceps delivery is done.

Treatment Consists of the Following:
- Immediate cesarean section for cephalopelvic disproportion
- Oxytocin stimulation if the pelvis is diagnosed as adequate
- Depending on the diagnosis and cause of the arrest, sedation for therapeutic rest, fluid and electrolyte therapy, and watchful waiting

Precipitous labor occurs when cervical dilatation is faster than 5 cm per hour (or 1 cm every 12 minutes) in nulliparas and 10 cm per hour (1 cm every 6 minutes) in multiparas. It is associated with the following:
- A normal latent phase in nulliparas
- Oxytocin administration
- Twice as many multiparous labors as nulliparous labors
- Uncomplicated and spontaneous vaginal deliveries

> Heavy sedation, minor fetal malpositions, and conduction anesthesia do not prevent precipitous dilatation from occurring.

Treatment: *The best treatment for precipitous labor is to anticipate the rapid descent of the fetus and a spontaneous delivery. Anticipate and prepare for the potential of a stressed newborn.*

Fetal Descent

▶ How does the pattern of descent appear on a graph?

Changes in the progressive descent of the fetus can be plotted by noting the fetal station. Friedman analyzed many labors to determine averages for descent of the fetus in nulliparas and multiparas. A definite relationship exists between dilatation and descent pattern.[15] *Descent in the nullipara occurs at approximately 1 cm per hour in the active phase.*

The *right side* of the graph in Figure 5.6 has the station marked from −1 to +5. The distance between each point is 1 cm. Notice that descent begins well before stage II of labor starts. The rate of descent increases late in the first stage of labor. By using the graph, you can determine whether the pattern of descent is normal or abnormal. The descent curve can also be divided into latent, accelerated, and maximum slope phases.

Figure 5.7 illustrates the normal dilatation and descent pattern in the multipara. *Descent in the multipara occurs at approximately 2 cm per hour or faster in the active phase.*

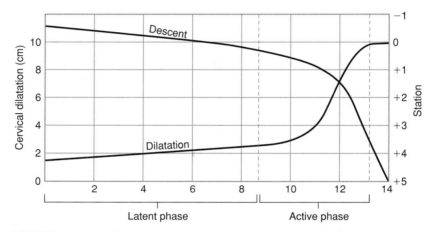

FIGURE 5.6 Dilatation and descent patterns in nulliparas. (Reproduced with permission from Friedman, E. A. [1970]. An objective method of evaluating labor. *Hospital Practice, 5*[7], 83. ©1970, The McGraw-Hill Companies. Illustration by Albert Miller.)

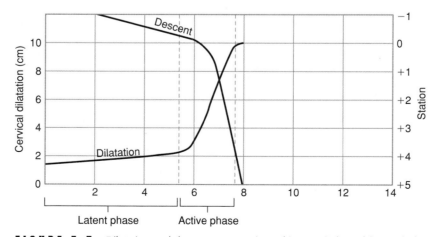

FIGURE 5.7 Dilatation and descent patterns in multiparas. (Adapted from Friedman, E. A. [1970]. An objective method of evaluating labor. *Hospital Practice, 5*[7], 82. Illustration by Albert Miller.)

THE TWO FRIEDMAN GRAPHS SHOWING PATTERNS OF DESCENT CLEARLY ILLUSTRATE THAT THE MOST PROGRESS IN DILATATION AND THE ONSET OF ACCELERATION IN DESCENT OCCUR DURING MAXIMUM SLOPE OF THE ACTIVE PHASE IN BOTH THE NULLIPARA AND THE MULTIPARA.

Both the rates of descent and dilatation are faster in the multipara than in the nullipara.

> Abnormal descent patterns occur twice as often in the nullipara as in the multipara.

Two major abnormal descent patterns can occur: protracted descent and arrest of descent.

A protracted descent pattern occurs when the rate of descent in the active phase is less than 1.0 cm per hour in the nullipara or less than 2.0 cm per hour in the multipara.

This Pattern is Associated With the Following:
• Protracted dilatation in the active phase
• Cephalopelvic disproportion
• Minor fetal malpositions, such as occiput posterior
• Excessive sedation
• Conduction anesthesia

Treatment Consists of the Following:
• Cesarean section is indicated if cephalopelvic disproportion is diagnosed.
• Avoid oxytocin stimulation because it is generally ineffective with this pattern.
• Provided the fetus is tolerating labor well, permit labor to continue with spontaneous vaginal delivery the goal. Avoid forceps delivery if possible.
• Careful attention must be given to hydration and electrolyte needs
  Emotional support for the woman, her family, and support team is essential

Arrest of descent occurs during the *active phase,* when there is no progress (as documented by two well-spaced vaginal examinations) for 1 hour or more in the nullipara or for 1/2 hour or more in the multipara. This pattern is associated with the following:
• Advanced gestational age
• Infants weighing more than 2,500 g (especially with infants weighing more than 4,000 g)
• Cephalopelvic disproportion
• Fetal malpositions (e.g., persistent occiput transverse or occiput posterior)
• Coexistent labor disorders (e.g., protraction disorders)

> When progressive descent of the fetal presenting part is interrupted late in labor, a serious problem can exist.

> Vaginal examination for assessment of descent must carefully distinguish between true descent and the occurrence of fetal scalp edema or molding of the cranial bones.

Treatment Consists of the Following:
• Careful assessment of the woman by vaginal examination should be done in all patterns of protraction or arrest.
• If cephalopelvic disproportion does not exist, rule out factors causing the problem that might be reversible (e.g., excessive sedation, conduction anesthesia).
• Cesarean section is performed on women with cephalopelvic disproportion.
• Careful oxytocin stimulation can be started in the woman with an adequate pelvis. This should be carried out for at least 2 hours in the case of arrested descent, beginning from the time of an established contraction pattern.

NOTE: If arrest of descent occurs during oxytocin stimulation, continued use of such stimulation is ineffective.

• Infrequently, allowing excessive sedation or conduction anesthesia to wear off or allowing therapeutic rest for the exhausted woman results in return of progressive labor.

Pain Control

Pain is a subjective experience. Pain is whatever someone says it is—for him or her. Physical, psychological, and cultural factors play important roles in the response women have to the childbirth experience. Pain control is managed in different ways and may vary according to the stage of labor; the rate of progress; the condition of the mother and fetus; the skill, experience, and attitude of members of the obstetric team; and the requests and attitudes of the mother and her family.

Methods of Pain Management Include the Following:
- Breathing and relaxation techniques
- Comfort measures
- Nonpharmacologic pain relief (e.g., water therapy)
- Analgesia
- Anesthesia

Comfort Measures

- *Do not leave a woman in active labor alone.*
- Promptly change soiled and damp linen.
- For mothers who are NPO status, provide frequent mouth care, give ice chips, lubricate lips, and/or encourage frequent mouth rinses.
- Suggest ambulation, position change, or the use of a shower or hot tub, if available.
- Apply massage to abdomen, back, and legs as desired.
- Ensure good ventilation in the room.
- Control the labor room environment according to the mother's wishes (e.g., lights, music, quiet, privacy).
- Promote the participation of a coach or significant family member.
- Offer support from a professional doula.

"*Doula* refers to a supportive companion professionally trained to provide labor support."[28] A doula is not trained to do clinical tasks and may provide support during labor and the postpartum period. Women who have a doula have been shown to have improved outcomes of birth with fewer epidurals and more positive feelings about their birth experience.[29] Doulas may be particularly useful in busy birthing units where individualized care by a nurse or midwife is not possible.

▶ **What causes pain in labor?**

Pain can be physical, physiologic, and psychological and is affected by a variety of factors, including level of anxiety, environment, support, and previous experience with painful stimuli.

Physical and Physiologic Causes Are Thought to Include the Following:
- Hypoxia of the uterine muscle because of diminished blood supply to the uterus during a contraction
- Stretching of and pressure on the cervix, vagina, and perineal floor muscles
- Distension of the lower uterine segment
- Traction on reproductive structures, such as the fallopian tubes, ovaries, and uterine ligaments
- Pressure on skeletal muscles
- Pressure on the bladder, urethra, and rectum
- Distension of the pelvic floor with tearing of the subcutaneous fascial tissue

NOTE: *Factors that undoubtedly influence the degree and character of pain include the following:*
- *Nature of contractions (intensity and duration)*
- *Degree of cervical dilatation*
- *Degree of perineal distension*
- *Maternal age, parity, and general health*
- *Maternal position*
- *Fetal size and position (e.g., posterior positions are usually accompanied by intense back pain)*

Other Factors That May influence a Mother's Response to Pain Include the Following:
- Anxiety and fear
- History of abuse or previous traumatic birth or hospital experience[16]
- Cultural influences and upbringing
- Value system and education level
- Lack of knowledge or preparation
- Absence of supportive significant person
- Lack of motivation

▶ **Can pain in labor have harmful effects on the mother or fetus?**

Pain May Have the Following Effects:
- *Hyperventilation,* or rapid breathing associated with pain, leads to oxygen and carbon dioxide imbalance in maternal blood and lungs. This results in decreased blood flow to the uterus and brain. Breathing changes may also lead to fetal acidosis.
- Poorly coordinated uterine activity, regulated by the sympathetic nervous system, worsens.
- When the mother is stressed, epinephrine is released and uterine blood vessels constrict, decreasing blood flow to the placenta and fetus.
- Epinephrine also causes high glucose levels in the mother's blood, leading to an increase of glucose in fetal blood and, therefore, in brain tissue. Such high glucose levels decrease the fetal brain cells' ability to handle hypoxia and render those cells susceptible to damage.
- Cardiac output and BP increase considerably during painful periods.
- Severe pain can change cardiac rhythms and decrease blood flow to the coronary arteries.
- Muscle tightening of the perineal floor makes delivery difficult.
- Fear, tension, and anxiety are greatly aggravated by pain.

▶ **What nonpharmacologic pain relief measures can be used with the laboring woman?**

Many techniques and therapies can be used to provide nonpharmacologic pain relief for labor and birth. These can be used alone or in combination with pharmacologic options or in an effort to delay the use of pharmacotherapy.

Commonly Used Therapies Include the Following:
- Acupressure
- Heat and cold therapy
- Hydrotherapy
- Massage
- Intradermal injections of sterile water

Nurses May Use the Following Techniques, Which Have Been Found to Be Useful for Women in Labor:
- Help mothers to identify the most comfortable position(s) and encourage frequent position changes.
- Provide hot and cold therapy with hot packs or ice packs.
- Use acupressure points.
- Encourage the use of a tub or shower.
- Provide or train a support person to use massage techniques.
- Apply counterpressure with tennis balls or other firm objects, particularly for women who have a baby in posterior position.
- Use the double hip squeeze to increase the outlet diameter and decrease pain. Hands are placed over the gluteus muscles with mothers assuming a position with hip joints flexed. Using the palms, pressure is given toward the center of the pelvis.[19]
- Use intradermal injections of sterile water for severe back pain.[30]
- Encourage support by a professional doula.

► **What measures should be taken to safely use hydrotherapy for women in labor and/or for birth?**[31]

Actions	*Remarks*
Rule out any contraindications for hydrotherapy in labor.	Any mothers requiring electronic fetal monitoring are not appropriate candidates. Dissatisfied mothers should be able to get out of the tub or shower quickly if necessary. Thick meconium is a contraindication to the use of tubs for labor and/or birth. Maternal fever is a contraindication.
Use established protocols for the following:	Jets must be cleaned according to infectious disease protocols.
• Cleaning of tubs	
• Use of long gloves for vaginal examinations	
• Fetal heart rate monitoring	Intermittent FHR monitoring can be accomplished when the mother is out of the water by using a waterproof Doptone or a fetoscope.
Use water at normal body temperature. Determine baseline FHR and maternal vital signs before initiation of hydrotherapy.	High water temperatures can result in elevated maternal temperatures and rapid FHR.
Cover IV lines or heparin locks with plastic.	
Provide a stool and/or pillow or a birth ball for maternal comfort.	Many women prefer to sit or lean in the shower.
Constant support must be available for women using hydrotherapy.	Neck pillows provide neck support for women using tubs.
Discontinue hydrotherapy at any time if requested by the mother or if unsafe conditions occur.	If water birth is anticipated, follow specific protocols established by a practice or institution. Care must be given to ensure that babies are lifted out of the water immediately after birth.

► **What measures should be taken when giving pain medication to the laboring woman?**

- Be sure that the mother has given informed consent to her health care provider.
- Know the mother's medical and obstetric history; check for allergies.
- Assess vital signs and FHR before and after administration of any medications.
- Know the status of labor and anticipated delivery at the time the medication is given.
- Consider the mother's requests.
- Be aware of the therapeutic effects, contraindications, and side effects of the drug being given.
- Use a large-bore (18-gauge) catheter when starting an IV infusion, which permits rapid fluid or blood administration if needed.
- Consider the mother's weight, the progress of labor, the maturity and size of the fetus, and the dosage of medicine being prepared.
- Reassess patient within 1 hour of medication administration to assess for desired effect.
- Use filtered needles with all medications drawn up from a glass ampules. Filters help to screen out glass particles and bacteria that are sometimes present in ampules after they have been broken open.

Nursing Responsibilities in Performing Subcutaneous/ Intracutaneous Injections of Sterile Water

Sterile water injections have been used to relieve acute pain such as pain associated with renal colic and other types of musculoskeletal pain. Possible theories that explain the reason for its effectiveness include blocked pain pathways according to the gate theory and release of endogenous endorphins.[30,32] This technique is particularly appropriate for women in labor who are experiencing acute back pain. A period of pain relief provided by this procedure gives an opportunity for rest and comfort and time for position changes to facilitate rotation of a posterior vertex to anterior.[33]

A c t i o n s
1. Secure informed consent.
2. Explain steps in the procedure.

3. Assist the obstetric provider
   with injection.

4. Document the time of injection
   and pain relief.

R e m a r k s

Emphasize to mothers that they will feel an acute
"stinging" sensation associated with injection.
Use 0.1 mL sterile water in four sites in the
lumbar-sacral region area adjacent to the
Michaelis rhomboid.[33]
Most women report relief soon after the injection
and for up to 60 to 90 minutes. Use this time
to reposition mothers to optimize rotation of
the fetus to an anterior position.

Figure 5.8 shows the location of the injection sites.

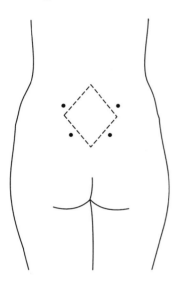

FIGURE 5.8   Location of injection sites in relation to the Michaelis rhomboid for intradermal injections of sterile water. (Adapted with permission from Martensson, L., & Wallin, G. [1999]. Labor pain treated with cutaneous injections of sterile water: A randomized controlled trial. *British Journal of Obstetrics and Gynecology 106*[7], 634.)

Nursing Responsibilities in Monitoring and Maintaining Epidural Anesthesia in the Laboring Woman

Epidural anesthesia involves threading a catheter into the epidural space to administer local anesthetics and or narcotics. Located between the dura mater and the enclosing vertebrae, the epidural space provides a passageway for nerve roots leaving the spinal cord. The nerves are bathed in the anesthetic being instilled via the epidural catheter, providing pain relief for the particular areas of the body that they innervate (Fig. 5.9).

Currently, there are no reliable statistically significant data showing a cause-and-effect relationship between the use of epidural anesthesia and adverse effects. This continues to be an area of controversy because of insufficient data. There is concern that epidural anesthesia may be associated with prolonged stages of labor, increased use of assisted techniques for delivery (e.g., vacuum extraction, forceps), and higher rates of cesarean births. Some clinicians believe that these effects may be related to individual styles of obstetric management (e.g., early labor assessment, pitocin augmentation) and these have just as much influence on the labor process as the epidural procedure.[15] The AWHONN evidence-based practice guideline, *Nursing Care of the Woman Receiving Regional Analgesia/Anesthesia in Labor*, includes accumulated research to suggest a model for practice.[34] There is no question that increased technology is associated with the use of epidurals, including IV therapy and electronic FHR monitoring.

Adequate nursing support is essential to the safe provision of an epidural. It is important that a registered nurse evaluate maternal and fetal status before, during, and intermittently after the epidural procedure. The AWHONN guidelines maintain that the insertion of epidural catheters and injection or rebolus of regional analgesic/anesthetic agents remains within the scope of the licensed, credentialed anesthesia care provider.[35]

Continuous low-dose lumbar epidural infusion is the anesthetic used most often. Sensory blockage gives uninterrupted pain relief with minimal motor blockade.

During the first stage of labor, anesthetic dosages are given to limit the block to the lower thoracic (T10) and upper lumbar segments. This allows perineal tone to be maintained to avoid interfering with internal rotation of the fetal head to the occiput anterior position. When stage II labor is reached, the block can be extended to the sacral area to promote perineal relaxation, delivery, and episiotomy repair.

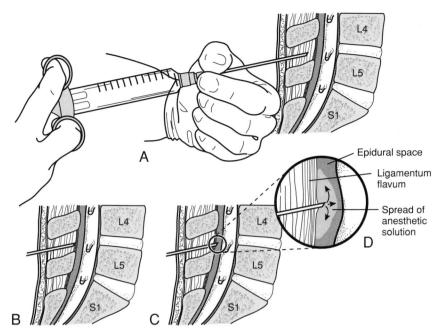

FIGURE 5.9 Technique of epidural block. **A.** Proper position of insertion. **B.** Needle in the ligamentum flavum. **C.** Tip of needle in epidural space. **D.** Force of injection pushing dura away from tip of needle. (Reprinted with permission from Taylor, T. [1993, March/April]. Epidural anesthesia in the maternity patient. *Maternal-Child Nursing Journal, 18*[2], 86.)

Levels of anesthesia for vaginal and cesarean deliveries are shown in Figure 5.10.

Nursing responsibilities for the epidural procedure have been adapted from AWHONN's *Evidence-Based Clinical Practice Guideline, Nursing Care of the Woman Receiving Regional Analgesia/Anesthesia in Labor.*[34] Readers are encouraged to read this document for further details and explanation of the scientific evidence surrounding this procedure.

Actions Before the Procedure[34,35]

1. Consult with anesthesia and obstetric providers when the decision is made to use epidural analgesia/anesthesia. Determine the woman's and support person's knowledge regarding the procedure and any concerns they may have.

2. Note contraindications, such as maternal fear or refusal, local infection at the injection site, coagulation defects, and maternal hypotension or shock.

Remarks

The anesthesiologist or nurse-anesthetist is responsible for explaining the procedure, its effect, and possible complications.

Sympathetic blockade worsens some of these.

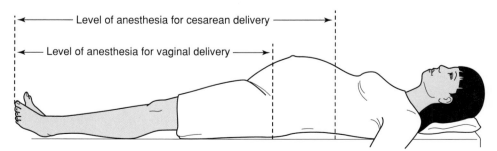

FIGURE 5.10 Levels of anesthesia for vaginal and cesarean deliveries. (Adapted with permission from Taylor, T. [1993, March/April]. Epidural anesthesia in the maternity patient. *Maternal-Child Nursing Journal, 18*[2], 92).

3. Obtain maternal baseline BP, pulse rate, respiratory rate, and fetal baseline heart rate and variability. Confirm a reassuring fetal heart tracing before the procedure.

4. Have the woman void before the procedure.

5. Administer an IV fluid bolus of 500 to 1,000 mL balanced saline or lactated Ringer's solution 10 to 30 minutes before the epidural procedure.

Anesthetic effects include vascular vasodilatation, decreased BP, and possible FHR accelerations that could exacerbate a preexisting problem.

The epidural block can reduce or eliminate bladder sensation. Urinary retention may occur.

A preprocedure bolus may help to prevent hypotension caused by vasodilatation from the anesthetic.

NOTE: *IV glucose solutions are not recommended because of the potential impact of fetal hyperglycemia with subsequent and rebound newborn hypoglycemia.*

> Never leave a mother unattended during the first 20 minutes after administration of the initial anesthetic or any bolus dose.

Actions During the Procedure[34,35]

6. Assist the woman to a side-lying position with legs slightly flexed or to a sitting position with the mother's head flexed forward, elbows resting on her knees, and feet supported on a chair.

7. Support the mother throughout the procedure of local infiltration and catheter threading.

8. Note maternal BP and pulse rate before and after the test dosage. Repeat at least every 5 minutes throughout administration of the anesthetic dose and for 15 minutes afterward. Thereafter, record BP, pulse, and respiration rate regularly based on institutional protocol and patient's status.

Remarks

This promotes moderate spinal flexion to assist in locating the appropriate vertebrae.

Breathing techniques appropriate to the phase of labor can be encouraged to promote relaxation.

Epinephrine is added to the test dosage. If the catheter is misplaced and is in the dilated epidural vein, maternal pulse rate increases by 20% to 30%. A normal rate reflects that the drug was not injected intravascularly. Systolic drops below 90 mmHg are considered inadequate to maintain uterine blood flow for fetal oxygenation.

Actions After the Procedure[34,35]

9. May need to reassure the mother if she feels a warm tingling sensation down her legs when the initial bolus loading dose is given.

10. Avoid maternal hypotension by promoting uterine displacement with a pillow/wedge or placing the mother in a full lateral position or in a supine position, with the head of the bed elevated. Assist the mother in turning every hour.

11. Evaluate the mother's bladder by palpation and observation at least hourly.

12. Periodically assess for level of anesthesia before administration of any bolus dose.

13. Determine the level of pain relief using institutional pain assessment scales.

Remarks

This is a normal preanesthetic effect.

This allows the drug to defuse bilaterally.

The woman can lose the sensation to void and may need to be catheterized. A full bladder not only is subject to trauma, but also can impede descent of the fetus.

This is important to avoid potentially high levels of anesthesia.

This is done to assess the fading of anesthesia. Avoid anesthesia receding too far before a "top off" (bolus dose) is needed.

14. Continually monitor for maternal complications.

Vital signs and monitoring should be done according to institutional guideline/protocols.

15. During stage II of labor, in preparation for delivery, assist the mother to a semiupright position, an upright position, or a side-lying position.

This allows the anesthetic to migrate into the sacral area. However, if the epidural is associated with a rapid second stage or if FHR decelerations occur, a lateral position may optimize blood flow to the fetus and prevent a rapid birth.

16. If narcotics are given via the epidural catheter, observe for potential side effects.

Nausea, vomiting, itching, and urinary retention are possible.

Side effects can be reversed by administering naloxone hydrochloride (Narcan) as ordered.

17. Document the following per institutional policy:
    • Maternal BP and pulse rates
    • Position changes
    • Oxygen administration
    • IV rate changes
    • Maternal response to procedure
    • Any complications
    • Use of oxygen
    • Other supportive interventions, should they be necessary

This documentation becomes part of the medical record.

Actions to Respond to Complications[34,35]

18. Evaluate and document maternal pain levels using standard assessment tools such as visual and verbal analog scales. Special techniques include the following:
    • Patient-controlled epidural anesthesia: allows the patient to self-titrate periodic amounts of anesthetic
    • Walking epidural: patients who have intentional motor function and mobility with a bolus or continuous infusion via an indwelling epidural catheter preceded by an injection of local anesthetic into the subarachnoid space

Remarks

19. *Maternal Hypotension*
    • Maternal hypotension is defined as a systolic BP less than 100 mmHg or a 20% decrease from preanesthesia levels.
    • Place the mother in a full lateral position.
    • Give oxygen by face mask.

Maternal hypotension may result in a fetal response such as fetal bradycardia and/or late decelerations. Interventions are intended to restore uterine blood flow.

Promote and maintain uterine displacement. Avoid the supine position.

Nausea and vomiting can occur in up to 50% of women having epidural anesthesia.

    • Give 250 to 500 mL IV bolus of non–glucose-balanced saline solution.
    • If vasopressors are needed, 5 to 10 mg IV ephedrine is recommended. Ephedrine should only be as ordered or according to established protocols. Notify providers (both anesthetic and obstetric) if hypotension does not resolve with position change and IV fluid bolus.

This is the vasopressor of choice because it targets cardiac muscle, thus increasing uterine blood flow by enhancing cardiac output.

20. Pruritus, a common and mild reaction to anesthetic, usually begins within 10 to 30 minutes of epidural initiation and medication administration.

The use of opioids may increase the risk of pruritus by 40% to 90%. Fewer than 20% of women require medication to alleviate it. Diphenhydramine or naloxone is used for treatment. Usually, the pruritus resolves within 1 hour of onset.

21. *Urinary retention* is a side effect of epidural anesthesia in a large percentage of women.

Assessment of bladder status is critical to avoid overdistension of the bladder, which the mother cannot feel. Urinary catheterization is necessary in some women.

> *Observe for signs of fetal bradycardia and/or late decelerations in response to maternal hypotension. Correction of maternal hypotension usually results in resolution of fetal bradycardia and/or late decelerations.*

---

22. *High spinal*
    - Prevailing symptom: profound motor and sensory block within 1 to 5 minutes of the epidural injection
    - Severe hypotension
    - Cessation of respirations
    - Cardiac arrest

    Take steps to do the following:
    - Establish a patent airway.
    - Give 100% oxygen at a high flow rate.
    - Intubate if necessary.
    - Administer vasopressors.
    - Manually push the gravid uterus to one side.

    Urinary displacement relieves pressure on the vena cava and aorta, promoting better venous return to the heart.

23. *Intravascular injection of local anesthetic*
    Signs of this include the following:
    - Change in maternal heart rate (tachycardia or bradycardia)
    - Maternal hypertension
    - Dizziness, tinnitus, or metallic taste
    - Loss of consciousness

    Inadvertent dural punctures occur in approximately 2% of pregnant women, in a blood vessel and inadvertent IV catheter placements can occur in up to 5% of pregnant women.

> Intravascular injection of a local anesthetic may result in seizure or cardiac arrest and requires an immediate response, including cardiopulmonary resuscitation, O_2 administration, and assisted ventilation.

---

24. *Spinal headaches*
    - If the dura is accidentally punctured, women may experience spinal headaches 24 to 48 hours after the puncture.

    Headaches develop in 1% to 3% of women who receive epidural anesthesia. As cerebrospinal fluid is lost, pressure is diminished throughout that compartment and the brain descends somewhat, especially when the mother is in an upright position.

    - Conservative treatment involves maintaining a flat position, hydration, and administering analgesics.
    - A blood patch may be used to seal the puncture site, using 15 mL of the patient's unanticoagulated blood. As the blood clots, it "patches" the area, usually affording quick relief.

121

*Actions During Recovery
From Epidural/Delivery*   *Remarks*

25. During the mother's recovery, keep the side rails up and the bed in a low position.

26. Remove the catheter once the placenta has been delivered and the mother begins her recovery period. It is preferable to remove the catheter with the mother in the same position used during placement. A registered nurse with training may remove the catheter if hospital policy and state regulations allow. Inspect the catheter carefully to make sure it is intact. If you suspect breakage, alert the anesthesiologist immediately and save the catheter for the anesthesiologist's inspection. Assess for motor and sensory return by asking the mother to move her legs up and down and side to side; perform plantar flexion and dorsiflexion of the feet. The mother must be able to support her knees in an upright position, as in a standing position before attempting ambulation.

The maternal position increases the intervertebral space.

*Actions to Assess Effects
on the Neonate*   *Remarks*

27. Monitor neonate for decreased motor tone and decreased respiratory effort.

Effects on the neonate may be observed up to 24 hours of age.
All neonatal care providers should be aware of anesthetic/analgesic agents used by a mother in labor.

PRACTICE/REVIEW QUESTIONS

After reviewing this module, answer the following questions.

1. There are many goals in intrapartum care. List at least four.

    a. _____

    b. _____

    c. _____

    d. _____

2. What steps can the caregiver take to promote achievement of the goals stated in question 1?

    a. _____

    b. _____

    c. _____

    d. _____

3. Name the two major techniques for monitoring fetal status during labor.

    a. _____

    b. _____

4. What is the appropriate nurse-to-patient ratio if FHR is being assessed every 15 minutes by auscultation? _____

    _____

5. What is the correct procedure for auscultating a FHR during any active labor contraction? Why? _____

    _____

    _____

6. How is the average fetal baseline assessed by auscultation?

    _____

    _____

7. How can a distinction be made between maternal and FHRs during auscultation?

    _____

    _____

8. State five situations in which FHR should be assessed.

    a. _____

    b. _____

c. _____

d. _____

e. _____

9. How might caregivers conduct a vaginal examination so that a laboring woman is empowered?

_____

_____

Give at least four elements of a sensitive vaginal examination.

a. _____

b. _____

c. _____

d. _____

10. What physical examination component should always precede your initial vaginal examination of a pregnant woman?

_____

11. For the low-risk woman in active labor who is dilated 8 to 10 cm, BP should be taken every _____ minutes; contractions should be monitored every _____ minutes; FHR, every _____ minutes; and show, every _____ minutes.

12. The best bed rest position for the laboring woman is probably the _____.

13. Maintaining the supine position for a long time sometimes results in _____.

14. Discuss six ways that you, as a nurse, can help make the laboring woman more comfortable.

a. _____

b. _____

c. _____

d. _____

e. _____

f. _____

15. What activities do caregivers engage in that laboring women perceive as "supportive"?

a. _____

b. _____

c. _____

d. _____

16. The nulliparous woman experiencing normal labor progress will achieve full dilatation after approximately _____ hours.

17. The multiparous woman having normal labor progress will achieve full dilatation after approximately _____ hours.

18. The dilatation curve can be divided into two major phases: _____ and _____.

19. At the end of the latent phase, the cervix is _____ and dilated approximately _____ cm in a normal labor pattern.

20. During the active phase of labor, the *rate* of cervical dilatation in nulliparas should occur at _____ cm or more per hour; in multiparas, cervical dilatation should occur at _____ cm or more per hour.

21. The *average* length of the first stage of labor for nulliparas is _____ hours; in multiparas, the average length of the first stage of labor is _____ hours.

22. Identify the dysfunctional cervical dilatation patterns in the following graph.

A. _____

B. _____

C. _____

D. _____

E. _____

23. The appropriate nursing intervention for a woman with prolonged labor in the latent phase is _____.

24. Protracted labor in the active phase can be associated with:

a. _____

b. _____

c. _____

d. _____

25. Secondary arrest of labor in the active phase occurs when _____ stops.

26. The outcome is good for babies born after secondary arrest of labor if delivered by _____ _____ _____.

27. Precipitous labor occurs when cervical dilatation is faster than _____ cm per hour in nulliparas and _____ cm per hour in multiparas.

28. Descent normally begins well before the _____ stage of labor starts in both nulliparas and multiparas.

29. The rate of descent and dilatation is _____ in the multipara than in the nullipara.

30. Abnormal descent patterns occur _____ as often in the nullipara as in the multipara.

31. Protracted descent occurs when the rate of descent in the active phase is _____ cm per hour in the nullipara or _____ cm per hour in the multipara.

32. It is important to avoid use of _____ and/or _____ when protracted descent occurs.

33. Arrest of descent occurs when there is no progress for _____ in the nullipara or for _____ in the multipara.

34. List four factors associated with arrest of descent.

a. _____

b. _____

c. _____

d. _____

35. What careful distinctions must be made when performing a vaginal examination of the presenting part for descent?

_____

_____

_____

36. If arrest of descent occurs while oxytocin stimulation is being given, it should be:

a. Continued.

b. Discontinued.

37. List at least five theories and/or factors thought to be related to causes of pain in labor.

a. _____

b. _____

c. _____

d. _____

e. _____

38. What are three therapies commonly used for nonpharmacologic pain relief in labor?

a. _____

b. _____

c. _____

39. Discuss the measures you should take when administering pain medication to the laboring woman.

_____

_____

_____

_____

_____

40. What are two reasons to provide sterile water injections in labor for women with a baby in a posterior position?

a. _____

b. _____

41. Epidural anesthesia is intended to provide complete blockade of _____ nerves and minimal blockade of _____.

42. During the first stage of labor, the anesthetic dose is given so that the sensory block is limited to the lower _____ and the upper _____ segments. This allows _____ to be maintained to avoid interfering with internal rotation of the fetal head.

43. Who is responsible for explaining to the mother the essentials of the epidural procedure and possible complications?

_____

44. State three contraindications to epidural anesthesia.

a. _____

b. _____

c. _____

45. Why are IV glucose solutions not recommended for fluid loading before epidural administration?

_____

46. Why is fluid loading done before epidural administration?

_____

47. The mother's bladder status should be evaluated every

_____ .

48. The most common complication with an epidural is

_____ .

49. List three steps to take in a maternal hypotensive episode with epidural anesthesia.

a. _____

b. _____

c. _____

50. What are three signs associated with intravascular injection of local anesthetic?

a. _____

b. _____

c. _____

51. The epidural catheter can be removed by a trained nurse if hospital policy and state practice act allow.

a. True

b. False

52. There are no known neonatal effects associated with maternal use of epidurals during labor and delivery.

a. True

b. False

PRACTICE/REVIEW ANSWER KEY

1. Any four of the following:
   a. Ensure a safe passage for mother and baby.
   b. Promote maternal coping behaviors.
   c. Support the mother and her family.
   d. Follow through on the mother's choices and desires whenever possible.
   e. Provide pain relief.
   f. Offer reassurance and information.

2. a. Create a quiet environment.
   b. Listen actively.
   c. Touch in a therapeutic manner.
   d. Integrate the support person.

3. a. Auscultation
   b. Continuous electronic fetal monitoring

4. 1:1

5. Count the FHR after uterine contractions and for at least 30 to 60 seconds. This is necessary to evaluate the fetal response to contractions.

6. Count between uterine contractions for 30 to 60 seconds.

7. Take the mother's radial pulse while counting FHR.

8. a. Before artificial rupture of membranes
   b. After artificial rupture of membranes
   c. Before and after ambulating the woman
   d. Before administering medication
   e. After procedures such as catheterizations

9. Explain why the examination is necessary, and ask the woman if you may perform the examination. Wait for her consent. Remain focused on the woman and maintain eye contact.
   a. Explain your findings.
   b. Acknowledge that the examination might be painful.
   c. Pay attention to what the woman says about any pain.
   d. Apologize for causing her any pain.

10. Leopold's maneuvers and FHR assessment

11. 30; 15; 15; 30

12. Lateral (right or left) position

13. Supine hypotensive syndrome (i.e., lowered BP and hypotension)

14. a. Do not leave the mother alone while she is in active labor.
    b. Give frequent mouth care: give ice chips, lubricate lips, and encourage mouth rinses.
    c. Massage abdomen, back, and legs.
    d. Be sure the room is well ventilated.
    e. Control the environment so that quiet, privacy, and appropriate lighting are provided.
    f. Promote participation of a support person.

15. a. Helping the woman feel that she can handle her contractions
    b. Showing her how to breathe or position herself
    c. Anticipating her information needs
    d. Reinforcing information and being concrete

16. 14

17. 8

18. Latent; active

19. Soft, well effaced; 3

20. 1.2; 1.5

21. 13.3; 7.5

22. B. Precipitous labor
    C. Prolonged latent phase
    D. Slow slope (protracted) active phase
    E. Secondary arrest of active phase

23. Emotional support and rest

24. a. Cephalopelvic disproportion
    b. Minor fetal malpresentations
    c. Amniotomy before or at onset of labor
    d. Administration of conduction anesthesia before active labor is well established

25. Cervical dilatation

26. Spontaneous vaginal birth

27. 5; 10

28. Second

29. Faster

30. Twice

31. Less than 1.0; less than 2.0

32. Oxytocin stimulation; forceps delivery

33. 1 hour or more; 1/2 hour or more

34. a. Advanced gestational age
    b. Large babies
    c. Fetal malpositions, such as occiput posterior
    d. Coexistent labor disorders, such as protraction disorders

35. Vaginal examinations must carefully distinguish between true descent of the fetal part and the occurrence of fetal scalp edema or molding of the cranial bones.

36. b. Discontinued

37. Any five of the following:
    a. Hypoxia of the uterine muscle because of diminished blood supply to the uterus during a contraction
    b. Stretching of and pressure on the cervix, vagina, and perineal floor muscles and perineum
    c. Traction on reproductive structures such as the fallopian tubes, ovaries, and uterine ligaments
    d. Pressure on the bladder, urethra, and rectum
    e. Nature of contractions (intensity and duration)
    f. Degree of cervical dilatation and perineal distension
    g. Maternal age, parity, and general health
    h. Fetal size and position (e.g., posterior positions are usually accompanied by intense back pain)
    i. Cultural influences and upbringing
    j. Value system and education level
    k. Anxiety and fear
    l. Lack of knowledge or preparation
    m. Absence of supportive significant person
    n. Lack of motivation

38. Any three of the following:
    a. Acupressure
    b. Heat and cold therapy
    c. Hydrotherapy
    d. Massage
    e. Intradermal injections of sterile water

39. Know the mother's medical and obstetric history; check for allergies. Take vital signs, BP, and FHR readings before administering any medications. Know the status of labor and anticipated delivery at the time medication is given. Consider the mother's request. Be aware of the therapeutic effects, contraindications, and side effects of the drug being given. Use a large-bore (18-gauge) catheter when starting an IV infusion, which permits rapid fluid or blood administration if needed. Consider the mother's weight, the progress of labor, the maturity and size of the fetus, and the dosage of medicine being prepared. Give all IV medications at the beginning of a contraction, when the blood vessels of the uterus and placenta are somewhat constricted. If possible, inject the medicine over a few minutes. Because the medication is concentrated in bolus form, this technique enables a smaller amount of the drug to cross the placenta during the first few minutes of circulation so that the fetus does not receive a large amount of the drug all at once. Aspirate the syringe before giving any medication. Use filters with all IV medications and epidural catheters. Filters help to screen out glass particles and bacteria that are sometimes present in ampules after they have been broken open. Do not give any drug with which you are unfamiliar. Assess pain relief. Allow the mother to assume other optimal positions for fetal rotation.

40. a. Blocked pain pathways according to the gate theory
    b. Release of endogenous endorphins

41. Sensory; motor

42. T10 (thoracic); lumbar; perineal tone

43. The physician and anesthesiologist

44. Any three of the following:
    a. Refusal
    b. Maternal fear
    c. Coagulation defects
    d. Maternal hypotension

45. Because of possible fetal hyperglycemia with subsequent and rebound newborn hypoglycemia

46. The epidural induces vascular vasodilatation with resultant decreased BP. Adequate plasma volume helps offset hypotensive effects.

47. 30 minutes

48. Hypotension

49. a. Place mother in a full lateral position.
    b. Give oxygen.
    c. Give 250 to 500 mL IV bolus non–glucose-balanced saline solution.

50. Any three of the following:
    a. Change in maternal heart rate
    b. Metallic taste
    c. Loss of consciousness
    d. Seizures
    e. Tinnitus
    f. Maternal hypertension

51. a. True

52. b. False

SKILL UNIT 1 | FRIEDMAN GRAPH: PLOTTING AND ANALYSIS

This section details how to plot and analyze dilatation and descent patterns of labor using the Friedman graph. Study this section and then attend a skill practice and demonstration session scheduled with your preceptor. You will need to demonstrate that you can plot various labor patterns and correctly analyze them.

ACTIONS	REMARKS

Prepare the Graph Paper

1. Use basic graph paper. Mark off time in hours, centimeters of dilatation, and fetal station (Fig. 5.11).

    The time is marked in 2-hour intervals on every other grid. Timing starts at the hour labor began.

Graphic recordings of cervical dilatation and fetal descent provide a guide for early detection of abnormal labor.

It is sometimes difficult to assign a definite time to the beginning of labor. It is generally determined from the point at which contractions occur at regular intervals, usually 3 to 5 minutes apart for the multipara. Sometimes it is necessary to assign a time to the beginning of labor in retrospect.

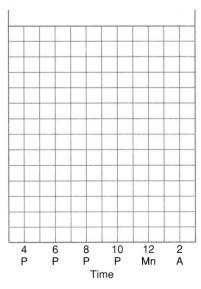

| 4 | 6 | 8 | 10 | 12 | 2 |
| P | P | P | P | Mn | A |

Time

FIGURE 5.11

2. Cervical dilatation is marked on the *left vertical side* of the grid using a key symbol, such as ⊙ (Fig. 5.12).
3. Station of the fetal presenting part is marked on the *right vertical side* of the grid using a key symbol, such as ×.

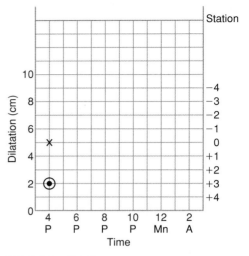

FIGURE 5.12

Plot the Graph

Mrs. Joy's contractions began occurring regularly 5 minutes apart at 12 noon. To prepare and plot the labor graph of Mrs. Joy, a nullipara, the following information is given:

Time	Cervical Dilatation (cm)	Station
12:00 noon	1	−1 to 0
4:00 PM	1	−1 to 0
6:00 PM	2–3	0
9:00 PM	3	0
10:00 PM	4	0 to +1
12:00 midnight	5	0 to +1
2:00 AM	6	0 to +1
3:00 AM	7	+1
4:00 AM	7	+1
4:30 AM	8	+2
5:00 AM	10	+3

4. *Station* at 12 noon is −1 to 0 and is indicated by × (Fig. 5.13).

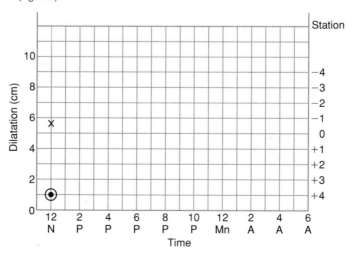

FIGURE 5.13

Dilatation at 12 noon is 1 cm and is shown by ⊙ *Time* labor begins at 12 noon, and 2 hours are marked on every other grid.

5. Mrs. Joy is not examined again until 4 PM and then again at 6 PM. Each finding is plotted and connected by a line (Fig. 5.14).

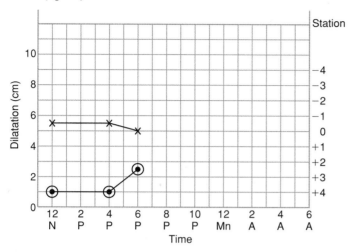

FIGURE 5.14

6. The findings from each vaginal examination are plotted (Fig. 5.15). Although this labor is slightly longer than the average 14 hours for a nullipara, the characteristic phases appear.

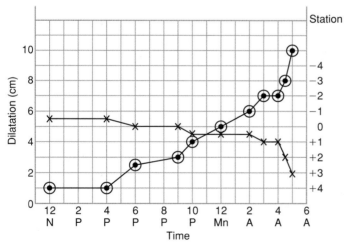

FIGURE 5.15

Latent phase is seen as straight line. If time is counted off to the point of the upward swing of dilatation, the latent phase lasts from 12 noon until 4 PM.

Active phase begins approximately 4 PM and lasts through full dilatation at 5 AM, approximately 13 hours.

Phase of maximum slope of dilatation occurs from 9 PM to 5 AM.

Note that the dilatation and descent lines cross, forming an "X" where the maximum slope begins (Fig. 15.15).

The *deceleration phase,* when dilatation slows, often goes unnoticed and cannot be seen.

The rate of *cervical dilatation* during the active phase can be calculated. At 4 PM, when the active phase begins, Mrs. Joy is dilated 1 cm. At the end of the active phase, 13 hours later, she is dilated 10 cm. She dilated 9 cm in 13 hours, or 9 ÷ 13 = 0.69 cm/hr. Mrs. Joy had an *abnormal protracted active phase.* The nullipara's normal rate of cervical dilatation during the active phase is 1.2 cm or faster.

The *rate of descent* of the presenting part during the active phase is slow as well. The normal descent rate in the nullipara during the active phase is 1 cm/hr or more, and in the multipara, 2 cm/hr or more.

At 4 PM, the station was −1 to 0 and by 5 AM, +3. If −1 is used as the starting station, a total of 4 cm of descent during the active phase is achieved in 13 hours, or 4 ÷ 13 = 0.3 cm/hr. *This is a protracted descent pattern.*

Practice Plotting Labor Patterns

7. Graph the labor data provided for a *nulliparous* patient.

Time	Cervical Dilatation (cm)	Station
1:00 AM	2	−2
6:30 AM	3	−1
7:00 AM	3	0
8:00 AM	7	+1
8:30 AM	9	+2
9:00 AM	10	+3

How would you interpret this labor? Check your answer with the answer key at the end of this Skill Unit.

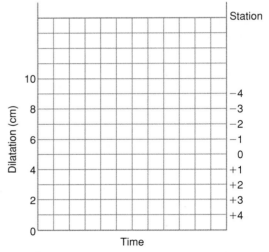

8. Graph the labor data provided for a *multiparous* patient. Contractions became fairly regular at approximately 3 PM.

Time	Cervical Dilatation (cm)	Station
3:00 PM	3	−1
4:00 PM	6	0
5:00 PM	7	0
7:00 PM	7	+1
8:00 PM	7	+1
9:00 PM	8	+2
10:00 PM	10	+3

How would you interpret this labor? Check your answer with the answer key at the end of this Skill Unit.

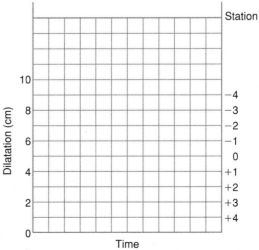

ANSWERS TO SKILL PRACTICE

7. Your graph pattern for the nulliparous patient should appear like Figure 5.16.

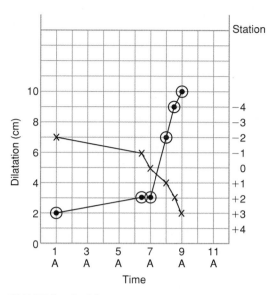

FIGURE 5.16

Interpretation

Assume that labor began at approximately 1 AM. Ordinarily, this is determined at the point when contractions begin to occur regularly. Because the average duration of labor for a nullipara is approximately 14 hours, this 8-hour labor is faster than usual. The *latent phase* occurred from 1 to 7 AM. The *active phase* began at 7 AM with a sharp maximum slope and ended at 9 AM when the patient reached 10 cm. There was no deceleration phase. The rate of cervical dilatation during the active phase was 7 cm in 2 hours, or 3.5 cm per hour. This rate is faster than the average of 1.2 cm per hour for the nullipara.

When looking at the descent pattern, note that the fetus descended during the active phase from 0 station to +3 station in 2 hours, or at a rate of 3 cm in 2 hours or 1.5 cm per hour. This is well within normal limits for the nullipara. A *protracted descent* occurs in the active phase when descent is less than 1 cm per hour in the nullipara.

This labor contained no protractions or arrests. Dilatation and descent occurred more rapidly than the average rates for the nullipara.

8. Your graph pattern of the multiparous patient should appear like Figure 5.17.

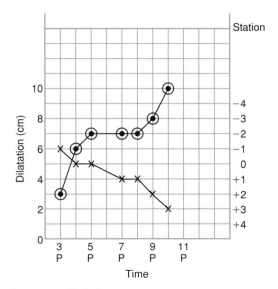

FIGURE 5.17

Interpretation

Assume that labor began at 3 PM. No latent phase was seen. Labor occurred over 7 hours with a cervical dilatation rate of 3 to 10 cm in a 7-hour period, or 7 cm in 7 hours = 1 cm per hour. This is slightly less than the average rate of 1.5 cm per hour for the multipara. Arrest of the active phase began at 7 cm at approximately 5 PM. Arrest is diagnosed when dilatation stops for 2 hours or more, as assessed by two vaginal examinations done 2 hours apart. It occurs more frequently in nulliparas than in multiparas.

Fortunately, this patient went on to dilate at a good rate after 8 PM. Descent of the fetus occurred from −1 station to +3 station in 7 hours. This is 4 cm per 7 hours or 0.57 cm per hour, a much slower rate than the normal 2 cm per hour for the multiparous patient.

You will need to attend a skill session(s) to practice this skill with the help of your preceptor. Mastery of the skill is achieved when you can demonstrate the following:
- Graphing of at least three different labors showing cervical dilatation and descent of the presenting part
- Accurate analysis of the graphed labor patterns

SKILL UNIT 2 | TECHNIQUES FOR BREATHING AND EFFLEURAGE

This section details two breathing techniques and a massage technique called effleurage, which can be taught to the laboring woman and her coach if they have had no childbirth preparation. Study this section and then attend a skill practice and demonstration session scheduled with your preceptor. You will need to demonstrate that you can perform and teach the techniques listed at the end of this section.

ACTIONS	REMARKS
Begin the Breathing Technique	
These techniques are done only during contractions. Rest and sleep between contractions is important. Instruct the laboring woman to do the following:	Every woman beginning labor must be taught simple techniques for coping with labor. The use of a specific breathing pattern during labor contractions has two objectives:
• Assume a comfortable position.	1. Helping the woman to relax by distracting her from the intense contraction sensations, and
• Try to maintain a relaxed state throughout the contraction.	2. Ensuring a steady, adequate intake of oxygen.
• Concentrate on a focal point while doing the breathing (e.g., a pretty picture, a button on someone's shirt).	
• Begin and end each breathing technique with a cleansing breath. This is simply a deep quick breath, like a big sigh. Inhalation is through the nose; exhalation is through slightly pursed lips.	

Slow Chest Breathing (Lamaze Technique: Slow-Paced Breathing)

This technique can be used in early labor and for as long as the mother is comfortable with it. For some women, this may last throughout the entire first stage of labor.
1. Take a cleansing breath as soon the contraction begins.
2. Breathe slowly and deeply in through the nose and out through slightly pursed lips or the nose over the duration of the contraction.
3. Maintain a steady rate of approximately 6 to 9 breaths during a 60-second contraction (the cleansing breaths do not count; Fig. 5.18).

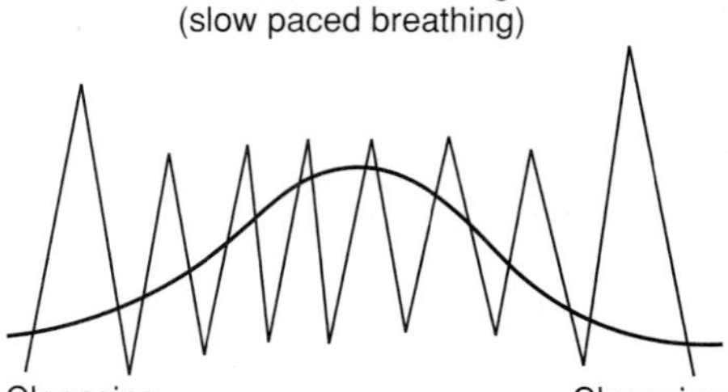

Slow chest breathing
(slow paced breathing)

Cleansing breath   6–9 per minute   Cleansing breath

FIGURE 5.18

4. Use a focal point throughout.

5. Finish the contraction with a cleansing breath.

This technique is suggested for early and active labor up to transition. However, some women use it throughout the entire labor.

In addition, the woman may gradually increase her rate of breathing as labor intensifies. This might work well for her as long as the intensification is not rapid.

Effleurage

This is a light massage over the abdomen with the fingertips. It can be done along with the breathing technique during a contraction.

1. Starting at the pubic bone, move the hands slowly up the sides of the abdomen in a wide circular sweep (Fig. 5.19).
2. During exhalation, move the fingertips down the center of the abdomen.
3. Effleurage can be done with one hand if a side-lying position is assumed.

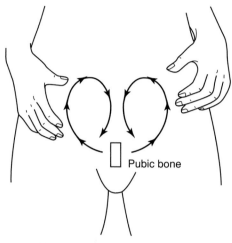

FIGURE 5.19

Effleurage often has a soothing effect and provides a distraction for the mother when she concentrates on a stimulus that is not painful. Coaches can be encouraged to do this for the mother. This technique can be used to help mothers slow their breathing and match the rhythm of effleurage.

Pant–Blow Breathing (Lamaze Technique: Patterned, Paced Breathing)

1. Begin with a cleansing breath.
2. Take four shallow breaths *through the mouth,* making a "hee" or "heh" sound. The exhalation is emphasized to give a sense of rhythm to this breathing.
3. Blow out through the mouth one time at the end of the four shallow breaths (Fig. 5.20). *The blow should be a short puff,* not a prolonged exhalation.
4. Keep an even and steady rhythm. The rate should not exceed 1 breath per second.

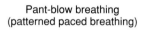

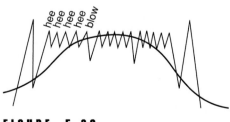

FIGURE 5.20

5. These rhythms can vary from two pants and one blow to three pants and one blow, or even six pants and one blow. Use whatever rhythm feels most comfortable.

6. Take a cleansing breath at the end of the contraction.
7. Effleurage is usually not used with this technique.

This is an effective technique to use during strong contractions and is particularly recommended for transition labor of 7 to 10 cm. However, some women might wish to begin using it earlier, especially those who experience a premature urge to push or those with rapid labor.

You will need to attend a skill session(s) to practice this skill with the help of your preceptor. Mastery of the skill is achieved when you can demonstrate the following:

- Slow chest breathing technique
- Effleurage
- Pant–blow breathing technique

SKILL UNIT 3 | TECHNIQUES FOR SECOND STAGE AND BIRTH

Stage II of labor is a normal physiologic event that is usually defined as the time from complete cervical dilatation to delivery of the fetus. Usually, stage II of labor occurs without intervention. However, many women experience an urge to push or begin spontaneous pushing before full cervical dilatation occurs, so this strict definition may need to be expanded to include these women.

When the pelvic floor is distended by the descending fetal presenting part, stretch receptors activate the release of endogenous oxytocin, resulting in the urge to push. This is called the "Ferguson reflex." It appears that the urge to push is influenced more by fetal station than by cervical dilatation. Women have given birth using a variety of positions for centuries and should be encouraged to use the position(s) of their choosing for stage II, provided they are not contraindicated for medical reasons. Although upright positions may be associated with an increase in blood loss, gravity may increase the pelvic diameter as much as 30% and facilitate descent and rotation, resulting in decreased use of vacuum and forceps and a shorter second stage; painful sensations may be minimized and the incidence of perineal trauma reduced. Maternal satisfaction with the birth experience may be enhanced.[36,37]

Laboring Down

"Laboring down" is a concept and clinical practice that promotes maternal rest and nondirected pushing once 10 cm of cervical dilatation is achieved. Instead of instructing the mother to push immediately upon reaching full dilatation, she is encouraged to rest until involuntary urges are experienced. During the maternal rest period, uterine contractions may facilitate further descent of the fetal head. If an epidural is used, the anesthetic effect may be allowed to taper down so that rectal pressure and the Ferguson reflex are eventually felt.[38,39]

Spontaneous maternal bearing-down efforts are found to be more effective and satisfying, resulting in less maternal fatigue.[40] As long as progress is being made and fetal signs are reassuring, no specific time limits or arbitrary rules related to duration of the second stage are deemed necessary.[38] The practice of "laboring down" is appropriate for women when fetal status is reassuring and there is no need to hasten delivery.

Guidelines for Second Stage

1. Let the mother rest if she does not feel any urge to push as she approaches full dilatation.

> Promote spontaneous pushing.

2. Respond to cues from the mother and support her short pushes if this occurs at approximately 8 or 9 cm of dilatation. Suggestions like "push when you feel the urge" help mothers to begin stage II with minimal coaching.

> Avoid prolonged bearing-down efforts. Encourage 4- to 6-second pushes.

Clinical studies show that when women rely on their own bodies, they tend to push for less than 6 seconds and often take several breaths between pushes. This applies to using breath holding (closed glottis) or short pushes with release of air (open glottis).

3. Encourage pushing from different positions (e.g., side-lying, hands and knees).

NOTE: When the fetal position is posterior, it may be useful to position a mother in alternate positions, such as on hands and knees, to facilitate rotation. By doing so, she can do pelvic rocks during the contraction to provide additional pressure on the heaviest presenting part (the head) to rotate. Other positions such as the lateral position, squatting, or sitting on the birth ball may also assist with rotation. An exaggerated side-lying position may assist with rotation of the presenting part for mothers with epidural anesthesia.[19]

4. Monitor fetal heart tones according to risk status and stage of labor.

5. Keep the mother hydrated, the perineal area clean, and the underpad dry. Perineal care remains an important comfort and hygiene measure.

6. When an epidural is used, the urge to bear down can diminish. More active coaching may be needed and/or the epidural effect allowed to wear off.[41]

   ***NOTE:** Although evidence regarding the benefits of perineal massage is conflicting, some women may receive comfort/benefit from warm compresses to the perineum. Using a mirror to view the perineum and encouraging the mother to touch the fetal head when it is visible at the perineum may promote effective pushing.[42]*

7. When no urge to push occurs after a rest period, the mother can be encouraged to move into an upright position in bed or sitting position. Use of a squat bar may be useful.

8. Keep the mother informed.
   • Let her know when she is being effective in her efforts.
   • Use terminology that she can understand (e.g., not all women understand "station +1").
   • Avoid negative statements (e.g., "That baby's head is way up there!").

9. Tell the mother when you are going to do a vaginal examination. Tell her your findings and avoid talking across the bedside (over the mother) when sharing results of the examination with another caregiver.

10. Avoid raising your voice when supporting a woman during the second stage.

ACTIONS	REMARKS (PICTORIAL)

Positions for Stage II

A woman may choose several positions during stage II, depending on the intensity of contractions, the urge to push, and the length of stage II. Stage II provides an opportunity for support person(s) to assist women as they move closer to birth and need reassurance and sensitivity.

1. **Semisitting**
   Head and shoulders should be elevated at least 30 to 45 inches (Fig. 5.21). The head of the bed can be rolled up. If in the delivery room, use pillows to prop up the mother.

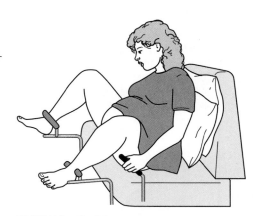

FIGURE 5.21

Mothers may grasp the legs with the hands behind or in front of the knees or have their partners sit behind them and hold their legs (Fig. 5.22).

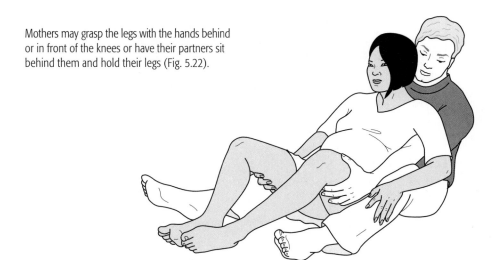

FIGURE 5.22

Flex the thighs on the abdomen by grasping the legs behind the knees, in front of the knees (Fig. 5.23), or at the ankles. Variation: Permit the legs to relax in a frog-leg position with pillows under each knee (Fig. 5.24).

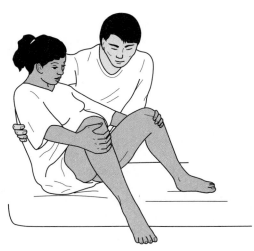

FIGURE 5.23

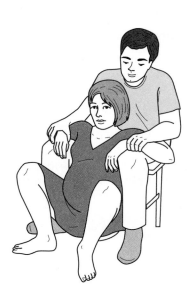

FIGURE 5.24

2. **Squatting**

   The squatting position is extremely effective. Pushing efforts are maximized in this position, and the force of gravity assists the mother's efforts (Fig. 5.25).

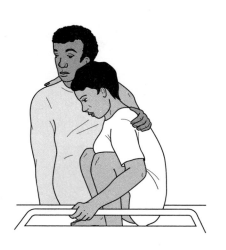

FIGURE 5.25

3. **Side-Lying**

The side-lying position (Fig. 5.26) is useful for women who need to lie on their side for medical reasons or who are experiencing a rapid second stage and benefit from increased spacing of contractions that can occur in a lateral position.

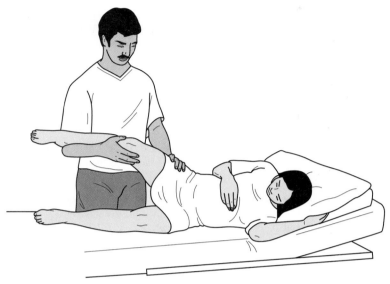

FIGURE 5.26

Technique for Physiologic Pushing (Open Glottis)

Encourage the mother to do the following:
1. Assume the position of choice.
2. Take two cleansing breaths.
3. Take a slow, deep breath in and begin to expel the breath slowly through slightly pursed lips.
4. Exhale slowly over 4 to 6 seconds. Grunting may occur toward the end of the exhalation. This is fine and provides effective effort in pushing. Remember to keep the perineal muscles relaxed.
5. Take a cleansing breath at the end of the contraction and relax.

Any breath-holding technique should be avoided!

Counteracting the Urge to Push

This method can be used before the second stage for intensive pelvic/rectal pressure or during the second stage as the fetal head is crowning. Less intense pushing may facilitate a slow delivery of the head and avoid tears and/or the need for an episiotomy.

Blow out with short, forceful exhalations. An equal amount of air is taken in after each exhalation. Take caution that this is not done too rapidly, causing dizziness and numbness in fingers and lips from hyperventilation. This is sometimes called "feather blowing."

Sometimes the urge to push is truly premature. If the cervix is not approaching 9 or 10 cm, pushing will only tire the mother. To push, the diaphragm is fixed and the breath held. Repeated blowing attempts help to counteract this tendency to push prematurely.

This technique is used only during that part of the contraction where the urge to push is felt.

You will need to attend a skill session(s) to practice this skill with the help of your preceptor. Mastery of the skill is achieved when you can demonstrate the following:
- A variety of positions appropriate for pushing during stage II of labor
- The technique for pushing using breath holding
- The technique for pushing using forceful exhalation
- Breathing to counteract the urge to push

REFERENCES

1. Mackey, M. C. (1998). Women's evaluation of the labor and delivery experience. *Nursing Connections, 11*(3), 19–32.
2. Gagnon, A. J., & Waghorn, K. (1996). Supportive care by maternity nurses: A work sampling study in an intrapartum unit. *Birth, 23*(1), 1–6.
3. Walker, J., Brooksby, A., McInerny, J., & Taylor, A. (1998). Patient perceptions of hospital care: Building confidence, faith and trust. *Journal of Nursing Management, 4,* 193–200.
4. Gennero, S. (1998). The childbirth experience. In Nichols F. H. & Hummenick S. S. (Eds.), *Childbirth education: Practice research and theory* (pp. 52–68). Philadelphia: WB Saunders.
5. Zeidenstein, L. (1998). Birth language: A renewed consciousness [editorial]. *Journal of Nurse-Midwifery, 43*(2), 75–76.
6. Mattson, S. (2000). Providing culturally competent care. *AWHONN Lifelines, 4*(5), 37–39.
7. Willis, W. O. (1999). Culturally competent nursing care during the perinatal period. *Journal of Perinatal and Neonatal Nursing, 13*(3), 45–59.
8. Rostant, D. M., & Cady, R. F. (1999). *AWHONN liability issues in perinatal nursing* (p. 101). Philadelphia: Lippincott Williams & Wilkins.
9. Feinstein, N. F., Sprague, A., & Trepanier, M. J. (2000). *Fetal heart rate auscultation* (p. 22). Washington, DC: The Association of Women's Health, Obstetric and Neonatal Nurses.
10. Friedman, E. A. (1978). *Labor: Clinical evaluation and management* (2nd ed.). New York: Appleton-Century-Crofts.
11. Albers, L. L., Schiff, M., & Gorwoda, J. G. (1996). The length of active labor in normal pregnancies. *Obstetrics and Gynecology, 87*(3), 355–359.
12. Malone, F. D., Geary, M., Chelmow, D., Stronge, J., Boylan, P., & D'Alton, M. E. (1996). Prolonged labor in nulliparas: Lessons from the active management of labor. *Obstetrics and Gynecology, 88*(2), 211–215.
13. Rojansky, N., Tanos, V., Reubinoff, B., Shapira, S., & Weinstein, D. (1977). Effect of epidural analgesia on duration and outcome of induced labor. *International Journal of Gynaecology and Obstetrics, 56*(3), 237–244.
14. Thorp, J. A., & Breedlove, G. (1996). Epidural analgesia in labor: An evaluation of risks and benefits. *Birth, 23*(2), 63–83.
15. Howell, C. J. (2000). Epidural versus non-epidural analgesia for pain relief in labour [Cochrane review]. In: *The Cochrane Library, 2.* Oxford: Update Software.
15a. Bergstrom, L., Roberts, J., Skillman, L., & Seidel, J. (1992). "You'll feel me touching you, sweetie": Vaginal examinations during the second stage of labor. *Birth, 19*(1), 10–18.
16. Holz, K. A. (1994). A practical approach to clients who are survivors of sexual abuse. *Journal of Nurse-Midwifery, 39*(1), 13–18.
17. Rhodes, N., & Hutchinson, S. (1994). Labor experiences of childhood sexual abuse survivors. *Birth, 21*(4), 213–219.
18. Hodnett, E. D. (2000). Caregiver support for women during childbirth (Cochrane review). In *The Cochrane Library, 4.* Oxford: Update Software.
19. Shermer, R. H., & Raines, D. H. (1997). Positioning during the second stage of labor: Moving back to basics. *Journal of Obstetric, Gynecologic, and Neonatal Nursing, 26*(6), 727–734.
20. Simkin, P. (1995). Reducing pain and enhancing progress in labor: A guide to nonpharmacologic methods for maternity caregivers. *Birth, 22*(3), 161–170.
21. Mendelson, C. L. (1946). Aspiration of stomach contents into the lungs during obstetric anesthesia. *American Journal of Obstetrics and Gynecology, 52,* 191–205.
22. American College of Nurse-Midwives (ACNM). (1999). Clinical bulletin No. 3: Intrapartum nutrition. *Journal of Nurse-Midwifery, 44*(2), 124–128.
23. American Society of Anesthesiologists. (1999). *Practice guidelines for obstetrical anesthesia care.* Park Ridge, IL: Author.
24. Sleutel, M., & Golden, S. S. (1999) Fasting in labor: Relic or requirement. *Journal of Obstetric, Gynecologic and Neonatal Nursing, 28*(5), 507–512.
25. Sommer, P. A., Norr, K., & Roberts, J. (2000). Clinical decision making regarding intravenous hydration in normal labor in a birth center setting. *Journal of Midwifery and Women's Health, 45*(2), 114–121.
26. Garite, T. J., Weeks, M. D., & Peters-Phair, K. (2000). A randomized trial on the influence of increased intravenous hydration on the course of nulliparous labor. *American Journal of Obstetrics and Gynecology, 182*(1 part 2), S37.
27. Bowes, W. A., & Thorp, J. M., (2004). Clinical aspects of normal and abnormal labor. In Creasy R. K. & Resnik R. (Eds.), *Maternal-fetal medicine principles and practice* (5th ed., pp. 671–705). Philadelphia: WB Saunders.
28. Doulas of North America (DONA). *What is a doula?* Available at: www.dona.org/faq.html.
29. Simkin, P., & Way, K. (1998). *Doulas of North America position paper: The doula's contribution to modern maternity care.* Available at: www.dona.org/positionpapers.html.
30. Reynolds, J. L. (2000). Sterile water injections relieve back pain of labor. *Birth, 27*(1), 58–60.
31. Bachman, J. A. (2001). Management of discomfort. In Lowdermilk, D. L., Perry, S. E., & Bobak I. M. (Eds.), *Maternity and women's health care* (7th ed., pp. 463–487). St. Louis: Mosby.
32. Martensson, L., & Wallin, G. (1999). Labour pain, treated with cutaneous injections of sterile water: a randomized, controlled

trial. *British Journal of Obstetrics and Gynecology, 106*(7), 633–637.

33. Hansson, B., & Wallin, G. (1990). Parturition pain treated by intracutaneous injections of sterile water. *Pain, 41*(2), 133–138.

34. Association of Women's Health. Obstetric and Neonatal Nursing (AWHONN). (2001). *Evidence-based clinical practice guideline: Nursing care of the woman receiving regional analgesia/anesthesia in labor.* Washington, DC: Author.

35. Taylor, T. (1993). Epidural anesthesia in the maternity patient. *Maternal-Child Nursing Journal, 18*(2), 86–93.

36. AWHONN. (2000). *Evidence-based clinical practice guideline, nursing management of the second stage of labor* (pp. 1–29). Washington, DC: Author.

37. Gupta, J. K., & Nikodem, V. C. (2000). Woman's position during second stage of labour. *Cochrane Database System Review, 2,* CD002006.

38. Roberts, J., & Woolley, D. (1996). A second look at the second stage of labor. *Journal of Obstetric, Gynecologic and Neonatal Nursing, 25*(5), 415–423.

39. Mayberry, L. J., Gennaro, S., Strange, L., Williams, M., & De, A. (1999). Maternal fatigue: Implications of second stage labor nursing care. *Journal of Obstetric, Gynecologic and Neonatal Nursing, 28*(2), 175–181.

40. Sampselle, C. M. (1999). Spontaneous pushing during birth. *Journal of Nurse-Midwifery, 44*(1), 36–39.

41. Mayberry, L. J., Hammer, R., Kelly, C., True-Driver, B., & De, A. (1999). Use of delayed pushing with epidural anesthesia: Findings from a randomized, controlled trial. *Journal of Perinatology 19*(1), 26–30.

42. Albers, L. L., Anderson, D., Cragin, L., Daniels, S. M., Hunter, C., Sedler, K. D., & Teaf, D. (1996). Factors related to perineal trauma in childbirth. *Journal of Nurse-Midwifery, 41*(4), 269–276.

MODULE

6

Intrapartum Fetal Monitoring*

DONNA JEAN RUTH

*This text is based on the module originally written by Meegan D. Page for the 3rd edition of the book. Her contribution is gratefully acknowledged.

Introduction to Fetal Monitoring

Introduction to Fetal Monitoring

▶ **What is fetal monitoring?**

Fetal monitoring consists of assessment tools used to evaluate fetal status both before and during labor. Information related to the fetal heart rate is obtained and evaluated to identify any abnormalities that may affect fetal well being. All laboring patients should have some type of monitoring to assist in identifying potential problems and planning for further care. The monitoring may be done by intermittent auscultation (IA) or by continuous electronic fetal monitoring (EFM).

Historically, monitoring of the fetal heart rate by auscultation has been in existence for over 200 years. The use of the electronic fetal monitor began in the late 1960s. The use of the electronic fetal monitor offered the hope of reduced perinatal morbidity and mortality. Over the last several decades the use of EFM has become common in many labor and delivery units.[1–3] During the 1980s and 1990s, a number of randomized, controlled clinical trials comparing IA with EFM were done and the results found that EFM did not decrease perinatal morbidity and mortality. In fact, the use of EFM was associated with increased cesarean delivery and instrumented vaginal deliveries.[4] Several potential reasons for why EFM failed to live up to its promise include:

- the use of an outcome measure that was not related to variant fetal heart rates.[5]
- the lack of standardized interpretation of fetal heart rate patterns.[5]

- disagreements regarding algorithms for interventions of specific fetal heart rate patterns.[5]
- inconsistent criteria and terminology used to describe fetal status.[6]
- the use of outcome variables for which there were insufficient sample sizes to determine a significant difference between IA and continuous EFM.[6]

Despite the finding that EFM does not offer significant benefits over IA, the use of continuous EFM remains very common in many labor and delivery units. Reasons for this include the fact that many practitioners find it hard to believe that intermittent assessment can be better than continuous recording of the same information.[7] Additionally, managing laboring women without continuous EFM is labor intensive. It is logistically and financially easier to use EFM than to provide one nurse for each laboring mother as is required with IA.[8]

In 1997, the National Institute of Child Health and Development (NICHD) of the National Institutes of Health gathered a panel of experts to look at some of the issues related to EFM. This group of experts proposed detailed, quantitative, and standardized definitions of fetal heart rate patterns.[9] The benefit of using such a system are twofold. First, these standardized definitions will serve as the basis for determining the reliability and validity of EFM in future studies. Additionally, the use of standardized definitions that are mutually agreed upon and used by all providers will enhance communication related to EFM.[10] This module uses the NICHD definitions that have been endorsed for use by both the American College of Obstetricians and Gynecologists (ACOG) and by the Association of Women's Health, Obstetric and Neonatal Nurses (AWHONN).

Ultimately, the decision as to which monitoring method is used should be a joint decision between patients and health care providers. Factors that influence this decision may include clinical situation and risk status, availability of equipment, unit staffing patterns, and knowledge and skill level of staff (in the selected monitoring method). It has been suggested that informed consent be obtained before the initiation of any type of fetal monitoring.[11]

Regardless of which method of monitoring is chosen, each unit should have written policies and guidelines for both IA and EFM that are in accordance with guidelines endorsed by professional organizations such as ACOG and AWHONN. Unit guidelines should clearly list the procedures to be followed when using the chosen monitoring technique, define the standard terminology to be used, and include the required frequency of assessments.[12] See Table 6.1 for the recommended frequency of assessment based on the phase and stage of labor. It is important to note that the recommended frequencies of assessments in latent phase of labor have not been established.

TABLE 6.1	GUIDELINES FOR ASSESSMENT OF FETAL HEART RATE[12]	
Low Risk		
Active phase	q30min	q30min
Second stage	q15min	q15min
High Risk		
Active phase	q15min	q15min
Second stage	q5min	q5min

Intermittent Auscultation

▶ What is intermittent auscultation?

Intermittent auscultation involves monitoring the fetal heart, through the use of either a fetoscope or Doppler, at specified intervals. IA allows for assessment of the fetal heart rate and also allows for greater maternal mobility. Therefore, IA may be much more comfortable for the laboring woman. IA has been found to be a safe and reasonable option for monitoring when performed by a practitioner who:

- Is experienced in the labor and delivery setting and competent in the use of IA
- Can discern, by auditory means, significant changes in the fetal heart rate (FHR)
- Is practiced in palpating uterine contraction and relaxation
- Is capable of initiating appropriate interventions when indicated[13]

(Review Module 4, Skill Unit 3 for a detailed discussion of how to perform IA)

► What can be assessed with intermittent auscultation?

In general, baseline rate and baseline rhythm can both be evaluated using IA. Baseline rate is assessed between contractions and during periods when the fetus is not active. In addition, baseline variations such as tachycardia (rate greater than 160 bpm) and bradycardia (rate less than 110 bpm) can be readily identified. If tachycardia or bradycardia is suspected, then more frequent assessments may be warranted to determine if a baseline change has occurred or if the increase or decrease in rate was temporary. Auscultation can also be used to detect abrupt changes in the FHR, both increases and decreases, if performed between contractions. The practitioner cannot distinguish the pattern of decelerations with auscultation alone.

Baseline rhythm (regular or irregular) can also be assessed with auscultation. Actual heart sounds can be heard using a stethoscope, fetoscope, or Pinnard device. Doppler can be used to identify baseline rhythm, but the sound produced by the Doppler device is a representation of and not the actual heart sounds. Auscultation may be used to verify the presence of a dysrhymia.[13] If an irregular rhythm is heard, alternative methods of assessment, such as ultrasound or fetal echocardiogram may be indicated to determine the type of dysrhythmia present, even though most dysrhythmias are benign and do not require further intervention.

Maternal and fetal heart rate can be differentiated using auscultation.[14–16] Palpation of the maternal pulse, while simultaneously auscultating the fetal heart rate, can be used to validate EFM findings.

► How is intermittent auscultation performed?

Follow these steps when performing IA (review Module 4, Skill Unit 3):
1. Explain the procedure to the laboring woman.
2. Determine fetal position using Leopold's maneuvers.
3. Palpate the uterus to assess for contractions and resting tone. This helps the practitioner to assess the FHR response to uterine activity.
3. Apply the fetoscope or Doppler device on the maternal abdomen over where the fetal back is located and where fetal heart sound will be heard best.
4. Auscultate the FHR between contractions, beginning immediately after the end of the contraction and listening for at least 30- to 60-second intervals to determine the fetal heart rate and rhythm and response to uterine activity.
5. Count the maternal pulse to differentiate between fetal and maternal heart rates.
6. Document your assessments.
7. Share your findings with the laboring woman.

Assessment of fetal heart rate should be performed **before:**
- Induction or augmentation of labor with oxytocin
- Initiation of anesthesia
- Administration of medications
- Ambulation
- Artificial rupture of membranes (amniotomy)
- Transfer or discharge

Assessment of the FHR should be performed **after:**
- Rupture of membranes (either spontaneous or artificial)
- Ambulation
- Vaginal examination
- Excessive uterine activity
- Change in oxytocin dosage
- Change in analgesia and anesthesia dosing
- On admission to the labor and delivery unit

Advantages/Benefits of Auscultation

Patient comfort—the woman may be up and about and may move easily in bed. Sometimes, the abdominal area and the lower back of a laboring woman are extremely sensitive. Belts and other equipment can cause irritation and discomfort and interfere with her ability to concentrate and relax.

Facilitation of ambulation—Ambulation often contributes to greater patient comfort and perhaps more rapid progress in labor. Freedom of movement (i.e., the ability to walk and stand) is supported by IA.

Requirement of caregiver to be at the bedside—This provides many benefits, such as comfort, support, and encouragement. A critical component of intrapartum care is support in labor. With IA, close, frequent contact between the patient and caregiver occurs.

Fewer interventions—Women who desire an atmosphere in which birth is viewed as a normal, natural event might prefer this method of monitoring.

Neonatal outcomes—Outcomes are comparable to those with EFM.

Lower cesarean birth rates—Cesarean birth rates are lower in comparison with EFM.

Technology—The technology used for IA allows for FHR assessments to be done even if the laboring woman is immersed in water.

Equipment—Equipment required for IA is less costly than that necessary for EFM.

No automatic paper is generated—No documentation is automatically produced with IA, in contrast with EFM, which produces a fetal monitor strip in which differences of opinion in interpretation of strips are often the source of debate in legal situations.

Disadvantages/Limitations of Auscultation

Practitioner skilled in auscultation—Auscultation skills are required to perform assessments. Competency in the performance of auscultation should be demonstrated before the provision of care.

Nurse-to-patient ratio of 1:1—The nurse-to-patient ratio must be 1:1. Nursing shortages and unit staffing patterns sometimes preclude this capability.

Invasion of personal space—Because very frequent, close personal contact is required to provide adequate assessment through IA, some women feel as if their personal space is being invaded.

Rapid heart rates (greater than 160 bpm)—These may be difficult to accurately count.

Inability to evaluate certain aspects of the FHR—Examples include variability and the ability to discern the type of deceleration heard.

Physical limitations of equipment—Maternal size (obesity), position, and polyhydramnios may interfere with the practitioner's ability to adequately assess the FHR by IA.

Documentation of FHR by Auscultation

Documentation of the findings must be done with each assessment. Each entry should include baseline rate and rhythm, the presence or absence of gradual or abrupt changes (increases or decreases) in the baseline rate. Other information that should be documented includes any change in patient status, all nursing interventions and patient responses, and any communication that occurs with health care providers.

Electronic Fetal Monitoring

▶ What is electronic fetal monitoring?

Electronic fetal monitoring (EFM) is an electronic method of providing a continuous visual record of the FHR and obtaining information about the laboring woman's uterine activity (Fig. 6.1). This information, which is recorded on *graph paper,* allows an ongoing minute-to-minute assessment of fetal well-being during labor. It also provides a permanent record for the medical chart. It is useful for screening or surveillance, but it is not intended as a diagnostic tool. There is general agreement that a normal, reactive EFM tracing is highly predictive of a well-oxygenated fetus. However, a nonreassuring tracing does not necessarily mean that the fetus is in trouble. In fact, the predictive value of a nonreassuring strip for poor fetal outcome is not strong.[9,17]

NOTE: At the onset of EFM, validation of the equipment should be performed by auscultation of the FHTs with a nonmechanical means such as the fetoscope and by testing of the internal circuitry by pushing the "test" button on the monitor and examining the test lines on the graph paper.[14]

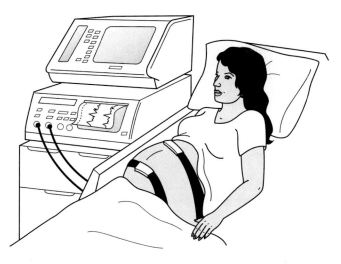

FIGURE 6.1 The electronic fetal monitor.

▶ What are indications for electronic fetal monitoring?

Many factors may influence the decision to use continuous EFM during labor. *Antepartal risk factors* are those that the woman either enters her pregnancy with (such as chronic hypertension or diabetes) or develops during the antepartum period. Other indications for monitoring may not appear until the woman is already in labor, these factors are considered *intrapartal risk factors*. IA may not be appropriate for all labors.[18] Most of the clinical trials that compared IA with EFM excluded those women at risk for adverse outcomes, so more studies are needed to assess whether IA and EFM are equivalent in the high risk patient.[18] Many factors may influence the decision to use continuous EFM during labor.

Antepartal Risk Factors Include the Following:

Hypertension
Pregnancy-induced hypertension
Diabetes mellitus
Chronic renal disease
Congenital or rheumatic heart disease
Sickle cell disease
Rh isoimmunization
Preterm infants (37 weeks' gestation)
Age factors (younger than 15 years of age or older than 35)

Postmature infants (more than 42 weeks' gestation)
Multiple gestations
Grand multiparity
Anemia
Intrauterine growth restriction (IUGR) or small for gestational age (SGA)
Genital tract disorders/anomalies
Poor obstetric history

Intrapartal Risk Factors Include the Following:

Prolonged rupture of membranes
Premature rupture of membranes
Failure to progress in labor or dysfunctional labor
Meconium-stained amniotic fluid
Abnormal FHR detected during auscultation
Abnormal presentations

Pitocin augmentation/induction
Premature labor
Possible cephalopelvic disproportion (CPD)
Previous cesarean section in labor
Hypotensive episodes in labor
Bleeding disorders—abruptio placentae, placenta previa

▶ Should the electronic fetal monitor be used routinely during labor?

Whether the fetal monitor should be used routinely during labor is controversial. Its use can limit mobility, interfere with the use of comfort techniques, and potentially contribute to the mother having negative feelings about the experience. Some women might believe that "something is wrong" even if an explanation is given about the routine use of the equipment. This is especially true for women whose pregnancies are low risk. Although EFM is an excellent means of predicting fetal well-being, it is much less accurate in predicting poor neonatal outcomes. In fact, routine use of EFM has contributed to the increased rates of cesarean sections and operative vaginal deliveries.[4] Ominous-looking FHR patterns may indicate a much worse picture of fetal condition than actually exists.[19] Another consideration is the change in the level of support of the laboring woman, which is widely recognized to play an extremely important role in labor. When EFM replaces IA, the nurse's focus shifts from the patient to machinery, reducing both physical contact and the level of intimacy between the laboring woman and caregiver. Research has shown that many factors are positively affected by the personal support given to the patient during labor, such as shorter labors, decreased need for oxytocin augmentation, fewer epidurals, and fewer operative deliveries both vaginal and cesarean section.[17,19] There is no doubt that support during labor has a significantly positive effect on both fetal and maternal well-being.

▶ How is the electronic monitor used to determine fetal well-being?

The electronic fetal monitor may be used in three different ways:

1. *External fetal monitoring* is also called *indirect fetal monitoring,* or *noninvasive fetal monitoring.* This method involves the use of an ultrasonic transducer to monitor the fetal heart while the contraction pattern is monitored with a tocodynamometer. Both are placed on the woman's abdomen and are secured in place by elastic belts (Fig. 6.2).

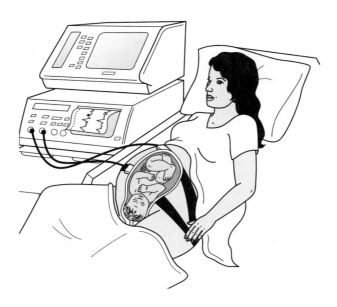

FIGURE 6.2 The external fetal monitor.

The *ultrasonic transducer,* more commonly known as an *ultrasound,* or *Doppler,* transmits high-frequency sound waves that detect movement within the fetal heart. The signal, which is similar to sonar used in submarines, is reflected back from moving structures and is recognized by the machine as a cardiac event. The movement detected is both ventricular contraction and the actual opening and closing of valves within the heart.

The *tocodynamometer,* more commonly known as a *toco,* provides information about the laboring woman's contraction pattern by detecting changes in the shape of the abdominal wall directly over the uterine fundus. These changes in shape are the direct result of the effects of the uterine contraction on the maternal abdomen.

As a result of the manner in which the data are obtained, these methods are referred to as *indirect* or external monitoring because the techniques are performed external to the fetus and uterus. Because the vagina, cervix, and uterus are not invaded when applying an external monitor, the technique is also termed *noninvasive.*

2. *Internal fetal monitoring* is also called *direct fetal monitoring,* or *invasive fetal monitoring.* With this method, the FHR is monitored by the use of a *helix/fetal spiral electrode* (*FSE*), which is applied directly to the presenting part of the fetus. The laboring

woman's contraction pattern is monitored by the use of an *intrauterine pressure catheter (IUPC),* which is inserted vaginally directly into the uterine cavity through the cervix (Fig. 6.3). Information is obtained *internally* from the laboring woman by the use of *invasive* methods, which *directly* monitor the fetus and the uterine activity.

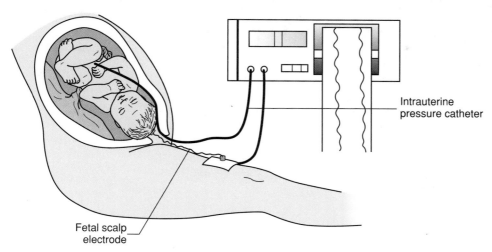

Intrauterine pressure catheter

Fetal scalp electrode

FIGURE 6.3 The internal fetal monitor.

3. *A combination of internal and external fetal monitoring* can be done. The FHR is monitored internally by the use of an *electrode,* and the laboring woman's contraction pattern is monitored externally by the use of a tocodynamometer (Fig. 6.4). However, the opposite may also be done. The FHR can be monitored externally by the use of an *ultrasound transducer,* and the laboring woman's contraction pattern can be monitored internally by the use of an *IUPC* (Fig. 6.5).

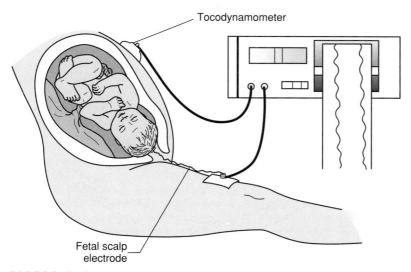

Tocodynamometer

Fetal scalp electrode

FIGURE 6.4 Combination of external and internal monitoring. The tocodynamometer and helix/fetal scalp electrode are used together.

▶ How does the fetal spiral electrode work?

The electrode tracks the FHR by picking up *R waves* on the fetal electrocardiogram (ECG). The interval between each R wave is measured and processed by internal circuitry and calculated to a rate in beats per minute (bpm); the result is printed on graph paper (Fig. 6.6).

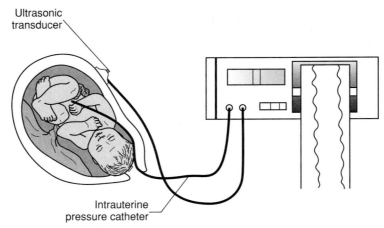

FIGURE 6.5   Combination of external and internal monitoring. The ultrasonic transducer and intrauterine pressure catheter are used together.

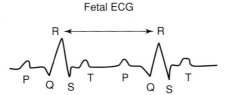

FIGURE 6.6   Determination of fetal heart rate with the use of a fetal scalp electrode.

During a vaginal examination, the examiner attaches the *spiral electrode,* or *fetal scalp electrode (FSE)*, directly to the presenting part of the fetus (Figs. 6.7 and 6.8).

The FSE is then secured to a leg plate/pad that has been attached to the woman's thigh and connected to the monitor. FSE may be used when continuous information is required and a satisfactory tracing cannot be accomplished with external monitoring. *Use of the FSE should be avoided in women who are HIV positive, have chronic or active hepatitis, have herpes simplex virus, or have a known and untreated sexually transmitted disease.*[6,20]

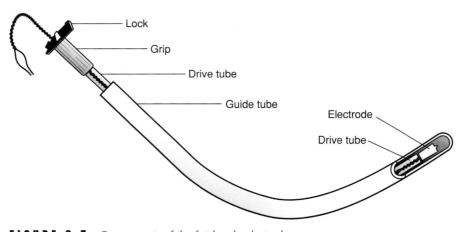

FIGURE 6.7   Components of the fetal scalp electrode.

▶ **How is the intrauterine pressure catheter used?**

During a vaginal examination, the intrauterine pressure catheter (IUPC), often called a *pressure catheter,* is inserted through the cervix into the uterus beside the presenting part of the fetus (Fig. 6.9). The catheter is used to measure the pressure in the uterus between contractions (uterine resting tone) and the amount of pressure generated during contractions.

The IUPC is used to determine the actual pressure inside the uterus during contractions (Fig. 6.10). Changes in pressure at the tip of the catheter (inside the uterus) are transmitted

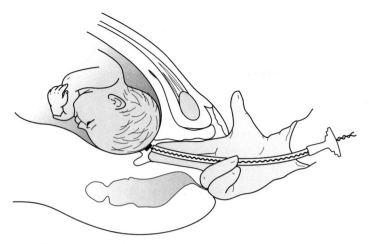

FIGURE 6.8 Application of a fetal scalp electrode to the presenting part of the fetus.

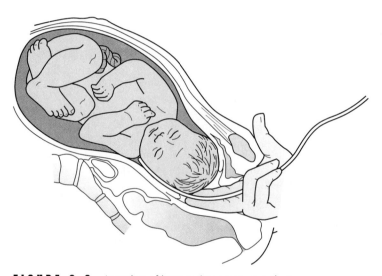

FIGURE 6.9 Insertion of intrauterine pressure catheter.

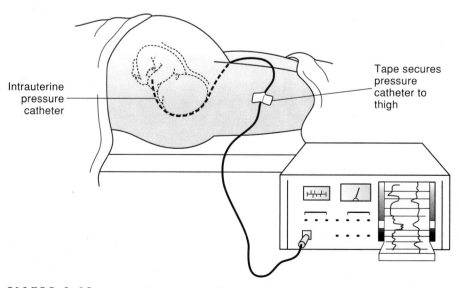

Intrauterine pressure catheter

Tape secures pressure catheter to thigh

FIGURE 6.10 Intrauterine pressure catheter.

along the catheter. These pressure changes are caused by the force or intensity of the contractions and are translated into an electrical signal that is converted to a pressure reading expressed in millimeters of mercury (mmHg). This measurement is then displayed on the monitor.

When clinical situations arise that require more precise measurements of uterine activity, an internal pressure catheter may be the preferred method of uterine monitoring. Examples of these situations *might* include the following:

- Induction/augmentation of labor with oxytocin
- Labor dystocias, including prolonged labors and arrested labors
- Suspected CPD
- The need to accurately define relationships between decelerations and contractions

Points to remember when using the IUPC include the following:

- When the IUPC is inserted, if resistance is met, the catheter must be slightly withdrawn and repositioned before insertion is attempted again.
- IUPCs must be "zeroed" to calibrate the instrumentation. (*Zeroing* means that the instrument is calibrated to air pressure so that pressure changes in the uterus can be compared against a baseline measurement.) Transducer-tipped catheters should be zeroed before insertion. Some of these catheters can be recalibrated after insertion. Water-filled catheters have the transducer outside the uterus and can be calibrated after insertion.

Advantages of External/Indirect Fetal Monitoring[16,21,22]

- The patient can be monitored at any time, regardless of whether the cervix has dilated or the membranes have ruptured.
- It is convenient.
- It is noninvasive (does not involve a vaginal examination).
- Minimal training is required to apply the external monitor.
- A continuous tracing allows health care providers to continuously assess uterine activity and fetal responses.
- Certain aspects of contractions are more easily assessed. Determination of frequency and duration of contractions is simpler and can be accomplished at a glance. Intensity, however, might not be fully appreciated with a tocodynamometer.
- Characteristic of the FHR, such as accelerations, decelerations, tachycardia, and bradycardia, can be easily identified.
- No fetal or maternal complications are associated with the use of an external fetal monitor.
- Relationships between some FHR patterns (decelerations) can be assessed earlier and more definitively than with auscultation alone.

Disadvantages of External/Indirect Fetal Monitoring[16,21,22]

- It maybe difficult to obtain a satisfactory tracing if the patient is obese or is moving and active during labor.
- The ultrasonic transducer may pick up and trace extraneous sounds. For example, the maternal pulse might be detected by the Doppler and traced instead of the FHR, causing the heart rate to appear bradycardic. Other sounds, such as bowel sounds, hiccups, fetal movement, or the rumpling of sheets, might also be detected by the machine, which can result in an inaccurate tracing. The tracing that these sounds cause is called "artifact"
- The FHR can temporarily be lost or difficult to follow continuously if the fetus is active or changes position.
- Sometimes the FHR is detected only when the laboring woman stays in one position. Not only is this uncomfortable for the woman, but some positions (e.g., the woman lying on her back) can adversely affect blood flow to mother and fetus.
- The contraction tracing *does not* give information about the quality or intensity of the contractions. Therefore, the fundus *must* be palpated during a contraction to determine contraction intensity.
- The baseline tone (resting tone between contractions) of the uterus cannot be determined so palpation *must* be done to assess uterine resting tone when external monitoring is used.

Advantages of Internal/Direct Monitoring[16,21,22]

- Internal monitoring allows the patient greater freedom of movement (e.g., standing, pushing alternatives, and sitting in a chair) without compromising the quality of the monitor tracing.
- Internal monitoring accurately measures the intensity of the contractions. Uterine pressure is measured in millimeters of mercury (mmHg).
- Internal monitoring measures the pressure of the uterus between contractions (baseline tone, resting tone).
- Internal monitoring is not usually affected by artifact.

Disadvantages of Internal/Direct Fetal Monitoring[17,22]

- Partial dilatation of the cervix and ruptured membranes are required for application of the FSE and IUPC.
- Application of the FSE and IUPC requires skill.
- Insertion of the IUPC is often uncomfortable for the woman because considerable pressure and cervical manipulation might be necessary for proper placement.
- Materials used must be sterile, and most are disposable, resulting in increased costs.
- Increased the risk of infection
- If the presenting part of the fetus is at a low pelvic station, it might not be possible to insert the IUPC.

Interpreting the Fetal Monitor Strip

▶ **How do you read a fetal monitor strip?**

Figure 6.11 illustrates monitor paper. This graph is marked in specific time intervals of 3 minutes to allow easy readability (paper speed should be set at 3 cm per minute). Each box represents 10 seconds.

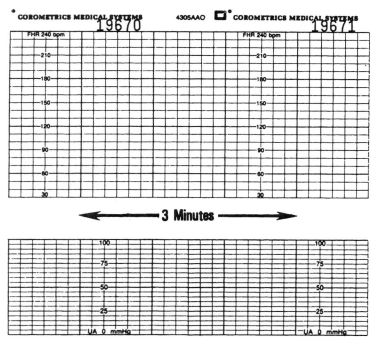

FIGURE 6.11 Graph monitor paper.

The numbers at the top of the strip in Figure 6.12 are reference numbers. They are sequential and appear at set intervals. On newer machines, these numbers may be located just above the uterine graph. These numbers assist in charting specific events by identifying their location on

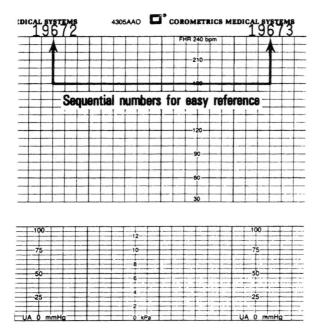

Sequential numbers for easy reference

FIGURE 6.12 Sequential numbering of strip graph paper.

the strip. They also assist in chronologically reassembling a strip that has been separated for closer inspection.

The strip is divided into two sections: an upper and a lower section (Fig. 6.13). The *upper* section is the portion of the graph on which the *FHR* appears. The *lower* section is the portion of the graph on which the *contractions,* or uterine activity, are recorded.

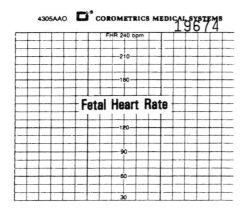

Fetal Heart Rate

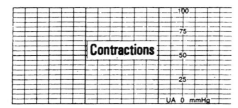

Contractions

FIGURE 6.13 Strip graph monitor paper provides sections for tracing fetal heart rate and uterine activity.

The FHR (upper) section of the graph is divided vertically by dark lines, with five light, vertical lines between every two dark lines (Fig. 6.14). The time interval between any two dark lines is *1 minute;* therefore, the time interval between any two light lines is *10 seconds.* This section of the graph is also divided *horizontally* by dark lines, with two light, horizontal lines between every two darker lines (Fig. 6.15). There is a horizontal column of numbers ranging from 30 to 240. These are reference numbers used in determining the FHR and are labeled *bpm*. The distance between any two darker lines is *30 bpm;* therefore, the distance between any two lighter lines is *10 bpm.*

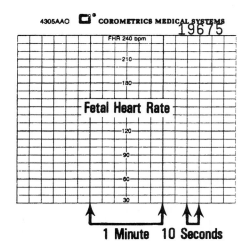

FIGURE 6.14 Division of fetal heart rate section into time intervals.

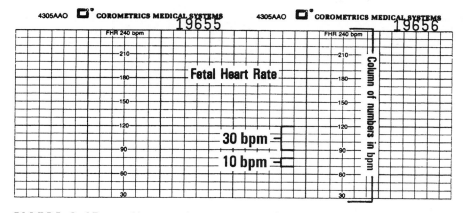

FIGURE 6.15 Fetal heart rate beats per minute (*bpm*).

The contraction or uterine activity (lower) section of the graph is divided *vertically* by dark lines, with five light, vertical lines between every two dark lines (Fig. 6.16). The time interval between any two dark lines is *1 minute;* therefore, the time interval between any two light lines is *10 seconds.*

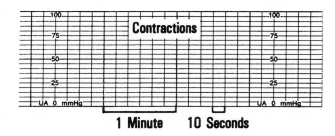

FIGURE 6.16 Division of uterine activity section into time intervals.

This portion of the graph is also divided *horizontally* by dark lines, with five light, horizontal lines between every two dark lines (Fig. 6.17). The numbers ranging from 0 to 100 in the horizontal column are reference numbers that are used to determine the intensity of contractions when a pressure catheter is used; they are labeled *mmHg*. The abbreviation *UA* stands for "uterine activity."

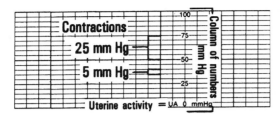

FIGURE 6.17 Uterine activity in millimeters of mercury (mmHg).

Fetal Heart Rate

▶ What is the baseline fetal heart rate, and how is it determined?

The baseline FHR is determined *between* contractions. It is defined (using the NICHD definitions) as the approximate mean FHR rounded to increments of 5 bpm during a 10-minute segment, excluding:

1. Periodic and episodic changes
2. Periods of marked variability
3. Segments of the baseline that differ by more than 25 bpm

In the 10-minute segment, the minimum baseline duration must be at least 2 minutes (Fig. 6.18). If you have less than 2 minutes of a baseline rate, the baseline is considered indeterminate. With this definition, the baseline rate is charted as one number representing the mean rate over the 10-minute period. It is not charted as a range.

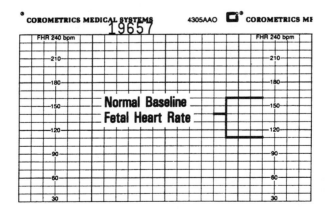

FIGURE 6.18 Normal baseline fetal heart rate.

On the strip in Figure 6.19, look at the FHR occurring between contractions. The baseline FHR is 155 bpm (this number represents the mean, rounded to the closest 5 bpm).

Characteristics of the Baseline Fetal Heart Rate

- Normal fetal heart baseline in a term or postterm fetus: 110 to 160 bpm
- Does not include periodic or episodic changes
- Decreases as the fetal nervous system matures and the parasympathetic nervous system becomes more dominant
- Is determined between contractions

In the absence of nonreassuring elements, a fetal heart baseline of 100 to 110 bpm is also usually considered normal.

Uterine Activity

▶ How are contractions assessed?

Uterine activity can be assessed by palpation, external tocodynamometer, or IUPC. The following parameters should be included in a complete assessment of uterine activity. These parameters are frequency, duration, baseline uterine tone, and contraction intensity. The type of information obtained depends on the type of monitoring method selected. Remember to use a 10-minute window when assessing the uterine activity (see Fig. 6.19).

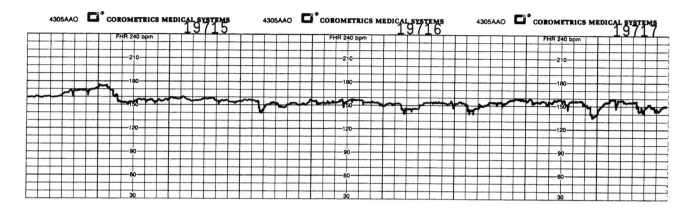

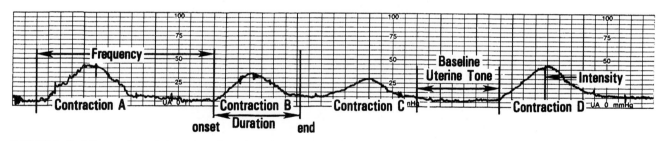

FIGURE 6.19 Pertinent information about the contraction pattern.

- **Frequency**—Frequency is the length of time from the beginning of one contraction to the beginning of the next contraction. In this strip, the contractions are occurring approximately every 2 minutes. *Normally, contractions should not occur more frequently than every 1½ to 2½ minutes.* Frequency is reported in a range because contractions are seldom uniform in frequency.

- **Duration**—Duration is the interval of time between the beginning (onset) and the end (offset) of the contraction. For *contraction B* on the strip graph in Figure 6.19, the duration is approximately 70 to 80 seconds. *Normally, a contraction should last no longer than 90 seconds.* (Uteroplacental blood flow decreases dramatically during the contraction, resulting in a reduction of available oxygen for the fetus. Contractions that last longer than 90 seconds might affect fetal oxygenation and reserve.) Contraction duration is also recorded in a range because duration is usually different from one contraction to the next.

- **Baseline uterine tone**—*Baseline uterine tone* (tone, tonus, baseline tone) is the (amount of tone, or) degree of muscular tension, and is assessed *between* contractions. *Normally, baseline uterine tone is 5 to 15 mmHg.* When palpation is used to assess uterine resting tone it should be described as either relaxed or not relaxed. If an IUPC is in place, the resting tone is described in terms of mmHg. A uterus that is not relaxed or has a persistently elevated uterine tone is abnormal and may represent a significant decrease in placental perfusion and fetal oxygenation. **Never accept as normal a uterine tone of greater than 30 mmHg.** If an IUPC is in place, it should be recalibrated and the resting tone assessed and verified with palpation. Blood flow to the placenta at this level of tension is significantly decreased (approximately 30% to 40%). A uterine pressure of 40 mmHg results in the complete cessation of blood flow through the uterus to the placenta. Increased tone can also indicate complications such as abruptio placentae or uterine hyperstimulation. The use of oxytocin for induction/augmentation can also increase baseline uterine tone. Baseline tone is determined by identifying the numerical range of uterine pressure between contractions. It is reported and documented as a range. Baseline tone can change between each contraction. In Figure 6.19, the baseline uterine tone is 5 to 10 mmHg.

- If the catheter reveals a baseline tone of 0 mmHg or a negative number, the system should be recalibrated according to manufacturer's specifications. A tone of 0 mmHg or less may be an indication of a malfunction in the system. When the system is not functioning as expected, one of the following situations may have occurred and needs to be corrected.
- The catheter may not be attached securely to the monitor. The internal pressure system should be checked to ensure proper attachment of all parts.
- The catheter may have curled on itself during insertion, with the tip coming near or out of the cervix in the vagina.
- The catheter may not have been accurately calibrated or zeroed before or after insertion.
- The catheter might be wedged against the uterine wall. Gently withdraw the catheter slightly to release any wedging.
- The catheter might have migrated from the uterine cavity into the vagina. The primary care provider should be notified so that a sterile vaginal examination can be performed to verify placement and/or to replace the catheter. Make no attempt to reinsert the catheter.
- **Intensity**—Intensity may be determined by palpation or by IUPC. If palpation is the method of assessment the contractions are described as mild, moderate, or strong. If an IUPC is in place, intensity is measured in mmHg. The intensity is calculated by subtracting the baseline tone from the peak pressure of the contraction. For *contraction A* in Figure 6.19, the contraction intensity is 40 mmHg. The strength of a mild contraction is approximately 15 to 30 mmHg, the strength of a moderate contraction is approximately 30 to 50 mmHg, and the strength of a strong contraction is 50 to 75 mmHg (Figs. 6.20 and 6.21).

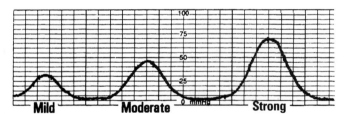

FIGURE 6.20 Contraction intensity.

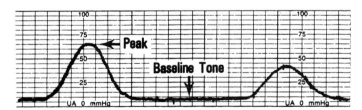

FIGURE 6.21 Determination of contraction intensity.

In Figures 6.22 and 6.23, notice the difference in appearance of the contraction curve using an external and internal monitor. The contractions are actually much stronger when internal monitoring is instituted than they appear in the external tracing.

An obese or multiparous patient with lax abdominal muscle tone and/or increased layers of tissue between the tocodynamometer and the abdominal muscles might be experiencing strong contractions that can appear mild when external monitoring is used. Conversely, a thin or nulliparous patient with good abdominal muscle tone may experience mild contractions, which, when monitored externally, appear strong. Remember that the external tocodynamometer is registering *only* changes in abdominal shape dependent on abdominal muscle tone as the fundus contracts. **When using a tocodynamometer, contraction intensity must be assessed by palpation.**

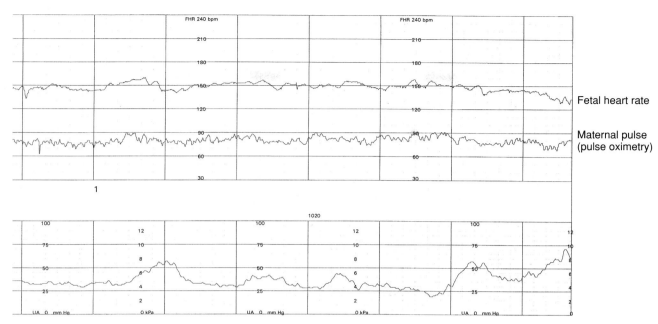

FIGURE 6.22 External (toco) contraction monitoring.

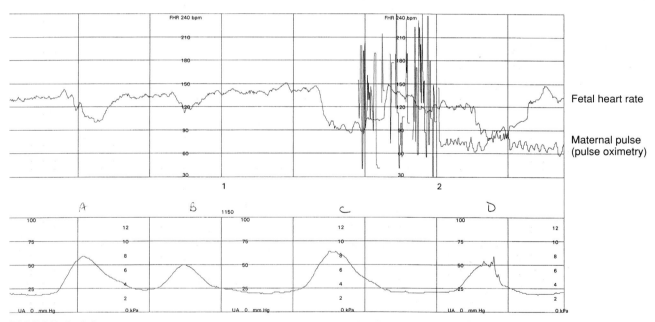

FIGURE 6.23 Internal (IUPC) contraction monitoring and FSE. Note the difference in the clarity of the contraction pattern with the IUPC as opposed to the contraction pattern in Fig. 6.22 using the toco.

To review terms associated with contraction pattern description of a normal contraction pattern, see Figure 6.24.

The uterine activity on the strip in Figure 6.25 should be interpreted as follows:

Interval (frequency)	Approximately 2 to 3 minutes
Duration	60 to 90 seconds
Tonus	10 mmHg
Intensity	40 to 60 mmHg

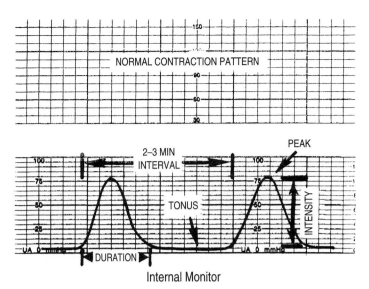

FIGURE 6.24 Normal contraction pattern.

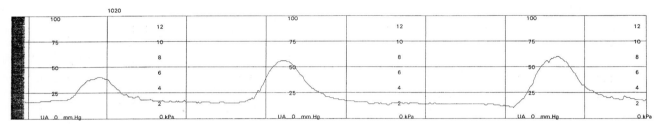

FIGURE 6.25 Internal contraction monitoring.

▶ How is contraction intensity documented during external monitoring?

Manual assessment of uterine contractions and baseline tone must be performed if the external mode of monitoring is used. This assessment is accomplished by palpating the fundus with the fingertips. The strength of the contraction is measured at its most intense point. In general, if the fundus is easily indented with the tips of the fingers, the contraction is considered "mild." If more pressure is needed to indent the fundus, the contraction is "moderate." The contraction is "strong" if the fundus cannot be indented at the contraction peak. **When contraction strength exceeds 40 mmHg, the uterine wall becomes difficult to depress with the fingertips.**

▶ How is uterine tone measured during external monitoring?

Manual assessment of the uterine tone is also an important consideration in external monitoring. The fingertips are sensitive to pressures beginning at approximately 15 mmHg so baseline tones above this level can be identified and appropriate action can be taken.

▶ When is labor adequate?

The simplest way to know that a contraction pattern is effective is to see progress in labor (the cervix dilates and the presenting part of the fetus descends further into the pelvis). Regardless of the characteristics of the contractions, if progress continues, labor is adequate.

If cervical dilatation is not progressing at the expected rate, another method of uterine monitoring using an IUPC may be employed to assess adequacy of labor. When contractions do not produce progression of labor, adequacy of the contraction pattern can be evaluated by a measurement standard called *Montevideo units* (*MVUs*). MVUs are calculated by identifying the peak pressure of each contraction (mmHg) in a 10-minute section (window) of the strip. All peak contraction pressures are added together. The baseline tone is determined by adding together the resting tone of the uterus between each contraction in the same 10-minute window. The final step is to subtract the sum of the baseline tone from the sum of the peak contraction intensity.

In simpler terms, the formula is as follows: sum of contraction intensities (in a 10-minute strip) minus the sum of baseline tone (in a 10-minute window) is a figure reported in Montevideo units.

MVUs may be calculated in a slightly different way by multiplying the average intensity by the contraction frequency in 10 minutes minus tone. Although other units of measurement exist, the most common measurement for quantification of uterine activity is MVUs.

MVU guidelines are as follows:

- Less than 150 MVUs indicates that the contraction pattern might be inadequate to affect labor progress.
- From 180 to 250 MVUs is usually sufficient to affect normal progress in labor.
- More than 300 MVUs indicates increased uterine activity; assessment of the fetal heart rate to this level of activity should be carefully monitored and assessed. If oxytocin is infusing, the dose may need to be decreased or discontinued.

PRACTICE/REVIEW QUESTIONS

After reviewing Part 1, answer the following questions.

1. List at least 10 risk conditions that may indicate a need for increased fetal surveillance in labor.

   a. _____

   b. _____

   c. _____

   d. _____

   e. _____

   f. _____

   g. _____

   h. _____

   i. _____

   j. _____

2. What is the normal FHR range in the term fetus?

   _____

3. Describe the parameters of IA for low-risk women and women with risk factors:

   Low-risk women: _____

   Women with risk factors: _____

4. Describe the advantages and disadvantages of IA.

   _____

   _____

   _____

   _____

5. What is recommended before beginning EFM with regard to validating the machine?

   _____

6. Clinically, what might indicate the need for internal monitoring?

   _____

   _____

   _____

7. What unit is used to measure uterine pressure with an IUPC? _____

8. List three disadvantages of the external fetal monitor.

   a. _____

   b. _____

   c. _____

9. Which of the following are advantages of external fetal monitoring?

   a. The mother may lie in any comfortable position.

   b. There are no fetal complications associated with its use.

   c. All necessary information can be obtained.

   d. Minimal training is necessary for application of equipment.

10. Define *uterine hypertonus.*

    _____

11. List three disadvantages of the internal fetal monitor.

    a. _____

    b. _____

    c. _____

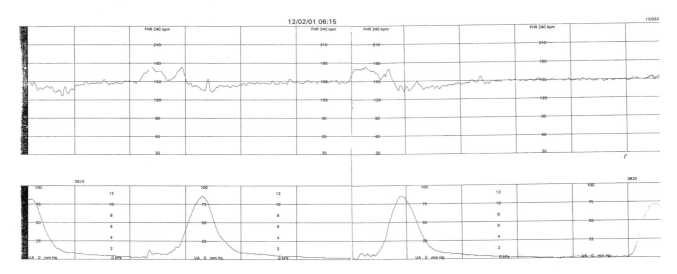

12. Study the strip above and then answer the following questions. This tracing was taken using internal fetal monitoring. The patient was receiving oxytocin (Pitocin).

   a. What is the baseline FHR? _____

      Is it in the normal range? _____

   b. What is the frequency of the contractions?
      _____

      Is it in the normal range? _____

   c. What is the duration of the contractions?
      _____

      Is it in the normal range? _____

   d. What is the baseline uterine tone? _____

      Is it in the normal range? _____

   e. What is the intensity of the contractions?
      _____

   f. Are these contractions mild, moderate, or strong?
      _____

13. How is the baseline FHR determined?

   _____

   _____

   _____

14. The tocodynamometer measures contraction duration, frequency, and intensity.

   a. True

   b. False

15. What uterine pressure is considered abnormal as a baseline tone? _____

16. What are Montevideo units, and how are they calculated?

   _____

   _____

   _____

PRACTICE/REVIEW ANSWER KEY

1. Any 10 of the following:
   a. Hypertension
   b. Pregnancy-induced hypertension
   c. Diabetes mellitus
   d. Chronic renal disease
   e. Congenital or rheumatic heart disease
   f. Sickle cell disease
   g. Rh isoimmunization
   h. Preterm infants (less than 37 weeks' gestation)
   i. Postmature infants (more than 42 weeks' gestation)
   j. Multiple gestations
   k. Grand multiparity
   l. Anemia
   m. Intrauterine growth-restricted infants or small-for-gestational-age infants
   n. Genital tract disorders/anomalies
   o. Poor obstetric history
   p. Age factors (younger than 15 years or older than 35 years of age)
   q. Prolonged rupture of membranes
   r. Premature rupture of membranes
   s. Bleeding disorders—abruptio placentae, placenta previa
   t. Premature labor
   u. Previous cesarean section in labor
   v. Hypotensive episodes in labor

2. 110 to 160 bpm

3. *Low-risk women:* FHTs obtained every 30 minutes during active labor and every 15 minutes during second stage. FHTs assessed during a contraction and for 30 seconds after its end.
   Women with risk factors: FHTs obtained every 15 minutes during active labor and every 5 minutes during the second stage. FHTs are assessed during a contraction and for 30 seconds after it is over.

4. *Advantages of IA:* Patient comfort; allows ambulation, which assists in labor progression; provides a more natural experience.
   Disadvantages of IA: A 1:1 nurse:patient ratio is needed; nurses must have extensive experience with auscultation to pick up subtle changes in the FHR; human error in counting the heart rate can be made; maternal movement might make it difficult to locate and follow the heart rate during contractions; it might take longer to detect subtle or early changes in the FHR.

5. Auscultation of FHR with a fetoscope and the pressing of the "test" button to check the internal circuitry of the monitor.

6. The presence of risk factors either antepartal or intrapartal might show the need for closer surveillance of the fetus by internal monitoring. Labors that do not progress at the expected rate might require assessment of contraction strength to help identify the cause of the delay.

7. Millimeters of mercury (mmHg)

8. Any three of the following:
   a. It is often difficult to obtain a readable tracing if the patient is obese or is active during labor.
   b. The ultrasonic transducer might pick up and trace artifacts.
   c. The FHR might be lost if the fetus is active or changes position. Sometimes, the FHR is picked up only when the laboring woman is on her back—this is not the preferred position for labor, and the woman might experience backache from continually lying on her back.
   d. The heart rate tracing does *not* give information about FHR variability.
   e. The contraction tracing does *not* give information about the quality or intensity of the contractions; therefore, the fundus *must* be palpated during a contraction to determine intensity.
   f. The baseline tone of the uterus cannot be determined.

9. b and d

10. Resting tone greater than 30 mmHg

11. Any three of the following:
    a. It requires partial dilatation of the cervix and ruptured membranes for application of the FSE and IUPC.
    b. It requires a skilled examiner to apply the FSE and pressure catheter.
    c. Insertion of the IUPC is often uncomfortable for the patient because much pressure and cervical manipulation might be necessary.
    d. It requires sterile, disposable equipment.
    e. If the presenting part of the fetus is at a low station, it might not be possible to insert the IUPC.
    f. Maternal and/or fetal morbidity is associated with the FSE and the pressure catheter.

12. a. 150 bpm, yes
    b. Every $3\frac{1}{2}$ to $4\frac{1}{2}$ minutes; yes
    c. 50 to 80 seconds; yes
    d. Approximately 2 to 5 mmHg; yes
    e. 70 to 80 mmHg; strong

13. Baseline FHR is determined by assessing a 10-minute FHR strip between contractions. It is reported as a mean rounded to the closest 5 bpm and should not include any periodic changes (accelerations or decelerations).

14. b, False

15. More than 30 mmHg

16. The MVU is a standard of measurement used to denote the strength and adequacy of the contraction pattern. It is calculated by the following method: sum of contraction intensities (in a 10-minute strip) minus the sum of baseline tone (in a 10-minute window) reported as Montevideo units.

2

Fetal Heart Rate Variability

Objectives

Objectives

After you complete Part 2 of this module, you should be able to:

1. Outline the regulatory factors of the fetal heart
2. Describe fetal heart rate variability
3. Explain the characteristics and significance related to changes in variability
4. Identify appropriate interventions for nonreassuring variability and describe the rationale for these interventions

Key Terms

When you have completed Part 2 of this module, you should be able to recall the meaning of the following terms as they relate to FHR. You should also be able to use the terms when consulting with other health professionals. The terms are defined in this portion of the module or in the glossary at the end of this book.

absent variability	minimal variability
baroreceptors	moderate variability
baseline variability	parasympathetic nervous system
chemoreceptors	pH
fetal reserve	sympathetic nervous system
marked variability	variability

Overview of Fetal Heart Rate Variability

▶ How is the fetal heart regulated?

The fetal heart is influenced by many factors, but it is primarily regulated by the autonomic nervous system (the parasympathetic and sympathetic branches), chemoreceptors, and baroreceptors.

▶ What are the effects of the autonomic nervous system on fetal heart rate?

The effect of the autonomic nervous system on the fetal heart rate depends on which of its branches is stimulated at a particular time. The two parts of the autonomic nervous system are the parasympathetic branch and the sympathetic branch. Their characteristics and effects are outlined in Display 6.1.

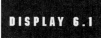

DISPLAY 6.1 CHARACTERISTICS OF THE PARASYMPATHETIC NERVOUS SYSTEM AND SYMPATHETIC NERVOUS SYSTEM

PARASYMPATHETIC NERVOUS SYSTEM (PSNS)

- It is the cardiodecelerator, slowing heart rate.
- Its influence on the FHR increases as gestation progresses. This means that, as gestational age increases, the FHR gradually decreases. The parasympathetic branch is not fully mature until relatively late in gestation at approximately 28 to 32 completed weeks' gestation. As a result of the late maturity of the PSNS, extremely premature infants (less than 20 weeks) can have a higher-than-normal heart rates.
- It is the primary factor that influences short-term variability.
- It is extremely sensitive to decreased levels of oxygen and lowered pH. *pH* is a measurement of acidity or alkalinity. A low pH indicates acidity, and high pH indicates alkalinity.

SYMPATHETIC NERVOUS SYSTEM

- It is the cardioaccelerator. It increases heart rate, cardiac output, and myocardial contractility.
- Its primary influence is on long-term variability.
- It matures earlier in gestation and therefore has more of an impact on FHR before 32 weeks' gestation.

► How do baroreceptors and chemoreceptors affect fetal heart rate?

Baroreceptors are located in the carotid arch and the aortic sinus. Cells in these areas are sensitive to the stretching of surrounding tissue (changes in arterial wall diameter) caused by increased or decreased blood pressure. When fetal blood pressure increases, it is sensed by the baroreceptors, which transmit the message to the brainstem, where the parasympathetic nervous system is stimulated to decrease or increase the fetal blood pressure.

Chemoreceptors are located in the aortic and carotid bodies and in the medulla oblongata. They are sensitive to changes in oxygen, carbon dioxide, and pH of fetal blood. Reduction in blood oxygen and pH and/or increases in CO_2 are recognized by the chemoreceptors. This causes an initial increase in heart rate in an attempt to increase circulation and thereby increase oxygen levels and stabilize pH. Prolonged stimulation of the chemoreceptors, along with hypoxia of the cardiac muscle, eventually results in a decrease in heart rate to bradycardic levels. *This drop can be gradual or it may be sudden.*

► What is fetal heart rate variability?

FHR variability represents the normal changes and fluctuations in the FHR and should be assessed between contractions and not include periodic or episodic changes. Variability is an important component of the baseline. The NICHD defines variability as follows:[9]
- fluctuations in the baseline FHR of two cycles per minute or greater
- these fluctuations are irregular in amplitude and frequency
- they are visually quantified as the amplitude of the peak to trough in beats per minute

It is important to note that in the NICHD report they did not distinguish between short-term and long-term variability, because clinically they are assessed as a unit, and instead used the term "baseline variability" to reflect this component of the fetal heart rate.[9]

Baseline variability may be assessed using external monitors. In the past, the older monitors used technology that greatly exaggerated variability, so much so that variability could only be assessed if a fetal scalp electrode was placed to measure the *r* to *r* intervals. With advances in Doppler technology, newer monitors are able to record the FHR with external devices that are able to represent the true variability.[6] With these newer monitors, the difference between the variability recorded with the external device and the FSE is minimal.

► What causes variability, and why is it important?

- Variability represents the balance and interplay of a normal sympathetic and parasympathetic relationship. Largely controlled by the autonomic nervous system, it indicates intact central nervous system (CNS) function and is the most important factor in characterizing the FHR.

Moderate variability indicates that the CNS of the fetus is well developed, well perfused, and well oxygenated. Moderate variability reflects adequate cerebral perfusion more than any other component of the FHR.[15] The presence of moderate variability is considered a reassuring finding and does not require any intervention other than continued surveillance.

- Variability is sensitive to hypoxia and decreased pH. The usual fetal heart response to hypoxia and decreased pH is a decrease in variability. Decreased variability occurs because of the fetus' limited ability to compensate for reduced oxygenation. The effect of oxygen deprivation is a decrease in the number of impulses from the cerebral cortex. The reduction of impulses results in decreased variability.
- *Variability represents a mature, intact nervous pathway through the brain, vagus nerve, and cardiac conduction system. It is believed to be the most significant indicator of fetal well-being. Variability also indirectly reflects fetal reserve.*
- Variability can be influenced by drugs, hormonal regulation, fetal sleep–wake states, oxygenation, hemodynamic changes, and abnormalities of the CNS (a fetus with anencephaly or hydrocephaly may exhibit absent or minimal variability). *Variability is an important marker for fetal acid-base balance.*

▶ What is fetal reserve?

The fetus uses a certain amount of oxygen to carry out basic metabolic functions. Normally, more oxygen is delivered to the fetus, by way of the placenta, than is required to meet these basic needs. The difference between the oxygen supplied and the oxygen required or consumed equals the *fetal reserve*. If there is only enough oxygen available to meet minimal needs, reserve quickly disappears. Fetal reserve illustrates fetal ability to deal with stress related to reduced oxygen levels in the tissues (hypoxia).

$$O_2 \text{ delivery} - O_2 \text{ required} = \text{Fetal } O_2 \text{ reserve}$$

Classifications of Variability

There are four classifications of baseline variability. They are:

Absent—amplitude of fluctuations is undetectable to the eye (Fig. 6.26). Absent variability appears as a flat line on the fetal monitor tracing. Absent variability may be seen when the level of hypoxia causes a loss of the normal regulatory mechanisms of the CNS and

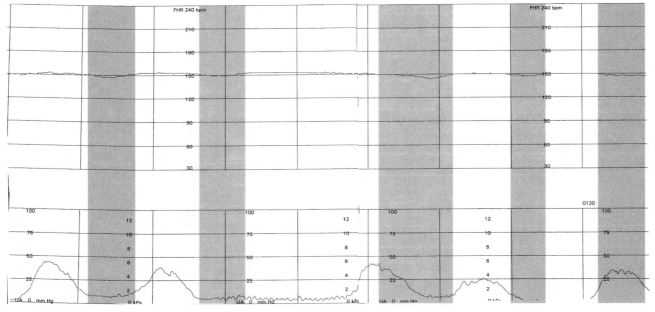

FIGURE 6.26 Absent variability.

direct myocardial depression. *It is an ominous sign that always requires attention from the provider.*

Minimal—amplitude range is greater than undetectable but less than 5 bpm (Fig. 6.27). Minimal variability may be related to premature gestation, administration of narcotics or other CNS depressants, and fetal sleep cycles. Minimal variability alone is usually not related to fetal acidosis.[23] Minimal variability that is accompanied by late or variable deceleration is a nonreassuring finding and requires intervention. *Loss of variability, in the presence of other periodic patterns during labor, is the most sensitive indicator of metabolic acidemia in the fetus.*[24] When minimal variability is noted it is important to watch for the return of moderate variability, which is a reassuring finding. It is also important to watch for the development of absent variability and late or variable decelerations, which are nonreassuring findings and require immediate intervention.

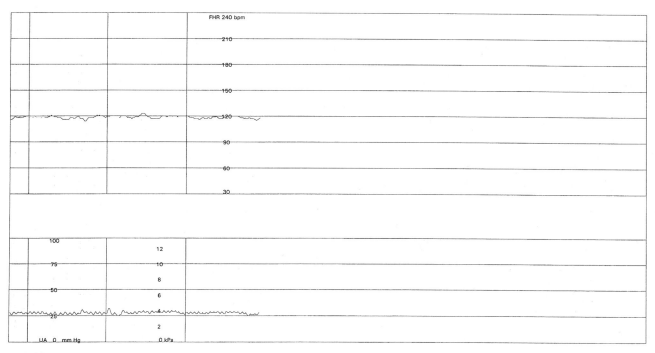

FIGURE 6.27 Minimal variability.

Moderate—amplitude range is 6 to 25 bpm (Fig. 6.28). The presence of moderate variability indicates that the fetus is well developed, well perfused, and well oxygenated. Moderate variability reflects adequate cerebral perfusion more that any other component of the FHR.[15] The presence of moderate variability is considered a reassuring finding and does not requires any interventions other than continued surveillance.

Marked—amplitude range is greater than 25 bpm (Fig. 6.29). Marked variability is usually observed in the intrapartum period, most often in the second stage of labor. Periods of marked variability generally do not persist and are not associated with severe or progressive hypoxia.[25]

NOTE: The use of alternative adjectives to describe variability should be discouraged as these alternative descriptors (e.g., good, average, and normal) may have different meaning for different providers and can lead to miscommunication and the potential for delay in treatment.

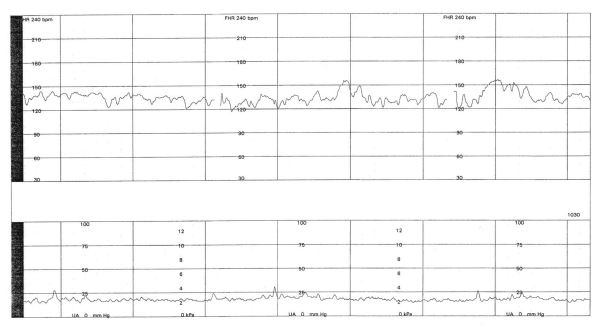

FIGURE 6.28 Moderate variability.

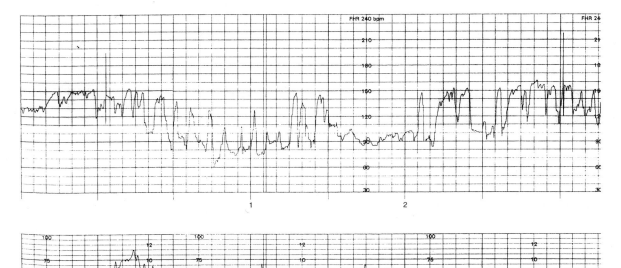

FHR = 120–155

FIGURE 6.29 Marked variability, also known as saltatory pattern. (Reprinted with permission from Menihan, C. A., & Zottoli, E. K. [2001]. *Electronic fetal monitoring: Concepts and applications.* Philadelphia: Lippincott Williams & Wilkins.)

Decreased and Increased Variability

Causes of Decreased Variability

It may be cause for concern if the fetus develops minimal (below 5 bpm) or absent (undetectable fluctuations) variability. There are many causes of decreased variability and the development of decreased variability should be assessed within the context of the total clinical picture in order to determine its meaning.[21] Causes of decreased variability include:

- **Hypoxia/acidosis**—this is the most worrisome cause. It is important to review the strip for the presence or absence of decelerations when decreased variability is noted. It is unlikely that the decreased variability is due to CNS depression unless decelerations are present.[20,23]

NOTE: The exception to this may be the fetus who presents with minimal/absent variability without decelerations. In this scenario, an hypoxic insult before admission cannot be ruled out.[20]

- **Drugs/medications**—CNS depressants such as narcotics, barbiturates, sedatives, tranquilizers, alcohol, magnesium sulfate, and anesthetic agents can all cause decreased variability. The effect on the fetus is generally temporary. The provider should monitor closely for the return of moderate variability.
- **Fetal sleep**—Decreased variability can occur during fetal sleep; however, fetal sleep is a transient state. Fetal sleep cycles last approximately 20 to 40 minutes. When the sleep cycle is over, moderate variability returns.
- **Congenital anomalies**—particularly anomalies that affect the CNS or a defect in the fetal cardiac conduction system such as heart block.
- **Extreme prematurity**—this is related to immaturity in the parasympathetic branch of the CNS. As the fetus matures, variability increases. It is important to remember that once a fetus has exhibited moderate variability, it should be expected to continue.[21]
- **Fetal tachycardia and other dysrhythmias**—with increased heart rate, cardiac control mechanisms may be affected.

Interventions for Decreased Variability

All interventions are aimed at increasing oxygen delivery to the fetus.

Decreased variability might be an indication of fetal stress, unless another cause can be identified as a potential factor in its appearance. It is especially worrisome when seen in conjunction with late, prolonged, or recurrent variable decelerations. Interventions are aimed at correcting the cause when known and increasing oxygen delivery to the fetus.

Interventions consist of the following:

Assessment of maternal vital signs—if the woman is either hypotensive or hypertensive, this may decrease perfusion to the placenta.

Lateral positioning—this maximizes blood flow to the placenta. Lateral positioning displaces the gravid uterus to the side, releasing compression on the vena cava and aorta, allowing for increased blood flow back to the heart and increased maternal cardiac output

Administer oxygen at 10 to 12 L per minute face mask. This optimizes the O_2 saturation in the woman's blood so that more oxygen is available to the fetus.

Discontinue/decrease oxytocin infusions—decreasing or discontinuing oxytocin alleviates the stress of uterine contractions.

Fetal scalp stimulation—fetal scalp stimulation may be done to elicit accelerations, which is a reassuring response.

Notify provider—notify provider of the interventions initiated and the fetal response. It may be necessary to request a bedside evaluation of the tracing especially with tracings that have absent variability.

Document—documents all interventions, fetal responses, and any communication with the provider, in the medical record.

Causes of Increased Variability

- **Increased fetal movement**—Greater oxygen demands and increased catecholamines for an extremely active fetus produce this variability change. When fetal activity returns to more moderate levels, moderate variability usually returns if this is the causal factor.
- **Hypoxia**—Variability is affected by a surge of catecholamines during stress (hypoxic episode). The fetus has some reserves at this point and is attempting to compensate somewhat for the insult. If the hypoxia is prolonged, variability decreases.
- **Vaginal examinations**—Stimulation of the fetal presenting part can elicit a catecholamine surge, causing increased variability. Excessively vigorous stimulation can cause a vagal response, resulting in a decreased FHR.
- **Second stage/pushing**—This is because of the reduced availability of oxygen with maternal breath holding. This is especially true when the closed glottis technique is used. Open glottis techniques should be encouraged.

PRACTICE/REVIEW QUESTIONS

After reviewing Part 2, answer the following questions.

1. FHR variability is defined as _____.

2. On the strips that follow, evaluate the baseline variability.

Strip A	Strip B

Strip A _____

Strip B _____

3. How should decreased variability in FHR be treated?

a. _____

b. _____

c. _____

d. _____

e. _____

f. _____

g. _____

4. List at least three possible causes for decreased variability and at least three possible causes of marked variability.

Decreased:

a. _____

b. _____

c. _____

Increased:

a. _____

b. _____

c. _____

5. Identify the branch of the autonomic nervous system (parasympathetic = P; sympathetic = S) that is responsible for the following:

a. _____ Cardioaccelerator

b. _____ Slows the heart rate

c. _____ Sensitive to low O_2 levels and low pH

d. _____ Matures earlier in gestation

6. _____ are located in aortic sinus and carotid arch and are sensitive to blood pressure changes.

7. _____ are located in the aortic and carotid bodies and medulla and are sensitive to oxygen and carbon dioxide content and pH of the blood.

8. _____ is a marker for acid-base balance.

9. What does *fetal reserve* mean?

_____

PRACTICE/REVIEW ANSWER KEY

1. The normal changes and fluctuations in the FHR over time

2. Strip A—moderate variability
   Strip B—minimal variability

3. a. Try to identify cause (medication?); check temperature.
   b. Begin oxygen therapy by face mask at 10 to 12 L per minute.
   c. Put the patient in the lateral position.
   d. Notify primary care provider.
   e. Chart time of occurrence, treatment, notification of primary care provider, and any associated factors such as decelerations or the presence of meconium.
   f. Attempt fetal stimulation.
   g. Ensure maternal hydration by giving a bolus of IV fluids.

4. Decreased (any three of the following):
   a. Hypoxia/acidosis
   b. Drugs
   c. Fetal sleep
   d. Congenital anomalies
   e. Extreme prematurity
   f. Fetal tachycardia and other dysrhythmias

   Increased (any three of the following):
   a. Increased fetal movement
   b. Hypoxia
   c. Vaginal examinations
   d. Second stage/pushing

5. a. S
   b. P
   c. P
   d. S

6. Baroreceptors

7. Chemoreceptors

8. Variability

9. The difference between the oxygen supplied and the oxygen required or consumed equals the fetal reserve.

Fetal Heart Rate Baseline, Periodic, and Nonperiodic Patterns

As you complete Part 3 of this module, you will learn:
1. To identify and name fetal heart rate baseline patterns
2. Causes of abnormal baseline fetal heart rate patterns
3. Nursing interventions appropriate for abnormal baseline changes
4. Effects of uterine contractions on fetal heart rate
5. To identify periodic patterns and explain the physiologic basis of each pattern
6. Characteristics of accelerations and their importance related to fetal well-being
7. Characteristics of early, variable, late, and prolonged decelerations
8. Interventions appropriate in the treatment of late, variable, and prolonged decelerations

When you have completed Part 3 of this module, you should be able to recall the meaning of the following terms. You should also be able to use the terms when consulting with other health professionals. The terms are defined in this portion of the module or in the glossary at the end of this book.

early decelerations

episodic heart rate changes

fetal accelerations

fetal bradycardia

fetal tachycardia

late decelerations

periodic heart rate changes

prolonged decelerations

sinusoidal pattern

uteroplacental insufficiency

variable decelerations

Characteristics of the Baseline Fetal Heart Rate

Fetal heart rate interpretation involves assessment and interpretation of the following parameters. These are baseline rate, baseline variability, presence of accelerations, presence of any periodic or episodic decelerations and changes in the fetal heart rate patterns over time.[9] It is important that any provider who is responsible for assessment and interpretation of fetal monitor tracings is properly educated, uses nationally standardized terminology in both written and verbal communication, and understands the technology used for fetal monitoring and its limitations.

Baseline Fetal Heart Rate

Baseline fetal heart rates will be one of the following:
Normal rate—between 110 and 160 bpm
Tachycardia—rate greater than 160 bpm
Bradycardia—rate less than 110 bpm
Sinusoidal—baseline rate is characterized by a smooth, undulating, wave-like pattern

Periodic and Episodic Changes

Periodic patterns are those that occur in response to a uterine contraction. Episodic patterns are those that occur randomly and are not associated with uterine contractions. Periodic and episodic changes include:

- accelerations
- early decelerations
- late decelerations
- variable decelerations
- prolonged decelerations

As labor progresses, regular assessments of the fetal heart rate should be done. These assessments help the provider to identify changes in the FHR, develop a plan of care, and initiate interventions in a timely manner.

Fetal Tachycardia

▶ What is fetal tachycardia, and what causes it?

Fetal tachycardia is an increase in the baseline FHR above 160 bpm for 10 minutes or longer (Fig. 6.30). It is important, when following baseline rates, that the providers pay attention to trends. A rising baseline, even when it is still within the normal range, may be an early sign of decreased oxygenation. Fetal tachycardia is associated with decreased variability when the FHR is especially rapid. It represents an increase in sympathetic tone and a decrease in parasympathetic tone.

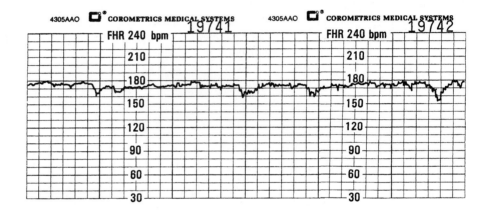
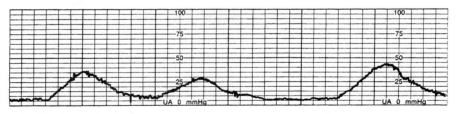

FIGURE 6.30   Fetal tachycardia.

Causes

- **Fetal hypoxia**—Tachycardia is often an *early* sign of hypoxia. The fetus attempts to increase heart rate to compensate for a decrease in oxygen supply.
- **Infection**—May be maternal infection, fetal infection or both.
- **Prolonged fetal activity or stimulation.**
- **Drugs**—Parasympatholytic drugs such as *atropine* and *scopolamine* block the parasympathetic nervous system, resulting in an increase in heart rate. Illicit drugs such as methamphetamine, cocaine, and PCP can also increase the heart rate. Drugs used to prevent or stop premature labor, such as *terbutaline* (β-adrenergics), have a stimulating effect on the fetal heart, which increases the rate.

- **Maternal anxiety**—During periods of maternal stress and anxiety, *epinephrine* is released into the mother's circulation. Small amounts of this epinephrine cross the placenta, resulting in an increase in FHR. The heart rate increase is usually only slight.
- **Maternal temperature elevation**—This is the most common cause of fetal tachycardia. During periods of maternal hyperthermia, both the mother's and the fetus' metabolism are elevated. The pH decreases as a result of lactic acid formation, and oxygen demands are increased. This, in turn, causes chemoreceptor stimulation and increased activity of the sympathetic nervous system. The effect of this process is to increase heart rate. Tachycardia can be an early sign of an intrauterine infection (chorioamnionitis), especially in the presence of decreased variability. Prolonged rupture of membranes can lead to uterine and/or fetal infection and temperature elevation.
- **Fetal anemia**—Reduced oxygen-carrying capacity of the fetal blood, resulting from anemia (decreased hemoglobin), can result in tachycardia. Causal factors for anemia might be related to placental abnormalities, such as partial abruption or previa and twin-to-twin transfusion.
- **Fetal cardiac tachyrhythmia**—This generally occurs intermittently, and most often is identified as supraventricular tachycardia (SVT) and atrial flutter. Cardiac rates of greater than 200 are almost always a result of a dysrhythmia.
- **Maternal hyperthyroidism**—Just as a patient with hyperthyroidism often exhibits an increased pulse rate, so does her fetus. Long-acting thyroid-stimulating hormones cross the placenta and stimulate the fetal thyroid, causing an elevated FHR.
- **Idiopathic causes**—Occasionally in some fetuses the tachycardia has no identifiable cause. Perhaps in these fetuses, the sympathetic nervous system becomes dominant in its regulatory action over the fetal heart.

Interventions

The treatment of fetal tachycardia is aimed at correcting the specific cause when known:

Assess the maternal temperature—this may help to identify an infectious cause.

Lateral positioning—this displaces the gravid uterus off the vena cava and aorta, which increases maternal cardiac output and placental perfusion.

Administration of an IV fluid bolus—administration of IV fluid enhances hydration and improves blood flow to the uterus. The usual bolus is 500 mL of a non–glucose-containing solution.

Validate the fetal heart rate—with a fetoscope. With some tachycardias, the monitor cannot count the rate accurately and it "halves" the rate. This may be suspected when the audible rates sound very rapid and the printed rate is much less. Verify the rate with an alternative method such as a fetoscope. Ultrasound examination can also be done to verify the rate.

Review the recent medication history—including over-the-counter medications and supplements that may increase heart rate.

NOTE: *If the tachycardia is accompanied by absent/minimal variability, late decelerations, or variable decelerations, the provider should be notified immediately. If oxytocin is infusing, it should be decreased or discontinued until reassuring fetal status returns.*[6]

Fetal Bradycardia

▶ What is fetal bradycardia, and what causes it?

Fetal bradycardia is a baseline rate below 110 bpm that persists for greater than 10 minutes (Fig. 6.31). Bradycardia may occur as a result of a variety of causes, both acute and chronic. Bradycardia presents a unique situation because the bradycardia may be the *result* of a hypoxic event or it may be the *cause* of the hypoxia. It is important for the provider to assess the rate, the duration, and whether variability is present. Assessment of these parameters helps to determine clinical management. Bradycardia that is associated with rates below 60, and absent or minimal variability are more often associated with poor fetal outcomes.[25–27] Bradycardia at rates between 80 and 100 bpm with moderate variability generally indicates the fetus is well oxygenated.[28] If bradycardia persists, the chances of inadequate oxygenation may increase because the fetus has only a limited ability to increase cardiac output. A sudden, profound bradycardia may signal a catastrophic event such as uterine rupture, cord prolapse, or placental abruption. These are emergencies that demand immediate attention. When the bradycardia is preceded by absent variability accompanied by late

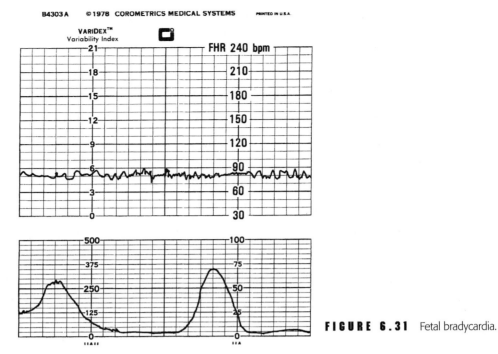

FIGURE 6.31 Fetal bradycardia.

and/ or variable deceleration that continues for a prolonged period may be referred to as *terminal bradycardia*. It is the result of severe fetal hypoxia and acidosis and precedes fetal death. Bradycardia that occurs during the second stage of labor immediately before delivery may be referred to as *end-stage bradycardia*. With end-stage bradycardia, variability is present and the fetal outcome is generally good. *These two terms are not interchangeable and should not be confused.*

Causes of Bradycardia

Fetal hypoxia—Bradycardia is a *late* sign of fetal hypoxia. The fetus, after initial attempts to normalize the oxygen level by increasing heart rate, can no longer compensate. The increased heart rate cannot be maintained in the presence of continued hypoxia and falling pH. The heart rate slows in response to these changes because they cause direct depression of heart muscle and sinoatrial (SA) node due to acidosis.

Cord compression/cord prolapse—prolonged cord compression can precipitate bradycardic episodes. Increased pressure in the fetal system owing to the obstructed blood flow leads to stimulation of the fetal baroreceptors, which in turn slows the heart rate. As long as the cord remains occluded, the heart rate will remain low.

Maternal hypotension—maternal hypotension leads to decreased placental perfusion. This decrease in perfusion leads to vagal stimulation in the fetus and a decrease in the fetal heart rate.

Uterine hyperstimulation—during periods of increased uterine activity, blood flow to the placenta is decreased. This decrease in perfusion leads to vagal stimulation in the fetus and a decrease in the fetal heart rate.

Abruptio placenta—this may result in sudden, profound bradycardia owing to the abrupt decrease in blood flow and oxygenation to the fetus.

Uterine rupture—bradycardia is the most common FHR change seen with uterine rupture.[29] In women who are attempting a vaginal birth after cesarean section, the development of a sudden bradycardia should prompt immediate assessment. If a uterine rupture has occurred, prepare for immediate cesarean delivery.

Second stage of labor—bradycardias are very common in the second stage of labor. As the fetus moves through the maternal pelvis, the vagal nerve is stimulated and the fetal heart rate slows. If moderate variability is present and the rate is above 80 bpm, interventions for immediate delivery are not usually necessary.[23]

Idiopathic causes—in some fetuses, bradycardia has no apparent cause. Perhaps in these fetuses, the parasympathetic nervous system becomes dominant in its regulatory action over the fetal heart. As long as variability is within normal limits, the fetal outcome is usually good.

Other, less common causes include the following:

Hypothermia—the temperature reduction decreases the metabolism of the fetal myocardium. The lowered myocardial activity lowers the oxygen requirements of the fetus resulting in bradycardia.

Medications—medications that decrease maternal heart rate also decrease the fetal heart rate. Medications used for paracervical blocks can produce bradycardia approximately 5 minutes after administration. The FHR may drop as low as 60 to 70 bpm.

Fetal cardiac dysrhythmias—bradycardia may be the result of congenital cardiac conditions. Congenital fetal heart block may be seen in the fetuses of women who have systemic lupus erythematosus.

Interventions for Bradycardia

The treatment of fetal bradycardia is aimed at correcting the specific cause when possible or preparing for an emergent delivery if the bradycardia cannot be corrected or hypoxia is suspected. Interventions include the following:

- **Verify** that the heart rate is fetal and not maternal
- **Lateral positioning** to optimize blood flow to the placenta/fetus and potentially release pressure on the umbilical cord
- **Administer oxygen** at 10 to 12 L per minute via face mask
- **Vaginal examination** to rule out prolapsed cord
- **IV fluid bolus** to increase hydration, increase intravascular volume, and blood flow. This may be especially important if the bradycardia is the result of maternal hypotension.
- **Prepare** for emergency cesarean delivery if uterine rupture or abruption is suspected
- **Limit pushing efforts** if the bradycardia occurs in the second stage of labor. Consider pushing with only every other contraction, avoid closed glottis pushing (holding breath while pushing), avoid supine positioning for pushing, and allow for passive descent of head when possible (labor down).
- **Monitor fetal heart rate variability** because decreasing variability may indicate a need for more expedient delivery.
- **Decrease or discontinue oxytocin infusions.** If/when the fetal heart rate returns to reassuring status, the oxytocin may be restarted.

Sinusoidal Patterns

Sinusoidal patterns are unusual. They are characterized by smooth, sine waves that are regular in frequency and amplitude (Fig. 6.32). The undulations are smooth and without variability. The

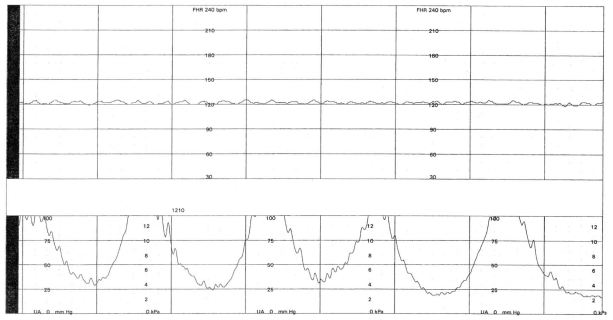

FIGURE 6.32 Sinusoidal pattern seen in a laboring patient with a partial placental abruption. Note uniform variability.

wave frequency is 2 to 5 cycles per minute with an amplitude of 5 to 15 bpm above and below the baseline.[9] *The sine waves should not be mistaken for variability.* The pattern may be intermittent or continuous. It has been suggested that intermittent sinusoidal baseline rate may be an early indicator of impending fetal compromise.[30]

Causes of a Sinusoidal Pattern

Severe fetal hypoxia—lack of oxygen with the resulting hypoxia and metabolic acidosis affect the autonomic nervous system and alter control of the fetal heart rate resulting in the sinusoidal pattern (Fig. 6.33).

Severe fetal anemia—can be caused by abruption placenta, placenta previa, maternal–fetal hemorrhage, vasa previa, and RH isoimmunization.

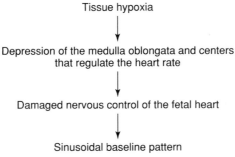

NOTE: If the fetal anemia is caused by Rh isoimmunization, the treatment may be intrauterine transfusion to correct the anemia. Once the anemia is corrected, the sinusoidal pattern resolves. The transfusion may need to be repeated at regular intervals during the pregnancy.

FIGURE 6.33 Physiology related to the sinusoidal pattern.

Interventions for Sinusoidal Patterns

- Notify provider and request immediate evaluation of the strip.
- Consider the potential causes of a sinusoidal pattern based on history and the clinical signs and symptoms.
- Administer oxygen at 10 to 12 L per minute via face mask.
- IV hydration—consider IV fluid bolus of 500 mL of a non–glucose-containing solution.
- Lateral positioning—to optimize blood flow to the placenta.
- Prepare for emergent delivery—notify the neonatal team; the fetus may be in need of resuscitation.

Pseudo-sinusoidal Patterns

A sinusoidal pattern may be the result of narcotic administration. The appearance is the same, but with a pseudo-sinusoidal pattern there may be periods of normal baseline, as well as accelerations and decelerations (Fig. 6.34).

Causes

Administration of narcotics particularly butorphanol, but also meperidine and morphine, cause pseudo-sinusoidal patterns. When associated with narcotic administration, this pattern does not seem to adversely affect fetal condition and the pattern disappears when the effect of the drug wears off.

Interventions

Before the administration of a narcotic, establish fetal reassurance. Once the medication has been given, monitor for the resolution of the sinusoidal pattern and a return of reassuring FHR patterns.

Effects of Uterine Contractions

Effect on Maternal–Fetal Blood Flow

Normal uterine contractions produce repeated stress on the fetus by interfering with placental blood flow from the mother to the fetus. Before a contraction, blood flow is at its greatest, moving freely between the mother and fetus. As a contraction begins, *veins* in the myometrium are compressed.

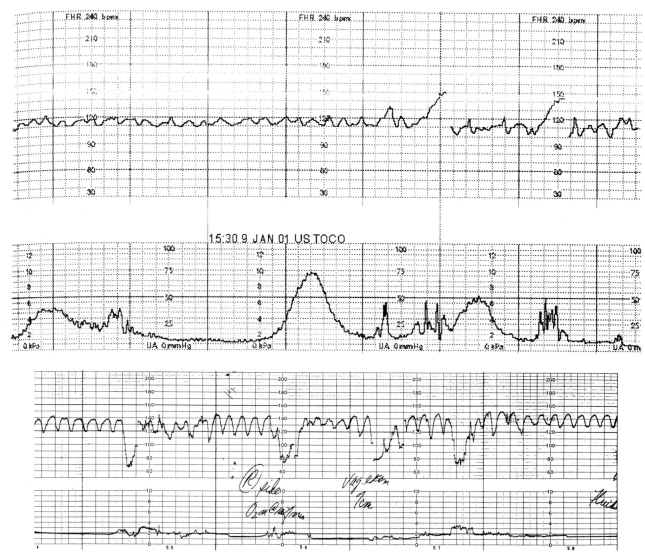

FIGURE 6.34 Sinusoidal pattern. (Reprinted with permission from Menihan, C. A., & Zottoli, E. K. [2001]. *Electronic fetal monitoring: Concepts and applications.* Philadelphia: Lippincott Williams & Wilkins; and Freeman, R. K., Garite, T. J., & Nageotte, M. P. [2003]. *Fetal heart rate monitoring* [3rd ed., p.86]. Philadelphia: Lippincott Williams & Wilkins.)

Compression of *arteries* in the myometrium occurs if the intensity of the contraction is greater than the mean arterial blood pressure of the mother. With the compression of the myometrial arteries, blood flow ceases and the fetus in essence "holds its breath." The point at which blood flow stops is at approximately 40 mmHg and is referred to as *physiologic isolation*. In a normal contraction, this physiologic isolation is brief, and the fetus is able to withstand this stress and maintain the heart rate. As the contraction subsides, the myometrial *arteries* open first, followed by an opening of the myometrial *veins*. Blood flow through the uterus to the placenta and fetus is restored.

Increased Uterine Activity

Tetanic contractions are contractions that last longer than 2 minutes. These contractions result in decreased blood flow through the uterus for an extended period. An already compromised fetus may not be able to tolerate these contractions. The degree of effect on the fetus is related to fetal health, the persistence of the contractions, and/or contraction length. Even the healthy fetus can be adversely affected under these circumstances.

In Figure 6.35, baseline is quickly affected by the contraction pattern. The first contraction lasts 130 seconds, and the second contraction lasts 190 seconds; both are tetanic contractions.

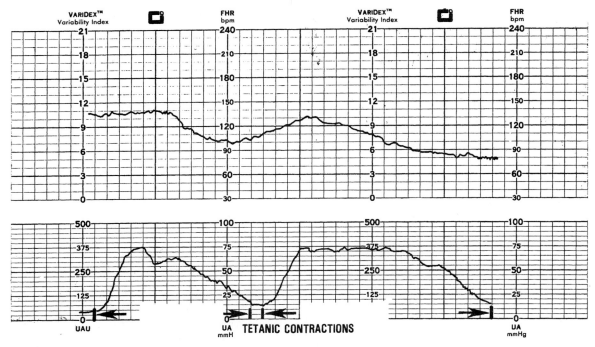

FIGURE 6.35 Effect of tetanic contractions on fetal heart rate.

The fetus has only a brief time for reoxygenation between the contractions and can no longer compensate for the hypoxic stress. The degree of compromise depends on the degree of fetal reserve and the persistence of the insult.

▶ What is uterine hyperstimulation?

There is no one universal definition of uterine hyperstimulation. Common themes appear in the literature when looking at the descriptions of uterine hyperstimulation. These common themes include the frequency of the contractions, duration of the contractions, and assessment of uterine resting tone. Commonly cited criteria for hyperstimulation include the following[31,32]:
- Contractions of normal duration occurring within 1 minute of each other
- A series of contractions lasting 2 minutes or more
- Contraction frequency of five or more in 10 minutes
- Increased uterine resting tone

When uterine activity or uterine tone is increased, blood flow through the uterus to the placenta is diminished. This decrease in blood flow may eventually lead to a tracing that reflects nonreassuring fetal status and the potential for the development of fetal hypoxia and acidosis.

NOTE: The administration of oxytocin is perhaps the most frequently identified cause of increased uterine activity (Fig. 6.36).

Interventions for Increased Uterine Activity

All interventions are directed at decreasing uterine activity and increasing uterine blood flow.
Interventions include the following:

Lateral positioning—displacement of the gravid uterus off the aorta and vena cava, promotes venous return, and increases maternal cardiac output; the result is improved uterine perfusion.

IV hydration—IV fluid bolus of 500 mL of a non–glucose-containing solution increases blood volume and increases placental perfusion.

Decrease or discontinue oxytocin infusions—this may decrease the excessive uterine activity. Removal of the uterine stimulants will allow for uterine relaxation.

NOTE: Do not restart or increase oxytocin unless the FHR pattern is reassuring.

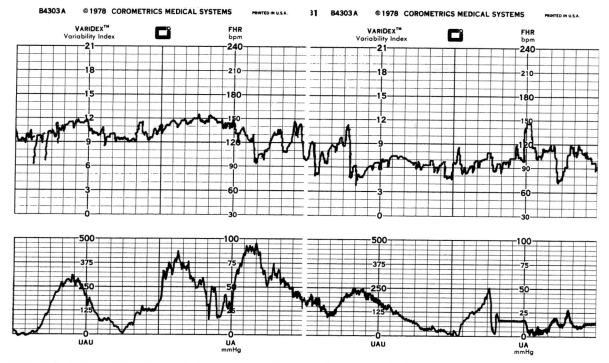

FIGURE 6.36 Effect of oxytocin-induced uterine hyperstimulation on the fetal heart rate.

Uterine relaxants—may consider the administration of a uterine relaxant if the above interventions do not result in a decrease in uterine activity.

Notify provider—notify the provider of assessments, interventions, and fetal and maternal responses.

Document—document your assessments, interventions, and maternal and fetal responses to interventions in the medical record. Also include in the documentation any communication with the provider.

Imagine holding your breath for a few seconds. This is a brief stress, but one that can be easily withstood. But what if you are ill? You might not be able to withstand the stress of holding your breath even for a few seconds. Whether or not you can withstand this stress depends on your reserve or status. The same holds true for the fetus. Normal uterine activity may prove too stressful in a fetus whose oxygen reserve is poor. A healthy fetus may tolerate increased uterine activity with no evidence of a nonreassuring tracing. However, an increase in uterine activity should prompt the provider to consider interventions, including decreasing or discontinuing oxytocin, before the development of a nonreassuring fetal tracing.

In summary, with each contraction, blood flow from the fetus to the mother is initially affected as the myometrial veins are compressed. If the contraction pressure is greater than the mother's mean arterial blood pressure, blood flow from the mother to the fetus ceases as the myometrial arteries are compressed. At this point, the mother and fetus are physiologically separated from each other. As the contraction begins to subside, the myometrial arteries reopen, allowing blood carrying oxygen and nutrients to flow from the mother to the fetus. As the contraction continues to subside, the myometrial veins open, allowing blood carrying fetal waste products to flow from the fetus to the mother.

▶ How do uterine contractions affect the fetal heart rate?

Uterine contractions can affect the FHR by increasing or decreasing that rate in association with any given contraction. The three primary mechanisms by which uterine contractions can cause a decrease in FHR (Fig. 6.37) are by compression of the following:

- Fetal head
- Umbilical cord
- Myometrial vessels

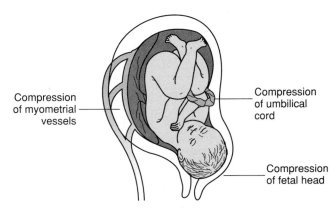

FIGURE 6.37 Three mechanisms by which uterine contractions may decrease fetal heart rate. (Adapted with permission from Barden, T. [1975]. *Intrapartum Labor Monitoring: A Slide/Lecture Series* [slide 4]. Wallingford, CT: Corometrics Medical Systems.)

Periodic and Episodic Patterns

▶ What are periodic and episodic heart rate patterns?

Periodic and episodic changes in the FHR are transient in nature. They may last from several seconds to several minutes. Periodic changes are those that are associated with contractions. Episodic changes can occur at anytime and are not related to uterine activity.

Periodic patterns—associated with contractions	**Episodic patterns**—not necessarily associated with contractions
Accelerations	Accelerations
Early deceleration	Prolonged decelerations
Late decelerations	Variable decelerations
Prolonged decelerations	
Variable decelerations	

Accelerations

▶ What are accelerations?

Accelerations are the most common type of periodic heart rate change. They are defined as a visually apparent abrupt increase in FHR (onset of acceleration to peak in less than 30 seconds; Fig. 6.38). The peak of the acceleration is 15 bpm above the most recently determined baseline and the acceleration lasts for at least 15 seconds. Before 32 weeks' gestation, acceleration must be 10 bpm above the baseline with a duration of 10 seconds.[9] Accelerations are one of the most reassuring signs of fetal well-being. Accelerations indicate central oxygenation and a low probability of fetal compromise. Accelerations may be periodic or episodic in nature. They may occur spontaneously or in response to fetal movement, maternal movement, acoustic stimulation, fetal scalp stimulation, or contractions. Regardless of the cause, accelerations are an indication of a normally oxygenated fetus.

Accelerations that are longer than 2 minutes but shorter than 10 minutes are considered prolonged accelerations. If the acceleration lasts longer than 10 minutes, it is not an acceleration but a change in baseline rate.

No treatment is necessary for accelerations. The presence of accelerations should be noted in the medical record.

Decelerations

▶ What are decelerations?

Decelerations are decreases in the FHR from the baseline. These decreases may be abrupt or gradual in nature. There are four main categories of decelerations: early decelerations, late decelerations, variable decelerations, and prolonged decelerations.

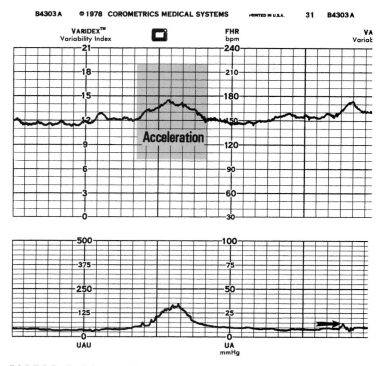

FIGURE 6.38 Fetal heart rate accelerations.

Early Decelerations

Early decelerations are defined as a visually apparent, *gradual* decrease (onset of deceleration to nadir greater than or equal to 30 seconds) and return to baseline associated with a contraction.[9] They occur with a contraction, so they are considered a periodic pattern. With early decelerations, the onset, nadir, and recovery from deceleration corresponds with the beginning, peak, and end of the contraction. Early decelerations are thought to be caused by pressure on the fetal head. The pressure alters cerebral blood flow and stimulates the vagal nerve, which slows the heart rate (Figs. 6.39 and 6.40). When the contraction lessens, the pressure decreases, and the FHR returns to baseline. This is a normal reflexive response. Early decelerations often occur in the active phase of labor as the fetal head begins descent into the pelvis.

Characteristics of Early Decelerations

- **Uniform shape**—Early decelerations have a uniform shape and appearance that changes little during labor. They are typically shallow in depth.
- **Timing**—"Mirrors the contraction." The deceleration begins with the onset of the contraction. It gradually deepens as the contraction gains intensity and then slowly

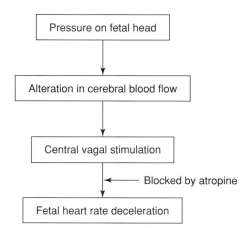

FIGURE 6.39 Mechanism of early deceleration (head compression). (Adapted with permission from Freeman, R. K., Garite, T. J., & Nageotte, M. P. [2003]. *Fetal heart rate monitoring* [3rd ed., p. 15]. Philadelphia: Lippincott Williams & Wilkins.)

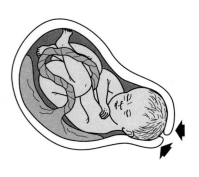

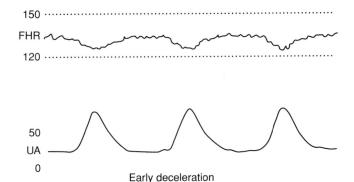

Head compression   Early deceleration

FIGURE 6.40   Head compression leading to early decelerations. (Adapted with permission from Hon, E. H. [1973]. *An Introduction to Fetal Heart Rate Monitoring* [p. 29]. Los Angeles: Postgraduate Division, University of Southern California.)

returns to baseline as the contraction intensity decreases. The deceleration mirrors the contraction. These decelerations *always* returns to baseline by the end of the contraction.

• **Variability**—FHR variability usually remains moderate.

No treatment is necessary for early decelerations. However, continue to watch the FHR pattern closely. *Assess to make sure the decelerations are truly early decelerations and not late decelerations, because implications and interventions for each of these are very different. Early decelerations are considered benign, require no interventions, and are not associated with hypoxia.* Document the presence of early decelerations in the patient's chart.

Late Decelerations

Late decelerations are defined as a visually apparent *gradual* decrease (defined as onset of deceleration to nadir as greater than or equal to 30 seconds) the decrease and return to baseline FHR is associated with a uterine contraction.[9] It is a periodic pattern. The deceleration is delayed in timing, with the nadir (or low point) of the deceleration occurring *after* the peak of the contraction. Late decelerations are late in onset (begin after the peak of the contraction). Late decelerations are late to return to baseline after the contraction is over. Late decelerations are always associated with a contraction.

Late decelerations may be the result of uteroplacental insufficiency. *Uteroplacental insufficiency* means that blood flow to the fetus had been compromised, resulting in a reduction in the amount of oxygen available for use by the fetus (Fig. 6.41). Late decelerations reflect the fact that the fetus is affected by the decrease in blood flow. The resulting hypoxia may adversely affect the fetal CNS and fetal myocardial tissues, resulting in a slowing of the heart rate, the late deceleration. This type of late deceleration is usually accompanied by minimal or absent variability. It is more common in a fetus with chronic placental insufficiency because the oxygen reserve may be diminished. The additional stress from contractions results in late decelerations. This type of late deceleration may also appear when there is an abnormal baseline rate. Late

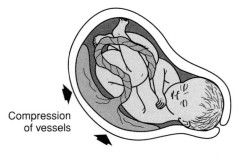

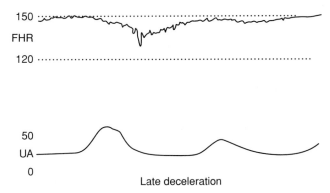

Compression of vessels

Uteroplacental insufficiency   Late deceleration

FIGURE 6.41   Uteroplacental insufficiency leading to late decelerations. (Adapted with permission from Hon, E. H. [1973]. *An Introduction to Fetal Heart Rate Monitoring* [p. 29]. Los Angeles: Postgraduate Division, University of Southern California.)

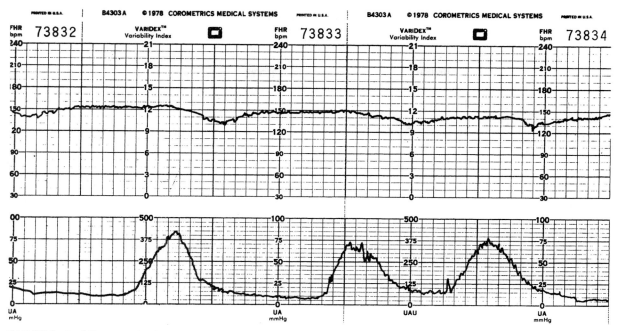

FIGURE 6.42 Late decelerations.

decelerations accompanied by an abnormal baseline rate and minimal or absent variability require immediate attention and intervention (Fig. 6.42).

Some late decelerations may have a different etiology. These late decelerations are the result of the transient decrease in oxygen during a contraction. Fetal chemoreceptors detect the transient decrease in oxygen and a reflex response is initiated. These so called "reflex lates" are not associated with hypoxia. The baseline variability is generally moderate and the baseline rate is normal (Fig. 6.43). These women can continue to labor, but close surveillance is required. Be

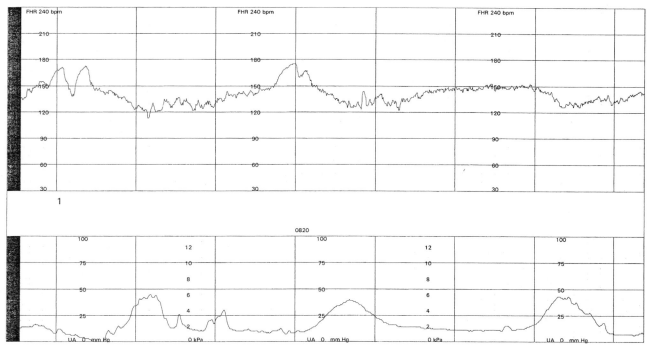

FIGURE 6.43 Reflex late decelerations. At 38 weeks' estimated gestation, this patient was a 29-year-old G2 P0 smoker who was lying in a supine position. When the patient was turned to the left lateral position, these decelerations resolved. At delivery, the placenta was small, with multiple infarcts and calcification.

alert to any change in status, such as decreased baseline variability or tachycardia. This represents a possible deterioration in fetal status and the provider should be notified immediately.

Regular and complete assessments of the FHR are very important at all times, but especially when decelerations are present. The baseline rate, baseline variability, and presence or absence of accelerations help to determine the true clinical picture and guide care.

Late decelerations may occur in the following clinical situations:

- **Uterine hyperstimulation**—produces extended periods of hypoxia related to vascular compression during contractions.
- **Hypertensive disorders**—interfere with oxygen transfer as a result of changes at the site of gas exchange in the placenta.
  - Chronic hypertension
  - Pregnancy-induced hypertension
- **Hypotensive problems**—reduced maternal cardiac output results in poor placental perfusion.
  - Supine hypotension syndrome
  - Complications from anesthetic procedures
  - Dehydration
- **Placental dysfunction**—contributes to fetal hypoxia through diminished sites for gas exchange.
  - Infarcted placentas
  - Postmature placentas
  - Placentas in the fetus with intrauterine growth restriction
  - Maternal smoking
  - Premature aging of placenta
  - Placental calcification
- **Bleeding disorders**—contribute to hypovolemia and resulting hypoxia.
  - Abruptio placenta
  - Placenta previa
- **Hematologic disorders**—affect the oxygen-carrying capacity of the blood, contributing to hypoxia.
  - Anemia
  - Sickle cell disease
  - Rh isoimmunization
- **Disorders affecting the blood vessels**—thickening of the walls of intervillous spaces diminishes the efficiency of gas exchange.
  - Diabetes mellitus
  - Arteriosclerotic heart disease
- **Maternal cardiac disease**—some maternal cardiac conditions may create the potential for reduced cardiac output and decreased blood flow to the placenta and fetus.

Characteristics of Late Decelerations (Fig. 6.44)

- **Uniform shape**—late decelerations have relatively the same uniform shape throughout labor. They begin with a gradual descent from the baseline and end with a gradual ascent back to the baseline.
- **Timing**—the deceleration begins after the peak of the contraction and *always* ends after the end of the contraction.
- **Variability**—it is very important to assess variability when late decelerations are present. Absent or minimal variability when late decelerations are present represent a nonreassuring finding.
- **Depth**—the depth of the deceleration is NOT proportional to the severity of the hypoxia and acidemia.
- **Frequency**—the presence of recurrent late decelerations, especially when combined with a loss of variability, is an ominous sign.

Interventions for Late Decelerations

- **Lateral position**—This position decreases pressure on the inferior vena cava and aorta, by displacing the pressure caused by the weight of the gravid uterus. The decrease in pressure improves blood flow, placental perfusion, and fetal oxygenation.
- **Decrease/discontinue oxytocin**—this action decreases uterine activity and as a result maximizes blood flow from the mother to the fetus.

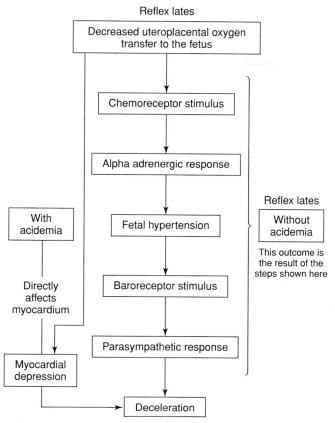

FIGURE 6.44 Physiology of late decelerations. (Adapted with permission from Freeman, R. K., Garite, T. J., & Nageotte, M. P. [2003]. *Fetal heart rate monitoring* [3rd ed., p.18]. Philadelphia: Lippincott Williams & Wilkins.)

- **Administer oxygen**—begin oxygen therapy by mask at 10 to 12 L per minute. This helps to increase the oxygen saturation of maternal blood, making more oxygen available for the fetus.
- **Administer IV fluids**—initiate IV fluid bolus (500 mL of a non–glucose-containing solution). This increases the woman's blood volume, which contributes to better placental perfusion.
- **Notify the primary care provider**—of all interventions and maternal and fetal responses. If the fetal status does not improve, you may request the presence of the provider at the bedside.
- **Document**—All assessments, interventions, maternal and fetal responses, and communication with the primary care provider in the medical record.
- **Consider performing a vaginal examination**—this examination provides information about progress in labor and provides the opportunity to perform a fetal scalp stimulation and assess for acceleration in response.

Variable Decelerations

Variable decelerations are the most common type of deceleration. They are defined as a visually apparent *abrupt* decrease (onset to nadir less than 30 seconds) below the baseline. The decrease in FHR is more than 15 bpm below baseline, lasts longer than 15 seconds and less than 2 minutes (Fig. 6.45). When associated with contractions, their onset, depth, and duration may vary.[9] They are called "variable decelerations" because they vary in timing, vary in depth, vary in duration, and vary in shape. They are thought to be caused by umbilical cord compression; when they occur in the second stage of labor, it may be a vagal response.

When variable decelerations are recurrent, it is also very important to assess baseline rate and baseline variability. Variable decelerations accompanied by a normal baseline rate and moderate

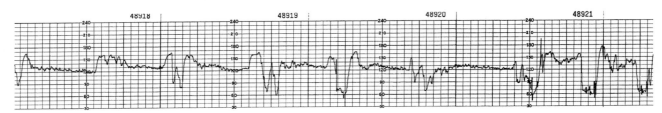

FIGURE 6.45 Variable decelerations. (Reprinted with permission from Freeman, R. K., Garite, T. J., & Nageotte, M. P. [1991]. *Fetal heart rate monitoring* [3rd ed., p.72]. Philadelphia: Lippincott Williams & Wilkins.)

variability require minimal interventions. Variable decelerations accompanied by an abnormal baseline rate and minimal or absent variability require more immediate intervention and assessment.

Characteristics of Variable Decelerations (Fig. 6.46)

- **Variable shape**—variable decelerations can assume *any* shape. They can appear V, W, or U shaped. It is not unusual for several variable decelerations on the same laboring woman's strip graph to appear different. *There is no consistent shape.*
- **Variable onset**—variable decelerations can begin at any time with or without the presence of contractions. If they do occur with a contraction, they can begin at the beginning, peak, or end of the contraction. There is no consistent timing of onset.
- **Variable offset**—variable decelerations can return to the baseline quickly, or the return can be gradual. If the deceleration occurs with a contraction, it can start at any point during the contraction and can return to baseline during or after the contraction ends. However, if the deceleration has occurred in relation to a contraction, it is often resolved by the contraction's end because the contraction might have been the cause of the cord pressure. There is no consistent offset.
- **Variable depth (amplitude)**—variable decelerations vary in the depth to which the FHR will drop. Often, they fall below 90 bpm. It is not unusual for variable decelerations on the same strip to vary in depth. This is because the depth of the deceleration is a reflection of the amount of pressure increase in the fetal system. The heart rate decreases as much as needed to prevent vascular pressure from becoming too great. There is no consistent depth.

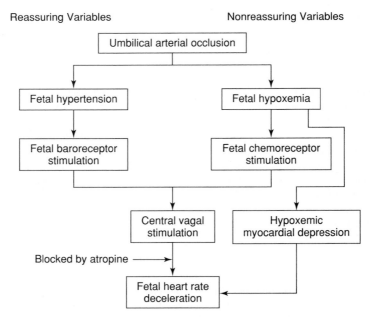

FIGURE 6.46 Physiology of variable decelerations. (Reprinted with permission from Freeman, R. K., Garite, T. J., & Nageotte, M. P. [2003]. *Fetal heart rate monitoring* [3rd ed., p. 17]. Philadelphia: Lippincott Williams & Wilkins.)

- **Variable duration**—variable decelerations can last for any length of time, from a few seconds up to 2 minutes. It is not unusual for variable decelerations on the same strip to have different durations. *There is no consistent duration.*
- **Variability**—the decelerations may be associated with normal or increased variability, which is a reassuring finding. Minimal or absent variability would be considered a nonreassuring characteristic.

Variable decelerations occur most frequently in the following clinical situations:

- **Second stage of labor**—as the fetus descends through the birth canal, the umbilical cord is more likely to be stretched and compressed.
- **Nuchal cord**—one or more loops of the umbilical cord can become wrapped around the fetal neck or shoulder.
- **Cord occlusion**—can be because of contractions, a true knot, or a cord around the body
- **After rupture of membranes**—there is no longer the protective fluid cushion of fluid surrounding the cord making it more vulnerable to compression.

Characteristics of Reassuring Tracing With Variable Decelerations (Fig. 6.47)

- **Resolves quickly**—a rapid return to baseline after the deceleration demonstrates that the fetus is able to return to its normal heart rate quickly, had minimal exposure to a hypoxic episode, and has good reserve.
- **Normal variability and baseline**—as stated, normal variability is always a reassuring strip characteristic and is indicative of normal oxygenation and normal pH, indicating a fetus that is maintaining homeostasis.
- **Short duration**—the deceleration lasts no more than 30 to 45 seconds. Variables of short duration yield minimal time of reduced oxygen and a shorter time for carbon dioxide buildup in the fetal blood.

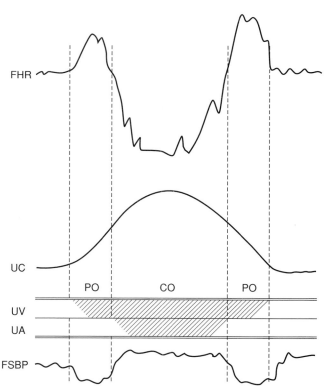

FIGURE 6.47 Blood pressure changes during variable decelerations. This figure represents fetal heart rate and fetal systemic blood pressure (*FSBP*) occurring during compression of the umbilical vein (*UV*) and the umbilical artery (*UA*). UC, uterine contraction. (Reprinted with permission from Lee, C. V., Loreto, P. C., & O'Lane, J. M. [1975]. A study of fetal heart rate acceleration patterns. *Obstetrics and Gynecology, 45,* 142.)

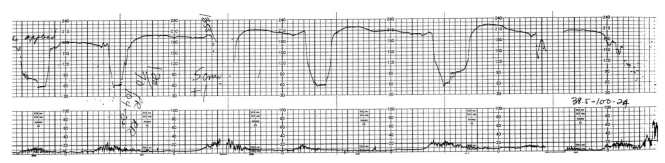

FIGURE 6.48 Variable decelerations with loss of variability (Reprinted with permission from Freeman, R. K., Garite, T. J., & Nageotte, M. P. [2003]. *Fetal heart rate monitoring* [3rd ed., p. 117]. Philadelphia: Lippincott Williams & Wilkins.

Characteristics of Nonreassuring Tracing With Variable Decelerations

- **Decreased variability**—minimal or absent variability may be associated with a high incidence of low Apgar scores and potentially poor neonatal outcomes.
- **Rising baseline**—a rising baseline often indicates decreasing fetal ability to tolerate hypoxic episodes. After the deceleration, the fetal heart may need to increase its rate to reoxygenate the tissues and maintain adequate level of homeostasis (Fig. 6.48).
- **Prolonged return to baseline and/or bradycardia after variable decelerations**—this lengthens the hypoxic episode, indicates that there is a problem resuming the original heart rate, is commonly associated with hypoxemia, and *is an ominous event.*
- **Development of tachycardia**—tachycardia may indicate that the fetal heart rate is increased to maintain adequate oxygen levels.
- **Recurrent decreases to less than 70 bpm and lasting longer than 60 seconds**—variable decelerations of this duration and frequency may increase stress on the fetus by decreasing the interval for reoxygenation

Interventions for Variable Decelerations

Many variable decelerations return to the FHR baseline quickly, and no interventions are necessary. The interventions for variable decelerations are aimed at alleviating the cause of the compression. Interventions for variable decelerations may include:

- **Change the laboring woman's position**—try side-lying, one side and then the other, followed by the semi-Fowler's position. The knee-chest position can also be used; however, it is generally reserved as the last position to be tried because it is uncomfortable for the laboring woman. *Remember to wait several seconds after each position change to assess whether the change has reduced cord compression and improved the heart rate.* This is sometimes difficult to do when the deceleration is especially severe and several seconds can seem like several minutes.
- **Perform a vaginal examination**—this is done to rule out a prolapsed cord, assess the stage of labor, and assist in estimating the time of delivery.
- **If the variables are recurrent or nonreassuring components are present, begin oxygen therapy by face mask at 10 to 12 L per minute**—although the blood flow to the fetus is compromised or stopped during cord compression, oxygen therapy improves the oxygen saturation of maternal blood. When the cord compression is relieved, the fetus has access to a richer oxygen supply, which can assist the fetus in a quicker recovery.
- **Decrease or discontinue oxytocin**—if variable decelerations are recurrent and nonreassuring components are present, oxytocin should be decreased or discontinued. Although oxytocin may not cause variable decelerations, it might be a contributing factor, especially if the decelerations are occurring with the contractions. Oxytocin may be restarted if the fetal tracing returns to reassuring status.
- **Notify the primary care provider**—of all interventions and maternal and fetal responses. If the fetal status does not improve, you may request the presence of the provider at the bedside.
- **Document**—all assessments, interventions, maternal and fetal responses, and communication with the primary care provider in the medical record.

• **Consider amnioinfusion according to protocols**—amnioinfusions are done to assist in relieving cord compression by reintroducing fluid into the uterus, thus providing a cushioning effect to the umbilical cord.

Prolonged Decelerations

Prolonged decelerations are defined as a visually apparent decrease in the FHR below the baseline. The decrease is more than 15 bpm and lasts longer than 2 minutes but less than 10 minutes. A decrease for longer than 10 minutes represents a change in baseline rate.[9] Prolonged decelerations may be an isolated event (episodic change) or associated with contractions (periodic change). Onset may be abrupt or gradual (see Fig. 6.36).

Prolonged decelerations have multiple causes, including:
• Isolated cord compression
• Maternal hypotension—supine position, and after placement of regional anesthetics
• Vagal stimulation—especially with vigorous scalp stimulation or with rapid descent of the fetal head
• Increase uterine activity—hyperstimulation or hypertonus
• Abruptio placenta
• Uterine rupture
• Cord prolapse, short cords, and true knots
  Less common causes include:
• Maternal seizure activity
• Maternal cardiovascular collapse

Characteristics of Prolonged Decelerations

• **Onset**—onset of the prolonged decelerations can be abrupt or gradual because these decelerations can be caused by many different factors. The onset of a particular deceleration might present a clue to the possible origin of the precipitating event (e.g., an abrupt drop in the FHR can indicate cord compression).
• **Duration**—this deceleration lasts at least 2 minutes (often lasts much longer), but no more than 10 minutes.
• **Offset**—the offset can be abrupt or gradual.

Interventions for Prolonged Decelerations

The interventions for a prolonged deceleration are to correct the cause if known. Rationale for interventions is the same as for variable decelerations. Interventions include:
• **Change position** to alleviate compression on the umbilical cord.
• **Administer oxygen** at 10 to 12 L per minute via face mask.
• **IV hydration**—500 mL of a non–glucose-containing solution.
• **Correct** maternal hypotension.
• **Decrease or discontinue oxytocin.**
• **Perform vaginal examination to rule out prolapsed cord**—Avoid vigorous scalp stimulation during a prolonged deceleration to avoid stimulating a vagal response (slows the FHR).
• **Administration of uterine relaxants**—if uterine hypertonus or hyperstimulation is suspected.
• **Notify provider**—of all interventions and maternal and fetal responses. May need to request presence at bedside, especially if deceleration does not resolve with above interventions.
• **Prepare for emergent delivery.**

NOTE: If the prolonged deceleration is an isolated event, and the FHR after the deceleration returns to a normal baseline rate and variability is present, the only intervention required is continued monitoring and fetal surveillance.

Following Trends in FHR Patterns

It is important to note that assessments and interpretation of the FHR are on-going and continues at regular specific intervals until delivery. The intervals for assessments should be outlined in unit policies that are based on national standards recommended by professional organizations.

Deterioration in fetal status can be the result of an acute event such as abruptio placenta or uterine rupture, but deterioration in fetal status may also be very gradual and occur slowly over the course of the labor. Abrupt changes are very dramatic and grab the attention of providers, but the more subtle changes occurring over time may be more easily missed simply *because* they are not so dramatic. Be very alert to changes in baseline rate and decreasing variability because these may be the first signals of fetal compromise. Providers should be assessing for and recognize changes that indicate a move from reassuring status to nonreassuring status. Early recognition of change in fetal status along with prompt and appropriate interventions are the goals of fetal monitoring.

Summary

Periodic or episodic changes in the FHR are transient excursions from the baseline. These changes may be part of a reassuring or nonreassuring tracing depending on the specific characteristics. These patterns provide clues to fetal oxygen status and reserve during labor. The data that these patterns provide should be used in planning and providing care.

PRACTICE/REVIEW QUESTIONS

After reviewing Part 3, answer the following questions.

1. Define *fetal tachycardia.*

   _____

2. Define *fetal bradycardia.*

   _____

3. For each of the following terms, indicate whether the condition might be a cause of fetal tachycardia (FT), fetal bradycardia (FB), or both (B).

   a. _____ Fetal hypoxia

   b. _____ Pitocin

   c. _____ Maternal anxiety

   d. _____ Prolapsed umbilical cord

   e. _____ Fetal infection

   f. _____ Maternal hypothermia

   g. _____ Prematurity

   h. _____ Fetal movement

   i. _____ Maternal fever

4. Describe the nursing interventions appropriate for fetal tachycardia.

   a. _____

   b. _____

c. _____

d. _____

e. _____

f. _____

5. Describe the nursing interventions appropriate for fetal bradycardia.

   a. _____

   b. _____

   c. _____

   d. _____

   e. _____

   f. _____

   g. _____

6. List the three primary ways in which uterine contractions can decrease FHR.

   a. _____

   b. _____

   c. _____

7. Study the following strip.

   a. Is the baseline rate normal? _____

   b. What periodic pattern is present? _____

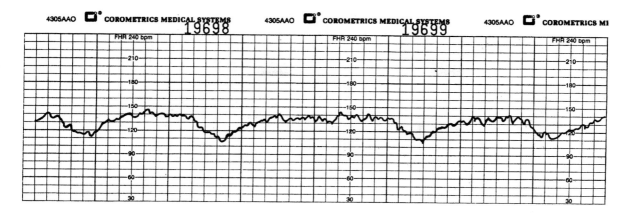

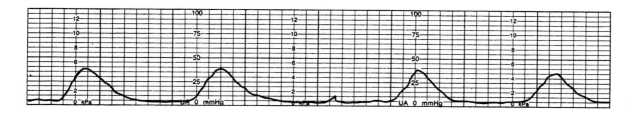

8. Describe the sinusoidal baseline pattern.

   _____

   _____

9. Name three possible causes of a sinusoidal pattern.

   a. _____

   b. _____

   c. _____

10. Identify and describe two kinds of abnormally increased uterine activity.

    a. _____

    b. _____

11. State the nonpharmacologic interventions for abnormally increased uterine activity.

    a. _____

    b. _____

    c. _____

12. Define *periodic heart rate changes.*

    _____

    _____

13. Indicate whether the following statements are true (T) or false (F).

    a. _____ Contractions have no effect on FHR.

    b. _____ Accelerations are a reassuring sign of fetal well-being.

    c. _____ Accelerations are a sign of fetal distress.

    d. _____ Early decelerations are *not* a sign of fetal distress.

    e. _____ Early decelerations usually do not fall below 100 bpm.

14. Define the following terms:

    a. Accelerations: _____

    b. Early decelerations: _____

15. List three situations in which early decelerations might occur.

    a. _____

    b. _____

    c. _____

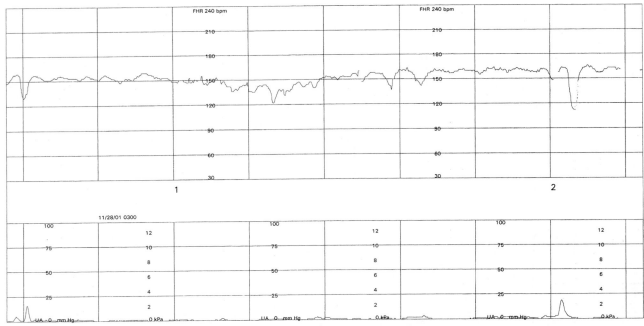

16. Study the strip above. What FHR pattern(s) is (are) present? _____

17. Variable decelerations are caused by _____.

18. Indicate whether the following statements are true (T) or false (F).

   a. _____ Variable decelerations always have the same shape and appearance.

   b. _____ Variable decelerations always begin at the peak of a contraction.

   c. _____ A variable deceleration might or might not occur with contractions.

   d. _____ There is no consistent depth to a variable deceleration.

   e. _____ It is unusual for several variable decelerations on the same patient's strip graph to have different durations.

   f. _____ Variable decelerations are commonly seen in labor.

19. List the actions used to alleviate variable decelerations.

   a. _____

   b. _____

   c. _____

   d. _____

   e. _____

20. Late decelerations are caused by _____.

21. Indicate whether the following statements are true (T) or false (F).

   a. _____ Late decelerations are a sign of fetal stress.

   b. _____ Late decelerations are uniform in shape throughout labor.

   c. _____ Labor may be allowed to continue when late decelerations are present if the variability is reassuring.

   d. _____ Late decelerations are often associated with a loss in variability.

22. List the treatment indicated for late decelerations.

   a. _____

   b. _____

   c. _____

   d. _____

   e. _____

   f. _____

23. Study the following strip graph. Describe the FHR pattern. _____

24. Describe the appearance of late decelerations.

   _____

   _____

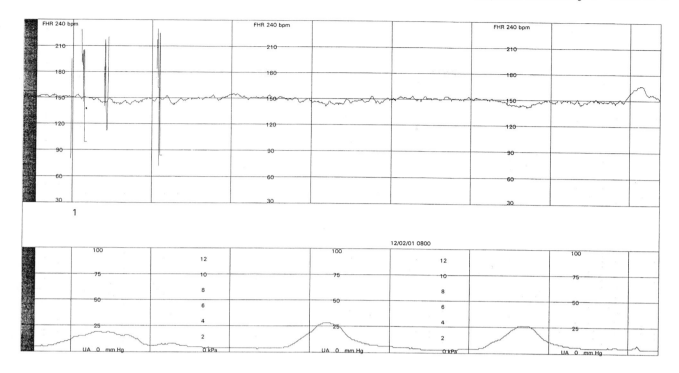

25. The deeper the late deceleration falls, the more ominous the tracing.

   a. True

   b. False

26. Name two nonreassuring characteristics of variable decelerations.

   a. _____

   b. _____

27. What are prolonged decelerations? _____

   _____

PRACTICE/REVIEW ANSWER KEY

1. Fetal tachycardia is a heart rate above 160 bpm that is sustained for 10 minutes or longer.

2. Fetal bradycardia is a heart rate below 110 bpm that is sustained for 10 minutes or longer.

3. a. B
   b. FB
   c. FT
   d. FB
   e. FT
   f. FB
   g. FT
   h. FT
   i. FT

4. a. Begin oxygen therapy via mask at 10 L per minute.
   b. Take the mother's vital signs, especially the temperature.
   c. Turn the patient to her side.
   d. Validate monitor with a fetoscope.
   e. Consider administering a bolus of IV fluids if patient is febrile.
   f. Notify the primary care provider immediately.

5. a. Begin oxygen therapy via mask at 10 L per minute.
   b. Take the mother's vital signs.
   c. Turn the patient to her side.
   d. Consider administering a bolus of IV fluids.
   e. Attempt to increase FHR by performing scalp stimulation.
   f. Listen to FHTs with a fetoscope.
   g. Notify the primary care provider immediately.

6. a. Compression of the myometrial vessels
   b. Compression of the fetal head
   c. Compression of the umbilical cord

7. a. Yes
   b. Early decelerations

8. A sinusoidal baseline is characterized by a regular, undulating baseline pattern that is within the normal heart rate range.

9. a. Severe fetal anemia
   b. Fetal asphyxia
   c. Drugs

10. Any two of the following:
    a. Tetanic contractions (i.e., contractions that last longer than 90 seconds)
    b. More than five contractions in 10 minutes
    c. Increased baseline tone of greater than 30 mmHg or not relaxed to palpation

11. a. Give bolus IV fluids.
    b. Turn the patient to her side.
    c. Administer oxygen per mask at 10 to 12 L per minute.

12. Periodic heart rate changes are FHR changes that are transient and associated with contractions.

13. a. F
    b. T
    c. F
    d. T
    e. T

14. *Accelerations:* brisk increases in the FHR of at least 15 beats above the baseline rate and lasting at least 15 seconds

    Early decelerations: caused by head compression, mirror the contraction, and always resolve by the end of the contraction

15. Any three of the following:
    a. In primigravidas
    b. During vaginal examinations
    c. In the late active phase and the second stage of labor during pushing
    d. During application of FSE or IUPC
    e. With CPD
    f. After amniotic sac has ruptured
    g. With occiput posterior presentations

16. Variable decelerations

17. Umbilical cord compression

18. a. F
    b. F
    c. T
    d. T
    e. F
    f. T

19. a. Change the patient's position.
    b. Perform a vaginal examination.
    c. Administer oxygen if variables are consistent or prolonged or if there is decreasing variability.
    d. Notify the primary care provider.
    e. Turn off oxytocin if decelerations are severe or prolonged or if there is decreasing variability.

20. Uteroplacental insufficiency

21. a. T
    b. T
    c. T
    d. T

22. a. Ask the patient to lie on her side.
    b. Turn off oxytocin if infusing.
    c. Administer oxygen.
    d. Correct hypotension (increase IV fluids).
    e. Perform a vaginal examination to estimate point in labor.
    f. Notify the primary care provider.

23. Early decelerations

24. Late decelerations usually start after contraction onset but *always* last longer than the contraction. They are uniform in shape and rarely drop below 100 bpm.

25. b. Subtle late decelerations are thought to mean the fetus is barely able to respond to the hypoxic insult.

26. Any two of the following:
    a. Overshoots
    b. Loss of shoulders
    c. Loss of variability
    d. Slow return to baseline

27. Prolonged decelerations are decelerations that last longer than 2 minutes and less than 10 minutes.

Fetal Acid–Base Balance and Dysrhythmias

As you complete Part 4 of this module, you will learn:

1. Normal fetal umbilical cord blood gas values
2. Cord blood gas results according to guidelines presented
3. Common terms used in acid–base analysis
4. To identify fetal heart rate patterns associated with abnormal and normal fetal cord gas results
5. To identify the clinical significance to the fetus and provider when abnormal tracings indicate acidosis
6. Common fetal dysrhythmias and their clinical significance
7. Necessary adjustments to monitoring equipment that allows documentation of fetal heart tones during dysrhythmic patterns

Fetal Homeostasis and Acid–Base Balance

▶ **What is the connection between the appearance of fetal heart tracings and the acid–base status of the fetus?**

The pH of the blood and tissues has an impact on all enzymes and proteins in the body, affecting organ function and infant status at birth. Acid–base status of the fetus is reflected in the characteristics of the fetal heart tracings. Certain patterns are associated with normal pH; other patterns are associated with pH reduction and acidosis. These relationships allow the practitioner to determine/predict fetal status by evaluating the characteristics of the tracing.

Terms Associated with Acid–Base Analysis

Acidemia—the buildup of acid (reduced pH) in the *blood*. (The pH of the tissues is generally lower than the pH found in the blood; as a result, the terms *acidosis* and *acidemia* are often used interchangeably. When blood values demonstrate a decreased pH, it can be assumed that the tissues are affected in the same manner.)

Acidosis—the buildup of acid (reduced pH) in the *tissues* (see above).

Base deficit (BD)—the amount of bases used by the body in an attempt to normalize a reduced pH (neutralize the acid); illustrates the degree of change in the bicarbonate concentration in the body; the more base used in attempting to normalize the pH, the larger the number becomes and the greater the deficit.

Hypoxemia—reduction of oxygen in the *blood*.

Hypoxia—reduction of oxygen in the *tissues*.

pH—a representation of the hydrogen ion concentration.

Pco_2—the partial pressure of carbon dioxide (quantity of CO_2 in the blood).

Po_2—the partial pressure of oxygen (quantity of O_2 in the blood).

▶ **What are the normal values for fetal blood gases?**[33]

Although blood gas values are often listed as a range, the values for the umbilical blood cord gases are listed here as single digits rather than ranges only to make recall easier. The values listed should be considered a guide and not an absolute. Normal umbilical cord gas values are as follows:

pH ≥ 7.10
Po_2 ≥ 20 mmHg
Pco_2 ≤ 60 mmHg
BD ≤ 10

Metabolic Acidemia/Acidosis

▶ What is metabolic acidemia/acidosis?

Each fetus reacts to periods of reduced oxygen in a unique way. "Healthy" fetuses with good reserves initially respond to the stress of hypoxia with little or no change in heart rate patterns. Fetuses with little or no reserve will often be quickly affected by even a small reduction in oxygen availability. Reduction of the pH in fetal blood below normal range (*acidemia*) can result when oxygen levels in fetal circulation fall below certain values. The pH values of the fetal blood are an indication of the pH found in the tissues; however, tissue pH tends to be even lower than the pH levels found in the blood. The kind of acidosis (decreased pH in the tissues) linked to decreased O_2 has its basis in metabolic processes and is called "metabolic acidosis."

At the cellular level, as glucose is used for energy, this metabolic process results in the formation of lactic acid. Normally, oxygen combines with lactic acid to produce CO_2 and H_2O, which are easily excreted by the fetus. If fetal oxygen is limited, the process stops at the formation of lactic acid, resulting in a buildup of this strong acid in the tissues and blood. The importance of oxygen in the acid–base schema is outlined in Figure 6.49.

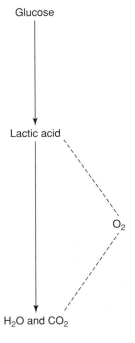

Glucose

All fetuses can perform this step no matter how hypoxic or acidotic they might be.

Lactic acid

O_2 is required for the conversion of lactic acid to harmless substances ($CO_2 + H_2O$), which can be excreted.

Without sufficient amounts of O_2, lactic acid builds up in the tissues and blood, causing acidosis and acidemia.

O_2

H_2O and CO_2

FIGURE 6.49 The importance of O_2 in normal metabolic processes.

▶ What acid-base values identify metabolic acidemia?[33]

Changes in values that identify the process of metabolic acidemia are as follows:

pH <7.10 **REDUCED**
Po_2 <20 mmHg **REDUCED**
Pco_2 <60 mmHg **NORMAL**
BD >10 **INCREASED**

▶ **What FHR monitor strip characteristics may indicate metabolic acidemia/acidosis?**

- **Absent variability**—as the fetus becomes more oxygen deprived and the pH falls, variability decreases and can vacillate between periods of minimal and absent variability. The periods of decreased variability become longer. Hypoxic effects on the autonomic nervous system, especially its parasympathetic branch, cause this change in variability, which may be indicative of metabolic acidosis. **If variability is absent, the provider should be prepared for the potential need of neonatal resuscitation at delivery.**
- **Late decelerations**—late decelerations may be associated with hypoxia and metabolic acidosis. They may occur simultaneously with minimal or absent variability. The presence of late decelerations alone does not mean that acidosis is present, but might indicate a shift in that direction (Fig. 6.50).

    A "shift" toward metabolic acidosis means that there is a reduction in the oxygen content of the fetal blood but that the pH remains within normal limits, as do the other blood gas values. If oxygenation does not improve, there is a risk of progression to metabolic acidosis. Evidence of this shift might be seen on the tracing in the following characteristics: normal variability with late decelerations (Fig. 6.51).

Blood gas values expected in a shift toward metabolic acidosis are as follows:

pH	**NORMAL**
Po_2	**REDUCED**
All other values	**NORMAL**

Respiratory Acidemia/Acidosis

▶ **What is respiratory acidemia/acidosis?**

Fetal acid-base status can also be affected by increased levels of CO_2. Because CO_2 is acidic, elevated levels of CO_2 in the fetal blood cause a reduction in pH and can result in acidosis and acidemia. This kind of acidemia is called "respiratory acidemia" because it is concerned with CO_2 buildup. Increased levels of CO_2 in fetal circulation are often associated with variable decelerations.

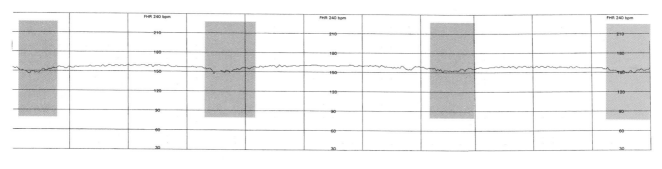

FIGURE 6.50 Recurrent late decelerations. Note decreased variability. If you look closely, the baseline appears to be sinusoidal. The patient, a 33-year-old G3 P1, had been diagnosed with partial placenta previa before the onset of labor. She was admitted in early labor at 36 weeks' estimated gestation with vaginal bleeding. This pattern is indicative of metabolic acidemia/acidosis. An emergency cesarean section was performed. Apgar scores were 1, 3, and 7.

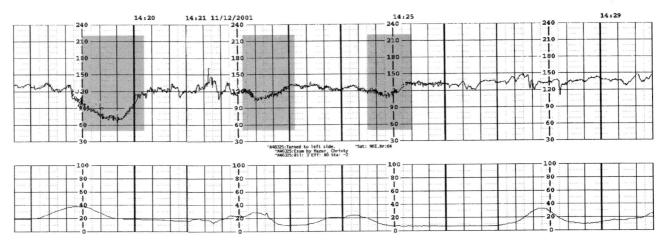

FIGURE 6.51 Late decelerations with moderate variability. A 26-year-old G1 P0 at 41 weeks' estimated gestation was admitted for induction of labor. The fetus demonstrated poor tolerance to mild contractions, which worsened as contractions became stronger. During the cesarean section, a very small placenta and abnormal cord were found. There was almost a complete absence of Wharton's jelly, with only a sheath covering cord vessels.

▶ What acid-base values may indicate respiratory acidemia?[33]

Changes in values that identify the process of respiratory acidemia are as follows:

pH	<7.10 **REDUCED**
P_{O_2}	Varies
P_{CO_2}	>60 mmHg **INCREASED**
BD	<10 **NORMAL** (no buildup of lactic acid)

▶ What FHR monitor strip characteristics indicate respiratory acidemia/acidosis?

- **Variable decelerations**—Variable decelerations, the pattern identified with cord compression, result in CO_2 buildup (lowers pH) in fetal circulation. When CO_2 levels rise high enough, fetal pH is affected and the outcome is an increase in acidity of tissues and blood (Fig. 6.52).

  At delivery, the infant with respiratory acidosis usually requires only the stimulation of neonatal respiration (i.e., crying, breathing) to rid the body of excess CO_2. Successful efforts most often are accomplished by tactile stimulation.

  A "shift" toward respiratory acidosis means that there is an increase in the level of CO_2 but that the pH and other values are within normal limits.

  Blood gas levels that indicate a shift toward respiratory acidosis are as follows:

P_{CO_2}	**INCREASED**
pH	**NORMAL**
Other values	**NORMAL**

Mixed Acidosis

▶ What is mixed acidemia/acidosis?

Mixed acidosis occurs when both metabolic and respiratory acidoses are present. The pH and P_{O_2} are reduced, and P_{CO_2} and base deficit are increased. **Be prepared:** A baby with both metabolic and respiratory acidosis may be depressed and need aggressive resuscitation.

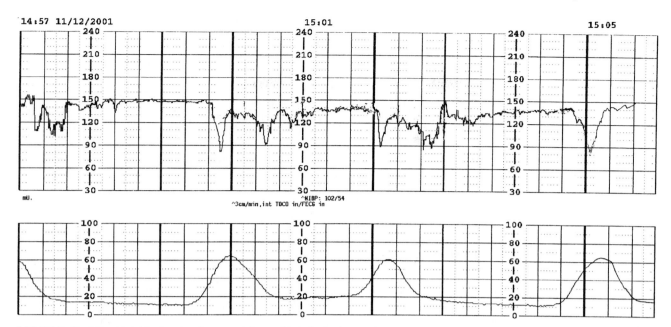

FIGURE 6.52 Variable decelerations. At delivery, this baby had a true knot in its cord. This strip most likely indicates respiratory acidosis in the fetus.

▶ **What acid–base values are associated with mixed acidosis?**[33]

All cord gas values are abnormal.

pH	<7.10	**REDUCED**
Po$_2$	>20 mmHg	**REDUCED**
Pco$_2$	>60 mmHg	**INCREASED**
BD	>10	**INCREASED**

▶ **What FHR monitor strip characteristics indicate mixed acidosis?**

The strip characteristics of the fetus with mixed acidosis might show the following (Fig. 6.53):
- **Absent variability**
- **Variable decelerations**
- **Late decelerations**

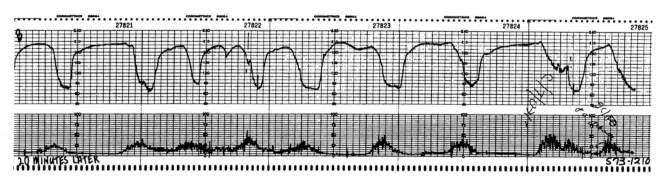

FIGURE 6.53 Mixed acidosis pattern. Note absent variability and variable decelerations. (Reprinted with permission from Freeman, R. K., Garite, T. J., & Nageotte, M. P. [2003]. *Fetal heart rate monitoring* [3rd ed., p. 117]. Philadelphia: Lippincott Williams & Wilkins.)

Interventions

Fetuses whose tracings are nonreassuring require interventions aimed at promoting oxygenation. The health care provider should:

- Change the maternal position to the lateral.
- Administer oxygen per mask at 10 to 12 L per minute.
- Administer a bolus of IV fluids if hypotension is suspected.
- Perform a vaginal examination to determine the status of labor and the estimated time of delivery. During the examination, it may be possible to elicit an acceleration which is a reassuring finding.
- Decrease uterine activity—stop oxytocin (if it is infusing).
- Notify the primary care provider and may need to request presence at bedside for evaluation.
- Document all assessments, interventions, maternal and fetal responses, and communication with the provider in the medical record.

Umbilical Cord Gases

Umbilical arterial cord gases represent the most objective measurements of fetal status at the time of delivery. It has been established that to define an acute intrapartum event sufficient to cause cerebral palsy, there must be evidence of metabolic acidosis in umbilical arterial cord blood obtained at delivery with a ph of less than 7.0 and base deficit of more than 12.[34] It is important to remember that despite having umbilical cord gases consistent with metabolic acidosis, most of these fetuses will develop normally.[35]

It is recommended that umbilical cord gases be obtained in the following clinical situations[35]:

- Cesarean delivery for fetal compromise
- Low 5-minute Apgar score
- Fetus with intrauterine growth restriction
- Abnormal fetal heart rate tracings
- Intrapartum fever
- Multifetal gestations
- Maternal thyroid disease

NOTE: *Both arterial and venous samples should be obtained (if possible) to prevent future debate over whether the specimen obtained was truly an arterial sample.[35]*

Procedure to Obtain Umbilical Cord Blood Samples[35]

- A segment of cord should be obtained and double clamped (one clamp at each end).

NOTE: *Clamped segments of cord and samples drawn up in a heparinized syringe are stable for up to 60 minutes.[36,37]*

- If the 5-minute Apgar score is satisfactory and the infant appears stable and vigorous, the sample does not need to be sent.
- If any concerns/problems persist at or beyond 5 minutes the cord gases should be sent to the laboratory for analysis.
- Be sure that the specimens are *clearly* labeled arterial and venous.

Fetal Heart Dysrhythmias

▶ **How can the presence of a fetal heart dysrhythmia be determined?**

Normally, the electrical impulse that governs heart rate and rhythm originates in the SA node located in the right atrium. Once initiated, the impulse then spreads downward to the atrioventricular (AV) node, the bundle of His, and Purkinje fibers. These impulses cause muscular contraction of the heart. Each part of this electrical system has the capacity for initiating cardiac contraction if the preceding mechanism fails. If abnormalities of the system exist, heart rate can be affected by

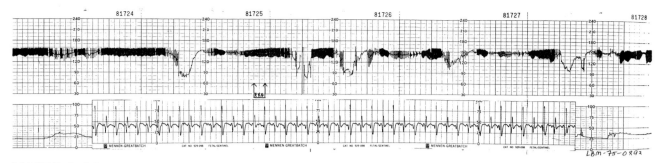

FIGURE 6.54   This tracing shows the fetal heart rate pattern above and fetal electrocardiograph below. (Reprinted with permission from Freeman, R. K., Garite, T. J., & Nageotte, M. P. [2003]). *Fetal heart rate monitoring* [3rd ed., p. 98]. Philadelphia: Lippincott Williams & Wilkins.)

dropped/skipped beats or premature contractions that can cause deviations in cardiac rhythm and rate. Deviations can also occur as a result of cardiac injury. These deviations are called "dysrhythmias." When the diagnosis of a fetal heart rate dysrhythmia is made in the antepartum period, follow-up examinations with ultrasound and fetal echocardiograms should be done to help establish the diagnosis. *The causal mechanism or type of dysrhythmia can be identified only by its characteristics on an ECG* (Fig. 6.54).

Dysrhythmic Patterns

▶ **What types of dysrhythmias are seen in the fetus, and what is their significance to fetal well-being?**

- **Premature atrial contractions (PACs) and premature ventricular contractions (PVCs)**—These are the most common sources of heart rate irregularity in the fetus. They are usually benign and require no intervention. They are not a sign of hypoxia (Fig. 6.55).
- **Supraventricular tachycardia (SVT)**—This is the most commonly encountered tachy-dysrhythmia and should be evaluated carefully because these dysrhythmias are associated with underlying cardiac disease. SVT is usually identified in the second trimester. The rate is often greater than 200 bpm but can exceed 250 bpm and can lead to fetal congestive heart failure, hydrops, and death. Management can include administration of medications such as digoxin, β-blocking agents, or calcium channel blockers to the mother to, hopefully, cause a conversion to a normal rhythm in utero.
- **Heart block**—approximately 50% to 60% of fetuses with complete heart block have mothers who have evidence of connective tissue disease. In mothers who have systemic

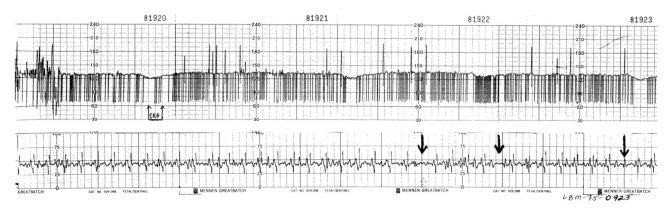

FIGURE 6.55   This tracing shows a series of downward deflections of the fetal heart rate in the upper tracing; the simultaneous fetal electrocardiograph in the lower tracing shows absent QRS complexes or dropped beats. (Reprinted with permission from Freeman, R. K., Garite, T. J., & Nageotte, M. P. [2003]. *Fetal heart rate monitoring* [3rd ed., p. 100]. Philadelphia: Lippincott Williams & Wilkins.)

lupus erythematosus, the antibodies that damage the heart's conduction system can cross the placenta and attack cardiac tissue. When diagnosed prenatally, arrangements need to be made for care of the baby after delivery. This may include the need for a pacemaker. Consultation with a maternal–fetal medicine specialist is recommended to devise a plan of care that includes a recommendation regarding location and mode of delivery.

Characteristics of Dysrhythmia

► What FHR monitor strip characteristics indicate that a dysrhythmia might be present?

The appearance of the tracing with a dysrhythmia is unique. It may have an organized appearance that can help to distinguish it from artifact because artifact tends to have a much disorganized appearance. When a dysrhythmia is suspected, the auscultation should be done to verify the rhythm. Placement of a FSE may also allow for a more accurate recording of the FHR, including the dysrhythmia.

The presence of dysrhythmias makes assessment and interpretation of the fetal monitor strip very challenging. Baseline rate and baseline variability may be impossible to assess accurately.

Summary: Dysrhythmias

Fortunately, most fetal dysrhythmias are benign.

However, it is important to understand that some can be potentially life threatening for the fetus, either during pregnancy or after delivery. The presence of a suspected dysrhythmia must be verified by auscultation of the FHT. The provider should be notified of these findings so that a comprehensive plan of care can be developed.

PRACTICE/REVIEW QUESTIONS

After reviewing Part 4, answer the following questions.

1. Determine the acid–base status demonstrated in the following fetal cord gases. (Acidosis or shift and kind [i.e., metabolic, respiratory, or mixed].)

   a. pH, 7.19; Po_2, 22 mmHg; Pco_2, 70 mmHg; BD, 7

   _____

   b. pH, 7.17; Po_2, 16 mmHg; Pco_2, 81 mmHg; BD, 11

   _____

   c. pH, 7.28; Po_2, 26 mmHg; Pco_2, 40 mmHg; BD, 5

   _____

   d. pH, 7.16; Po_2, 24 mmHg; Pco_2, 78 mmHg; BD, 12

   _____

2. Evaluate the following strips in terms of your expectations of the acid–base status of the fetus.

   a. _____

      _____

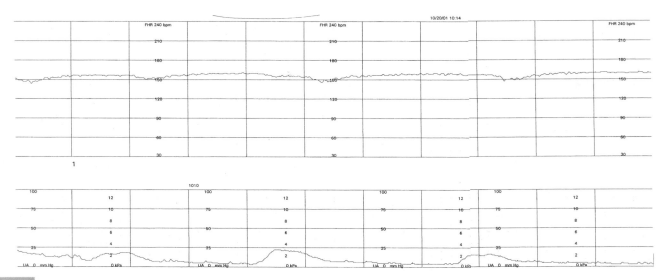

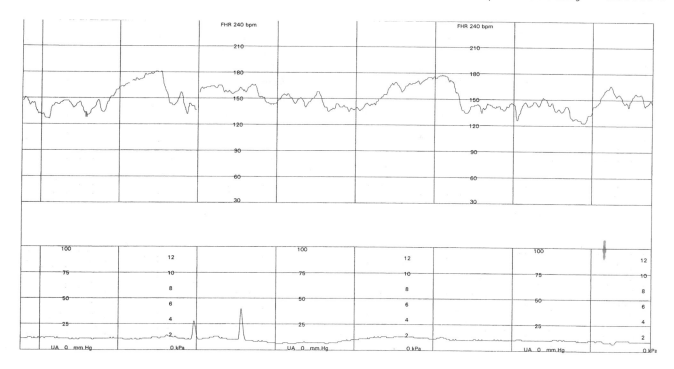

b. _____

_____

3. Describe the necessary interventions if you suspect that a fetus has metabolic acidosis.

a. _____

b. _____

c. _____

d. _____

4. Where would you expect the pH to be lower (more acidic): in the blood or in the tissues?

_____

5. State the identifying characteristic of the fetus with respiratory acidosis.

_____

6. State the identifying characteristic of the fetus with metabolic acidosis.

_____

7. What is the primary cause of metabolic acidosis?

_____

8. What is the primary cause of respiratory acidosis?

_____

9. What is meant by a "shift" toward acidosis?

_____

_____

_____

10. Match the following terms in Column A with their meanings in Column B.

Column A

1. _____ Hypoxia
2. _____ Acidemia
3. _____ Acidosis
4. _____ Hypoxemia
5. _____ pH
6. _____ Po_2
7. _____ Pco_2
8. _____ Base deficit

Column B

a. Used by the body in an attempt to normalize a reduced pH

b. Buildup of acids in the tissues

c. Partial pressure of oxygen

d. Reduced amount of oxygen in the blood

e. Representation of the hydrogen ion concentration

f. Partial pressure of carbon dioxide

g. Buildup of acids in the blood

h. Reduction of oxygen in the tissues

11. Explain the importance of pH in the biologic function of the body.

    _____

    _____

12. If you suspect a fetal cardiac dysrhythmia, how can you confirm this assessment?

    a. _____

    b. _____

13. What is the only definitive method available for diagnosing the kind of dysrhythmia that is present? _____

14. Most fetal dysrhythmias represent grave consequences for the baby when it is born.

    a. True

    b. False

15. What is the most common dysrhythmia, and what are the implications of the dysrhythmia for the fetus?

    _____

    _____

PRACTICE/REVIEW ANSWER KEY

1. a. Respiratory acidosis
   b. Mixed acidosis
   c. Normal
   d. Respiratory acidosis

2. a. Potential for metabolic acidosis—late decelerations, minimal variability
   b. Normal gases—moderate variability and accelerations present

3. a. Administer O_2 per mask at 10 to 12 L per minute.
   b. Place the mother in the lateral position.
   c. Give bolus of IV fluids.

d. Notify the provider (also consider discontinuation of oxytocin if infusing).

4. In the tissues

5. Variable decelerations

6. Absent STV

7. Hypoxia (i.e., insufficient oxygen supply to the fetus)

8. CO_2 buildup

9. A shift toward acidosis means that the pH is normal but other characteristics are present that are associated with developing acidosis. Compensation is possible at this time because reserve is present; however, the body is utilizing necessary resources to maintain a normal pH.

10. 1. h
    2. g
    3. b
    4. d
    5. e
    6. c
    7. f
    8. a

11. The pH of the blood and tissues has an impact on all enzymes and proteins in the body, affecting tissue, enzymes, and organ function.

12. a. Auscultation with a fetoscope
    b. ECG

13. ECG

14. b. False

15. Premature atrial contractions (PACs). They are usually benign and require no intervention.

Documentation

As you complete Part 5 of this module, you will learn:

1. The rationale for complete documentation in the medical record
2. To list the types of documentation systems
3. To describe why documentation on fetal monitor strips is no longer recommended

Documentation

Documentation of the care provided in the intrapartum period is vitally important. The medical record should provide a complete, factual, and objective record of the care provided and include only clinically relevant data. These goals for documentation are much easier to discuss than to accomplish. Concerns related to inaccuracies and omission have forced providers to spend increasing amounts of time *documenting* care rather than *providing* care, which may be frustrating and unsatisfying for both patients and providers. The ideal documentation system should be easy to use, time and cost efficient, and most comprehensive so that it accurately reflects the care provided.

Problem With Inaccurate and Incomplete Documentation

Despite the emphasis that many providers and institutions place on documentation, inaccuracies and omissions remain common. The results of these problems are many and include the following[38]:

- decreased communication among members of the health care team, because an incomplete or inaccurate medical record may be used to plan care
- lost information for both statistical purposes and outcome data for quality surveillance
- denial of reimbursements by insurance carriers, resulting in lost revenue
- during litigation, difficulty for the defense to prove its case because of an incomplete or inaccurate record; additionally, omissions and inaccuracies may leave the impression of a provider who is careless and imprecise

Because litigation may occur several years following an event the medical record is often the only source of information related to the event. Most providers may only have limited recall and have to rely on the information documented in the medical record. A record that is full of omission and inaccuracies is not a very powerful tool. Without a complete medical record, many providers may find themselves in the position of being unable to defend their care.[39,40]

Types of Documentation

Several types of documentation systems may be used to chart care. These include flowsheets (electronic and written), clinical pathways, checklists, narrative notes, and electronic documentation systems. Each system may have benefits, but no one system has been proven to be superior.

Flowsheets

Flowsheets may be either written or electronic. These are a popular choice because they can be customized for each institution. Flow sheets should include information related to the following:

- Fetal assessments
- Maternal assessments
- Nursing interventions
- Response to interventions
- Type of monitoring, external or internal, if EFM is being utilized
- Vaginal examination

- Intake and output
- Procedures—such as artificial rupture of membranes or epidural placement
- Communication with providers

One of the benefits of flowsheets is that use of flow sheets can facilitate timely and accurate documentation.[41] Flowsheets provide a streamlined system that may help to prevent errors, improve quality, and decrease the amount of time spent on documentation.[42] Flow sheets can be designed to include standardized terminology, such as the NICHD recommended terminology related to EFM. The use of standardized terminology is recommended to enhance communication among members of the health care team.[12] This is very important, because communication issues have been identified as one of the most common barriers to teamwork.[43]

Narrative Notes

Narrative notes may be used to document the course of a labor. Narrative documentation can be very time consuming and also may encourage delays in documentation. Use of flowsheets with narrative notes as an adjunct is a very common combination of documentation systems. Commonly, narrative notes are used to clarify or expand on events that are not easily captured in with a flowsheet.

Electronic Systems

The capabilities and usage of electronic documentation systems have expanded over the last decade. In addition to their documentation capabilities, many of these systems also allow for central fetal monitoring surveillance, remote review of the fetal heart rate tracings, and electronic storage of both the fetal monitor tracings and medical records. One of the concerns related to use of this technology is that more time will be spent watching the computer monitors and the amount of time spent at the bedside will decrease. However, if the systems are designed for easy use, they may free the provider from time spent in documentation and allow for increased time at the bedside.

Documentation on the Monitor Strip

Historically, documentation on the FHR monitor strip was recommended because it was generally thought that the monitor strip should contain enough information that it should be able to "stand alone," independent of any other documentation. This practice is no longer recommended for the following reasons[34,41,42]:

- Duplicate documentation increases the amount of time spent documenting care and decreases the amount of time providing care. This is unsatisfying for both patient and providers.
- This practice was thought to encourage a delay in documentation in the medical record.[41]
- It could lead to errors in transcription to the medical record. This could be very problematic, because the information on the fetal monitor strip would not match the information in the medical record.
- If handwritten notes are on a tracing that is electronically stored, the information written on the strip does not become part of the medical record.

Notes recorded on the strip in an emergency do not replace documentation of the event required in the medical record. The strip may be used to reconstruct the timing of the event and interventions, but care should be taken that times documented in the medical record match times on the tracing. Additionally, the documentation of the emergency and the interventions initiated should be recorded in the medical record as soon as possible after the event.

NOTE: Some electronic systems have become very sophisticated and notes entered on the flow sheet are automatically recorded on the fetal monitor strip.

General Guidelines for Institutional Documentation and Continuing Education Related to Fetal Heart Rate

- Use uniform terminology based on national standards and definitions to describe FHR patterns and uterine activity. When all members of the health care team are using the same terminology, it enhances both communication and teamwork.

- Follow written guidelines for documentation. Formulate institutional guidelines with respect to meeting national standards.
- Ensure that *all caregivers and providers* are current in their knowledge of standards, terminology, and interpretation of fetal monitoring by requiring competency validation at set intervals and by providing resources and opportunities for both formal and informal continuing education.
- Encourage staff consultation for nonreassuring and/or questionable patterns. Document these consultations. Good documentation is the best defense available for all staff members if a lawsuit occurs. Make sure correct terminology is used and that it represents a thorough accounting of what occurred during labor, delivery, and recovery.

PRACTICE/REVIEW QUESTIONS

After reviewing Part 5, answer the following questions.

1. List four potential problems with inaccurate and incomplete documentation.

   a. _____

   b. _____

   c. _____

   d. _____

2. List some of the kinds of information that should be included in the medical record.

   a. _____

   b. _____

   c. _____

   d. _____

   e. _____

   f. _____

   g. _____

   h. _____

3. List three types of documentation systems.

   a. _____

   b. _____

   c. _____

4. What are the benefits of a flowsheet?

   _____

   _____

   _____

5. Why is the practice of documenting on the fetal monitor tracing no longer recommended?

   _____

   _____

   _____

PRACTICE/REVIEW ANSWER KEY

1. a. Decreased in communication among members of the health care team
   b. Lost information
   c. Denied reimbursements
   d. Difficult to defend care in litigation

2. Flowsheets, narrative notes, electronic systems

3. a. fetal assessments
   b. maternal assessments
   c. interventions
   d. response to interventions
   e. type of monitoring
   f. vaginal examinations
   g. intake and output
   h. communication with provider
   i. procedures

4. Timely and accurate documentation
   Prevent errors
   Improve quality
   Decrease amount of time spent in documentation

5. It was duplicate documentation.
   It delayed charting in the medical record.
   The potential for transcription errors.
   Handwritten notes on a monitor strip that is stored electronically will not become part of the medical record.

Practice with Strip Graph Interpretation

Objectives

For each of the strip graphs presented, you should be able to:

1. Determine the baseline fetal heart rate and evaluate variability
2. Determine frequency, duration, and intensity of the contraction patterns
3. Determine the baseline tonus of the uterus
4. Correctly identify any periodic heart rate patterns
5. Describe the appropriate treatment for any abnormal tracings
6. Estimate cord gases

For each strip represented, answer the set of questions following the strip. **The monitoring mode for both FHR and contractions is internal unless otherwise stated.**

Practice Strip 1

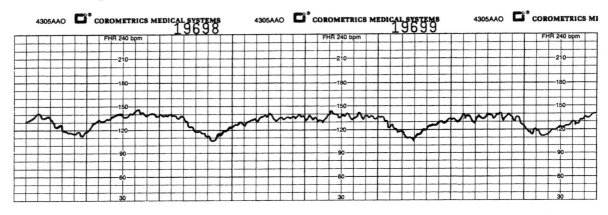

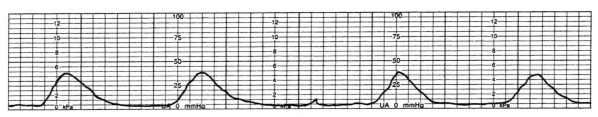

FIGURE 6.56 Practice strip 1.

1. What is the baseline FHR? _____

   Is it within normal limits? _____

2. Describe frequency, duration, and intensity of the contraction pattern.

   Frequency: _____

Duration: _____

Intensity: _____

Is the contraction pattern within normal limits? _____

_____

3. What is the baseline tonus of the uterus? _____

   Is the tonus within normal limits? _____

4. What is the heart rate variability? _____

   Is the variability considered:

   a. Absent

   b. Moderate

   c. Minimal

   d. Unable to be assessed

5. Are any periodic or nonperiodic changes present? _____ If so, are they:

   a. Accelerations

   b. Early decelerations

   c. Variable decelerations

   d. Late decelerations

   e. Prolonged deceleration

6. Based on your interpretation of **practice strip 1,** what treatment, if any, would you administer?

   _____

   _____

7. Estimate blood gas results, if done at this time.

   _____

   _____

Practice Strip 2

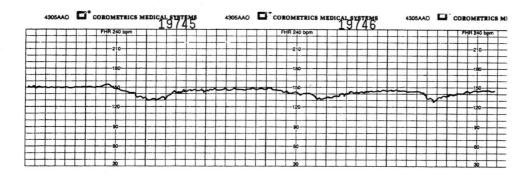

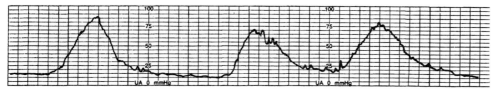

FIGURE 6.57 Practice strip 2.

1. What is the baseline FHR?

   _____

   Is it within normal limits? _____

2. Describe frequency, duration, and intensity of the contraction pattern.

   Frequency: _____

   Duration: _____

   Intensity: _____

   Is the contraction pattern within normal limits?

   _____

3. What is the baseline tonus of the uterus? _____

   Is the tonus within normal limits? _____

4. What is the heart rate variability? _____

   Is the variability considered:

   a. Marked

   b. Minimal

c. Increased

d. Unable to be assessed

5. Are any periodic changes present? _____ If so, are they:

a. Accelerations

b. Early decelerations

c. Variable decelerations

d. Late decelerations

e. Prolonged deceleration

6. Based on your interpretation of **practice strip 2,** what treatment, if any, would you administer?

_____

_____

Practice Strip 3

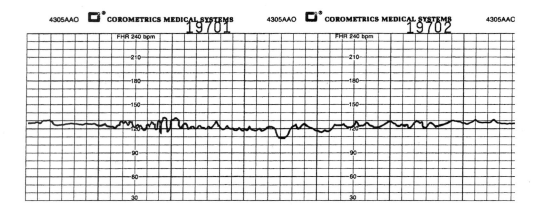

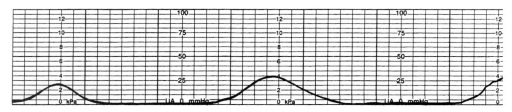

FIGURE 6.58 Practice strip 3.

1. What is the baseline FHR? _____

   Is it within normal limits? _____

2. Describe frequency, duration, and intensity of the contraction pattern.

   Frequency: _____

   Duration: _____

   Intensity: _____

   Is the contraction pattern within normal limits? _____

   _____

3. What is the baseline tonus of the uterus? _____

   Is the tonus within normal limits? _____

4. What is the heart rate variability? _____

   Is the variability considered:

   a. Absent

   b. Minimal

   c. Moderate

   d. Unable to be assessed

5. Are any periodic or nonperiodic changes present? _____ If so, are they:

   a. Accelerations

   b. Early decelerations

   c. Variable decelerations

d. Late decelerations

e. Prolonged deceleration

6. Based on your interpretation of **practice strip 3,** what treatment, if any, would you administer?

_____

_____

7. Estimate fetal blood gases, if done at this time.

_____

_____

Practice Strip 4

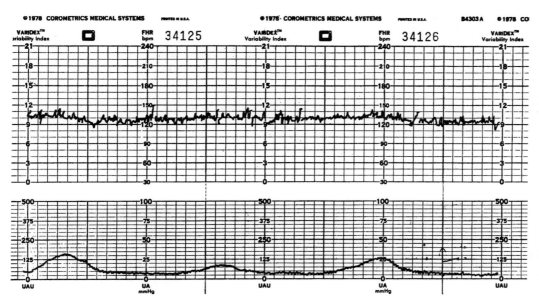

FIGURE 6.59 Practice strip 4.

1. What is the baseline FHR? _____

Is it within normal limits? _____

2. Describe frequency, duration, and intensity of the contraction pattern.

Frequency: _____

Duration: _____

Intensity: _____

Is the contraction pattern within normal limits? _____

_____

3. What is the baseline tonus of the uterus? _____

Is the tonus within normal limits? _____

4. What is the heart rate variability? _____

Is the variability considered:

a. Absent

b. Minimal

c. Moderate

d. Marked

5. Are any periodic or nonperiodic changes present? _____ If so, are they:

a. Accelerations

b. Early decelerations

c. Variable decelerations

d. Late decelerations

e. Prolonged deceleration

6. Based on your interpretation of **practice strip 4,** what treatment, if any, would you administer?

_____

_____

7. Estimate fetal blood gases, if done at this time.

_____

_____

Practice Strip 5

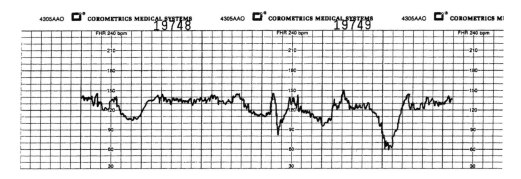

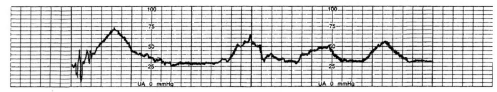

FIGURE 6.60 Practice strip 5.

1. What is the baseline FHR? _____

   _____

   Is it within normal limits? _____

   _____

2. Describe frequency, duration, and intensity of the contraction pattern.

   Frequency: _____

   Duration: _____

   Intensity: _____

   Is the contraction pattern within normal limits? _____

   _____

3. What is the baseline tonus of the uterus? _____

   _____

   Is the tonus within normal limits? _____

   _____

4. What is the heart rate variability? _____

   _____

   Is the variability considered:

   a. Decreased

   b. Normal

   c. Moderate

   d. Unable to be assessed

5. Are any periodic or nonperiodic changes present?

   _____ If so, are they:

   a. Accelerations

   b. Early decelerations

   c. Variable decelerations

   d. Late decelerations

   e. Prolonged deceleration

6. Based on your interpretation of **practice strip 5,** what treatment, if any, would you administer?

   _____

   _____

7. Estimate fetal blood gases, if done at this time.

   _____

   _____

Practice Strip 6

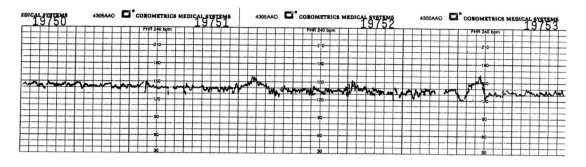

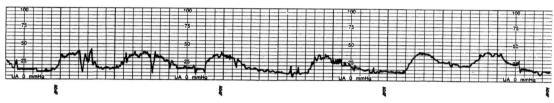

FIGURE 6.61 Practice strip 6.

1. What is the baseline FHR? _____

   _____

   Is it within normal limits? _____

   _____

2. Describe frequency, duration, and intensity of the contraction pattern.

   Frequency: _____

   Duration: _____

   Intensity: _____

   Is the contraction pattern within normal limits? _____

   _____

3. What is the baseline tonus of the uterus? _____

   _____

   Is the tonus within normal limits? _____

   _____

4. What is the heart rate variability? _____

   _____

   Is the variability considered:

   a. Absent

   b. Normal

   c. Moderate

   d. Unable to be assessed

5. Are any periodic or nonperiodic changes present? _____

   _____ If so, are they:

   a. Accelerations

   b. Early decelerations

   c. Variable decelerations

   d. Late decelerations

   e. Prolonged deceleration

6. Based on your interpretation of **practice strip 6,** what treatment, if any, would you administer?

   _____

   _____

7. Estimate fetal acid–base status at this time.

   _____

   _____

Practice Strip 7–External Monitor

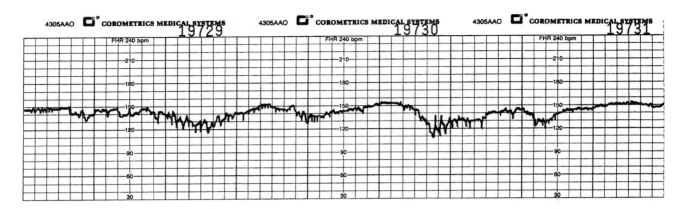

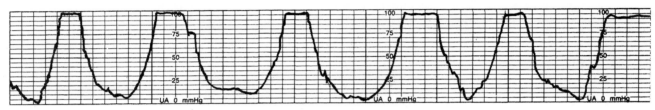

FIGURE 6.62 Practice strip 7 (external monitor).

1. What is the baseline FHR? _____

    _____

    Is it within normal limits? _____

    _____

2. Describe frequency, duration, and intensity of the contraction pattern.

    Frequency: _____

    Duration: _____

    Intensity: _____

    Is the contraction pattern within normal limits? _____

    _____

3. What is the baseline tonus of the uterus? _____

    _____

    Is the tonus within normal limits? _____

    _____

4. What is the heart rate variability? _____

    _____

    Is the variability considered:

    a. Moderate

    b. Minimal

c. Increased

d. Marked

5. Are any periodic or nonperiodic changes present? _____ If so, are they:

    a. Accelerations

    b. Early decelerations

    c. Variable decelerations

    d. Late decelerations

    e. Prolonged deceleration

6. Based on your interpretation of **practice strip 7,** what treatment, if any, would you administer?

    _____

    _____

7. Estimate fetal acid–base status at this time.

    _____

    _____

Practice Strip 8—External Monitor

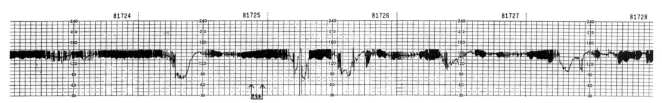

FIGURE 6.63 Practice strip 8 (external monitor).

1. What is the baseline FHR? _____

   _____

   Is it within normal limits? _____

2. What is the heart rate variability? _____

   _____

   Is the variability considered:

   a. Decreased

   b. Normal

   c. Increased

   d. Unable to be assessed and why

3. Are any periodic or nonperiodic changes present?

   _____ If so, are they:

   a. Accelerations

   b. Early decelerations

   c. Variable decelerations

   d. Late decelerations

   e. Prolonged decelerations

4. Based on your interpretation of **practice strip 8,** what treatment, if any, would you administer?

   _____

   _____

5. Estimate fetal acid–base status at this time.

   _____

   _____

6. What do you think is happening in this strip? How would you confirm this?

   _____

   _____

PRACTICE STRIP REVIEW ANSWER KEY

Practice Strip 1

1. 135 bpm
   Yes

2. Frequency: 2 to 3 minutes
   Duration: 50 to 60 seconds
   Intensity: 35 to 40 mmHg
   Yes

3. 3 to 5 mmHg
   Yes

4. c

5. Yes
   b

6. No treatment is necessary. May consider a vaginal examination if this is a new pattern, if it has become more pronounced, or if the woman feels vaginal or perineal pressure, because fetal descent might be occurring. Continue to watch tracing.

7. Within normal limits.

Practice Strip 2

1. 145 bpm
   Yes

2. Frequency: 2 to 3 minutes
   Duration: 70 to 90 seconds
   Intensity: 70 to 85 mmHg
   Yes

3. 10 to 20 mmHg
   Yes

4. a

5. Yes
   d

6. Start oxygen therapy per face mask at 10 L per minute. Turn woman to the lateral position. Administer a bolus of IV fluids. Turn off oxytocin, if on. Notify primary care provider.

Practice Strip 3

1. 125 bpm
   Yes

2. Frequency: 3 to 3½ minutes
   Duration: 60 to 90 seconds
   Intensity: 20 to 30 mmHg
   Yes

3. 0 mmHg
   No; below lower limit (calibrate or replace pressure catheter)

4. b

5. No
   Not applicable

6. Look for cause of decreased variability—medications, and so on. Change maternal position to the side-lying. Perform scalp stimulation—watch for acceleration. If no cause can be isolated and variability does not improve with these interventions, begin oxygen therapy per face mask at 10 L per minute and notify primary care provider.

7. Within normal limits but shift toward metabolic acidosis

Practice Strip 4

1. 130 bpm
   Yes

2. Frequency: 2½ minutes
   Duration: 70 to 80 seconds
   Intensity: 18 to 37 mmHg
   Yes

3. 5 to 10 mmHg
   Yes

4. c

5. No
   Not applicable

6. Possibly vaginal examination to stimulate fetus for better assessment

7. Within normal limits

Practice Strip 5

1. 135 bpm
   Yes

2. Frequency: 1 to 2½ minutes
   Duration: 50 to 70 seconds
   Intensity: 65 to 70 mmHg
   No; hyperstimulation, last three contractions occur too frequently

3. 25 to 30 mmHg
   No; tone is increased, hypertonus

4. c

5. Yes
   c

6. Change position (preferably to the side to attempt to alleviate pressure on the cord, improve perfusion, and decrease contraction frequency). Begin oxygen therapy per face mask at 10 L per minute. Discontinue oxytocin, if infusing, to decrease frequency of contraction pattern and to decrease baseline uterine tone. Notify primary care provider. Perform vaginal examination to assess for cord prolapse. Administer a bolus of IV fluids.

7. Progression to respiratory acidosis; loss of preshoulder with the last deceleration

Practice Strip 6

1. 135 bpm
   Yes

2. Frequency: 1 to 2 minutes
   Duration: 50 to 80 seconds
   Intensity: 35 to 40 mmHg
   No; contractions too frequent, hyperstimulation

3. 10 to 20 mmHg
   Yes

4. c

5. Yes, accelerations

6. No treatment is necessary at this point for fetal heart pattern; however, that could quickly change if this contraction pattern continues. Discontinue oxytocin. Turn the patient

to her side to increase cardiac output, improve uterine perfusion, and decrease the frequency of contractions. Notify the primary care provider.

7. Normal cord pH

Practice Strip 7

1. 140 bpm
   Yes

2. Frequency: 80 to 110 seconds
   Duration: 70 to 90 seconds
   Intensity: cannot interpret without palpating fundus
   No; most of the contractions are too frequent

3. Cannot interpret on external monitor
   Cannot interpret

4. b

5. Yes
   Probably b, but is somewhat difficult to assess

6. No treatment for diagnosis of early decelerations. Consider vaginal examination for assessment of labor progress. Early decelerations and flattening at the top of contractions can indicate fetal descent and pushing. If labor is early or progress is abnormal, consider applying an internal monitor to more accurately assess contraction strength and FHR pattern.

7. Normal cord gases (pH)

Practice Strip 8

1. Difficult to determine based on this strip, appears to be within normal range
   Yes

2. d; unable to assess; because there is almost no portion of the strip that is without dysrhythmia, variability cannot be assessed

3. c

4. Auscultate with a fetoscope, reposition to promote fetal oxygenation, and notify the primary care provider.

5. Variable decelerations. However, because variability cannot be assessed, there is a potential for problems with metabolic acidosis and respiratory acidosis or mixed acidosis.

6. Fetal cardiac dysrhythmia
   Auscultate with a fetoscope and/or obtain a fetal ECG.

R E F E R E N C E S

1. Curtin, S. C., & Park, M. M. (1999). Trend in the attendant, place and timing of births, and in the use of obstetrical interventions: United States, 1989–97. *National Vital Statistics Reports, 47*(27), 1–12.
2. Parer, J. T., & King, T. L. (1999). Whither fetal heart rate monitoring. *Obstetrics, Gynecology and Fertility, 22*(5), 149–192.
3. Thacker, S. B., Stroup, D. F., & Peterson, H. B. (1995). Efficacy and safety of intrapartum electronic fetal monitoring: An update. *Obstetrics and Gynecology, 86*(4, Pt. 1), 613–620.
4. Alfirevic, Z., Devane, D., & Gyte, G. M. L. (2006). Continuous cardiotocography (CTG) as a form of electronic fetal monitoring (EFM) for fetal assessment during labour. *Cochrane Database of Systemic Reviews, 3*, 1–30.
5. Parer, J. T., & King, T. L., (2000). Fetal heart rate monitoring: Is it salvageable? *American Journal of Obstetrics and Gynecology, 182*(4), 982–987.
6. King, T. L., & Simpson, K. R., (2001). Fetal assessment during labor. In Simpson K. R. & Creehan P. A. (Eds.), *Perinatal Nursing*. Philadelphia: Lippincott Williams & Wilkins.
7. Cibils, L. A. (1996). On intrapartum fetal monitoring. *American Journal of Obstetrics and Gynecology, 174*(4), 1382–1389.
8. Morrison, J. C., Chez, B. F., Davis, I. D., Martin, R. W., Robert, W. E., & Martin, J. M. (1993). Intrapartum fetal heart rate assessment: monitoring by auscultation or electronic means. *American Journal of Obstetrics and Gynecology, 168*(2), 63–66.
9. National Institute of Child Health and Human Development Research Planning Workshop. (1997). Electronic fetal heart rate monitoring: Research guidelines for interpretations. *American Journal of Obstetrics and Gynecology, 177*(6), 1385–1390, and *Journal of Obstetrics, Gynecology and Neonatal Nursing, 26*(6), 635–640.
10. Simpson, K. R., & Knox, G. E. (2000). Risk management and EFM: Decreasing risk of adverse outcomes and liability exposure. *Journal of Perinatal and Neonatal Nursing, 14*(3), 44–58.
11. Wood, S. H. (2003). Should women be given a choice about fetal assessment in labor? *MCN, The American Journal of Maternal and Child Nursing, 28*(5), 292–298.
12. American Academy of Pediatrics & American College of Obstetricians and Gynecologists. (2002). *Guidelines for Perinatal Care* (5th ed.). Washington, DC: Author.
13. Feinstein, N., Sprague A., & Trepenier, M. J. (2000). *Fetal Heart Rate Auscultation: Symposium*. Washington, DC: Association of Women's Health, Obstetric and Neonatal Nurses.
14. Society of Obstetrician and Gynecologists of Canada. (1995). Fetal surveillance in labor. *Journal of the Society of Obstetricians and Gynecologists of Canada, 17*, 865–901.
15. Parer, J.T. (1997). *Handbook of Fetal Heart Rate Monitoring* (2nd ed.). Philadelphia: W.B. Saunders.
16. Murray, M. (1997). *Antepartum and intrapartum fetal monitoring* (2nd ed.). Albuquerque, NM: Learning Resources International.
17. Haggerty, L. A. (1999). Continuous electronic fetal monitoring: Contradictions between practice and research. *Journal of Obstetric, Gynecologic and Neonatal Nursing, 28*(4), 409–417.
18. American College of Obstetricians and Gynecologists. (2005). *Intrapartum Fetal Heart Rate Monitoring* (Practice Bulletin Number 70). Washington, DC: Author.
19. Vintzileos, A. M., Nochimson, D. J., Guzman, E. R., Knuppel, R. A., Lake, M., & Schifrin, B. S. (1995). Intrapartum electronic fetal heart rate monitoring versus intermittent auscultation: A meta-analysis. *Obstetrics and Gynecology, 85*(1) 149–155.

20. Freeman, R. K., Garite, T. J., & Nageotte, M. P. (2003). *Fetal Heart Rate Monitoring* (3rd ed.). Philadelphia: Lippincott Williams & Wilkins.

21. Menihan, C. A., & Zottoli, E. K. (2001). *Electronic Fetal Monitoring Concepts and Applications.* Philadelphia: Lippincott Williams & Wilkins.

22. Murray, M. L., & Urbanski, P. (2000). *Essentials of Fetal Monitoring.* Albuquerque, NM: Learning Resources International.

23. Parer, J. T., & Livingston, E. G. (1990). What is fetal distress? *American Journal of Obstetrics and Gynecology, 162*(6) 1421–1425.

24. Low, J. A., Victory, R., & Derrick, E. J. (1999). Predictive value of electronic fetal monitoring for intrapartum fetal asphyxia with metabolic acidosis. *Obstetrics and Gynecology, 93*(2), 285–291.

25. Westgate, J. A., Bennet, L., & Gunn, A. J. (1999). Fetal heart rate variability during brief repeated umbilical cord occlusions in near term fetal sheep. *British Journal of Obstetrics and Gynecology, 106*(7), 664–671.

26. Dellinger, E. H., Boehm, F. H., & Crane, M. M. (2000). Electronic fetal heart rate monitoring: Early neonatal outcomes associated with normal rate, stress and fetal distress. *American Journal of Obstetrics and Gynecology, 182*(1, Pt. 1), 214–220.

27. Larma, J. D., Anadir, M. S., Holcroft, C. J., Thompson, R. E., Donohue, P. K., & Graham, E. M. (2007). Intrapartum electronic fetal heart rate monitoring and the identification of metabolic acidosis and hypoxic-ischemic encephalopathy. *American Journal of Obstetrics and Gynecology, 197*(3), 301–308.

28. Gull, I., Jaffa, A. J., Oren, M., Grisaru, D., Peyser, M. R., & Lessing, J. P. (1996). Acid accumulation during end stage bradycardia: How long is too long? *British Journal of Obstetrics and Gynecology, 103*(11), 1096–1101.

29. Menihan, C. A. (1998). Uterine rupture in women attempting a vaginal birth following prior cesarean birth. *Journal of Perinatology, 18*(6, Pt. 1), 440–443.

30. Kang, A. H., & Boehm, F. H. (1999). The clinical significance of intermittent sinusoidal fetal heart rate patterns. *American Journal of Obstetrics and Gynecology, 180*(1), 151–153.

31. American College of Obstetricians and Gynecologists. (1995). *Dystocia and the Augmentation of Labor* (Technical Bulletin Number 218). Washington, DC: Author.

32. American College of Obstetricians and Gynecologists. (1999). *Induction of Labor* (Practice Bulletin Number 10). Washington, DC: Author.

33. Cypher, R. L., & Adelsperger, D. (2003). Assessment of fetal oxygenation and acid-base status. In Feinstein, N., Torgersen, K. L., & Atterbury, J. (Eds.). *Fetal Heart Monitoring Principles and Practice* (3rd ed) Washington DC: Association of Women's Health, Obstetric and Neonatal Nurses.

34. American College of Obstetricians and Gynecologists. (2006). *Umbilical Cord Blood Gas and Acid-Base Analysis.* (Committee Opinion Number 348). Washington, DC: Author.

35. American Academy of Pediatrics & American College of Obstetricians and Gynecologists. (2003). *Neonatal Encephalopathy and Cerebral Palsy: Defining the Pathogenesis and Pathophysiology.* Elk Grove, IL: American Academy of Pediatrics; Washington, DC: American College of Obstetricians and Gynecologists.

36. Duerbeck, N. B., Chaffin, D. G., & Seeds, J. W. (1992). A practical approach to umbilical artery pH and blood gas determinations. *Obstetrics and Gynecology, 79*(4), 959–962.

37. Strickland, D. M., Gilstrap, L. S., Hauth, J. C., & Widmer, K. (1984). Umbilical cord pH and PCO_2: Effects of interval from delivery to determination. *American Journal of Obstetrics and Gynecology, 148*(4), 191–194.

38. Simpson, K. R., & Chez, B. F. (2001). Professional and legal issues. In Simpson, K. R., & Creehan, P. A. (Eds.). *Perinatal Nursing* (2nd ed). Philadelphia: Lippincott William & Wilkins.

39. Rommel, C. (1996). Risk management issues in the perinatal setting. *Journal of Perinatal and Neonatal Nursing, 10*(3), 1–31.

40. Berry, M. C. (1999). Changes in the nursing environment create new liability exposures. *MMI Advisory, 15*(3), 1–4.

41. Simpson, K. R., & Poole, J. H. (1999). *Cervical Ripening, Induction, and Augmentation of Labor: AWHONN Symposium.* Washington DC: Association of Women's Health, Obstetric and Neonatal Nurses.

42. Chez, B. F. (1997). Electronic fetal monitoring: Then and now. *Journal of Perinatal and Neonatal Nursing, 10*(4), 1–4.

43. Joint Commission on Accreditation of Healthcare Organizations. (2004). *Preventing Infant Death and Injury During Delivery.* Sentinel Event Alert #30. Oakbrook Terrace, IL: Author.

MODULE

7 Induction and Augmentation of Labor

MARCELLA T. HICKEY ■ DONNA JEAN RUTH

Skill Unit 1

Oxytocin Induction and Augmentation

Objectives

As you complete this module, you will learn:

1. The indications for labor induction/augmentation
2. The role of oxytocin in the active management of labor
3. Contraindications for labor induction/augmentation
4. Conditions necessary for the safe administration of oxytocin
5. Preinduction preparation of an "unfavorable" cervix using prostaglandins
6. To anticipate potential problems associated with the use of prostaglandins
7. The recommended method of oxytocin administration
8. To anticipate potential problems of oxytocin administration
9. The recommended nursing interventions when problems arise with the use of oxytocin or prostaglandins
10. The safe method of administering oxytocin for inducing/augmenting labor

Key Terms

When you have completed this module, you should be able to recall the meaning of the following terms. You should also be able to use the terms when consulting with other health professionals. The terms are defined in this module or in the glossary at the end of this book.

active management of labor (AML)   oxytocin
amniotomy   cervical ripening
augmentation   prostaglandins
cephalopelvic disproportion (CPD)   uterine dystocia
induction

Induction and Augmentation of Labor

▶ What is induction of labor?

Induction of labor is the deliberate initiation of uterine contractions before they begin on their own with the goal of a vaginal birth. Induction of labor may be accomplished using a variety of methods, which are discussed later this Module.

▶ What is augmentation of labor?

When uterine contractions are ineffective (not frequent enough or do not have the necessary power to cause cervical dilatation, effacement, or descent of the baby) it may be desirable to augment or increase the contractions to help labor progress.

▶ What is oxytocin?

Oxytocin is a hormone, normally released by the posterior pituitary gland, causing the uterus to contract. Oxytocin is released in response to breast stimulation, cervical stretching, and stimulation of the lower genital tract. Oxytocin released in response to vaginal and cervical stretching results in uterine contractions.[1] Oxytocin is the most common pharmacologic agent used for both induction and augmentation of labor. It is also the hormone responsible for the "let down" of milk from alveolar cells in the breast during the postpartum period.

▶ How does oxytocin function in labor?

Oxytocin increases free intracellular calcium, which is essential for smooth muscle activity. To exert its effect, oxytocin must bind with the oxytocin receptors. Oxytocin receptors in the uterus increase throughout gestation to reach their maximal levels at term.[2] In fact, oxytocin receptors at term are increased 300 times over nonpregnant level. As well as having increased numbers of receptor sites at term, this increase is accompanied by an increase in uterine responsiveness to oxytocin at term.[3] It is interesting to note that although some aspects of oxytocin and its actions are well known, many questions remain to be answered. One question still to be answered is why some women have decreased numbers of oxytocin receptor sites and seem almost "oxytocin resistant."[4]

▶ What is the half-life of oxytocin?

The pharmacokinetic half-life of oxytocin is generally accepted to be between 10 and 15 minutes. Three to four half-lives of oxytocin are needed to reach steady-state plasma concentrations.[5] Uterine response to IV oxytocin administration occurs within 3 to 5 minutes of IV administration, and within 40 minutes steady state plasma level is achieved. This information led Seitchik et al.[6] to recommend at least a 40-minute interval between increases of oxytocin to allow time for the oxytocin to reach steady state and exert it's full effect on the uterus. This dosing regime is intended to prevent women from receiving higher doses of oxytocin than are necessary.[6]

Common Techniques for Induction and Augmentation of Labor

Common methods of inducing or augmenting labor include the following:
- *Amniotomy*—occurs when the membranes are deliberately ruptured. It is used more often for augmentation with women in active labor. It is very successful in multiparous women with cervical dilation of 3 cm or more. For some women, this may be enough stimulation and no other medications are necessary.

Amniotomy is done when the cervix is effaced and dilated. The head of the fetus should be against the lower uterine segment and at least dipping into the pelvis. Rupturing the membranes can cause the uterus to begin contracting, especially if the cervix is favorable.

- **Nipple stimulation**—When the woman stimulates her nipples, oxytocin is released, causing the uterus to contract. Overstimulation of the nipples can result in uterine hyperstimulation, so the contractions should be monitored closely. Nipple stimulation can be accomplished manually by the woman or may be accomplished by application of a warm compress to the breast.
- **Ambulation**—Mild or ineffective uterine contractions may be stimulated by walking. In the upright position, pressure from the presenting part is maintained against the cervix and contractions become more efficient.
- **Stripping membranes**—is less commonly used to induce labor. Stripping the membranes involves separating the membrane from the wall of the cervix and lower uterine segment during a vaginal examination. It is assumed that this action causes a release of prostaglandins and may also stimulate oxytocin release.[7] It appears to be most beneficial in women who are pregnant for the first time and have an unripe cervix at term.[8]
- **Use of oxytocin infusion**—Intravenous administration of oxytocin stimulates the smooth muscle of the myometrium of the uterus to contract. Oxytocin administration is covered in detail in Skill Unit One.

Medical Indications for Induction/ Augmentation of Labor

The following are examples of maternal and fetal conditions that are indications for induction of labor:
- Abruptio placentae
- Preeclampsia/pregnancy-induced hypertension (PIH)

- Maternal disease state—including but not limited to diabetes mellitus, renal disease, chronic pulmonary disease, and chronic hypertension
- Fetal compromise—including but not limited to severe fetal growth restriction or isoimmunization
- Premature rupture of membranes (PROM)
- Chorioamnionitis
- Postterm
- Biophysical profile less than 6 or oligohydramnios
- Intrauterine fetal death (induction of labor can also be accomplished by using prostaglandins)
- *Uterine dystocia*—usually described as poor-quality contractions that do not cause the proper cervical changes
- Prevention of prolonged labors (active management of labor)

Labor may also be induced for logistical reasons, such as history of rapid labor, distance from the hospital or psychosocial indications. In such instances, there should be a frank discussion between the woman and her care provider regarding the risks and benefits of induction. If such an induction is undertaken the following dating criteria should be followed or fetal lung maturity established before the induction begins[9]:

1. Fetal heart tones have been documented for 20 weeks by nonelectric fetoscope or for 30 weeks by Doppler.
2. It has been 36 weeks since a positive serum or urine human chorionic gonadotropin pregnancy test was performed by a reliable laboratory.
3. An ultrasound measurement of crown–rump length, obtained at 6 to 12 weeks' gestation, supports a gestational age of at least 39 weeks.
4. An ultrasound examination performed between 13 and 20 weeks of gestation confirms the gestational age of at least 39 weeks by clinical history and physical examination.

Prerequisites for Induction/Augmentation of Labor

▶ What are some prerequisites for an induction/augmentation to be safe and effective?

The woman should not have any of the contraindications for induction/augmentation. In addition it is recommended that the following occur[9]:

1. Gestational age, cervical status, pelvic adequacy, fetal size, and fetal presentation should be assessed before the administration of any cervical ripening agents or oxytocin.
2. Any potential risk to the mother and fetus should be considered.
3. The medical record should document that a discussion was held between the pregnant woman and her health care provider about the indications, the agents, and the methods of labor induction and cervical ripening, including the risks, benefits, alternative approaches, and the possible need for repeat induction (if first attempt fails) or cesarean delivery.

> Initiating an elective induction of labor for reasons of convenience, although very common, should not be encouraged by health care providers or hospitals.

▶ Can every woman be safely induced/augmented?

No, although induction and augmentation have become a safer procedure for both women and their fetuses, there are some women for whom induction and augmentation carry an unacceptable risk.

Contraindications for Induction/ Augmentation of Labor

Listed in Display 7.1 are clinical situations in which induction/augmentation should not be attempted.[6]

DISPLAY 7.1 CONTRAINDICATIONS TO INDUCTION/AUGMENTATION

Transverse fetal lie
Previous fundal or prior classical uterine incision
Nonreassuring fetal heart rate patterns
Pelvic structural abnormalities
Umbilical cord prolapse
Complete placenta previa
Vasa previa
Active genital herpes infection

- **Transverse fetal lie**—fetus is not in the proper position for delivery and cannot be delivered vaginally.
- **Previous fundal incision or prior classical uterine incision**—contractions induced or augmented might be too powerful and may rupture the scar.
- **Nonreassuring fetal status**—with each contraction of the uterus, there is a normal decrease in blood circulation and oxygen supply to the placenta and baby. Because oxytocin increases the intensity of the contractions, there can be an even greater loss of oxygen to the baby. If the fetus already shows signs of distress, it might not be able to survive the additional intensity of induced/augmented contractions.
- **Pelvic structural abnormalities**—abnormalities in the normal structure of the pelvis prevent a vaginal birth so labor should not be induced.
- **Umbilical cord prolapse**—when the umbilical cord presents before the presenting part, blood flow to the fetus may be compromised. This is an emergency that requires immediate Cesarean delivery.
- **Complete placenta previa and vasa previa**—the cervical os is completely covered by the placenta with a complete placenta previa. This can be a life-threatening condition. Labor should be avoided and the fetus delivered by cesarean birth. A vasa previa occurs when the umbilical arteries and veins cross the cervical os in front of the presenting part. It is a life-threatening complication for the fetus.
- **Active genital herpes infection**—in the presence of an active genital herpetic lesion, a cesarean birth is recommended to prevent transmission to the fetus

Conditions That Require Special Attention During Induction/Augmentation

There are some situations in which induction/augmentation of labor might present problems. These women require careful and close monitoring (Display 7.2).

DISPLAY 7.2 RELATIVE CONTRAINDICATIONS TO INDUCTION/AUGMENTATION

Trial of labor after a previous cesarean
Presenting part not engaged in pelvis
Severe maternal hypertension
Grand multiparity
Multiple gestations
Polyhydramnios
Abnormal fetal heart rate patterns (not requiring emergent intervention)
Maternal heart disease

- **Trial of labor after a previous cesarean birth**—spontaneous labor appears to decrease the risk of uterine rupture in women attempting a vaginal birth after cesarean (VBAC). If induction of labor is done in this situation, a complete discussion of the increased risk of uterine rupture must be documented in the medical record. Prostaglandin preparation for cervical ripening are contraindicated for these women.[10]

- **Presenting part not engaged in pelvis**—there is space between the presenting part and the bony pelvis. With forceful contractions, the bag of waters can rupture and the umbilical cord has room to prolapse. Also, if the presenting part is not engaged, it might indicate that the fetus is too large for the pelvis.
- **Severe maternal hypertension**—control of maternal blood pressure should be the priority before induction of labor is initiated.
- **Grand multiparity**—in a woman who has had several children (five or more), the uterus is more likely to rupture with the powerful contractions caused by the induction/augmentation of labor.
- **Multiple gestations**—caution must be taken to prevent overstimulation of a uterus already overly distended.
- **Polyhydramnios**—the uterus is overly distended and might not respond well. The possibility of an amniotic fluid embolus is increased.
- **Abnormal fetal heart rate patterns** (not requiring emergent birth)—close monitoring of the fetal heart rate is necessary to rapidly identify any deterioration in fetal status.
- **Maternal heart disease**—these women may be induced, but require careful monitoring of maternal hemodynamic status throughout the labor and delivery process.

▶ What is active management of labor?

Active management of labor (AML) is an augmentation protocol used in many institutions as a strategy to decrease cesarean births for labor dystocia. The goal is to establish effective contractions and accomplish a vaginal delivery within 12 hours of admission. Although active management is often considered a high-dose oxytocin protocol, it is really a labor management protocol and oxytocin administration is just one component of a whole program of labor.

The term *active management of labor* is interpreted differently from one institution to another. Many of the protocols are based on the belief that **once labor had been diagnosed, the rate of cervical dilatation should be 1 cm per hour.** This rate of labor progress is actively supported by performing an amniotomy and using oxytocin, when necessary.[11]

The original protocol was developed in Dublin, Ireland, to shorten labor and conserve resources in maternity hospitals. All aspects of their protocol are not included in many U.S. hospitals. The following criteria are used for identification of patients for inclusion in AML protocols.
- Nulliparity
- More than 37 weeks' gestation
- Single fetus in no distress
- Spontaneous labor

Cervical Ripening

Cervical ripening is the process of effecting physical softening in preparation for labor and delivery. A variety of different methods may be used to induce cervical ripening. These include mechanical devices and several different prostaglandin preparations. Before beginning any cervical ripening or induction, assessment of the cervix should be done and a Bishop's score assigned. This score helps to identify those women who would benefit from cervical ripening before beginning an induction of labor.

▶ What is a Bishop's score?

A Bishop's score is a method of evaluating how favorable or "ripe" the cervix is. A vaginal examination is done to evaluate cervical *dilatation, effacement, consistency* (i.e., softness or firmness), and *cervical position,* as well as *station* of the presenting part. The findings are scored on a scale that was developed based on studies of many women undergoing labor induction (Table 7.1). Successful inductions are more likely to occur when a woman's cervix has undergone certain biochemical changes. Based on the findings and using a scoring system for these changes, it is possible to predict which women are the best candidates for labor induction.

TABLE 7.1	BISHOP'S SCORE				
	SCORE[a]				**Subtotals**
	0	**1**	**2**	**3**	
Dilatation (cm)	0	1–2	3–4	5–6	
Effacement (%)	0–30	40–50	60–70	80	
Station (cm)	−3	−2	−1	+1	
Cervical consistency	Firm	Medium	Soft		
Cervical position	Posterior	Midline	Anterior		
				Total	_____

[a] A multiparous woman (one who has delivered a child previously) can best be induced at a score of ≥5. A nulliparous woman (one who has *not* delivered a child previously) can best be induced at a score of ≥7.

> Bishop developed this score based on observations of multiparous women. Over time, it was applied to nulliparous women. Best outcomes for multiparous women are seen with a score of 5 or higher. The nulliparous woman has the best response with a score of 7 or greater.

Mechanical Methods of Cervical Ripening

These methods should be limited to women who have a clear indication for induction and have little or no cervical effacement.[12] The devices used are placed in the endocervical canal by the health care provider. The most common methods include:

Laminaria—made from seaweed and absorbs fluid from the cervical tissues. They absorb fluid from the cervix and vagina, causing the seaweed to swell resulting in mechanical dilation of the cervix and prostaglandin release, which may stimulate contractions.

Synthetic osmotic dilators—made from polymer sponges and soaked in magnesium sulfate. They absorb fluid from the cervix and vagina causing the sponge to swell, resulting in mechanical dilation of the cervix and prostaglandin release.

Foley bulbs—large-gauge Foley catheter balloons are inflated above the internal cervical os using sterile saline or sterile water. The catheter is secured to the maternal leg. The inflated bulb puts direct pressure on the cervix and causes stretching of the lower uterine segment, resulting in prostaglandin release.

> ▶ **If the cervix is not favorable but a woman otherwise meets the criteria for induction, can prostaglandin preparations be used to ripen the cervix?**

There are a variety of prostaglandin preparations that may be used for cervical ripening before the induction of labor. These include both prostaglandin E_2 preparations, such as Prepidil gel and Cervidil vaginal inserts, as well as prostaglandin E_1 preparations such as misoprostol tablets. Health care providers should be aware that use of these preparations may lead to the onset of labor. However, this result is usually not a concern because the intent of the cervical ripening process is to prepare for labor.

> ▶ **What are the potential concerns for the health of the mother and fetus when cervical ripening is achieved with prostaglandin preparations?**

Concerns for the mother include the following:
- Uterine hyperstimulation
- Gastrointestinal upset (e.g., nausea, vomiting, diarrhea)

Concerns for the fetus include the following:

- Fetal heart rate abnormalities—which are usually related to uterine hyperstimulation. The most common abnormalities are late decelerations, variable decelerations, and abnormal baseline rates, either tachycardia or bradycardia.

Contraindications for Cervical Ripening Using Prostaglandin Preparations

Prostaglandins are not recommended in the following situations:

- If labor or oxytocin are contraindicated, prostaglandins for cervical ripening should be avoided.
- The presentation is abnormal.
- Contraction patterns are hyperactive or there is an increase in uterine tone.
- Membranes are ruptured (**gel** contraindicated; **insert** may be placed).
- Placenta previa or unexplained vaginal bleeding occurred during this pregnancy.
- A vaginal delivery is not indicated (e.g., vasa previa or active herpes genitalia).
- There is a nonreassuring fetal heart rate tracing.

Administration of Prostaglandins

▶ **What precautions should be taken to provide safe administration of PGE$_2$ using endocervical or vaginal routes?**

To ensure the greatest safety for mother and fetus, it is recommended that:

- Fetal heart tones and uterine activity be monitored electronically for 20- to 30-minutes to establish baseline assessments before administration.
- After endocervical instillation, the mother should assume a side-lying position for 1 to 2 hours to help prevent leaking of the gel from the endocervix.
- Fetal heart tones and uterine activity should be electronically monitored for at least 2 hours after instillation or placement.
- After placement for a vaginal insert, the mother remains supine for 2 hours and then may ambulate.
- The vaginal insert should be removed with onset of active labor or 12 hours after placement.
- Maternal blood pressure, pulse rate, and temperature should be monitored every 30 minutes for the first hour, then every 4 hours.

GEL PLACEMENT. Proper placement of the gel **in the endocervical canal** just below the internal os (**away from the membranes**) decreases complications. It is placed by a physician or nurse-midwife in the hospital. The appropriate-sized shielded endocervical catheter (10 or 20 mm) is selected and is attached to the prefilled, room temperature Prepidil (dinoprostone 0.5 mg) prostaglandin E$_2$ syringe. Air is expelled from the syringe. With the use of a sterile speculum, the cervix is visualized and the selected catheter is inserted through the external os *into the endocervix* (Fig. 7.1). It is critical to avoid intrauterine placement or placement against the amniotic membranes. Prepidil gel is contraindicated for use with ruptured membranes.[13]

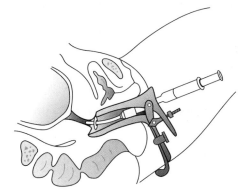

FIGURE 7.1 Prepidil Gel syringe and catheter. Application of gel for preinduction cervical ripening at or near term.

CERVIDIL VAGINAL INSERT (Fig 7.2). Proper placement of the insert (dinoprostone 10 mg, released at 0.3 mg per hour over 12 hours) does not require visualization of the cervix or warming. Remove the insert from the foil package using sterile gloves and a very small amount of K-Y jelly. Place the insert transversely in the posterior fornix (**not in the endocervical canal**). Tuck the end of the retrieval system into lower vaginal space. This may be used with ruptured membranes.[14]

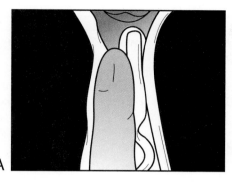

A

The Cervidil Vaginal Insert system is inserted into the vagina, up to the posterior fornix.

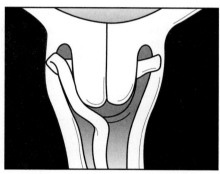

B

The system is left in place, transverse to the posterior surface of the cervix.

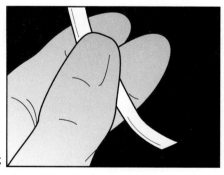

C

The Cervidil Vaginal Insert system can be easily grasped for gentle removal and discontinuation of drug administration.

FIGURE 7.2 Cervidil Vaginal Insert.

▶ **If uterine hyperstimulation, fetal bradycardia, or decelerations in fetal heart rate occur, what actions should the nurse take?**

The woman should be placed on her left side, oxygen administered, uterine and fetal heart rate monitoring continued, and the woman's health care provider notified if no immediate improvement is observed. *If the Cervidil Vaginal Insert is in place, it must be removed.* IV fluids, tocolytic therapy, and cesarean section might be indicated. Specific protocols regarding nursing management of prostaglandin-related emergencies should be developed by each hospital using PGE$_2$ endocervical gel or vaginal inserts.

▶ **Can more than one dose of Prepidil Gel be administered if inadequate ripening occurs?**

A repeat dose of Prepidil Gel 0.5 mg can be administered after 6 hours. The maximum cumulative dose in a 24-hour period is 1.5 mg.[13]

▶ **Can more than one dose of Cervidil Vaginal Insert be administered if inadequate ripening occurs?**

NO. The manufacturer does not currently recommend more than one application of the Cervidil because adequate studies have not been conducted on repeat dosing. Maximum overall time of administration is 12 hours.[14]

▶ **With adequate cervical ripening and no labor, how soon after prostaglandin administration can oxytocin be administered for labor induction?**

It is recommended that 6 to 12 hours lapse between the last dose of Prepidil Gel and starting the IV oxytocin. It is recommended that the Cervidil Vaginal Insert be removed at least 30 minutes before IV oxytocin is started.

Use of Misoprostol for Cervical Ripening

Although not FDA approved for this indication, misoprostol is widely used in many settings for cervical ripening. Misoprostol has been administered intravaginally in the posterior fornix using doses ranging from 50 μg every 6 hours to 25 μg every 3 hours. The higher dosage has been associated with increased incidence of uterine hyperstimulation and nonreassuring fetal heart patterns. When used for cervical ripening, 25 μg placed in the posterior vaginal fornix should be considered for the initial dose.[9] Health care providers should be alert; even with 25 μg intravaginally every 4 hours, uterine hyperstimulation may still occur.[15]

▶ **Are there additional restrictions or concerns for the use of misoprostol?**

It is recommended that the woman be admitted to a hospital where continuous electronic monitoring is available. *Women with a history of prior uterine surgery, including a low transverse cesarean section, should not receive the drug.* Redosing is withheld if, adequate cervical ripening is achieved, the woman enters active labor, or the fetal heart rate is nonreassuring. Hyperstimulation is a common side effect so the health care provider should monitor closely and oxytocin should not be given until 4 hours after the last dose. The medication is only available in 100-μg tablets. It is recommended that the hospital pharmacy prepare the 25-μg tablets before administration.[16]

Recommendations for Safe Use of Misoprostol

To ensure the greatest safety for mother and fetus, it is recommended that *the following be true before administering misoprostol:*

- The Bishop's score is less than 6.
- The woman is experiencing fewer than 12 contractions in an hour.
- The fetus has a reactive nonstress test (RNST) before the drug is placed.
- There is no history of uterine surgery.
- There is no concern for CPD.
- The pharmacist uses a 100-μg tablet and quarters it using a pill cutter to obtain a consistent dose of 25 μg.
- Terbutaline or magnesium sulfate is available if needed to treat hyperstimulation.
- IV access is in place.
- Electronic monitoring is done for 2 hours after each dose is inserted in the vagina.
- If membranes rupture after placement of misoprostol, the labor pattern and fetal response are observed for 2 hours before an additional dose is placed.
- Oral intake is restricted for 2 hours before and after placement.
- The facility has the capability of offering urgent/emergency cesarean delivery.
- Protocols are developed by the department and include guidelines for misoprostol use, evaluation of outcomes, and documentation of adherence to guidelines.

Oxytocin for Induction and Augmentation of Labor

Oxytocin remains the most common pharmacologic agent used to accomplish both induction and augmentation of labor. It is more fully discussed in Skill Unit One.

PRACTICE/REVIEW QUESTIONS
After reviewing this module, answer the following questions.

1. Define *induction of labor.*

   _____

   _____

2. Define *augmentation of labor.*

   _____

   _____

3. What are four common ways to induce or augment labor?

   a. _____

   b. _____

   c. _____

   d. _____

4. Oxytocin is a _____ secreted by the _____ gland. Oxytocin causes the uterus to _____.

5. Using commercially prepared FDA-approved products, how is PGE_2 administered?

   _____

6. Why is it necessary to carefully control the rate of oxytocin administration?

   _____

   _____

7. Describe the best way to administer oxytocin so that the rate of administration is controlled.

   _____

   _____

8. List at least five medical indications for the induction or augmentation of labor.

   a. _____

   b. _____

   c. _____

   d. _____

   e. _____

9. What should be considered when a woman requests an induction for reasons of convenience?

   _____

   _____

10. Why are some institutions implementing active labor management protocols?

    _____

    _____

11. List four criteria used to select women who might benefit from active labor management.

    a. _____

    b. _____

    c. _____

    d. _____

12. List at least five additional concerns of adverse effects for the mother who is experiencing induction/augmentation of labor.

    a. _____

    b. _____

    c. _____

    d. _____

    e. _____

13. List at least three concerns of adverse effects for the fetus during induction/augmentation.

    a. _____

    b. _____

    c. _____

14. List four situations that are absolute contraindications for induction of labor.

    a. _____

    b. _____

    c. _____

    d. _____

15. What are relative contraindications to induction of labor?

    _____

16. List four relative contraindications to the induction/augmentation of labor.

    a. _____

    b. _____

    c. _____

    d. _____

17. List at least three prerequisites for a safe and effective induction/augmentation.

    a. _____

    b. _____

    c. _____

18. What is Bishop's score used to determine?

    _____

19. Mrs. J. is being assessed for induction of labor. Her cervix is dilated 1.5 cm and is 60% effaced. The vertex is at −1 station, cervical consistency is medium, and cervical position is midline. What is her Bishop's score?

    _____

20. Match the definitions in Column B with the items in Column A.

    Column A

    1. _____ Labor
    2. _____ Complete placenta previa
    3. _____ Hypertonic uterus
    4. _____ Premature rupture of membranes
    5. _____ Used to evaluate cervical status

    Column B

    a. Bishop's score
    b. Indication for induction
    c. Contraindications to induction/augmentation
    d. Uterine contractions causing desired changes to cervix
    e. Relative contraindications to induction/augmentation
    f. Too rapid birth

21. Oxytocin should always be administered using:

    _____.

22. What evaluative/assessment technique is strongly recommended when using oxytocin?

    _____

23. List three items to be included in the written procedures for oxytocin administration?

    a. _____

b. _____

c. _____

24. List at least two concerns of effects for the fetus during preinduction cervical ripening.

    a. _____

    b. _____

25. Which one of the following dosages of misoprostol is recommended in the ACOG Committee Opinion?

    a. 50 μg every 6 hours in the posterior vaginal fornix
    b. An initial dose of 25 μg in the posterior vaginal fornix
    c. 50 μg every 6 hours by mouth
    d. 25 μg every 3 hours in the posterior vaginal fornix

26. The ACOG Committee Opinion on the use of misoprostol indicates that it is not recommended for women with a history of a low transverse cesarean section.

    a. True
    b. False

PRACTICE/REVIEW ANSWER KEY

1. Deliberately starting uterine contractions before they begin on their own

2. The act of helping increase contractions that have already started on their own

3. a. Amniotomy
   b. Use of oxytocin
   c. Ambulation
   d. Nipple stimulation

4. Hormone; posterior pituitary; contract

5. Instilled into the endocervical canal or placed in the posterior fornix of the vagina

6. Because it causes more powerful and frequent contractions than normal

7. Using an IV catheter in the arm, with a two-bottle system and the fluid flow rate controlled by an infusion control pump

8. Any five of the following:
   a. Life-threatening vascular disease
   b. Preeclampsia
   c. Rh incompatibility
   d. Diabetes
   e. Premature rupture of membranes
   f. Chorioamnionitis

g. Postterm
h. Intrauterine fetal death
i. Uterine dystocia
j. History of rapid labor
k. Living a great distance from hospital or having psychosocial problems
l. Prevention of prolonged labor
m. Biophysical profile less than 6 or oligohydramnios

9. An induction for convenience may not be supported when evaluated in terms of maternal and/or fetal risk.

10. In an attempt to decrease the rate of cesarean deliveries for dystocia

11. a. Nulliparity
    b. More than 37 weeks' gestation
    c. Single fetus in no distress
    d. Spontaneous labor

12. Any five of the following:
    a. Hypertension or stroke
    b. Postpartum hemorrhage
    c. Embolism (amniotic fluid embolism)
    d. Too-rapid birth
    e. Lacerations to vagina, vulva, perineum, and rectum
    f. Water intoxication
    g. Increased fear

13. Any three of the following:
    a. Hypoxia
    b. Bradycardia
    c. Increased trauma
    d. Bilirubinemia

14. Any four of the following:
    a. Cephalopelvic disproportion
    b. Some previous uterine surgical procedures
    c. Severe fetal distress
    d. Soft tissue masses
    e. Lack of willingness
    f. Central or total placenta previa

15. Conditions that *might* or *might not* present severe problems for mother and baby

16. Any four of the following:
    a. Unfavorable cervix
    b. Presenting part not engaged in pelvis

c. Abnormal presentation
d. Grand multiparity
e. Multiple gestation
f. Hydramnios
g. Hypertonic or incoordinate uterus
h. Maternal exhaustion
i. Previous classical uterine incision

17. a. The woman should not have any of the contraindications for induction/augmentation.
    b. Gestational age of the fetus should be accurate.
    c. The woman's health care provider should supervise the procedure.

18. Whether the cervix is "favorable" for induction

19. 7

20. 1. d
    2. c
    3. e
    4. b
    5. a

21. An infusion pump

22. Fetal/uterine monitoring

23. Any three of the following:
    a. Evaluation of cervical effacement and dilatation before administration
    b. Immediate availability, during administration, of a physician who has privileges to perform cesarean surgery
    c. Use of an IV catheter, infusion pump, two-bottle system
    d. Maximum concentration of solution and maximum rate of administration
    e. Monitoring of contractions, flow rate, and blood pressure at least every 30 minutes

24. Any two of the following:
    a. Hypoxia
    b. Heart rate abnormality
    c. Sepsis

25. b. An initial dose of 25 µg in the posterior vaginal fornix

26. a. True

SKILL UNIT 1 | OXYTOCIN LABOR INDUCTION/AUGMENTATION

This skill unit instructs you on how to set up for an induction/augmentation of labor with oxytocin, how to identify the appropriate equipment needed, and how to regulate the infusion.

Remember, induction or augmentation with oxytocin is a procedure that stimulates regular uterine contractions. The procedure must *always* be ordered by the health care provider managing the woman's labor. There must be no absolute contraindications present for the induction/augmentation to proceed.

After you study this section, your preceptor should demonstrate the procedure and then give you an opportunity to demonstrate your skill.

Please remember that types of equipment and supplies vary from hospital to hospital, depending on the manufacturer and surgical supply houses used.

Administration of Oxytocin

▶ What is the recommended method of oxytocin administration?

Oxytocin should always be administered as a secondary infusion. There should be a mainline IV that does not contain medications with the oxytocin "piggybacked" into this mainline. Oxytocin infusions should always be controlled using an infusion pump. This IV set up allows the provider to discontinue the oxytocin infusion while allowing the mainline infusion to continue.

> INFUSION CONTROL PUMPS. Pumps provide a very carefully controlled flow of fluids. Many models are available on the market. It is critical to be aware of the manufacturer's guidelines for operation.

Every hospital should have written protocols or guidelines for oxytocin infusions that include:
- Evaluation of the patient by a physician or a nurse qualified to assess the woman before administration of oxytocin.
- Immediate availability, during oxytocin administration, of a physician qualified to perform a cesarean delivery should problems arise.
- Documentation of fetal heart rate, resting uterine tone, frequency and characteristics of contractions, oxytocin dosage, and maternal vital signs. Frequency of assessments is based on risk assessments and stage of labor (continuous electronic fetal monitoring is recommended).
- Guidelines for maximum dosage and interval for increases for both induction and augmentation.

> MULTIPLE PROTOCOLS FOR OXYTOCIN ADMINISTRATION EXIST. IT IS ESSENTIAL FOR EACH INSTITUTION TO HAVE GUIDELINES FOR INDUCTION, AUGMENTATION, OR ACTIVE MANAGEMENT OF LABOR THAT ARE SPECIFIC FOR THE INSTITUTION.

> COMPREHENSIVE PROTOCOLS THAT ADDRESS NURSING RESPONSIBILITY IN OXYTOCIN ADMINISTRATION SHOULD INCLUDE CRITERIA FOR PATIENT SELECTION, RESPONSIBILITY FOR AND INFORMATION TO BE COVERED IN THE INFORMED CONSENT, DRUG PREPARATION AND ADMINISTRATION, PATIENT MONITORING, POTENTIAL SIDE EFFECTS, AND THERAPEUTIC GOALS.

ACTIONS	REMARKS

Assemble the Equipment

Set up mainline IV. Connect the infusion with the oxytocin to the port most proximal (closest) to the patient.

Piggyback setups vary from hospital to hospital, depending on IV products used. Refer to your hospital procedure manual for recommended procedures for piggyback infusions.

Mainline IV fluid

Solution should be a balanced solution (lactated Ringer's or 0.9% sodium chloride). Discourage the routine use of glucose-containing solutions.

1,000 mL of aqueous solution without medication

To decrease the possibility of water intoxication, avoid use of D_5W.

10 units of oxytocin in a 1,000-mL solution
20 units of oxytocin in a 1,000-mL solution
15 units of oxytocin in a 250-mL solution
Filter needle (for use if oxytocin is drawn from a glass ampule)

The labor unit protocols need to specifically state which dilution is to be used.

If the pharmacy does not supply prepackaged bags of oxytocin. The filter needle is then exchanged for another regular needle to add oxytocin to the IV solution.

Infusion control pump (Fig. 7.3)

Need to be familiar with the operation of the infusion control pump.

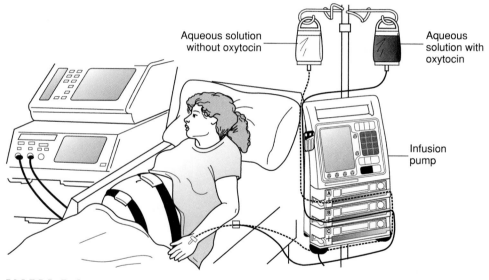

Aqueous solution without oxytocin

Aqueous solution with oxytocin

Infusion pump

FIGURE 7.3 Infusion control pump: setup for oxytocin administration.

Prepare for IV Administration

Obtain informed consent.

The woman must give permission with full awareness of the effects and side effects to herself and her baby. She needs your support and encouragement.

Start IV infusion. Use aqueous solution without oxytocin.
Set flow rate at 125 mL/h.
Apply external fetal and uterine monitor.

The woman must be evaluated before drug administration.
This provides the woman with adequate hydration.
The monitor can be external or internal. **Do not start oxytocin in the presence of a nonreassuring strip.**

Record baseline fetal heart rate and uterine contraction information for 20 minutes before administration of medication. Maternal temperature, pulse, respirations, blood pressure should be assessed before the administration of medication.

Document all findings in the medical record. Follow up with health care provider if there are any deviations from normal parameters.

Start the Administration of Oxytocin

Connect the oxytocin infusion to the pump and start the piggyback infusion.

Adjust the dose until satisfactory contractions are established.

The woman's health care provider should order the initial dose. Maximum dose and interval of dose increases should be according to institutional guidelines (Table 7.2).

Evaluate fetal and uterine response before all dose increases. As the uterus begins to contract and the cervix starts to dilate, the dose might need to be adjusted. The process of titrating oxytocin dosage is dynamic—assessment of the fetal heart rate, contraction pattern, and progress in labor guide the titration of the medication.

Discontinuing Oxytocin Infusions

Discontinue oxytocin in the presence of
- Nonreassuring fetal heart rate patterns
- Contractions that are more frequent than every two minutes
- Contractions that last >90 seconds
- Uterine resting tone that is not relaxed to palpation

Notify the health care provider of nonreassuring fetal status.

Often these problems are related to uterine hyperstimulation and resolve with decreasing or discontinuing the oxytocin infusion.

Record the Procedure

> Documentation is required and should be according to institutional and unit guidelines

Document in the medical record the following:
- date and time for each entry
- vital signs
- fetal heart rate
- resting uterine tone
- frequency, duration, and intensity of contractions and response to contractions
- vaginal findings: dilatation, effacement, station
- oxytocin infusion rate
- mainline IV infusion rate
- fluid intake and output

Uterine Hyperstimulation

Uterine hyperstimulation is the most common complication of induction and augmentation of labor, yet much confusion exists regarding what defines excessive uterine activity. Uterine hyperstimulation, tachysystole, and hypertonus are all terms that may be used in reference to excessive uterine activity. Common themes emerge when reviewing definitions of uterine hyperstimulation and include the frequency of contractions, duration of contractions, and the resting tone of the uterus between contractions. Some definitions of uterine hyperstimulation exist that require evidence of a nonreassuring fetal response before uterine activity can be labeled as excessive. Such definitions may not be appropriate; it may encourage increases in oxytocin dosage **until** there is a nonreassuring fetal response. Each institution should develop clinical guidelines that include a clear definition of uterine hyperstimulation and the expected interventions to be initiated when excessive uterine activity is noted.

You will need to attend a skill session(s) to practice this skill with the help of your preceptor. Mastery of the skill is achieved when you can do the following:
- Assemble all of the necessary equipment
- Prepare the IV solution administration setup including the mainline and piggyback infusions
- Regulate the oxytocin dose, using the infusion pump
- Apply the fetal and uterine monitor and interpret the findings
- Document findings and observations according to unit and hospital standards

TABLE 7.2 OXYTOCIN CONVERSIONS

Rate (mU/min)	SOLUTION CONCENTRATION		
	10 U Oxytocin/1,000 mL (10 mU/mL) (mL/hr)	20 U Oxytocin/1,000 mL (0 mU/mL) (mL/hr)	15 U Oxytocin/250 mL (60 mU/mL) (mL/hr)
0.5	3	1.5	0.5
1	6	3	1
2	12	6	2
3	18	9	3
4	24	12	4
5	30	15	5
6	36	18	6
7	42	21	7
8	48	24	8
9	54	27	9
10	60	30	10
11	66	33	11
12	72	36	12
13	78	39	13
14	84	42	14
15	90	45	15
16	96	48	16
17	102	51	17
18	108	54	18
19	114	57	19
20	120	60	20

Adapted with permission from Poziac, S. (1999). Induction and augmentation of labor. In L. K. Mandeville & N. H. Troiano (Eds.). *High-risk and critical care intrapartum nursing* (2nd ed., pp. 139–158). Philadelphia: Lippincott Williams & Wilkins.

REFERENCES

1. Association of Women's Health, Obstetric and Neonatal Nurses. (2002). *Cervical ripening and induction and augmentation of labor* (2nd ed.). Washington, DC: Author.
2. Kimura, T., Takemura, M., & Nomura, S. (1996). Expression of oxytocin receptors in human pregnant myometrium. *Endocrinology, 137*, 780–785.
3. Fuchs, A.R., Periyasamy, S., & Alexandrova, M. (1983). Correlation between oxytocin receptor concentration and responsiveness to oxytocin in the pregnant rat myometrium. *Endocrinology, 113*, 743–749.
4. Smith, J., & Merrill, D. (2006). Oxytocin for induction of labor. *Clinical Obstetrics and Gynecology, 49*(3), 594–608.
5. Stringer, J. L. (1996). *Basic concepts in pharmacology*. St. Louis: McGraw-Hill.
6. Seitchik, J., Amico, J., Robinson, A. G., & Castillo, M. (1984). Oxytocin augmentation of dysfunctional labor. IV Oxytocin pharmacokinetics. *American Journal of Obstetrics and Gynecology, 150*, 225–228.
7. Norwitz, E. R., Robinson, J. N., & Repke, J. T. (2002). Labor and birth. In Gabbe, S. G., Niebyl, J. R., & Simpson, J. L. (Eds.). *Obstetrics: Normal and problem pregnancies* (4th ed.). New York: Churchill-Livingstone.
8. Krammer, J., & O'Brien, W. F. (1995). Mechanical methods of cervical ripening. *Clinical Obstetrics and Gynecology, 38*, 280–286.
9. American College of Obstetricians and Gynecologists. (1999). *Induction of labor* (Practice Bulletin No. 10). Washington, DC: Author.
10. American College of Obstetricians and Gynecologists. (1999). *Vaginal birth after previous cesarean birth* (Practice Bulletin No. 5) Washington, DC: Author.
11. Socol, M. L., & Peaceman, A. M. (1999). Controversies in labor management: Active Management of Labor. *Obstetrics and Gynecology Clinics, 26*(2), 287–294.
12. Ramsey, P. S., Ramin, K. D., & Ramin, S. M. (2000). Labor induction. *Current Opinions in Obstetrics and Gynecology, 12*, 463–473.
13. Upjohn Company. (1987). Prepidil gel. Kalamazoo, MI: Author.
14. Forest Pharmaceuticals. (1995) Cervicil. St. Louis, MO: Author.
15. American College of Obstetricians and Gynecologists. (1999). *Induction of labor with misoprostol* (Committee Opinion No 228). Washington, DC: Author.
16. Wing, D. A., & Paul, R. H. (1999). Misoprostol for cervical ripening and labor induction: The clinician's perspective and guide to success. *Contemporary OB/GYN, 44*(4), 46–61.

M O D U L E

8

Caring for the Woman at Risk for Preterm Labor or With Premature Rupture of Membranes

ELIZABETH A. FRITZ ■ NANCY WEBSTER SMITH

Objectives

As you complete this module, you will learn:

1. The definition of *preterm labor*
2. Strategies to identify women at risk for preterm labor
3. The limitations of risk appraisal
4. How to recognize and treat early symptoms of preterm labor
5. Care-seeking behaviors of expectant women
6. Management of preterm labor, including the following:
   a. Indications
   b. Contraindications
   c. Pharmacologic agents
   d. Nursing implications
   e. Controversies
7. The side effects of tocolytic agents and initiation of appropriate supportive measures
8. Appropriate education and counseling for women at risk for preterm labor to enhance their chances of delivering a mature infant
9. Decision making in telephone triage
10. The definition of *premature rupture of membranes*
11. Risks to the mother and fetus associated with premature rupture of membranes
12. Management methods when premature rupture of membranes occurs in a term pregnancy
13. Management methods when premature rupture of membranes occurs in a preterm pregnancy, including the following:
    a. Chorioamnionitis
    b. Expectant management options
    c. The role of antibiotics for these patients
14. Priorities for nursing interventions in caring for the woman with premature rupture of membranes
15. The role of steroid therapy in the prevention of neonatal complications

Key Terms

When you have completed this module, you should be able to recall the meanings of the following terms. You should also be able to use the terms when consulting with other health professionals. The terms are defined in this module or in the glossary at the end of this book.

17-α-hydroxyprogesterone
  caproate (17P)
Bacterial vaginosis
β-adrenergic agonist
β-adrenergic receptor
Braxton Hicks contractions
Chorioamnionitis
Corticosteroid
Corticotropin-releasing hormone
  (CRH)

Fetal fibronectin (fFN)
Home uterine activity monitoring
Late preterm birth
Premature rupture of membrane (PROM)
Preterm birth
Preterm premature rupture of membranes
  (preterm PROM)
Prostaglandins
Tocolytic therapy
Very preterm birth

This module reviews current information regarding preterm labor and premature rupture of membranes. Continuing research is constantly changing our understanding of the process leading to these events. There is very little evidence that any of the medical strategies or behavioral interventions that have been widely used in the past 20 years have had any significant impact on the prevention of preterm labor or reduction in the number of preterm births. The clinician must stay informed of the current evidence so that the health care provider can base practice decisions on proven strategies, better utilize resources, and avoid potentially harmful interventions.

Epidemiology of Preterm Labor[1]

Despite the millions of dollars spent on research related to preterm labor and the development of programs to prevent preterm birth, the incidence of preterm birth in the United States continues to rise. A *preterm birth* is defined as the delivery of an infant at less than 37 weeks of gestation. The incidence of preterm birth in the United States has increased from 9.6% of all live births in 1983 to 12.5% of all live births in 2004. In fact, in 2004, one out of eight babies was born preterm. *Late preterm births*, or infants delivered between 34 and 36 weeks of gestation, account for approximately 8.9% of all preterm deliveries and this is a 15% increase in the past 10 years alone. *Very preterm births* have been defined as infants delivering before 32 completed weeks of gestation. These births account for 2% of all preterm births.

The majority of preterm births are to mothers at the age extremes, either older than 35 years or younger than 20 years. When statistics are further broken down by race, major differences are also present. From 2002 to 2004, African-American preterm births accounted for the greatest number of preterm births, at 17.8% of all preterm births. Caucasian preterm births occurred at a rate of 11.3% and Hispanic preterm births at a rate of 11.8%. The preterm birth rate for Native Americans was 13.4%. Asian preterm births occurred at the lowest rate of 10.5%.

Preterm deliveries account for at least 85% of all perinatal morbidity and mortality. The very preterm deliveries are the most costly. In the United States in 2004, the estimated cost to society for preterm births, including medical expenditures, lost wages, and educational expenses, amounted to approximately $26.2 billion.

► **How is preterm labor defined?**

There are essentially three types of preterm births:
- Medically indicated preterm births for maternal or fetal reasons
- Preterm births due to preterm premature rupture of membranes
- Preterm births due to spontaneously occurring preterm labor

In this section, spontaneously occurring preterm labor, which accounts for approximately 50% of preterm births, is discussed. Spontaneous preterm labor is usually defined as regular uterine contractions occurring between 20 and 37 weeks of gestation that are accompanied by one or more of the following:

- Progressive cervical change (cervical dilatation or effacement changes detected by serial examination)
- Cervical dilatation of 2 cm or more
- Cervical effacement of 80% or more

Another definition sometimes used for research purposes includes contractions occurring between 20 and 36 weeks of gestation at a rate of four in 20 minutes with at least one of the following:

- Cervical change over time
- Dilation of 2 cm or more

> These definitions, although important, do not always predict which women will deliver prematurely. In many women with presumptive preterm labor and even hospitalization for this preterm labor, preterm delivery will not occur.[2]

In recent years, efforts have been made to develop diagnostic tests that reliably differentiate between "true" and "false" labor, between preterm labor that will lead to delivery and preterm contractions. If clinicians could use standardized criteria to more accurately identify those women truly at risk for having a preterm delivery, they could significantly reduce unnecessary hospitalizations and medical treatments, as well as the stress related to these interventions. To find such tests, the pathophysiology of preterm labor and the risk factors associated with it have to be examined and better understood.

Pathophysiology of Preterm Labor

The physiology of the onset of labor in humans at term or preterm is not fully understood. However, there are four main pathways currently being researched in an effort to explain why some women deliver before full term. The ultimate cause of an early delivery is most likely some combination of these physiologic pathways.

Inflammation and Infection

Infection and inflammation are associated with the maternal or fetal cytokine response, which in turn produces prostaglandins and can stimulate the breakdown of fetal membranes.[3] Prostaglandins are key components to the labor process. They not only increase the number of contractions by stimulating the influx of calcium ions into smooth muscle cells, but they also improve coordination of uterine muscle contraction by increasing the number of gap junctions between the individual myometrial (uterine muscle) cells. Prostaglandins are also important to cervical ripening because they are used in the production of proteases necessary for this ripening.[4]

It is still unclear exactly how infection and inflammation in particular can lead to preterm deliveries, but the infectious process has been strongly linked in many studies to preterm deliveries, especially very preterm deliveries. Of the births that occur at less than 30 weeks of gestation, about 80% can be linked to chorioamnionitis or some infectious organism in the placental membrane. Unfortunately, practically every vaginal organism has been tied to a preterm delivery in at least one study. Treating these organisms associated with both lower and upper genital tract infections does not consistently prevent preterm birth. The more infectious causes are studied, the less likely it seems that vaginal colonization with any *one* organism, other than bacterial vaginosis, is associated with a preterm delivery.[5]

Bacterial vaginosis, the most commonly diagnosed vaginal infection in women of child-bearing age, is the only organism consistently connected to preterm births in studies. This infection is especially prevalent in African-American women. And, in studies, women who had bacterial vaginosis were two times more likely to have a spontaneous preterm birth, especially one precipitated by rupture of membranes. Despite this information, most trials have failed to show with any statistical significance, that the treatment of bacterial vaginosis can prevent preterm birth.[5] For this reason, the American College of Obstetricians and Gynecologists (ACOG) does not recommend routine screening for bacterial vaginosis to prevent preterm birth. However, women who are symptomatic and diagnosed with bacterial vaginosis should be treated appropriately for this infection.[6]

Maternal or Fetal Stress

It has been suggested that stress stimulates the maternal–fetal hypothalamic–pituitary–adrenal axis. This, in turn can cause increased production of corticotropin-releasing hormone (CRH). CRH is linked to cytokine release and prostaglandin production, which can facilitate uterine contractions. Abnormal or early elevations of these hormone levels in maternal plasma have been documented in preterm labor. However, studies have not consistently shown the connection between stress, increased levels of CRH, and preterm deliveries.[7] Further studies are needed to explain how stress may affect different women or why some women in very stressful situations still deliver at term.

Decidual Hemorrhage or Abruption

This pathway involves disruption in uterine tone as well as the initiation of the coagulation cascade, ensuring the increased production of thrombin. This thrombin production encourages cervical ripening, uterine contractions, and a breakdown of the membranes resulting in premature rupture of the fetal membranes.[3]

Mechanical Stretch of the Uterus

This pathway explains why multifetal pregnancies or the development of polyhydramnios can lead to preterm delivery. The abnormal uterine stretching can stimulate prostaglandin production, thereby creating contractions.

Risk Assessment for Preterm Labor

Even though there is no specific mechanism to accurately identify women who will experience preterm labor, certain factors appear to increase the risk for its occurrence. Most preterm birth prevention programs have been based on risk assessment tools designed to identify women at risk for preterm labor, with specific interventions aimed at reducing identified risk factors. Most of these programs have proven ineffective at reducing the rate of preterm birth. Risk assessment tools have had low detection rates, especially for primigravid women, and seem to be population specific. Until the cause of preterm birth is better understood, it will be difficult to improve the detection rate of risk assessment tools.

In most cases, the cause of preterm labor is probably related to an interplay of various factors related to socioeconomic status, clinical history, and behavioral and biologic factors.

DISPLAY 8.1 RISK FACTORS ASSOCIATED WITH PRETERM LABOR

DEMOGRAPHIC RISKS

Maternal age ≤20 or ≥35 years
African-American race
Low socioeconomic status
Unmarried
Low level of education

MEDICAL RISKS IN CURRENT PREGNANCY

Multiple gestation
Poor weight gain
Short interpregnancy interval
Infection (especially bacterial vaginosis)
First or second trimester bleeding
Placental problems, such as previa
    or abruption
Hyperemesis
Hypertension: chronic or pregnancy induced
Polyhydramnios/overdistended uterus
Abnormal hemoglobin
Fetal anomalies
Incompetent cervix
Premature rupture of membranes

MEDICAL RISKS PREDATING PREGNANCY

Previous preterm birth
Multiparity ≥5
Low prepregnant weight for height
Uterine or cervical abnormalities or
    surgery
Nonimmune status for certain infections
Repeated second trimester abortions
Diethylstilbestrol (DES) exposure
Maternal genetic factors
Chronic medical conditions, such as diabetes,
    hypertension, or heart disease

ENVIRONMENTAL/BEHAVIORAL/PSYCHOSOCIAL RISKS

Smoking
Alcohol or other substance abuse
Poor nutritional status
High altitude
Domestic abuse
Strenuous job activity
High stress
Lack of or inadequate prenatal care

THE SINGLE GREATEST RISK FACTOR FOR PRETERM LABOR IS A PREVIOUS HISTORY OF PRETERM LABOR. HOWEVER, IN A REVIEW OF OVER 100,000 WOMEN, 79% OF THE WOMEN WITH VERY PRETERM DELIVERIES HAD NO HISTORY OF A PRETERM BIRTH.[9]

Some of the conditions that seem to predispose women to preterm labor and low birth weight infants are outlined in Display 8.1.[8]

Screening for Preterm Labor Risk

► What other methods are used to identify women at risk for preterm delivery?

Methods that have been used to identify woman at risk for preterm delivery include cervical assessment, transvaginal ultrasound, studies of biochemical markers, and home uterine activity monitoring.

Cervical Assessment

Routine digital assessment of dilation of the cervix by itself has not been proven to be an effective screening tool to detect women at high risk for preterm delivery. However, using *all* components of the Bishop score helps to correlate this finding more closely with preterm delivery. With a Bishop score of 6 or more, the likelihood of a delivery is increased.[10]

Transvaginal Ultrasound

The normal cervical length in the midtrimester of pregnancy varies from 10 to 50 mm (median, 35 mm). Several studies have shown that the shorter the cervix, the higher the risk of preterm birth. A cervix of 25 mm or less at 16 to 24 weeks of gestation has been consistently predictive of early delivery in a variety of populations, including asymptomatic low- and high-risk women, women with multiple gestational pregnancies, and symptomatic women. Measuring cervical length by transvaginal ultrasound can be a valuable tool to predict preterm labor.[11]

However, there are limitations to transvaginal ultrasounds. The accuracy of measurements depends on the ultrasonographer; factors such as bladder distension and maternal position can affect measurements. Furthermore, many women (up to 60% in some studies) who have a short cervix will not deliver preterm. Despite this finding, transvaginal ultrasound is still very useful for its negative predictive value.[12,13] If the cervix is found to be of an appropriate length, there is very little chance that the patient will deliver preterm. This result can be very reassuring for many women who are at high risk for a preterm delivery.

Biochemical Markers

Biochemical markers to accurately identify those truly at risk for preterm birth would offer supplemental information that could help clinicians to avoid unnecessary and costly treatment for those patients who, despite contractions, will have a term delivery. Some of the biochemical markers that have been studied include CRH, salivary estriol, and fetal fibronectin (fFN). fFN is the only biochemical marker that has an excellent predictive value for preterm delivery, allowing it to *guide clinical interventions.*[5,12]

fFN assays have been approved by the U.S. Food and Drug Administration (FDA) for clinical use in identifying women at risk for preterm labor. The fFN immunoassay is a qualitative test for the detection of this protein *in cervicovaginal secretions.* fFN is a glycoprotein produced by the chorion (fetal membranes). It is found at the junction of the membranes and the uterus. fFN can be found in cervicovaginal secretions in early pregnancy and at term, *but is rarely detectable between 21 and 37 weeks unless there is a disruption in the membrane–uterine junction.* The clinician can test for the presence of fFN in symptomatic and asymptomatic pregnant women who may be at high risk for early delivery. A negative test provides a 99% negative predictive value for delivery, indicating that these patients will most likely not deliver within 14 days of the negative test. Although a negative test appears to be useful in ruling out imminent preterm birth, the clinical implications of a positive result are not fully understood. For this reason, it is not recommended as a routine screening tool for asymptomatic women.

Although the collection of fluid for fFN testing is very simple, there are some contraindications:
- Vaginal examination within the past 24 hours
- Cervical dilation greater than 3 cm
- Ruptured membranes
- Cerclage in place
- Vaginal bleeding or placenta previa
- Sexual intercourse within the past 24 hours

All of these findings may result in a false-positive result. For this reason, a thorough history should be obtained from the patient and fFN testing should be performed before a vaginal examination is done.

Home Uterine Activity Monitoring

The role of *home uterine activity monitoring* in preventing preterm birth has been controversial. It was hoped that the monitoring of uterine activity using a portable external fetal monitoring system and telephone modem to transfer data to a monitoring center would hold promise for reducing the rate of preterm birth. Although it has been demonstrated that women who eventually deliver at preterm gestation have more uterine activity than other women at the same gestational age who eventually deliver at term, the difference is not reliable enough to be used effectively in screening for high-risk women. *The research to date shows no proven maternal, fetal, or neonatal benefit from the use of home uterine activity monitoring.*[13]

Signs and Symptoms of Preterm Labor

▶ **What are the warning signs of preterm labor?**

The early warning signs of preterm labor are often subtle and can be difficult to differentiate from routine discomforts of pregnancy. These warning signs can often go unrecognized until labor is advanced. The key to treating preterm labor and preventing some of the morbidity associated with an early delivery is early recognition and treatment. *Pregnant women should be educated to recognize the following symptoms:*

- **Uterine contractions**—Frequent uterine contractions, occurring every 10 minutes or less (more than five in an hour), might indicate preterm labor. Irregular uterine contractions, called "Braxton Hicks contractions," occur normally as pregnancy progresses; however, frequent or regular contractions should not be ignored. Preterm labor contractions are *often painless* and might be described as a tightening of the uterus or as "the baby balling up."
- **Menstrual-like cramps**—These cramps in the lower part of the abdomen or upper thighs can be intermittent or constant.
- **Low, dull backache**—Backaches during pregnancy are not uncommon, but low backaches that are not relieved by rest or changes in position should be investigated. The pain may be described as "toothachy" or throbbing below the waistline, which can be intermittent or constant, and can radiate to the front of the abdomen.
- **Pelvic pressure**—Many women describe this as a heaviness in the lower abdomen, pelvis, back, or thighs, which feels as if the baby is pushing down. This is often a rhythmical pelvic pressure not relieved by rest.
- **Abdominal cramping**—Intestinal cramps with or without diarrhea, sometimes described as "gas pains," can be associated with preterm labor.
- **Increase or change in vaginal discharge**—A milky white discharge is normal during pregnancy. However, a sudden increase or *change* in discharge, whether mucousy, watery, or tinged with blood, can be associated with preterm labor.

A woman in preterm labor may have only one or all of these signs. The woman experiencing one or more of the signs of preterm labor must be examined and evaluated promptly.

In addition to educating women and their families, all personnel who might have contact with pregnant women should be knowledgeable about the early symptoms of preterm labor and the appropriate response. It is important to ensure that the expectant woman understands the terms used and can describe her symptoms. The importance of prompt reporting of these symptoms should be emphasized. The risks of delaying evaluation and treatment should be made clear, and women should be made to feel comfortable reporting symptoms or coming in for further evaluation, even when they are found not to be in labor.

Management of the Woman at Risk for Preterm Labor

▶ **What is the appropriate response to telephone calls from women with symptoms of preterm labor?**

Pregnant women who have symptoms of preterm labor for more than 1 hour or who are having difficulty describing the symptoms should be evaluated in a clinical setting.

If a pregnant patient calls with symptoms that began while the woman was physically active and have been present for less than 1 hour, she should be instructed to do the following:

- Empty her bladder
- Rest on her left or right side
- Drink fluids (2 to 3 glasses of a noncaffeinated beverage, such as water or juice)
- Palpate for uterine contractions
- Call back in 1 hour if symptoms persist or if symptoms recur with resumption of normal activities
- Call back immediately for
  - Leaking of clear fluid from vagina, such as amniotic fluid
  - Frequent, strong contractions (every 5 minutes or less)
  - Changes in vaginal discharge
  - Vaginal bleeding

All personnel in hospital clinics or private practice offices who have contact with pregnant women need to be well sensitized to the dilemmas and subtleties of preterm labor. Secretaries and medical receptionists are often the first contact when an inquiry is made by a pregnant woman confused by what she is experiencing. The woman needs to know from the person on the other end of the line that her call is welcomed and important. Pregnant women delay seeking care because they do not interpret what they feel as anything abnormal. They also delay because they fear subtle "put downs" or being stereotyped as fearful and overanxious. (See Module 15 for a complete discussion related to telephone triage.)

> Before giving instructions, the woman's knowledge level of preterm labor, her pregnancy history, and distance from the hospital should be ascertained.

Considerations About Care-Seeking Behaviors of Pregnant Women[14,15]

> Keep in mind as you review this section that risk appraisal fails to identify 50% of women who enter preterm labor.

- Preterm labor is usually not in the thinking of most expectant women.
- Women have difficulty bringing a meaningful interpretation to symptoms because pregnancy itself brings unexpected similar physical discomforts. Even a previous preterm delivery does not make it easier to distinguish the symptoms of preterm labor.
- The focus of women's advocacy groups and society in general is on the normalcy of pregnancy.
- Many women do not receive education about recognizing symptoms of preterm labor.
- The expectant woman attempts to make sense out of what she is feeling by taking several different steps. Studies have shown that she fights a tug of war between not wanting to ignore symptoms that might lead to harm for her baby and not wanting to overreact. This process often delays treatment for her symptoms.
  - She gathers data and seeks information by comparing with her own expectations and here she will often attempt to "normalize" her symptoms.
  - She compares what she is feeling with the experiences of others (e.g., her mother, sister, friend).
  - She self-manages her symptoms as long as she can. Women rarely interpret sensations as preterm labor, but they think they "worked too hard," "got extra tired," "are coming down with the flu," or "strained their back."

Guidelines for Assessment and Intervention

▶ **What should be included in the initial assessment of preterm labor?**

- Health history
- Reproductive history
- Prenatal course of this pregnancy—obtain records if possible
- Determination of precise fetal age, based on last menstrual period (LMP), early sonograms, fundal height measurements, date of quickening, and first date of audible fetal heart tones
- Routine obstetric clinical parameters
- Assessment of signs/symptoms of preterm labor

> Document the occurrence of symptoms, onset, duration, and severity. Ask what activities preceded their onset and what relief measures have been tried.

Nursing and Provider Interventions

- Bed rest—lateral position for maximum placental perfusion
- Hydration—oral or intravenous

- Urine and cervical cultures
- Treat any infections noted such as bacterial vaginosis
- Monitor maternal vital signs
- Monitor fetal status using external fetal heart rate monitor
- Monitor contraction pattern. Use external monitoring system to document the frequency and quality of uterine contractions. Intensity of contractions should be assessed by palpation.
- Baseline cervical examination—should be done gently with minimal manipulation of the cervix

> Preterm contractions often stop with rest and hydration.

> Instruct the woman to report continuation or change in symptoms of preterm labor, even in the absence of documentation of uterine contractions on the external monitor. *Do not depend on the monitor alone in assessing uterine contractility.*

> Serial gentle cervical examinations should be done by the same examiner, when possible, to improve reliability of assessing early or subtle cervical change. Evaluate and record the following during cervical examination:
> - Position of the cervix
> - Dilation
> - Effacement (estimated length in centimeters)
> - Station of the presenting part
> - Consistency of cervix (firm, soft)

NOTE: If there is suspicion of amniotic membrane rupture or leakage, a sterile speculum examination should be done.

- Prepare patient and family for the possibility of the following:
  - Ultrasound
  - Amniocentesis
  - Tocolytic therapy
  - Steroid therapy
  - Baseline laboratory work including complete blood count (CBC)
- Provide comfort measures and emotional support.
- Consistently reevaluate symptoms of preterm labor.

> Preterm labor can be an extreme crisis for a family. Common responses might be guilt, fear, and/or anger. It is important to provide reassurance and support in an atmosphere that encourages expression of feelings.

▶ What measures can be recommended to help prolong pregnancy?

The provider can:
- Teach the expectant mother and her family about the signs and symptoms of preterm labor and the importance of seeking obstetric care immediately when they occur.
- Teach the expectant mother about palpating contractions and paying close attention to uterine contractions. She can monitor for contractions through palpation, twice a day or if symptoms occur.
- Schedule women for regular (weekly or bimonthly) prenatal visits to allow ongoing assessment of cervical status and uterine activity.

Further teaching should be given to these women regarding lifestyle modification such as:
- Modifying activities depending on type of employment, the occurrence of symptoms of preterm labor, and cervical status. Bed rest may not be necessary.

- Restricting travel.
- Maintaining an adequate diet and hydration, taking prenatal vitamins and iron, and performing good hygiene.
- Avoiding smoking and other substance abuse.
- Avoiding stressful situations when possible.

Information to Consider Regarding Smoking During Pregnancy

Smoking during pregnancy is strongly associated with preterm birth. Smoking is also related to placenta previa, placental abruption, premature rupture of membranes, spontaneous abortion, and decreased birth weight and infant stature. Tobacco smoke contains more than 2,000 chemicals, most of which easily cross the placenta. Nicotine and carbon monoxide are two of the main chemicals thought to be responsible for poor fetal outcomes as the result of decreased oxygenation to the mother and fetus.

Because of the difficulty with stopping smoking and the high rate of relapse, tobacco dependence should be viewed as a chronic condition requiring repeated intervention. Smokers often view smoking as a stress reducer or coping tool in their lives, so interventions to encourage cessation should address this aspect, as well as the impact that stopping smoking will have on the woman and her family. The most successful smoking cessation programs for pregnant women have addressed five important areas of concern[16]:

1. Risks of smoking
2. Benefits of quitting
3. Recommendation to quit
4. Feedback about fetal status
5. Teaching cognitive–behavioral strategies for quitting

Management of Preterm Labor

▶ Does Anything Really Work?

Despite intense medical intervention designed to treat contractions early in pregnancy, women continue to deliver preterm. Bed rest and hydration, both orally and intravenously, are the two traditional first-line treatments for preterm labor. Although many preterm contractions stop with these interventions, preterm labor itself may not. In the case of bed rest, there are some negative consequences to its use in the long term.

Information to Consider Regarding Bed Rest[17]

Traditionally, throughout history, when complications developed in pregnancies and treatment was uncertain, bed rest was prescribed. Bed rest was used both antenatally and in the postpartum period for a variety of complications. To this day, bed rest is still prescribed by more than 90% of obstetricians when patients are faced with miscarriage, preterm labor, and other complications.

The assumptions that bed rest is effective in preventing adverse pregnancy outcomes and is safe for the woman and her fetus are now being challenged. There have been multiple studies about the effects of bed rest on nonpregnant patients and these studies indicate that almost every bodily system is negatively affected by the bed rest. Although studies in pregnancy are limited, they do suggest that pregnant women on bed rest suffer similar physical and emotional complications. Bed rest in pregnancy can be associated with these complications:

- Thromboembolic disease
- Muscle atrophy
- Bone loss
- Weight loss
- Cardiovascular deconditioning (decreased plasma volume, total blood volume, cardiac output, and red cell mass)
- Endocrine system changes

These effects can remain for a prolonged period after delivery also. Many women who were prescribed bed rest during pregnancy reported significant mobility issues during the postpartum period. The severity of adverse effects while on bed rest appears to be related to the amount of activity restriction and may be reduced by exercise.

The severe emotional and economic effects of bed rest on women and their families also need to be taken into consideration. Studies show that women treated during pregnancy with bed rest, both in the hospital and at home, report a significant amount of stress related to their experience. They feel lonely, bored, and often depressed. These women report a loss of control and a perception that health care providers do not understand the consequences related to the bed rest they prescribe.

Because there is a lack of evidence that bed rest can prevent preterm deliveries and, in fact, evidence that bed rest causes both physical and emotional harm to women, ACOG does not recommend routinely prescribing bed rest.[13] If bed rest is ordered, even for a short time, the following issues need to be taken into consideration:

- Balancing maternal and fetal risks and benefits
- Involving the woman in decision making and planning regarding activity levels
- Discussing potential stressors for the whole family
- Including exercise in the plan of care while on bed rest

▶ What about tocolytic therapy?

Past treatment methods for preterm labor have included not only bed rest and hydration, but also the use of drugs such as ethanol, narcotics, progesterone, and sedatives to inhibit uterine contractions. More recently, drugs that have a quieting or depressant effect on the myometrium (muscle) of the uterus have been used. The depressant effect on the myometrium is called a *tocolytic effect*. The process of administering a drug for the purpose of inhibiting uterine contractions is called *tocolytic therapy*. It should be noted that the widespread use of tocolytics has not reduced the incidence of preterm deliveries. However, clinical studies indicate that tocolytics may prolong gestation for 24 to 48 hours.[13] This can improve neonatal outcomes by allowing time for administration of corticosteroids to facilitate fetal lung maturity and time to transfer the pregnant woman to a hospital where appropriate neonatal care is available.

▶ What are the indications for tocolytic therapy?

Labor inhibition is generally indicated when:

- The diagnosis of preterm labor is made
- Gestation is beyond 23 to 24 weeks but less than 34 weeks
- There is a live fetus without signs of severe distress or congenital anomalies incompatible with life

Aggressive obstetric and neonatal interventions may have a minimal effect on the survival of infants at 22 to 23 weeks or before. Always involve the woman and her family in the decision to start or stop tocolytic therapy.

ANTENATAL CORTICOSTEROIDS SHOULD ALWAYS BE ADMINISTERED WHEN TOCOLYTIC THERAPY IS INITIATED.

▶ What are the contraindications to tocolytic therapy?

Factors that threaten maternal and fetal status are contraindications to labor suppression. Some examples include[13]:

- Preeclampsia or eclampsia
- Placental abruption or acute hemorrhage
- Intrauterine infection
- Lethal congenital or chromosomal abnormalities
- Evidence of fetal compromise or intrauterine demise
- Advanced cervical dilatation
- Maternal hemodynamic instability or complications

Medications Currently Used for Tocolysis

Four classes of tocolytic agents are in use or under study (Table 8.1):

1. β-Adrenergic agents
2. Magnesium sulfate
3. Calcium channel blockers
4. Nonsteroidal anti-inflammatory drugs (NSAIDs)

β-Adrenergic Agonists

There are two types of β-adrenergic receptors in humans:
1. β_1-Adrenergic receptors are found in the heart, liver, pancreas, kidney, small intestine, and adipose tissue.
2. β_2-Adrenergic receptors are found in smooth muscle of the uterus, blood vessels diaphragm, and bronchioles.

By binding to these receptor sites, β-adrenergic agonists initiate a series of reactions resulting in reduced levels of calcium and reduced sensitivity of the actin–myosin contractile unit to calcium. With lowered intracellular calcium levels, smooth muscle contraction is less effective and uterine contractions may cease. However, continued exposure to these medications can lead to desensitization as the number of β-adrenergic receptors decrease.

Because β-adrenergic receptors are present in multiple sites, side effects can be seen in various organ systems and the probability of maternal risk is higher than with some of the other tocolytics. Some of these effects are as follows:

Cardiovascular	• Increases heart rate, systolic blood pressure, pulse pressure, stroke volume, and cardiac output.
	• Decreases diastolic pressure and peripheral vascular resistance.
	• Cardiac dysrhythmias have been reported.
	• Increased heart rate and myocardial contractility can predispose patients to myocardial ischemia.
Pulmonary	• Increases plasma renin and arginine vasopressin, which is associated with sodium and water retention. This predisposes patients to pulmonary edema, especially in multiple gestations. Excessive intravenous fluids combined with the antidiuretic effect of high dosages of these medications can result in fluid overload.
Metabolic	• Increases maternal blood glucose levels and insulin levels. This effect is enhanced by concomitant administration of corticosteroids. Lipolysis can also be included, which can lead to severe metabolic acidosis in diabetic women.

Magnesium Sulfate

Magnesium sulfate is an inexpensive alternative to β-adrenergic therapy. It is often used as the first-line tocolytic agent, even though randomized studies have not proven it to be effective for tocolysis. The side effects of parenteral magnesium for the treatment of preterm labor appear to be less severe and less frequent than those of β-adrenergic therapy. Magnesium sulfate is also safer to use with insulin-dependent diabetic patients because it decreases the risk of uncontrolled hyperglycemia, which can occur with β-adrenergic medications. The mechanism by which magnesium sulfate inhibits uterine contractions is not fully understood, but is thought to be related to its ability to inhibit the reuptake of acetylcholine at the nerve synapse. In this way, magnesium sulfate blocks neuromuscular transmissions and depresses the central nervous system.

Calcium Channel Blockers

Calcium channel blockers, such as procardia, have shown promise in inhibiting smooth muscle contractions, although the exact mechanisms are unknown. They produce vasodilatation and decreased peripheral vascular resistance, resulting in flushing of the skin and a transient increase in maternal and fetal heart rates. Postural hypotension can occur with sudden position changes. However, in most women, the side effects of procardia are minimal. Procardia should not be used concurrently with magnesium sulfate due to increased risks of cardiovascular collapse.

Nonsteroidal Anti-Inflammatory Drugs

NSAIDs, such as indomethacin, decrease the synthesis of prostaglandin. As stated, prostaglandins play an important role in both preterm and term labors. Prostaglandins increase the frequency of contractions, help to coordinate contractions, and ripen the cervix. When used

TABLE 8.1 DRUGS MOST COMMONLY USED IN THE TREATMENT OF PRETERM LABOR

DRUG	ACTION	DOSAGE/ROUTE	MATERNAL SIDE EFFECTS	FETAL SIDE EFFECTS	NURSING IMPLICATIONS
Magnesium sulfate	CNS depressant	*IV:* 4–6 g loading dose diluted and infused over 20–30 min, then 1–3 g/h maintenance dose until contractions stop (usually 2 g/h); maintenance dose is based on serum magnesium level, reflex response, and patient response (serum therapeutic range is 5–8 mg/100 mL)	Drowsiness, lethargy, slurred speech, blurred vision, ptosis, flushing, decreased GI motility, headache, nausea, vomiting, muscular weakness, urinary retention, shortness of breath, pulmonary edema	Decreased FHR variability, neonatal hypotonia, and drowsiness; possible bone abnormalities and congenital rickets have been associated with prolonged exposure	Closely monitor: 1. Maternal vital signs, including BP, HR, respiratory rate, and oxygen saturation levels. 2. FHR tracing 3. Intake and output 4. For signs of toxicity including absence of DTRs, increased lethargy, decreased urinary output, respiratory depression, cardiac arrhythmias and cardiac arrest. Obtain serum magnesium levels as ordered Medication should be discontinued if maternal respirations ≤12 breaths/min, urinary output ≤25 mL/hr, and patellar reflexes absent Have antidote (10% calcium gluconate) and resuscitation equipment immediately available
Nifedipine (procardia)	Calcium channel blocker	10 mg PO every 4–8 h	Transient hypotension, tachycardia, palpitations, headache, dizziness, facial flushing, nausea, peripheral edema	Intrauterine growth restriction	Closely monitor blood pressure; serial ultrasounds may be ordered to monitor fetal growth Avoid in diabetes; avoid concomitant use of magnesium sulfate
Terbutaline	β-Adrenergic agonist	*Oral:* 2.5–5 mg every 4 to 6 h *Subcutaneous:* 0.25 mg every 2–4 hours for 12 h *IV:* 1 mg/min initially; increase by 0.5 mg/min every 10 min to maximum of 8 mg/min or contractions stop. The FDA has issued an alert regarding the potential dangers associated with terbutaline pump therapy and the lack of evidence supporting the efficacy of this treatment.	Tachycardia, hypotension, hyperglycemia, hypokalemia, pulmonary edema	Hypoglycemia, lactic acidosis, ileus, death	Monitor 1. vital signs including respiratory rate, BP, HR. Hold medication for maternal HR >120. 2. Breath sounds for signs of pulmonary edema (dyspnea, coughing, crackles, wheezing). 3. FHR tracing 4. Intake and output

Drug	Classification	Dosage	Maternal Side Effects	Fetal/Neonatal Effects	Nursing Implications
Ritodrine hydrochloride	β-Adrenergic agonist	*IV:* 0.05–0.1 mg/min; may be increased every 10 min to maximum of 0.35 mg/min or contractions stop. *Oral:* 10 mg every 2 hr up to maximum of 120 mg/24 hr (first dose administered 30 min before IV infusion discontinued)	Palpitations, nervousness, tremors, tachycardia, sweating, headache, nausea, vomiting, thirst, chest pain, ECG changes and cardiac dysrhythmia, hyperglycemia, hypocalcemia, pulmonary edema	Tachycardia, neonatal hypoglycemia	Same implications as for terbutaline administration. Before initiating IV therapy Serum potassium Serum glucose Baseline ECG
Indomethacin	Prostaglandin inhibitor	50–100 mg rectal suppository loading dose, then 25 mg orally every 6–8 h for up to 72 h	GI irritation including peptic ulcer, GI bleeding, GI upset, nausea or vomiting, decreased renal blood flow, dizziness, postpartum hemorrhage, prolonged bleeding time	Oligohydramnios Transient constriction of ductus arteriosus—prolonged use may cause premature closure of the fetal ductus arteriosus and can lead to neonatal bowel ischemia and intraventricular hemorrhage	Review history for contraindications: peptic ulcer disease, aspirin sensitivity, renal or liver disease, bleeding abnormalities, pregnancy beyond 32 weeks' gestation, IUGR and oligohydramnios. Treatment should be used for 48–72 h only. After 72 h, fetal echo should be performed weekly and ultrasound for amniotic fluid index twice weekly.

in appropriate pregnant patients at less than 32 weeks gestation and for a short-term course (less than 72 hours; see table 8.1), indomethacin can be very effective in delaying preterm birth with minimal side effects.[4]

▶ How effective are tocolytics for the treatment of preterm labor?

Although tocolytic therapy often temporarily stops contractions, it has not been proven to prevent preterm births. *The use of tocolytics in a maintenance capacity following an episode of acute tocolysis has not been shown to be effective. Also, the repeated use of tocolytics in women with a recurrence of preterm labor is usually not recommended except for maternal transport.*[13] Therefore, tocolytics should be used in the short term to provide time for steroid administration and, if necessary, maternal transport to a facility with appropriate neonatal care.

> THERE IS NO EVIDENCE THAT OUTPATIENT USE OF TOCOLYTICS PROLONGS GESTATION.[13]

▶ When preterm labor is advanced or is unresponsive to tocolysis, what preparations should be made for delivery?

- If possible, women who are at less than 34 weeks' gestation should be transported to a tertiary care center *before delivery* so that intensive care facilities will be immediately available for the infant. This intervention in itself has been proven to decrease perinatal morbidity and mortality. (See Module 16, Maternal transport.)
- Assess the family's understanding of the rationale for starting or stopping tocolytic therapy and their expectations for the preterm infant's appearance, needs, and care.
- Provide contact information for the neonatal care unit to facilitate communication.

Progesterone

Recently, a lot of attention has been given to progesterone as another means of treating preterm labor. *17-α-Hydroxyprogesterone caproate* (17P) is a naturally occurring metabolite of progesterone. Both 17P and progesterone itself are produced in large quantities during pregnancy. In 1998, the National Institute of Child Health and Human Development (NICHD) conducted a multicenter trial to investigate progesterone. In this study, women who had experienced a previous preterm birth, received 250 mg of 17P intramuscularly each week from 15 to 20 weeks of gestation until 36 completed weeks of gestation. This administration of 17P was able to reduce the rate of a recurrent preterm birth, as compared with patients receiving placebo, in many of the participants, regardless of race. Women with a very preterm birth in their prior pregnancy showed the greatest benefit.[18,19]

Despite the positive results noted in this study, there are still many questions surrounding this treatment option. First, the mechanism of action of progesterone in preventing preterm birth is not clearly understood. In addition, this study focused on a particular population of women, namely, those at risk owing to a previous preterm birth and who also had singleton pregnancies. Further studies are being done on women with multiple gestations, and so far, the data suggest that progesterone may not prolong those pregnancies. Furthermore, the rate of preterm births in the NICHD study remained high, despite the 17P administration, and data analysis shows that on average the pregnancies were prolonged by only 1 week more than the untreated control subjects. For these reasons, at this time ACOG recommends that 17P be considered only for the treatment of women who have experienced a previous preterm birth.

Definitions, Etiology, and Risk Factors for Premature Rupture of Membranes

▶ What is premature rupture of membranes?

Premature rupture of membranes (PROM) is the spontaneous rupture of membranes *before the onset of labor, regardless of gestational age.* This occurs in about one third of preterm labor cases.[20]

▶ **What is preterm premature rupture of membranes?**

Preterm premature rupture of membranes (*preterm PROM*) is rupture of membranes *before term* (i.e., before the completion of 37 weeks' gestation), with or without the onset of labor. Preterm PROM remains a major cause of preterm birth and can lead to significant perinatal morbidity and mortality.

▶ **What is the cause of PROM?**

Although risk factors that appear to be related to PROM have been identified, the exact cause is unknown and probably results from a variety of factors. At full term, physiologic changes and the forces produced by contractions often lead to weakening of membranes and then to PROM. The causes for preterm PROM are more complicated. Intramniotic infections have been found in anywhere from 13% to 60% of women with preterm PROM depending on the studies.[20] However, preterm PROM often occurs in women without recognized risk factors.

Risk factors related to PROM include the following[20]:
- Prior preterm PROM or preterm delivery
- Smoking
- Infection
- Cerclage or cervical procedures
- Chronic abruption or vaginal bleeding
- Low socioeconomic status
- Sexually transmitted infections
- Uterine distension

Diagnosis, Management, and Nursing Interventions With PROM

▶ **How is PROM diagnosed?**

Symptoms suggestive of PROM should be evaluated promptly. An accurate diagnosis is essential to the appropriate management of suspected PROM. Usually, ruptured membranes can be diagnosed on the basis of the history and physical examination. When confirming this diagnosis, a sterile speculum examination should be performed rather than a digital examination. A sterile speculum examination minimizes the risk of infection and allows the clinician to inspect for cervicitis and umbilical cord prolapse, to do cervical cultures as indicated, and to assess cervical dilation and effacement.
- Observation of amniotic fluid coming through the cervix is the best method to confirm the diagnosis.
- If the diagnosis is still in question, Nitrazine paper can be used to test the pH of the fluid. The pH of vaginal fluids is usually 4.5 to 6.0. Amniotic fluid has a higher pH of 7.1 to 7.3 and therefore turns Nitrazine paper blue—a positive result. False positives may occur if blood, semen, or infections such as bacterial vaginosis are present.
- Ferning is another test that can be done. Fluid from the posterior vaginal vault is placed on a glass slide and allowed to dry. Under microscopic examination, the presence of a ferning pattern is suggestive of amniotic fluid.
- The measuring of amniotic fluid volume by ultrasound may also be of value, but should not be used to diagnose PROM.

Risks Associated With PROM at Term

At term, maternal risks of ruptured membranes are low. Risks to the fetus from term PROM include fetal umbilical cord compression and ascending infection. *Maternal and fetal risks rise with the duration of time before delivery and with the number of digital vaginal examinations.*

Risks Associated With Preterm PROM

Risks associated with preterm PROM are as follows:
- Intrauterine infection (*chorioamnionitis*)
- Fetal malpresentation
- Umbilical cord accident
- Placental abruption
- Complications of prematurity

Infection is evident in many women with preterm PROM, especially those with very early gestational ages. The incidence of infection rises with the number of cervical examinations done. Most women with preterm PROM deliver within 1 week regardless of management, leading to significant neonatal complications owing to prematurity.[20]

▶ What nursing interventions should be taken when a woman is admitted with PROM?

- Confirm membrane status and document the time of rupture, the time of onset of labor, and the color and odor of amniotic fluid. Avoid a digital examination—wait for the primary care provider unless an emergent situation presents (e.g., variable decelerations with a prolapsed cord suspected).
- Review dating criteria for the pregnancy. Review data on LMP, early assessment of uterine size, and early sonograms.
- Monitor fetal heart rate and assess fetal status.
- Evaluate uterine activity.
- Observe for signs of infection.
- Determine the need for transport to a tertiary care center based on gestational age and fetal status. If less than 34 weeks' gestation and not in active labor, the woman should be transferred to a facility capable of providing intensive neonatal care.
- Assess the woman's understanding of the implications of PROM and management options. Provide psychosocial support.
- PREPARE FOR A HIGH-RISK INFANT IF INDICATED.
  - *Neonatal resuscitation team should be notified and present for delivery.*
  - *Resuscitation equipment should be in working order and in the delivery area.*
  - *Nursery should be notified of possible high-risk infant.*

▶ What is the management of PROM?

Numerous controversies exist regarding optimal management and treatment of PROM, whether preterm or at term. Management decisions should be based on the following:
- Gestational age
- Presence or absence of labor
- Presence or absence of maternal infection
- Presence or absence of fetal reassurance
- Fetal presentation
- Cervical examination
- Availability of neonatal intensive care

At term women with PROM should be induced at the time of presentation to decrease their risks of chorioamnionitis. Gestational age and fetal well-being play important roles in the decision about how to best care for women with preterm PROM. Women with preterm PROM who are at 34 weeks' gestation or more and who are hospitalized where neonatal intensive care is available may be best managed by prompt induction of labor. ACOG recommends that labor can be induced for patients at gestational ages of 32 to 33 weeks only with documented fetal lung maturity.[20] At these gestational ages, the risks of prematurity are considerably less than the risks, such as infection, for the undelivered patient and fetus with preterm PROM.

▶ What is expectant management of preterm PROM?

When the potential complications associated with prematurity outweigh the risk of maternal and neonatal complications, expectant management is recommended. Hospitalization is usually required after preterm PROM, if fetal viability is present. Women with preterm PROM who are at less than 34 weeks' gestation or who have an immature fetal lung profile should be managed expectantly.[20] If the woman is not in active labor, she should be transferred to a high-risk medical center. Prophylactic tocolysis is not recommended, but may be used in the short term to administer corticosteroids.

Expectant management protocols may include the following:
- Modified bed rest
- Pelvic rest (e.g., avoid intercourse, sexual stimulation)
- Assessment for infection (chorioamnionitis)
  - Maternal or fetal tachycardia
  - Temperature higher than 100.4°F
  - Uterine tenderness
  - Foul-smelling, purulent amniotic fluid
- Surveillance for fetal compromise
  - Nonstress test
  - Ultrasound/biophysical profile
- Prophylactic antibiotics
- Administration of corticosteroids
- Limited course of tocolytics if necessary

> Maternal tachycardia usually precedes a rise in maternal temperature and subsequent fetal tachycardia.
> Elevated white blood cell counts are not a reliable indicator of infection in women with PROM, especially if corticosteroids have been administered. During labor, even in the absence of infection, white blood counts can become elevated to levels of 25,000/mm[3] or more.

> Digital cervical examinations should not be done on women with PROM who are not in labor and in whom immediate induction of labor is not planned.

Recommendations for Antibiotics[13,20]

Although inflammation and infection have been linked to both preterm labor and preterm PROM, the benefits of antibiotics for these patient populations have been frequently debated. Because infection of the upper genital tract has been associated with preterm deliveries, there has been speculation that treatment with antibiotics could perhaps prevent delivery in these patients. However, for patients with preterm labor, without rupture of membranes, treatment with antibiotics has not been proven successful in preventing a preterm delivery. Therefore, antibiotics are not recommended in women with preterm labor, except for group B streptococcus prophylaxis before delivery.

On the other hand, in women with preterm premature rupture of membranes, antibiotics have been shown to delay delivery and reduce neonatal morbidity. In large multicenter studies, treatment with antibiotics was able to delay delivery for 7 days to up to 3 weeks. These studies also found that newborns had a reduced need for oxygen and a reduced incidence of respiratory distress syndrome, necrotizing enterocolitis (NEC), and sepsis. ACOG recommends the use of ampicillin and erythromycin IV for 48 hours, followed by amoxicillin and erythromycin orally for 5 days during expectant management of the preterm PROM patient.

Recommendations for Antenatal Corticosteroids[21]

The appropriate use of corticosteroids to accelerate lung maturation in the fetus is one of the most effective ways to improve the outcomes of preterm births. Evidence from clinical trials since the 1970s has proven that antenatal corticosteroid administration is effective in reducing infant mortality by 30% and neonatal respiratory distress by 50%. Since 1994, the National Institutes of Health has recommended that **all women at risk for preterm delivery between 24 and 34 weeks' gestation are candidates for corticosteroid therapy** (Display 8.2). Studies have shown a decrease in the risk and severity of respiratory distress syndrome, intraventricular hemorrhage, and mortality in the neonate. The decrease in these complications also lowers the cost and duration of neonatal care. The optimal benefit of antenatal corticosteroid therapy is greatest more than 24 hours after starting therapy. In a randomized, placebo-controlled trial done in conjunction with 13 academic centers, repeated courses of antenatal corticosteroids given to women at risk for preterm delivery did not reduce neonatal morbidity when compared with a single course.

DISPLAY 8.2 CORTICOSTEROID TREATMENT REGIMENS

Betamethasone 12 mg intramuscularly every 24 hours for two doses
OR
Dexamethasone 6 mg intramuscularly every 12 hours for four doses

---

Antenatal corticosteroid therapy is one of the most effective strategies in the prevention of mortality and disability in preterm infants. A single course of corticosteroids should be given to all pregnant women between 24 and 34 weeks' gestation if at risk for preterm delivery.[21]

PRACTICE/REVIEW QUESTIONS

After reviewing this module, answer the following questions.

1. *Preterm labor* is labor occurring after _____ and before _____ completed weeks' gestation.

2. The diagnosis of preterm labor is made when contractions less than 10 minutes apart are accompanied by:

   a. _____

   b. _____

   c. _____

3. The majority of perinatal morbidity and mortality in the United States are the result of _____

   _____.

4. A very preterm birth is defined as a delivery of an infant of less than _____ completed weeks' gestation.

5. Five *demographic* risk factors related to preterm labor are:

   a. _____

   b. _____

   c. _____

   d. _____

   e. _____

6. The single greatest risk factor for preterm labor is

   _____.

7. List two of the four physiologic pathways related to the onset preterm labor.

   a. _____

   b. _____

8. Five *behavioral* risk factors related to preterm labor are

   a. _____

   b. _____

   c. _____

   d. _____

   e. _____

9. List six warning signs of preterm labor.

   a. _____

   b. _____

   c. _____

   d. _____

   e. _____

   f. _____

10. List three things to consider before giving telephone instructions to women complaining of vague symptoms of preterm labor.

   a. _____

   b. _____

   c. _____

11. A knowledgeable patient with an uncomplicated pregnancy who experiences symptoms of preterm labor with physical activity might be instructed to do the following:

    a. _____

    b. _____

    c. _____

    d. _____

    e. _____

12. The ultimate diagnosis of true labor progress is

    _____.

13. _____ is the only biochemical marker with an excellent predictive value for preterm delivery.

14. Contraindications to collecting this biochemical marker (in question 13) are:

    a. _____

    b. _____

    c. _____

    d. _____

    e. _____

    f. _____

15. List five parameters used to determine fetal age.

    a. _____

    b. _____

    c. _____

    d. _____

    e. _____

16. About half the time, preterm contractions will stop with

    _____ and _____.

17. List complications patients may develop when placed on bed rest.

    a. _____

    b. _____

    c. _____

    d. _____

    e. _____

    f. _____

    g. _____

18. Well-controlled studies confirm that bed rest is an effective therapy for preterm labor.

    a. True
    b. False

19. List five clinical observations that should be noted when doing a cervical examination on a woman at risk for preterm labor.

    a. _____

    b. _____

    c. _____

    d. _____

    e. _____

20. Women often react to their preterm labor by feeling

    _____ and _____.

21. List the initial nursing interventions when caring for the woman being admitted for preterm labor.

    a. _____

    b. _____

    c. _____

    d. _____

    e. _____

    f. _____

    g. _____

    h. _____

    i. _____

22. Risk appraisal (does) (does not) identify approximately 90% of women who will eventually experience preterm labor.

23. The expectant woman usually appreciates that preterm labor is a risk for her.

    a. True
    b. False

24. Drugs that have a depressant effect on the myometrium of the uterus are called_____

    _____.

25. The process of administering a drug for the purpose of inhibiting uterine contractions is called _____

    _____.

26. List seven contraindications to tocolytic therapy.

    a. _____

    b. _____

    c. _____

    d. _____

    e. _____

    f. _____

    g. _____

27. Two of the drugs that are commonly used for tocolysis

    are _____ and _____.

28. List seven side effects of β-adrenergic drugs.

    a. _____

    b. _____

    c. _____

    d. _____

    e. _____

    f. _____

    g. _____

29. During tocolytic therapy with terbutaline, the physician should be notified if the maternal pulse exceeds

    _____ bpm.

30. The nurse should listen to the patient's breath sounds before tocolytic therapy begins and should monitor for

    signs of pulmonary edema, including _____,

    _____, _____, or _____.

31. MgSO$_4$, a central nervous system depressant, should

    never be administered in the absence of _____.

32. Seven potential side effects of MgSO$_4$ administration are:

    a. _____

    b. _____

    c. _____

    d. _____

    e. _____

    f. _____

    g. _____

33. Define *premature rupture of membranes*.

    _____

34. A vaginal infection known to have a strong relationship to preterm delivery, especially in African-American

    women, is called _____.

35. List eight nursing interventions when a woman is admitted with PROM.

    a. _____

    b. _____

    c. _____

    d. _____

    e. _____

    f. _____

    g. _____

    h. _____

36. List three possible complications resulting from PROM.

    a. _____

    b. _____

    c. _____

37. Name four signs of chorioamnionitis.

    a. _____

    b. _____

    c. _____

    d. _____

38. The management of PROM is determined by the gestational age of the fetus and the presence or absence

    of _____, _____, _____, and

    _____.

39. If the fetus is less than 34 weeks and the mother is not in

    active labor, her care should take place at _____.

40. Every fetus between 24 and 34 weeks' gestation at risk for preterm delivery should be considered a candidate for

    antenatal treatment with _____.

41. If chorioamnionitis develops or if there is evidence of

    fetal distress, _____ is indicated.

42. The benefits of antenatal administration of corticosteroids to the fetus at risk of preterm delivery include a

    reduction in the risks of _____, _____ and

    _____.

PRACTICE/REVIEW ANSWER KEY

1. 20; 37

2. a. Progressive change in the cervix
   b. Cervical dilatation of 2 cm or more
   c. Cervical effacement of 80% or more

3. Preterm births

4. 32

5. a. Age ≤ 20 or ≥ 35
   b. Race—African American especially
   c. Low socioeconomic status
   d. Unmarried
   e. Low level of education

6. Previous preterm birth

7. Any two of the following:
   a. Inflammation and infection
   b. Maternal or fetal stress
   c. Decidual hemorrhage or abruption
   d. Mechanical stretch of the uterus

8. Any five of the following:
   a. Smoking
   b. Alcohol and other substance abuse
   c. Poor nutritional status
   d. High altitude
   e. Domestic abuse
   f. Strenuous job activity
   g. High stress
   h. Lack of prenatal care
   i. Diethylstilbestrol (DES) exposure and other toxic exposures

9. a. Uterine contractions—five or more in hour
   b. Menstrual-like cramps
   c. Low, dull backache
   d. Pelvic pressure
   e. Abdominal cramping
   f. Increase or change in vaginal discharge

10. a. The patient's knowledge level of preterm labor
    b. Her pregnancy history
    c. Distance from the hospital

11. a. Empty her bladder
    b. Rest on her side
    c. Drink two to three glasses of water or juice
    d. Palpate for contractions
    e. Call back in 1 hour if symptoms persist or if symptoms recur with resumption of normal activities.

12. Cervical change

13. Fetal fibronectin (fFN)

14. a. Vaginal examination within past 24 hours
    b. Cervical dilation greater than 3 cm
    c. Ruptured membranes
    d. Cerclage in place
    e. Vaginal bleeding or placenta previa
    f. Sexual intercourse within the past 24 hours

15. a. LMP
    b. Early sonograms
    c. Fundal height measurements
    d. Date of quickening
    e. First date of audible fetal heart tones

16. Bed rest; hydration

17. a. Thromboembolic disease
    b. Muscle atrophy
    c. Bone loss
    d. Weight loss
    e. Cardiovascular deconditioning
    f. Endocrine changes
    g. Increased anxiety, depression, and somatic complaints

18. b. False

19. a. Position
    b. Consistency
    c. Effacement
    d. Dilation
    e. Station

20. Anger; guilt

21. a. Assessment of signs and symptoms of preterm labor
    b. Monitor uterine status.
    c. Monitor fetal status.
    d. Monitor maternal vital signs.
    e. Instruct patient on initial bed rest and hydration.
    f. Prepare for collection of urine/cervical cultures.
    g. Baseline cervical examination.
    h. Provide comfort measures and emotional support.
    i. Prepare for the possibility of ultrasound, amniocentesis, tocolytic drug therapy, steroid therapy, baseline blood chemistry (CBC). Educate patient and family about these procedures/therapies.

22. Does not

23. b. False

24. Tocolytic drugs

25. Tocolytic therapy or tocolysis

26. a. Severe preeclampsia/eclampsia
    b. Placental abruption, acute hemorrhage, or active vaginal bleeding
    c. Intrauterine infection
    d. Lethal congenital or chromosomal abnormalities

e. Evidence of fetal compromise or intrauterine demise
f. Advanced cervical dilation
g. Maternal hemodynamic instability or complications

27. Terbutaline; magnesium sulfate

28. a. Tremors
    b. Maternal and fetal tachycardia
    c. Headache
    d. Palpitations
    e. Anxiety/nervousness
    f. Nausea and/or vomiting
    g. Hypotension

29. 120

30. Dyspnea; wheezing; coughing; rales

31. Patellar reflexes

32. a. Drowsiness
    b. Decreased sensorium
    c. Slurred speech
    d. Heavy eyelids
    e. Flushing
    f. Decreased gastrointestinal motility
    g. Respiratory depression

33. The spontaneous rupture of membranes before the onset of labor, regardless of gestational age

34. Bacterial vaginosis

35. a. Confirm membrane status.
    b. Review dating criteria.
    c. Monitor fetal heart tones.
    d. Evaluate uterine activity.
    e. Observe for signs of infection.
    f. Determine the need for transport.
    g. Assess woman's understanding of the implications of PROM and provide support and education.
    h. Prepare for delivery of a high-risk infant.

36. a. Intrauterine infection (chorioamnionitis)
    b. Preterm labor
    c. Prolapsed umbilical cord

37. a. Maternal or fetal tachycardia
    b. Temperature higher than 100.4°F
    c. Uterine tenderness
    d. Foul-smelling, purulent amniotic fluid

38. Labor; chorioamnionitis; fetal distress; fetal lung maturity

39. A high-risk regional medical center

40. Corticosteroids (betamethasone)

41. Immediate delivery

42. Respiratory distress syndrome; intraventricular hemorrhage; mortality

R E F E R E N C E S

1. PeriStats. (2007). Available at: www.marchofdimes.com/peristats/.
2. McPheeters, M. L., Miller, W. C., Hartmann, K. E., Savitz, D. A., Kaufman, J. S., Garrett, J. M., & Thorp, J. M. (2005). The epidemiology of threatened preterm labor: A prospective cohort study. *American Journal of Obstetrics and Gynecology, 192* (4), 1325–1329.
3. March of Dimes. (2006). *The compendium on preterm birth.* (2006). Available at: www.marchofdimes.com/prematurity/21329_21509.asp.
4. Vermillion, S. T., & Robinson, C. J. (2005). Antiprostaglandin drugs. *Obstetrics and Gynecology Clinics North America, 32* (3), 501–517.
5. Goldenberg, R. L., Goepfert, A. R., & Ramsey, P. S. (2005). Biochemical markers for the prediction of preterm birth. *American Journal of Obstetrics and Gynecology, 192* (5 Suppl.), 36–46.
6. American College of Obstetricians and Gynecologists. (2001). *Assessment of risk factors for preterm birth* [ACOG Practice Bulletin No. 31]. Washington, DC: Author.
7. Rich-Edwards, J. W., & Grizzard, T. A. (2005). Psychosocial stress and neuroendocrine mechanisms in preterm delivery. *American Journal of Obstetrics and Gynecology, 192* (5 Suppl.), S30–S35.
8. Moos, M. K. (2004). Understanding prematurity: Sorting fact from fiction. *AWHONN Lifelines, 8,* 32–37.
9. Mercer, B., Milluzzi, C., & Collin, M. (2005). Periviable birth at 20 to 26 weeks of gestation: Proximate causes, previous obstetric history and recurrence risk. *American Journal of Obstetrics and Gynecology, 193*(3 pt 2), 1175–1180.
10. Volumenie, J. L. (2004). Ultrasonographic cervical length measurement is not a better predictor of preterm delivery than digital examination in a population of patients with idiopathic preterm labor. *European Journal of Obstetric and Gynecologic Reproductive Biology, 117*(1), 33–37.
11. Grimes-Dennis, J., & Berghella, V. (2007). Cervical length and prediction of preterm delivery. *Current Opinion in Obstetrics and Gynecology, 19*(2), 191–195.
12. Bernhardt, J., & Dorman, K. (2004). Preterm birth risk assessment tools. *AWHONN Lifelines, 8*(1), 38–44.
13. American College of Obstetricians and Gynecologists. (2003). *Management of preterm labor* [ACOG Practice Bulletin, No. 43]. Washington, DC: Author.
14. Weiss, M. E., Saks, N. P., & Harris, S. (2002). Resolving the uncertainty of preterm symptoms: Women's experiences with the onset of preterm labor. *Journal of Obstetric, Gynecologic, and Neonatal Nursing, 31*(1), 66–76.
15. Patterson, E. T., Douglas, A. B., Patterson, P. M., & Bradle, J. B. (1992). Symptoms of preterm labor and self-diagnostic confusion. *Nursing Research, 41*(6), 367–372.
16. Lumley, J., Oliver, S., & Waters, E. (2001). Interventions for promoting smoking cessation during pregnancy. *Cochrane Database System Review, (2),* CD001055.
17. Sprague, A. E. (2004). The evolution of bed rest as a clinical intervention. *Journal of Obstetric, Gynecologic, and Neonatal Nursing, 33*(5), 542–549.
18. Armstrong, J. (2007). 17 progesterone for preterm birth prevention: A potential $2 billion opportunity. *American Journal of Obstetrics and Gynecology, 196*(3), 194–195.

19. Meis, P. J. (2005). 17 hydroxyprogesterone for the prevention of preterm delivery. *Obstetrics and Gynecology, 105*(5, Part 1), 1128–1135.

20. American College of Obstetricians and Gynecologists. (2007). *Premature rupture of membranes* [ACOG Practice Bulletin, No. 80]. Washington, DC: Author.

21. National Institutes of Health Consensus Development Panel. (2000). Antenatal corticosteroids revisited. *National Institutes of Health Consensus Development Conference Statement.* Available at: http://consensus.nih.gov/2000/2000 AntenatalCorticosteroidsRevisited112PDF.pdf.

SUGGESTED READINGS

Azria, E. (2004). Magnesium sulfate in obstetrics: Current data. *Journal de Gynecologie, Obstetetrique, et Biologie de al Reproduction (Paris), 33*(6 pt 1), 510–517.

Effect of corticosteroids for fetal maturation on perinatal outcomes. NIH Consensus Development Panel on the Effect of Corticosteroids for Fetal Maturation on Perinatal Outcomes. (1995). *Journal of the American Medical Association, 273,* 413–418.

Goldenberg, R. L. (2002). The management of preterm labor. *Obstetrics and Gynecology, 100*(5 pt 1), 1020–1037.

Goldenberg, R. L., Mercer, B. M., Meis, P. J., Copper, R. L., Das, A., & McNellis, D. (1996). The preterm prediction study: Fetal fibronectin testing and spontaneous preterm birth. *Obstetrics and Gynecology, 87,* 643–648.

Kovacevich, G. J., Gaich, S. A., Lavin, J. P., Hopkins, M. P., Crane, S. S., Stewart, J., Nelson, D., & Lavin, L. M. (2000). The prevalence of thromboembolic events among women with extended bed rest prescribed as part of the treatment for premature labor or preterm premature rupture of membranes. *American Journal Obstetrics and Gynecology, 182*(5), 1089–1092.

Meis, P. J., Klebanoff, M., Thom, E., Dombrowski, M. P., Sibai, B., Moawad, A. H., Spong, C. Y., Hauth, J. C., Miodovnik, M., Varner, M. W., Leveno, K. J., Caritis, S. N., Iams, J. D., Wapner, R. J., Gabbe, S.; National Institute of Child Health and Human Development Maternal–Fetal Medicine Units Network. (2003). Prevention of recurrent preterm delivery by 17 alpha-hydroxyprogesterone caproate. *New England Journal of Medicine, 348,* 2379–2385.

Palmer, L., & Carty, E. (2006). Deciding when it's labor: The experience of women who have received antepartum care at home for preterm labor. *Journal of Obstetric, Gynecologic, and Neonatal Nursing, 35*(4), 509–515.

Stevens, A. O., Chauhan, S. P., Magann, E. F., Martin, R. W., Bofill, J. A., Cushman, J. L., & Morrison, J. C. (2004). Fetal fibronectin and bacterial vaginosis are associated with preterm birth in women who are symptomatic for preterm labor. *American Journal of Obstetrics and Gynecology, 190*(6), 1582–1587.

Wadhwa, P. D. (2004). Placental corticotrophin-releasing hormone (CRH), spontaneous preterm birth, and fetal growth restriction: A prospective investigation. *American Journal of Obstetrics and Gynecology, 191*(4), 1063–1069.

Yost, N. P. (2005). Hospitalization for women with arrested preterm labor: A randomized trial. *Obstetrics and Gynecology, 106*(1), 14–18.

M O D U L E

9

Caring for the Laboring Woman With Hypertensive Disorders Complicating Pregnancy

E. JEAN MARTIN ■ JUDITH H. POOLE

When you have completed this module, you should be able to recall the meaning of the following terms. You should also be able to use the terms when consulting with other health professionals. Terms are defined in this module or in the glossary at the end of this book.

antiphospholipid antibodies
clonus
disseminated intravascular coagulation (DIC)
endothelin-derived releasing factor (EDRF)
endothelium (endothelial lining)
epigastric pain
gestational hypertension
hydatidiform mole
hydralazine (Apresoline)
hydrops

iatrogenic
microangiopathy
oliguria
prostacyclin (PGI$_2$)
proteinuria
scotomata
thrombocytopenia
thromboxane
vasopressor

Introduction

Hypertension is the most common medical risk factor for pregnant women.[1,2] A diagnosis of hypertension complicating pregnancy challenges the care provider, who must weigh the risks, benefits, and alternatives of treatment as related to maternal, fetal, and neonatal well-being. Everyone caring for the woman during her pregnancy must be aware of the significance of the disease process, current diagnostic criteria, and management recommendations to decrease risk to the woman and her newborn.

Hypertension associated with pregnancy complicates 6% to 8% of all pregnancies. Preeclampsia, one form of hypertension complicating pregnancy, is a significant contributor to maternal and perinatal morbidity and mortality, complicating approximately 5% to 8% of all pregnancies not terminating in first-trimester abortions.[1,2] The incidence of this serious disorder can vary greatly among racial and ethnic groups and is influenced by age and parity.

Among the four leading causes of maternal mortality in the United States—thromboembolic disease, hypertension, hemorrhage, and infection—hypertension during pregnancy is second only to thromboembolic disease. Current estimates attribute 12% to 18% of all pregnancy-related maternal deaths to hypertension disorders (i.e., approximately 70 maternal deaths in the United States and 50,000 maternal deaths worldwide occur each year).[1] Because the fetus is exposed to maternal pathophysiologic alterations underlying a hypertensive disorder, pregnancy outcomes include stillbirths and neonatal morbidity and mortality. The main causes of neonatal death are placental insufficiency and abruptio placentae. Intrauterine growth restriction (IUGR) is common in infants of women with preeclampsia.[3]

Although the etiology and pathophysiology of hypertension in pregnancy have been intensively researched over the years, a great deal is still unknown. This module presents what is currently reflected in the literature as well as guidelines from the National High Blood Pressure Education Program Working Group Report on High Blood Pressure in Pregnancy.[4,5] The Working Group uses evidence-based findings and consensus in providing guidelines for management to clinicians.

Studying this module will perhaps involve repeated reading and a "letting go" of previous concepts and understanding. Diagnostic criteria have changed. For the nurse, nurse-midwife, and physician, astute and early assessments are critical to appropriate diagnosis and early intervention.

Terminology and Classification

Many classification schemes and terminology have been proposed by various authors, agencies, and even countries, resulting in imprecise usage and confusing, nonstandardized diagnostic categories. A concise and clinically useful classification is needed. The National High Blood

Pressure Education Program, Working Group Report on High Blood Pressure in Pregnancy (Working Group) published through the National Institutes of Health, and the National Heart, Lung, and Blood Institute, outlines current accepted terminology for the hypertensive disorders of pregnancy.[4–6]

The most important issue in the classification of disorders of blood pressure (BP) in pregnancy is differentiating those hypertensive disorders occurring before pregnancy from those occurring during pregnancy with potentially serious consequences, specifically preeclampsia. Preeclampsia is peculiar to pregnancy and comprises a specific syndrome of the following:

- Reduced organ perfusion (brain, kidney, and liver), which is caused by the following:
  - Vasospasm of tiny arteries (arterioles) occurring at the organ(s) site and elsewhere in the body's vasculature
  - Activation of a coagulation process leading to abnormal fibrin deposition and platelet consumption (i.e., platelets are "used up")[5]

These pathophysiologic processes result in signs and symptoms in the pregnant woman that have degrees of significance and importance. Issues in making a diagnosis of a hypertensive disorder as complicating pregnancy have to do with the importance attached to the:

- Timing of the hypertensive disorder in relation to gestational age
- Timing of signs and symptoms in relation to gestational age
- Reliability of the sign or symptom (diagnostic criteria)

Diagnostic criteria or **diagnostic markers** are used in developing classification systems. A great deal of research has been done on behalf of substantiating the authenticity (reliability, reproducibility, and degree of predictability) of the diagnostic criteria used in the classification system presented by the Working Group.[5] The classification system is based on terminology and definitions similar to those developed by the American College of Obstetricians and Gynecologists (ACOG) in 1972 and modified by the ACOG in 1986, 1996, and most recently in 2002.[7]

Clarification of Terms

Pregnancy-Induced Hypertension

A number of authors have used the term *pregnancy-induced hypertension* (PIH) broadly to describe all new onsets of hypertension in pregnancy, including hypertension not accompanied by proteinuria as well as hypertension with proteinuria (i.e., preeclampsia). Currently, key obstetric textbooks and journal articles are dropping the term; *pregnancy-induced hypertension* is no longer being used.[3–9] The Working Group Report on Hypertensive Disorders of Pregnancy has proposed a simplified classification system and defined terminology that might serve as a standard guideline. This module incorporates this new classification system.

Gestational and Transient Hypertension

Gestational hypertension is defined as a blood pressure elevation (as defined above) detected for the first time after midpregnancy, generally after 20 weeks. This term is nonspecific and is considered an umbrella term for the continuum of hypertensive disorders unique to pregnancy. This term has replaced pregnancy-induced hypertension or PIH. *Transient hypertension* describes the group of women who have gestational hypertension that resolves during the postpartum period.[5]

NOTE: Gestational and transient hypertension previously fell under the broad category of PIH. The new classification system arranges these terms for the purpose of diagnosis somewhat differently.

Classification of Hypertensive Disorders Complicating Pregnancy

Each hypertensive disorder complicating pregnancy has distinguishing characteristics, diagnostic criteria, and risks of perinatal morbidity and mortality. This discussion follows the Working Group Classification System:

1. Gestational hypertension
2. Preeclampsia/eclampsia

NOTE: HELLP syndrome—a serious extension of preeclampsia—is discussed within this category.

3. Preeclampsia superimposed upon chronic hypertension
4. Chronic hypertension

Important observations that reflect current understanding of the hypertensive disorders in pregnancy include the following:

- Pregnancy can induce hypertension in normotensive women *or* aggravate existing hypertension.[5]
- Hypertensive states are classified according to certain signs or symptoms and time of occurrence in relation to the pregnancy.
- The term *pregnancy-induced hypertension* has sometimes been used to designate women with elevated BP but no proteinuria or edema. It is not a diagnostic category in the classification system presented by the Working Group Report.[5]
- The presence of hypertension before or very early in pregnancy increases the incidence of complications for both the mother and fetus, with a 10-fold higher risk of fetal loss.[5]
- When hypertension is documented before conception or before 20 weeks' gestation, it is more likely to be chronic hypertension that is either essential hypertension from unknown causes or secondary hypertension with an identified cause (e.g., renal disease).[2]
- Elevated BP seen at midpregnancy (20 to 28 weeks) may be due to either early preeclampsia, which is rarely seen before 24 weeks; transient hypertension, which resolves quickly after delivery; or chronic hypertension that has not been recognized in the woman and will remain beyond 12 weeks postpartum.[5]
- HELLP syndrome does not appear in the classification system because it is considered an extension of the pathophysiologic process of preeclampsia. HELLP syndrome is addressed later in this module.
- Fetal risks in a pregnancy complicated by hypertension include growth restriction, abruptio placentae, fetal distress, preterm birth, and low birth weight with subsequent perinatal morbidity and mortality.[3]
- The perinatal mortality rate increases as maternal BP and proteinuria increase.[3–5]
- Chronic hypertension and preeclampsia **do not** have the same etiology or pathophysiology and must be carefully differentiated.

NOTE: *Although pregnancy-related hypertensive disorders are discussed as separate diagnoses, it must be remembered that gestational hypertension and chronic hypertension may coexist and that progression from mild disease to severe disease can occur rapidly. Because the classification system is not precise and a missed diagnosis may lead to increased risk of adverse maternal and perinatal outcomes, a more prudent approach for clinical management of pregnancy-related hypertension is to overdiagnose preeclampsia.*

Gestational Hypertension

- Formerly called PIH or transient hypertension, in clinical practice, *gestational hypertension* is a retrospective diagnosis
- Onset of hypertension, generally after the 20th week of pregnancy, appearing as a marker of a pregnancy-specific vasospastic condition[3–5]
- Can progress to preeclampsia with development of proteinuria and other diagnostic indicators
- Is referred to as **gestational hypertension of pregnancy** *if hypertension is first diagnosed during pregnancy, is transient, does not progress into preeclampsia, and the woman is normotensive by 12 weeks postpartum*

OR

Is diagnosed as **chronic hypertension** *if BP elevation persists beyond 12 weeks postpartum*

NOTE: *The diagnosis of gestational hypertension is used during pregnancy until criteria (signs and symptoms) arise that define a more specific diagnosis. The practitioner must keep in mind that hypertension during pregnancy represents a continuum of disease processes. Hypertension may be the first sign, but the underlying pathophysiology can involve all major organ systems.*

Preeclampsia/Eclampsia

- Usually occurring after 20 weeks' gestation, preeclampsia is characterized by renal involvement, as evidenced by the onset of proteinuria and represents a pregnancy-specific

syndrome of reduced organ perfusion including the utero–placental–fetal unit, secondary to cyclic vasospasms, and activation of the coagulation cascade[5,6]
- Occurs earlier in hydatidiform mole or hydrops (diseases of the trophoblast placenta)
- Determined by hypertension as defined above and proteinuria
- **Eclampsia**—the onset of seizure activity or coma in the woman diagnosed with preeclampsia, with no history of preexisting neurologic pathology[5,6]

Preeclampsia Superimposed Upon Chronic Hypertension (Superimposed Preeclampsia)

- Occurrence of preeclampsia in a woman who enters pregnancy with known hypertension

Chronic Hypertension

- Hypertension that is present and observable before pregnancy

OR

- Hypertension that is diagnosed for the first time during pregnancy and persists beyond the 84th day postpartum[3]

Diagnosis

▶ **How are the various hypertensive disorders diagnosed?**

Screening Criteria

In the past, noninvasive screening procedures were used to predict a woman's risk of developing hypertension or preeclampsia. The tests are mentioned here because their use needs to be put to rest once and for all. The three most commonly used tests were the following:
- Calculating the second trimester mean arterial pressure (MAP) to predict risks and associated perinatal morbidity and mortality
- Noting the absence of a decline in late second trimester BP, which might be interpreted as a pathophysiologic response predicting maternal or fetal risk
- Using the roll-over test (supine pressure test)—performed at 28 to 32 weeks' gestation to detect a woman's unique sensitivity to vasopressor substances in her circulatory system by assessing BP on her side and then on her back

    These screening tests do not contain consistently predictable, reproducible, and reliable results and should not be used in screening women to predict a risk for preeclampsia.[5]

> Because reliable screening criteria are unavailable, the emphasis in clinical practice should be on timely and accurate assessment of *diagnostic criteria*. The goal of management should target the prevention of maternal and perinatal morbidity and mortality by the initiation of palliative therapy and timely birth of the infant.

Diagnostic Criteria

Using evidence-based medicine, the Working Group Report on High Blood Pressure in Pregnancy and others[5,6] identify reliable *diagnostic criteria* and guidelines to be used in the evaluation of hypertensive states in pregnancy. Table 9.1 illustrates the diagnostic criteria for each.

Gestational Hypertension

- Gestational hypertension is hypertension only, without proteinuria, with normal laboratory test results, and in the absence of symptoms.
- It has been defined and explained in terms of *criteria* and *timing* under the classification listing on page 261.
- This classification no doubt includes women with hypertension of different etiologies. Some women may develop essential hypertension later in life.

TABLE 9.1	DIAGNOSTIC CRITERIA USE IN THE DIAGNOSIS OF HYPERTENSIVE DISORDERS COMPLICATING PREGNANCY

TYPE OF HYPERTENSION	DIAGNOSTIC CRITERIA	SIGNIFICANCE
Gestational hypertension	• New onset of hypertension, generally after 20 weeks of gestation • Hypertension defined as: • SBP ≥140 mmHg, **OR** • DBP ≥ 90 mmHg	• Replaces PIH • A retrospective diagnosis • BP normalizes to prepregnancy values by 12 weeks postpartum • Think oxygenation and perfusion
Preeclampsia	• Gestational hypertensive plus gestational proteinuria in a previously normotensive woman • Gestational proteinuria defined as • >300 mg on random specimen • ≥1+ on dipstick	• In absence of proteinuria, suspect if any of the following are present: • Headache • Blurred vision • Abdominal pain • Abnormal laboratory tests
Severe	• Diagnosis of preeclampsia plus at least one of the following: • SBP ≥160 mmHg • DBP ≥110 mmHg • Proteinuria >2 g/24 hr • Serum creatinine >1.2 mg/dL (unless known to be previously elevated) • Platelets <100,000 • ↑ LD (hemolysis) • ↑ ALT or AST • Persistent HA, cerebral/visual disturbances • Persistent epigastric pain	• One of sickest patients on unit • At increased risk for complications • Additional criteria for diagnosis may include: • Oliguria defined as <500 mL/24 hrs • Pulmonary edema • Impaired liver function of unclear etiology • IUGR • Oligohydramnios • Grand mal seizures (eclampsia)
HELLP syndrome	• Diagnosis based on presence of: • Hemolysis • Elevated liver enzymes • Low platelets • Hemolysis • Abnormal peripheral smear • LD >600 U/L • Total bilirubin ≥1.2 mg/dL • Elevated liver enzymes • Serum AST >70 Units/L • LD >600 U/L • Low Platelets <150,000	• Form of severe preeclampsia • Laboratory diagnosis • Impairs oxygenation and perfusion • Severity of disease, morbidity/mortality, and recovery related to platelet levels • <150,000 BUT >100,000 • <100,000 BUT >50,000 • <50,000
Eclampsia	• Diagnosis of preeclampsia • Occurrence of seizures • No other possible etiology for seizure	• Critically ill patient • At risk for cerebral hemorrhage and aspiration • Foley's rule of 13: • 13% mortality • 13% abruption • 13% seize after MgSO$_4$ therapy • 13% seize >48 hours postpartum
Chronic hypertension	• Hypertension defined as: • SBP ≥140 mmHg, **OR** • DBP ≥90 mmHg • Hypertension • Present and observable before pregnancy • Diagnosed before 20 weeks gestation • Persist beyond 12 weeks postpartum	• Diagnosis not known prior to pregnancy • Places pregnancy at increased risk for abruption

table continues on page 264

TABLE 9.1	DIAGNOSTIC CRITERIA USE IN THE DIAGNOSIS OF HYPERTENSIVE DISORDERS COMPLICATING PREGNANCY *(Continued)*

TYPE OF HYPERTENSION	DIAGNOSTIC CRITERIA	SIGNIFICANCE

Superimposed preeclampsia	• Diagnosis based on presence of ≥1 of the following in the woman with chronic hypertension:
	  • New onset of proteinuria
	  • Hypertension and proteinuria before 20th week gestation
	  • Sudden ↑ in proteinuria
	  • Sudden ↑ BP (previously well controlled)
	  • ↑ ALT or AST to abnormal levels
	  • Thrombocytopenia
		• Prognosis worse for woman and fetus
		• Mandates close observation
		• Timing of delivery indicated by overall assessment of maternal–fetal well-being rather than fixed end-point

Abbreviations: ALT (SGPT), alanine amino transferase; AST (SGOT), aspartate aminotransferase From National Blood Pressure Education Program (2000). *Working Group report on high blood pressure in pregnancy.* Bethesda, MD; National Heart, Lung, and Blood Institute.[6]

- A rise of BP in the latter half of pregnancy should be watched carefully. Both the mother and fetus could be in danger. Overdiagnosing preeclampsia is preferable to missing the diagnosis until the disease process has worsened.[5,6]
- Transient hypertension
  - *Is diagnosed in retrospect (when BP elevation resolves with no adverse sequelae)*
  - Is not accompanied by poor birth outcomes
  - Is sometimes seen in normotensive mothers within the first few hours after delivery, with subsequent return to baseline BP levels within 24 hours[5,6]

Preeclampsia

Preeclampsia is a progression of gestational hypertension characterized by renal involvement as evidenced by the onset of proteinuria. Preeclampsia is either said to be mild or severe, based on maternal or fetal findings.[5]

> Gestational BP elevation is defined as BP 140 mmHg or higher systole or 90 mmHg or higher diastole in a woman who has been normotensive before 20 weeks' gestation.

Remember, when distinguishing gestational hypertension from preeclampsia, *preeclampsia is more than hypertension—it is a syndrome.*

NOTE: Preeclampsia is actually a syndrome that occurs only in the presence of pregnancy (the placenta plays a key role). Preeclampsia is caused by reduced perfusion of one or more organs, which results from vasospasm of arterioles and damage to the lining (endothelium) of the arterioles. It resolves with delivery of the fetus and placenta.

While acknowledging that the cause of this disorder is unknown and most likely has no one single cause, Norwitz and Repke[10] state that preeclampsia is a multisystem disorder specific to the placenta. They cite the primary pathology as being a defect in placental development. The normal physiologic process involves embryo/fetal-derived cells of the trophoblast, which invade the uterine lining (decidua) and its vasculature, specifically the arteriole walls of uterine blood vessels. This invasion appears to play a critical role in the progressive and marked enlargement of the spiral arterioles in the endometrial lining. "The fetus is anchored to the mother." *The result ensures an adequate blood supply to the growing placenta and fetus.* Preeclampsia is characterized by a restriction of this process in which 30% to 50% of the placenta's spiral arteries show no evidence of trophoblastic invasion.[10]

According to Norwitz and Repke, "the end result in preeclampsia is an inability of the uterine vasculature to accommodate the necessary increase in blood flow with increasing gestational age…clinical manifestations of the disorder become apparent when the fetal placental unit outgrows its blood supply."[10] Underperfusion of the placenta is believed to produce chemical factors that enter the maternal circulation and eventually affect the vascular endothelium (the endothelial lining of the body's widespread arteriolar system). More of the pathophysiology is discussed later in this module.

Other important facts related to preeclampsia include the following:
- Preeclampsia can occur before the 20th gestational week, when there are pathologic changes in the placenta, and with the development of a hydatidiform molar pregnancy. In the United States and Europe, molar pregnancies occur in 1 per 1,000 expectant women and are typically characterized by the following:
  - Severe nausea and vomiting
  - Elevated BP
  - Elevated human chorionic gonadotropin (hCG) levels
  - Absence of fetal movement or fetal heartbeat
  - Uterine size larger than dates by last menstrual period
  - Vaginal bleeding
  - Passage of grapelike clustered vesicles

> Preeclampsia before 24 weeks' gestation necessitates evaluation to rule out a complete or partial molar pregnancy.

- Preeclampsia occurs in approximately 5% of pregnant women, but this incidence is highly variable, with a higher incidence in women younger than 20 or older than 35 years of age, in nulliparous women, and in women with multiple fetuses.[5]
- Preeclampsia complicates approximately 20% of teenage pregnancies (younger than 20 years of age).
- It exists as a disease for weeks or even months before signs or symptoms are evident.
- It is often not accompanied by proteinuria until late in the disease (late third trimester or intrapartum period).
- Significant proteinuria means:
  - 300 mg/L in a 24-hour specimen

OR

  - 2+ or greater on dipstick (tested twice 4 hours apart) in the absence of a urinary tract infection

> Bacterial invasion of the vaginal or urinary tract mucosal lining causes tissue breakdown, releasing protein metabolites. Thus, protein found in the urine of a woman with a urinary tract or vaginal infection does not necessarily indicate kidney malfunction.

CLINICAL SIGNS OF PREECLAMPSIA CAN OCCUR SUDDENLY. NEVER UNDERESTIMATE THE IMPORTANCE OF EVEN MILD BLOOD PRESSURE ELEVATIONS COMPLICATING A PREGNANCY.[5]

Preeclampsia is usually categorized as mild or severe, based primarily on the degree of hypertension or proteinuria and whether other organ systems are involved.

Mild preeclampsia occurs when the following are found:
- BP has reached 140/90 mmHg or greater but is less than 160/110 mmHg on two different occasions 4 hours apart.
- Proteinuria, trace to +1 or about 300 mg in a 24-hour urine specimen, is noted.
- Signs that preeclampsia may be present are as follows:
  - Weight gain of more than 5 pounds per week during the second trimester or more than 2 pounds per week during the third trimester
  - Slight edema throughout the body

Severe preeclampsia occurs when the following are found:
- Systolic blood pressure of 160 mmHg or higher or diastolic blood pressure 110 mmHg or higher
- Proteinuria is persistent 2+ or more (500 mg or greater per 24 hours).
- Urine output decreases to less than 500 mL in 24 hours (i.e., less than 30 mL/h).

NOTE: Differentiating between mild and severe preeclampsia is not always clinically helpful because mild disease can rapidly progress to severe illness.

In severe preeclampsia, the kidneys can go into failure with little output. This is a serious situation that can lead to permanent renal injury.

Symptoms of severe disease include:

Severe headaches
Visual problems (scotoma or blurring)
Epigastric pain
Nausea or vomiting

Thrombocytopenia

Irritability, restlessness, or apprehension
Pulmonary edema with respiratory distress

Signs of severe disease include[5,7]:

Severe proteinuria (3+ dipstick or greater)
Oliguria (less than 500 mL per 24 hours)
Low platelet count (less than 100,000/mm^3)
Elevated hepatic enzymes (alanine amino-
    transferase [ALT] or aspartate
    aminotransferase [AST])
Increased serum creatinine (greater than
    1.2 mg/dL unless known to be previously
    elevated)
Fetal IUGR
Coagulation abnormalities

Early identification of worsening preeclampsia in a patient at a Level I or II hospital is critical. Transport to a high-risk regional center should be done while the patient is stable and before a critical state is reached. Both the mother and fetus are at risk.[4,11]

When severe preeclampsia occurs before 32 weeks' gestation, the incidence of serious complications in the mother is high and fetal outcome may be poor, often as a result of growth restriction and/or asphyxia at birth.

WATCH FOR SIGNS OF THE FOLLOWING:

- Abruptio placentae
- HELLP syndrome
- Eclampsia
- Disseminated intravascular coagulation (DIC)
- Acute renal failure

▶ **Are certain pregnant women at risk for developing preeclampsia?**

Predisposing factors to preeclampsia exist in women[5]:

- Who are young and pregnant for the first time
- Who are young and experiencing a second pregnancy but with a new father
- With a partner who has fathered a preeclamptic pregnancy in another woman
- With a history of chronic hypertension or renal disease (renal vascular hypertension, nephrotic syndrome, adult polycystic kidney disease)
- With a twin pregnancy
- With diabetes
- With a history of preeclampsia
- Who are black and older than 35 years of age
- With collagen vascular disease (i.e., lupus or antiphospholipid antibody syndrome)

Pregnancies in which placental size is increased (e.g., multiple fetuses, diabetes, syphilis, isoimmunized pregnancies, hydatidiform moles) carry a higher risk because the placenta plays an important role in pathophysiologic processes.

Careful assessment should be done on women identified as at risk:

- Teenagers or women over 35 years of age
- African-American and other minority women 35 years of age and older
- Women with a multiple gestation
- Women with a history of chronic hypertension
- Women who were hypertensive during a previous pregnancy

HELLP Syndrome

- HELLP syndrome, a multisystem disease, *is a form of severe preeclampsia*
- It is named for its primary laboratory abnormalities—**H**emolysis, **E**levated **L**iver enzymes, and **L**ow **P**latelets (HELLP)[3,4,8]
- Experts agree that hemolysis, liver dysfunction, and thrombocytopenia must be present for the diagnosis, but no agreement has been reached regarding specific criteria.
- HELLP syndrome involves a group of clinical/pathologic manifestations resulting from arteriolar vasospasm, which lead to the development of microangiopathic hemolytic anemia. Microvascular endothelial damage and intravascular platelet activation can be documented with laboratory studies. No one precipitating cause of this syndrome has been found.[3,8]
- The incidence of HELLP syndrome in preeclamptic women is reported to be 2% to 12%. An accurate rate of occurrence is unknown because of difficulties with agreement on diagnostic criteria.[3,8]
- HELLP syndrome occurs before term (late second or early third trimester) in more than 80% of women, with 11% of the cases occurring before 27 weeks; approximately one third of cases become evident during the postdelivery period.
- A significant risk of maternal mortality, approaching 1.0% to 3.5%, is seen with HELLP syndrome.

NOTE: Women with HELLP syndrome often present with nonspecific symptoms or subtle signs. The woman is usually white and in her second or third trimester.

A common scenario is a woman complaining of "just not feeling good," "a flulike feeling," nausea, epigastric pain, or right upper quadrant pain. She may have no hypertension (15% of cases) or only mild hypertension (16% of cases). In addition, proteinuria may be absent or only 1+ on a urine dipstick. These women are very ill but are often misdiagnosed with the flu, gastroenteritis, appendicitis, viral hepatitis, gallbladder disease, or pyelonephritis.

- The *maternal* mortality rate approaches 1.0% to 3.5%.
- Maternal mortality and morbidity are consequences of the following:
  - Spontaneous and postpartum hemorrhage
  - Development of superimposed DIC
  - Abruptio placentae
  - Renal failure
  - Pulmonary edema
  - Hepatic rupture
- The *perinatal* mortality rate ranges from 56 to 637 per 1,000 births.[12] Fetal death often occurs at gestational ages near the limit of viability because of the following:
  - Severe growth restriction
  - Abruptio placentae
- Many patients initially worsen after delivery and then begin to improve.

Eclampsia

- Eclampsia is defined as the onset of seizure activity or coma in the woman diagnosed with gestational hypertension or preeclampsia, with no history of preexisting neurologic pathology.[4-7]
- It represents a worsening of preeclampsia, with rapid deterioration of function in several organs and systems.
- The incidence is estimated at 1 in 3,250 for women in the United States.
- It is seen both in women without HELLP syndrome and in those with HELLP.
- Eclamptic women with HELLP syndrome often experience the following:
  - Preterm labor
  - Earlier gestational ages
  - Lower birth weights
  - Lower Apgar scores
  - Greater perinatal morbidity and mortality
  Maternal mortality is most often due to the following:
- Abruptio placentae

- Cerebral hemorrhage
- Acute renal or cardiac failure
- DIC

NOTE: Eclamptic convulsions can occur in women who have mildly elevated BP and mild proteinuria and in women who show few warning signs of a worsening condition.

Eclamptic seizures are generally self-limited, lasting 1 to 2 minutes.[13] Immediate care during a seizure is to provide supportive therapy and ensure a patent airway. Once this has been attained, adequate oxygenation must be maintained by use of supplemental oxygen. Supportive therapy is continued and focuses on minimizing the risk of aspiration, minimizing the risk of recurrent seizure activity, and controlling blood pressure. Once the patient has become stable, management is directed to delivery of the infant.

Despite the rapid onset of convulsions characterizing eclampsia, ideally, no woman should experience eclampsia in a hospitalized setting. Signs, symptoms, and risk factors should indicate the woman's deterioration to medical and nursing personnel. However, a woman presenting to the labor unit with limited or no prenatal care can progress quickly to eclampsia.

▶ What distinguishes eclampsia from preeclampsia?

The distinguishing characteristic of eclampsia is the presence of convulsions. Before convulsions, the BP often rises and the woman complains of a severe headache and epigastric pain. The convulsive state involves the following:

- Initial twitching of facial muscles
- Alternating muscle contraction, with hands and teeth clenching and then relaxing
- Respirations that stop and then begin again with deep, heavy, and noisy breathing
- Coma, which can follow and last from 2 to 3 minutes to several hours

> Aspiration is a leading cause of maternal morbidity after an eclamptic seizure. The woman should be in a lateral decubitus position to minimize the risk of aspiration if vomiting occurs. Emergency airway equipment, including suctioning, should be readily available.

REMEMBER: Preeclampsia need not be severe to progress to eclampsia. Also, eclampsia can occur in the absence of proteinuria.

Rapid assessments of maternal status, uterine activity, cervical status, and fetal status are performed immediately after an eclamptic seizure. During the seizure, membranes may rupture, and the cervix may dilate because the uterus becomes hypercontractile and hypertonic. If birth is not imminent, the timing and route of delivery and the induction of labor versus cesarean birth depend on maternal and fetal status. All medications and therapy are merely temporary measures.

Preeclampsia Superimposed on Chronic Hypertension

- Preeclampsia superimposed upon chronic hypertension is defined as the occurrence of preeclampsia in women who have chronic hypertension.[5,7]
- *The prognosis for both the mother and fetus is much worse than with either chronic hypertension or preeclampsia alone.*
- The diagnosis is highly likely with the following findings:
  - New-onset proteinuria (300 mg or greater or +1 or greater dipstick in 24 hours) in women at less than 20 weeks' gestation with hypertension but no proteinuria
  - Hypertension and proteinuria before 20 weeks' gestation
  - Sudden increase in proteinuria
  - Sudden increase in BP in a woman whose hypertension has previously been well controlled
  - *Thrombocytopenia* (platelet count less than 100,000 cells/mm^3)
  - Increase in ALT or AST to abnormal levels
- The incidence of superimposed preeclampsia is about 25% in women with chronic hypertension.

- The combination of hypertension and proteinuria in pregnancy significantly increases the risks of perinatal morbidity and mortality.
- The disease can progress to eclampsia.
- The risk of abruptio placentae is increased in these women.
- The fetus is at even greater risk of growth restriction than with preeclampsia or chronic hypertension alone.

Chronic Hypertension

- Chronic hypertension is defined as hypertension that is present and observable before pregnancy or that is diagnosed before the 20th week of gestation.[3,5,14,15]
- The distinction between chronic hypertension, gestational hypertension, and preeclampsia can be complex in the clinical setting. Even more difficult is the differentiation between the exacerbation of preexisting hypertension and the development of superimposed preeclampsia.[3]

***NOTE:** When hypertension is diagnosed for the first time during pregnancy and does not resolve by 84 days postpartum, it is diagnosed as chronic hypertension.[5,16]*

- The prevalence of chronic hypertension in women of reproductive age varies according to age, race, ethnicity, and body mass index.
- Women are experiencing pregnancies at a later age in the United States. Given the trend of childbearing at an older age, it is expected that the incidence of chronic hypertension in pregnancy will continue to rise.[15]
- Of all chronic hypertensive pregnant women, 90% have primary (or essential) hypertension (hypertension with no known cause).
- Many women have secondary hypertension, the cause of which lies in a pathologic process of an organ system (e.g., renal disease).
- Chronic hypertension occurs in 1% to 5% of pregnancies, depending on the population and diagnostic criteria used (Table 9.2).

TABLE 9.2	PREVALENCE OF HYPERTENSION IN WOMEN OF REPRODUCTIVE AGE		
	18–29 YEARS (%)	**30–39 YEARS (%)**	**40–49 YEARS (%)**
African American	2.0	22.3	30.5
Caucasian	0.6	4.6	12.7
Mexican American	1.0	6.2	10.6

Data from AHRQ. (2000). *Management of chronic hypertension in pregnancy* [Evidence Report/Technology Assessment Number 14]. (p. 12). Rockville, MD: U.S. Department of Health and Human Services.

- The prevalence of essential hypertension is two to three times higher in African-America women than in white women.
- Pregnancies complicated by chronic hypertension are associated with increased rates of adverse outcomes such as fetal deaths, fetal growth restriction, small-for-gestational-age infants, premature delivery, and placental abruption. This is especially seen in women with superimposed preeclampsia, severe hypertension, and long-standing hypertension, as well as in women with preexisting cardiovascular renal disease.[5,16]
- When pregnant women experience mild, uncomplicated chronic hypertension, perinatal morbidity and mortality do not increase significantly.
- When renal disease is present, the woman has an increased risk of perinatal mortality and can experience reduced renal function during her pregnancy.
- During pregnancy, women with chronic hypertension but no complicating illnesses require careful surveillance for high BP and other signs or symptoms of preeclampsia. Prenatal visits may be scheduled more frequently.

***NOTE:** Sodium restriction in pregnant women with mild or moderate chronic hypertension is not advocated because many of these women will have a lower plasma volume than normotensive women. Sodium restriction might lead to an even lower plasma volume.*

Evidence-Based Findings on Clinical Management of Chronic Hypertension[9–11]

- Specific preconception BP management strategies to ascertain beneficial or adverse effects on conception or pregnancy outcomes *have not been studied in trials.*
- Women with stage 1 or stage 2 hypertension (defined as systolic blood pressure of 140 to 179 mmHg or diastolic blood pressure of 90 to 109 mmHg) are at low risk for cardiovascular complications during the pregnancy.[5]
- Women with essential hypertension, stage 1 or stage 2, with normal renal function are candidates for nondrug therapy; currently there are no data to support improved perinatal outcomes in this group with antihypertensive therapy.[5]
- If the woman is on antihypertensive therapy at the initial prenatal visit, there is a lack of consensus on whether the antihypertensive agent should be continued or discontinued. The use of antihypertensive agents may be beneficial for the woman to lower blood pressure; however, the lower pressure may impair uteroplacental perfusion leading to fetal compromise.[17]
- Care of the woman who has chronic hypertension parallels routine antenatal management, with an emphasis on assessments to identify exacerbation of the hypertension or end-organ dysfunction.
- The use of ACE inhibitors are contraindicated because of their association with IUGR, oligohydramnios, neonatal renal failure, and neonatal death. Although data are not available on the use of angiotensin II receptor antagonists during pregnancy, adverse effects are likely to be similar to ACE inhibitors; these agents should be avoided. See Table 9.3 for the antihypertensive agents used for chronic hypertension complicating pregnancy.[5,14]

TABLE 9.3 ANTIHYPERTENSIVE AGENTS FOR CHRONIC HYPERTENSION					
AGENT	**MECHANISM OF ACTION**	**CARDIAC OUTPUT**	**RENAL BLOOD FLOW**	**MATERNAL SIDE EFFECTS**	**NEONATAL SIDE EFFECTS**
Methyldopa	False neurotransmission, CNS effect	Unchanged	Unchanged	Lethargy, fever, hepatitis, hemolytic anemia, positive Coombs	
Hydralazine	Direct peripheral vasodilatation, arterial predominant	Increased	Unchanged or increased	Flushing, headache, tachycardia, palpitations, lupus syndrome	
Labetalol	α- and β-adrenergic blockade	Unchanged	Unchanged	Tremulousness, flushing, headache	Depressed respirations, hypoglycemia, bradycardia
Nifedipine	Calcium channel blocker	Unchanged	Unchanged	Orthostatic hypotension, headache, tachycardia	None demonstrated in humans
Clonidine	CNS effects	Unchanged or increased	Unchanged	Rebound hypotension, little information on use in pregnancy	
Propranolol	β-Adrenergic blockade	Decreased	Decreased	Increased uterine tone with possible decrease in placental perfusion	Depressed respirations
Thiazide	Initial: decreased plasma volume and cardiac output Later: decreased total peripheral resistance	Decreased	Decreased	Electrolyte depletion, serum uric acid increase, thrombocytopenia, hemorrhagic pancreatitis	Thrombocytopenia

Abbreviation: CNS, central nervous system.

Major Theories Regarding the Etiology of Preeclampsia/Eclampsia

Preeclampsia has been called the "disease of theories." Epidemiologic evidence suggests that an immune maladaptive response is involved in the etiology of preeclampsia/eclampsia. Pregnancy normally involves degrees of maternal inflammatory responses. The presence of preeclampsia may be the result of an abnormal or exaggerated intravascular response to the presence of foreign genetic material (i.e., fetal and especially placental tissue).[5,10,14]

Paternity may also play a significant role in the pathogenesis of preeclampsia. Women conceiving with men from a different racial group have a higher incidence of preeclampsia. In addition, the multiparous woman appears to return to the nullipara's (first pregnancy) risk for developing preeclampsia when she conceives with a new partner. Immune mechanisms explaining these relationships have not been identified.[5,10,14]

Genetic disposition is thought to play a fairly strong role, and there is a significant amount of evidence supporting familial disposition to preeclampsia/eclampsia. Increased evidence is seen in the obstetric histories of mothers, daughters, and granddaughters. There may be maternal inheritance of single-gene recessive trait or a dominant gene with incomplete dominance.

▶ What are the major pathophysiologic and anatomic changes that occur during preeclampsia or eclampsia?

Many experts consider the placenta the pathogenic focus (primary origin point of pathology) for all manifestations of preeclampsia because delivery is the only definitive cure. Understanding the pathophysiologic and anatomic changes that lead to preeclampsia and eclampsia can make medical management and nursing care for women far more insightful. The underlying disease process is one of widespread arteriolar vasospasm that probably results from abnormal sensitivity of a woman's vascular smooth muscle to vasoconstrictor substances produced in her body. The vasospastic episode leads to injury of the endothelial lining of blood vessels, with a subsequent platelet deposition and fibrin adherence to damaged cell walls. A damaged vascular endothelium results in capillary leakage of protein and fluid (referred to as *vascular permeability*). Intravascular fluid moves to the extravascular space.[3,5] The pathogenesis of preeclampsia remains incompletely understood, despite years of research. Hypertension is the primary clinical feature of the disease, but it is neither the cause nor the earliest symptom.[3,5]

Preeclampsia is a complex clinical syndrome that can involve one system or all organ systems. It is thought to develop early in pregnancy, perhaps as early as implantation, but is expressed late in the disease process as a vasospasm of arteriolar beds.

Remember that what seems to be involved here is a pathologic process that precedes the development of diagnostic signs by several weeks or months. Because vasospasms can occur within the placental bed, fetal circulation can be compromised long before warning signs are evident.

> The rationale for nursing interventions and medical management is directly related to the pathophysiologic and anatomic changes that occur in preeclampsia.

▶ Why do some pregnant women experience arteriolar vasospasm and hypertension?[3,5]

Women with pregnancy-induced hypertensive disorders fail to experience certain homeostatic, physical, and biochemical changes that are characteristic of normal pregnancy. Generally, homeostasis in humans is maintained between vasopressor (vasoconstriction) and vasodilator (vasodilatation) tendencies, resulting in "normal" BP. This finely tuned balance is mediated by complex chemical and neurogenic controls, many of which are not completely understood. The following are a few of the more widely accepted findings that explain pathophysiologic processes in pregnant woman that lead to increased sensitivity to circulating vasoconstricting substances.

Preeclamptic women have an imbalance in two potent vasoactive substances:

Prostacyclin (PGI₂)
- A hormone synthesized in the endothelial lining of blood vessels
- A potent vasodilator
- An inhibitor of platelet aggregation
- Appropriate levels important for resisting circulating vasoconstrictors, such as angiotensin II and norepinephrine

Thromboxane
- Produced primarily by platelets
- A potent vasoconstrictor
- A stimulator of platelet aggregation

Studies indicate that, although the blood levels of both substances are increased in pregnancy, preeclamptic women demonstrate much higher levels of thromboxane.

Preeclamptic women have an increased sensitivity to a chemical substance called angiotensin II. This vasoconstrictor is produced by a complex conversion system that begins with renin production by the kidneys, ovaries, uterus, and placenta. Renin acts on the precursor angiotensinogen in the liver to convert it to an inactive chemical, angiotensin I. In turn, angiotensin I becomes biologically active angiotensin II, which effects smooth muscle contractions, stimulates aldosterone production and sodium retention, and enhances the reactivity of the smooth muscles of the vascular system to norepinephrine. In normal pregnancies, the vasoactive responses to angiotensin II are moderate and vascular tone is not unduly increased.

Recently, investigators have theorized that the vasoconstricting potential of some vasopressor substances such as angiotensin II and endothelin (produced in endothelial cells) is magnified in preeclampsia as a result of diminished nitric oxide synthase and endothelin-derived releasing factor (EDRF)—both substances playing a role in mediating delicate vasopressor/vasoconstrictor mechanisms.

Therefore, preeclamptic women appear to experience a deficiency of certain protective substances thought to be found in these prostaglandins. This deficiency predisposes the woman to increased vasopressor sensitivity, which leads to increased vascular tone and hypertension.

Preeclamptic women tend to have an abnormal placental implantation process, resulting in incomplete invasion of the uterine spiral arteries. Normally, as the developing placenta (called the trophoblast) implants in the uterine wall, it literally erodes into the spiral arteries found in the endometrium (the inner lining of the uterus). This process of erosion or migration into the spiral arteries converts small, narrow arteries to widened uteroplacental arteries that accommodate a generous blood supply that empties into the intervillous spaces of the placenta.

In preeclampsia, this process does not happen completely and is thought to lead to arterial vasoconstriction at the uteroplacental site.

Currently, many studies are underway to explore more completely the pathogenesis of this puzzling disorder. The etiology of the disease remains unknown.

The following are major areas affected by arteriolar vasoconstriction and vasospasm that give rise to symptoms.

- Kidney
- Cerebrum
- Uteroplacental unit
- Liver

▶ How does the vasospastic process lead to pathophysiologic alterations?

Understanding the vasospastic process is critical for appreciating the diagnostic signs and symptoms in hypertensive disorders of pregnancy.

***NOTE:** Microangiopathy is a disease of small blood vessels—as in diabetic microangiopathy, in which the basement membrane of capillaries thickens, or as in thrombotic microangiopathy, in which thrombi form in the arterioles and capillaries.*

An example using a visual life experience might aid in grasping the significance of microangiopathic changes in the vascular system.

Imagine a solid but flexible pipe, 4 inches in diameter. Fluids flow through it at a moderate pace. Because the pipe walls are intact, the volume of fluid flowing in and out remains unchanged.

Now imagine the pipe being subjected, for long periods, to great stress, such as severe vibrations or immense pressure on all sides. The pipe, initially whole and intact, begins deteriorating. The walls might begin to collapse, and/or small cracks or openings appear.

If the pipe narrows, the volume of fluid flowing through at a certain rate is reduced. If the pipe walls begin to crack, some of the fluid and its contents are lost through the tiny openings.

Now apply this imagery to a blood vessel—an arteriole or capillary. When subjected to intense vasopressor substances, the vessel might constrict and/or spasm. This stress can also cause the blood vessel to lose its integrity. Intense vasospasm causes injury to the endothelial cells, which make up the lining of the arterioles. Several changes can occur:

- Pressure within the arteriole is increased.
- Fluid or fluid components can seep out of the blood vessel. These components could be protein substances (e.g., albumin), fluid, or both.

- Perfusion to the tissues that the arterioles supply is reduced not only in amount but possibly in content. Perfused components that could potentially be reduced are blood with its oxygen-carrying capacity and proteins.

When applying these activities to the blood supply of a body system such as the kidney, the overall result would be as follows:

- Hypertension within the kidney
- Reactive vasospasm in arterioles
- Breakdown in the endothelial lining of the arterioles
- Loss of blood and plasma content from the kidney vasculature
- Hemorrhage
- Change in oncotic pressures
- Poor perfusion leading to accumulation of extracellular fluid in kidney tissue and/or ischemia and necrosis

Imagine these alterations occurring at cerebral, hepatic, or uteroplacental sites. The result is poor perfusion to the site, as well as edema and the formation of hemorrhagic areas throughout the tissue of the particular target organ.

▶ What about other pathophysiologic changes?

Arteriolar spasm leading to damage of the endothelial layer of small blood vessels remains the basis on which other changes occur.

1. The endothelial layer forms lesions (cracks in the pipe, so to speak), activating the body's immune system. Platelets accumulate at lesion sites and a fibrin network forms. Because blood continues to course through the damaged vessels, red blood cells are forced through the network under high pressure and are fragmented or "chopped up." This fragmentation of red blood cells results in hemolysis and is referred to as *microangiopathic hemolytic anemia.* It is a unique sign of the severest form of preeclampsia: HELLP syndrome.
2. Platelets are used up in this pathologic process, leading to thrombocytopenia.
3. As a consequence of vessel narrowing and changes in the coagulation process, microemboli form in the vasculature. The coagulation process leads to ischemia (diminished tissue perfusion) with subsequent tissue damage (e.g., the liver or kidney) and serious organ malfunction. When these pathologic alterations progress to the extreme, dire consequences that lead to maternal death occur from the following:
   - Abruptio placentae
   - Cerebral hemorrhage
   - Acute renal or cardiac failure
   - DIC

Figure 9.1 relates pathophysiologic alterations in severe hypertensive disease in pregnancy to their evolved signs and symptoms in the patient. Nursing and medical interventions make eminent sense when seen in this context.

Expert Clinical Assessment

Measuring Blood Pressure

There is no substitute for BP appropriately measured using a calibrated mercury sphygmomanometer.[4,5,18–22] This is noted despite the recent rise in the use of automated BP equipment, including the newer ambulatory BP monitoring devices.

Appropriate use of electronic devices requires periodic validation for accuracy in measurements. Electronic BP machines systematically underestimate diastolic pressures and overestimate systolic pressures. The main point is that the measurements should be taken using a consistent method that tracks trends.

Measurement of blood pressure is important in the evaluation, diagnosis, and management of hypertension. In the past, Korotkoff 4 (K4; muffling of sound) has been used to identify the diastolic pressure. However, current recommendations are to use Korotkoff 5 (K5; disappearance of sound). It is also important to keep in mind that the diagnosis of hypertension is not made on one blood pressure evaluation. In an ambulatory setting, the diagnosis of hypertension is based on two determinations, generally within a week. The degree of suspected hypertension determines the interval between blood pressure determinations.

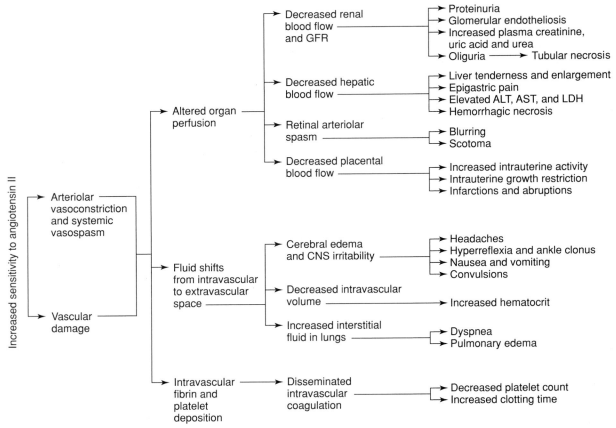

FIGURE 9.1 Pathophysiologic alterations occurring in severe hypertensive disease in pregnancy. *Abbreviations:* ALT, serum alanine aminotransferase (formally known as SGPT); AST, aspartate amino-transferase (formally known as SGOT); GRF, glomerular filtration rate; LDH, lactose dehydrogenase. (Adapted with permission from Koniak-Griffen, D., & Dodgson, J. [1987]. Pathophysiologic alterations occurring in severe PIH. *Heart and Lung, 16*[6], 664.)

In addition to the recommendation of using K5, patient position also influences blood pressure readings. Historically, blood pressure determinations were obtained in a left lateral position using the right arm. However, this position falsely lowers systolic, diastolic, and mean pressures. Current recommendations are to evaluate the blood pressure with the woman in a sitting position, using the left arm with the cuff at heart level. If reevaluation is required, the patient should be in the same position as the initial evaluation. If the left lateral position is being maintained by the patient, the blood pressure will still be taken in the left arm; the arm should not be under the patient or below the level of the heart.[18]

> Keep in mind that the clinical onset of preeclampsia can be insidious and might not be accompanied by overt symptoms.

Previous criteria of an increase of 30 mmHg systole or 15 mmHg diastole over baseline readings have limited diagnostic value. Recent studies have revealed that increases in systolic and diastolic BP can be either normal physiologic changes or signs of developing pathology. Some pregnant women develop preeclampsia with either systole or diastole elevations, but a certain percentage do not. For example:[6]

- From 67% to 73% of normotensive pregnant women experience a greater than 30 mmHg systole increase or a greater than 15 mmHg diastole increase. This is often a gradual increase during the second or third trimester.
- Women who develop preeclampsia might have higher baseline BP measurements in the first trimester than women who remain normotensive. Given the elevated first trimester

BP, women with preeclampsia might never demonstrate any further significant increase in BP.
- Women with a diastolic BP of 85 mmHg at 9 to 12 weeks' gestation have a 95% chance of remaining normotensive throughout pregnancy.

NOTE: *Relative gradual increases in BP throughout a pregnancy should never be ignored or interpreted as "normal." Rather, they signify a need to remain alert to risk factors, to the possibility of an increase in the presence of existing hypertension, and to the development of additional signs and symptoms.*

Evaluating Proteinuria

> Until recently, the diagnosis of preeclampsia required the presence of proteinuria or edema. Edema is no longer considered a reliable criterion.

The presence of protein in urine is key to the identification of preeclampsia and tends to develop late in the disease (or might not occur at all). Detection of protein in the hypertensive woman is considered a hallmark of the pathology occurring in the kidney. When renal arteriolar pressure is elevated, endothelial trauma results; vasospasms occur as a protective mechanism in the arterioles. Lesions of the endothelial lining develop, altering the glomerular filtration process. Protein normally retained within the renal artery is lost into the filtrate and appears in the urine in varying amounts.

Clinical Significance of Proteinuria
- Protein might be the most ominous sign of preeclampsia.
- When protein is 2+ or greater in the presence of hypertension, the perinatal mortality increases appreciably.
- In *mild preeclampsia,* the usual protein content in a 24-hour specimen is 300 mg to 2 g/L.
- Proteinuria reaching 2 g or greater in a 24-hour specimen serves as a standard criterion for a diagnosis of *severe preeclampsia.*

Guidelines for Technique
Urinary dipstick analysis is only moderately reliable. Readings can be falsely positive or falsely negative based on the accuracy of the dipstick performance by the individual. In addition, a dipstick analysis of proteinuria on a urine specimen may not accurately represent protein excretion over a 24-hour period.[23]
- Interpretation when using a multiple reagent strip (dipstick) is as follows:
  Trace = 0.1 g/L
    1+ = 0.3 g/L
    2+ = 1.0 g/L
    3+ = 3.0 g/L
    4+ = 10.0 g/L

> Avoid "rounding up" of color assignments when reading the dipstick. This can lead to inaccurate readings.[23]

- "Significant" proteinuria should be based on either:
  - A 24-hour urine collection

OR

  - A random clean-catch or catheter specimen
- Specimens showing 2+ proteinuria or 300 mg or greater are "significant."
- When obtaining a trace or more of proteinuria, do a repeated test of either a clean-catch or catheter specimen.
- Avoid using diluted urine because it can give false-negative results.
- Obtain clean urine samples. Do not use urine that has been collected in a Foley catheter collection bag; aspirate fresh urine from the tubing.
- When using a multiple reagent strip, always test for specific gravity (SG) and pH.

NOTE: *If SG is less than 1.010, beware of false-negative values resulting from diluted urine. If SG is 1.030 or more, beware of false-positive values resulting from concentrated urine. When using sulfosalicylic acid (very alkaline) or when pH is 8.0 or higher, beware of false-negative tests.*

- Vaginal and urinary tract infections can result in proteinuria because of the presence of bacterial activity. Exercise, posture, and urinary contamination with blood can also influence proteinuria.

A 24-hour urinary protein measurement is recommended for all pregnant women with hypertension.[5]

Pathologic Alterations and Assessment of Signs or Symptoms Reflecting Pathologic Alterations

- BP of 140/90 mmHg or higher—BP elevation to this extent in a woman beyond 20 weeks' gestation on two occasions 4 hours or more apart may indicate early preeclampsia, transient hypertension, or chronic hypertension.

Look for the following
- BP of 140/90 mmHg or higher
- Significantly rising BP—should be watched carefully
- Development of other signs and symptoms—BP and laboratory values must be scrutinized

---

- Decreased oxygen and glucose delivery to all body tissues.
- Shift of fluids (especially blood plasma) from inside the circulatory system to the tissues of the body, resulting in decreased intravascular volume. Women with preeclampsia do not have the expanded blood volume normally experienced in pregnancy. This poses a great risk of hemorrhage at delivery. In addition, the intravascular space is contracted as a result of vasospasm. Therefore, the severe preeclamptic or eclamptic woman is sensitive to vigorous fluid therapy and even to normal blood loss at delivery.

Look for the following
- Generalized edema (facial, digital, abdominal, sacral, and lower extremities)
- Large, sudden weight gain

NOTE: *Plasma volume is lower than that of normal pregnancy, even in the presence of marked edema.*

NOTE: *Some of the most severe forms of preeclampsia occur in the absence of edema.*

- Hemoconcentration within the circulatory system as the plasma content decreases.

Look for the following
- Elevated or rising hematocrit values

OR
- Falling hematocrit values if hemolysis is occurring

- Thrombocytopenia—the rates of change in platelet counts and lactate dehydrogenase (LDH) seem to correlate significantly with severity of the preeclampsia syndrome.[24]

> **Look for the following**
> - Decreasing platelets; thrombocytopenia is present when platelets are[3]:
>   Low = less than 100,000/mm^3
>   Severe = less than 50,000/mm^3

NOTE: Currently, in hypertensive states, intracranial hemorrhage is one of the leading causes of maternal death. The presence of thrombocytopenia adds to this risk.[3,11]

- Proteinuria owing to renal arteriolar vasospasm with resulting failure in the kidney's filtering process—Proteinuria usually develops late in the disease.
- **In normal pregnancies,** renal blood flow increases by 25% and glomerular filtration by 50%. This leads to an *increase* in *urinary* creatinine and urea nitrogen levels with a concomitant *decrease* in *blood* values. *Serum* (or plasma) creatinine, blood urea nitrogen (BUN), and uric acid levels *decrease.*
- With **preeclampsia,** renal perfusion and glomerular filtration are reduced. *Urinary levels of creatinine and urea nitrogen levels decrease and plasma levels increase.* Plasma uric acid concentration tends to be high in women with severe disease. The pathologic plasma volume reduction seen in preeclampsia also contributes to plasma creatinine levels being elevated.

> **Look for the following**
> - Proteinuria greater than 300 mg/L per 24 hours
> - Elevated BUN
> - Elevated uric acid
> - Elevated plasma creatinine (in severe disease, plasma values can be up to several times nonpregnant values).
>
> *NOTE: As urine BUN, uric acid, and creatinine levels fall, plasma levels rise.*

- Spasm of the blood vessels and possibly edema in the brain or the optical vascular bed. Precise effects of preeclampsia and eclampsia on cerebral blood flow are unknown. Changes in cerebral perfusion and cerebral arterial wall damage may play a role in the development of headaches and altered consciousness. Cerebral hemorrhage can occur as a result of ruptured arteries in severe hypertension and is more common in older women with chronic hypertension.[1]

> **Look for the following**
> - A complaint of visual disturbances, such as blurred vision, scotomata, and dizziness
> - Persistent, sometimes severe headache

- Spasm of the blood vessels with subsequent hemorrhages in the liver capsule.

> **Look for the following**
> - Changes in the liver enzymes with elevated AST or ALT more than two times the upper limit of normal
> - A complaint of *epigastric pain*—pain in the upper right quadrant of the abdomen. (This is a late and serious symptom of preeclampsia caused by hemorrhaging in the liver capsule, which leads to subcapsular hematoma and/or necrosis, or rupture, which is usually fatal.)
> - Liver enlargement

- Irritation of the central nervous system.

Look for the following
- Changes in level of consciousness or behavior
- Focal neurologic deficits (e.g., blurred vision, slurred speech, seizures)

NOTE: Hyperreflexia is not considered diagnostic for preeclampsia or a risk factor for eclampsia. In healthy young women, hyperreflexia can be a common finding. Deep tendon reflexes are evaluated once magnesium sulfate therapy is begun to assess for early signs of magnesium toxicity.[3]

- Decreased blood supply to the placental vascular bed, which reduces uteroplacental blood flow—Decreased blood supply can result in inadequate placental growth and function, thus compromising the fetus.

Look for the following
- Signs of intrauterine growth restriction (IUGR), reflected in fundal height measurements below expected norms
- Ultrasonic verification of fetal size if IUGR is suspected from fundal height measurement
- Reduced amniotic fluid volume verified with ultrasonography

---

Look for the following
- Signs of fetal hypoxia in electronic fetal monitoring tracings

NOTE: Nonstress testing (NST), ultrasound assessment of fetal activity, and amniotic fluid volume (BBP) are recommended antenatal fetal surveillance methods that may provide important fetal risk factors before admission.[5]

BE PREPARED FOR A HIGH-RISK INFANT. When possible, stabilize the mother and transport her to a Level III hospital if severe preeclampsia or HELLP syndrome is suspected.

Detecting Preeclampsia While Admitting the Laboring Woman

- Look at all aspects of the laboring woman's record, as well as her present state.
- Review her past medical and obstetric history to note predisposing factors.
- Review her prenatal history during this pregnancy.

Assess the following:
- Baseline BP
  - Compare baseline BP with the BP ranges recorded throughout the woman's pregnancy. Ideally, a baseline BP was documented before the woman became pregnant.

BP readings taken within the first 8 weeks of pregnancy are often the only "baseline" BP readings obtainable. Keep in mind that in women predisposed to developing preeclampsia, BP can be somewhat elevated during the early weeks of gestation.

- Proteinuria at any time in the pregnancy (usually a late sign in preeclampsia)
- Weight gain
  - Note sudden, considerable weight gain or excessive overall weight gain.

> SUDDEN, EXCESSIVE WEIGHT GAIN IS SOMETIMES THE FIRST SIGN OF IMPENDING PREECLAMPSIA. A weight gain of 2 pounds or more per week in the third trimester can precede signs of preeclampsia. This sudden weight gain is usually caused by fluid retention, regardless of whether it shows up as edema.

- A history of or current complaints of headache or blurred vision and/or severe edema of the hands, legs, feet, and face

> Some edema of the hands, feet, and pretibial area is normal in pregnancy. The severity of edema in these areas, as well as facial, abdominal, and sacral edema, should alert you to the possibility of preeclampsia.

At the time of admission, assess the woman's status through questioning and physical examination.
- Take her BP.
- Check for edema in all body areas (including hands and feet) and especially facial, abdominal, and sacral areas.
- Check deep tendon reflexes (knee-jerk reflex). This serves as a baseline to determine an early sign of magnesium sulfate toxicity.
- Evaluate a clean-catch or catheterized urine specimen.
- Question her about recent:
  - Headaches
  - Blurred vision
  - Loss of consciousness
  - Nausea and vomiting
  - Worsening of edema
  - Epigastric pain
  - General sick feeling

Detecting Severe Preeclampsia

Mild preeclampsia occurs when the following are found:
- BP has reached 140/90 to 160/110 mmHg on two different occasions 4 hours apart.

> An increase in the diastolic reading is a more reliable indication of preeclampsia.

- Proteinuria is 2+ or between 300 mg and 5 g in a 24-hour urine specimen.

Be alert when you see the following:
- Weight gain of more than 5 pounds per week during the second trimester or more than 2 pounds per week during the third trimester
- Slight edema throughout the body

Severe preeclampsia occurs when the following are found:
- BP rises to 160/110 mmHg or higher on two different occasions 4 hours apart.
- Proteinuria is 2 g or higher in a 24-hour urine specimen.
- Urine output decreases to less than 400 mL in 24 hours (i.e., less than 30 mL/h).

NOTE: *Clinical signs of preeclampsia can appear suddenly. Never underestimate the importance of even mild BP elevations complicating a pregnancy.*

> In severe preeclampsia, the kidneys can go into failure with little output. This is a serious situation that can lead to permanent injury.

Symptoms Develop and Include the Following:
- Severe headaches
- Visual problems

- Epigastric pain
- Nausea or vomiting
- Thrombocytopenia
- Irritability, restlessness, or apprehension
- Pulmonary edema with respiratory distress

> Early identification of worsening preeclampsia in a patient at a Level I or II hospital is critical.

When severe preeclampsia occurs before week 32 of gestation, the incidence of serious complications in the mother is high and the fetal outcome is poor, often as a result of growth restriction and/or asphyxia at birth.

Signs to watch for include the following:
- Abruptio placentae
- HELLP syndrome
- Eclampsia
- DIC
- Acute renal failure

Detecting HELLP Syndrome

Follow the same steps as described for detecting preeclampsia in the laboring woman. Particular care should be taken when obtaining the admission history.

Specifically Question the Woman About Recent:	*The Expectant Mother Might Be Assigned One of the Following Differential Diagnoses:*
Nausea and vomiting	Viral hepatitis
General sick feeling	Gastroenteritis
Epigastric or right upper quadrant pain	Gallbladder disease
Worsening edema	Kidney stones
Diarrhea	Pyelonephritis
Hematuria	Peptic ulcer
Bleeding gums	Idiopathic thrombocytopenia
Abdominal, flank, or shoulder pain	Appendicitis
	Acute fatty liver of pregnancy
	Encephalopathy
	Pancreatitis
	When in fact she has HELLP syndrome.

NOTE: Experts recommend that all pregnant women showing any of these signs or symptoms during the second half of pregnancy have a complete blood cell count with platelets, a peripheral blood smear, and determination of liver enzymes taken, irrespective of maternal BP level.[3,5]

These women are critically ill and must be rigorously and constantly assessed. Remember what is happening:
- Arteriolar vasospasms damage the endothelial layer of small blood vessels, forming lesions.
- Platelets accumulate at lesion sites and a fibrin network forms.
- Red blood cells are forced through the fibrin network under high pressure, resulting in hemolysis with damaged erythrocytes (schistocytes, Burr cells).

> **Look for the following**
> - Falling hematocrit
> - Hyperbilirubinemia
> - Increased LDH
> - Jaundice including sclerae

> **H**—hemolysis as detected with the following:
> - Abnormal red blood cells on a peripheral smear
> - Bilirubin greater than 1.2 mg/dL

- Maternal liver failure results from microemboli in the hepatic vasculature, which causes ischemia and tissue damage within the liver.

Look for the following
- Increased LDH
- Increased AST/ALT
- Feelings of malaise
- Viral-like syndrome
- Right upper quadrant pain

EL—elevated liver enzymes
- AST greater than 70 IU/L (also elevated ALT)
- LDH greater than 600 IU/L

- Thrombocytopenia occurs because of increased platelet consumption.

Look for the following
- Falling platelet count
- Abnormal coagulation and fibrinolytic values

LP—low platelets
- Low = less than 100,000/mm^3
- Severe = less than 50,000/mm^3

- Obstruction of hepatic blood flow and the continual deposit of fibrin cause hepatic distention.

Look for the following
- Complaints of epigastric or right upper quadrant pain
- Complaints of nausea and vomiting
- Decreased blood glucose

IT IS IMPORTANT TO REMEMBER THAT THE PHYSICAL SYMPTOMS OF HELLP SYNDROME MIGHT NOT INITIALLY CORRELATE WITH PREECLAMPSIA. THE SIGNS AND SYMPTOMS OF HELLP SYNDROME CORRELATE WITH THE PATHO-PHYSIOLOGY. THE CLASSIC TRIAD OF HYPERTENSION, PROTEINURIA, AND EDEMA NEED NOT BE PRESENT TO DIAGNOSE HELLP SYNDROME.

If appropriate for timing, distance, and her medical condition, a woman with HELLP syndrome needs to be referred to a tertiary care center for both maternal and fetal safety.

Priorities for Treatment and Nursing Management

Management of Preeclampsia

The primary goals in the management of the preeclamptic woman are as follows:
1. To prevent convulsions through the use of magnesium sulfate
2. To ensure adequate kidney function
3. To monitor fetal status continuously for signs of uteroplacental insufficiency
4. To stabilize the woman so that a vaginal or cesarean birth can be accomplished

The *definitive treatment* for preeclampsia is delivery.

In mild preeclampsia, clinical management usually involves a conservative approach, with office visits as frequent as twice a week, judiciously prescribed rest periods, and frequent laboratory and physical assessment. Fetal surveillance includes tests for fetal well-being, such as fetal movement counting, nonstress testing, contraction stress testing, and biophysical profiles. Hospitalization might be required for the woman who is uncooperative or whose condition does not improve. Along with bed rest, a regular diet with no salt restriction is promoted. A woman with preeclampsia might experience a reduced plasma volume; salt restriction can worsen the situation.

In severe preeclampsia, management is quite focused. Hospitalization facilitates the following:

- Intense maternal monitoring
- Administration of the anticonvulsant medication magnesium sulfate
- Administration of an antihypertensive medication, such as hydralazine or labetalol
- Delivery of the fetus by vaginal or cesarean birth depending on maternal and fetal conditions
- Electronic fetal monitoring

Nursing care for the laboring woman with severe preeclampsia includes the following:

- Maintain a nurse-to-patient ratio of 1:1.
- Assess vital signs based on maternal-fetal status to determine worsening of the disease and response to therapy.
- Obtain standardized BP readings by practicing the following steps:
  - Use the left arm throughout. If pressure readings differ in each arm by more than 10 mmHg, use the arm with the higher reading.
  - Keep the arm horizontal and at the level of the heart.
  - Fit a sphygmomanometer cuff appropriately sized for the woman's arm.
  - Ensure that BP readings are taken with the woman in the same posture each time.
  - Use the sitting position. If the blood pressure is taken in the lateral position, the left arm is still used for the measurement.
  - To minimize compression of the inferior vena cava (and thus risk increasing BP), encourage a semirecumbent position at a 45-degree angle and on the same side as the arm used in measuring BP. A left or right side-lying position with a 15- to 30-degree tilt will give similar BP readings in pregnant women. Consistent positioning minimizes false high or low readings. **Readings taken in different positions are not comparable.**

BP readings are:
- Highest when supine or standing
- Intermediate when sitting (recommended when possible)
- Lowest in the lateral recumbent position

- Personnel on the unit should be consistent in the methods used for recording the diastolic reading. Consider the following:
  1. Using the fifth phase disappearance of the sound (the K5 sound) places diastolic measurements abnormally low or even at the zero level in some women. Use of the fifth phase (K5 sound) was recommended for pregnant women in 1992 by the National Heart, Lung, and Blood Institute and in 2000 by the Working Group Report on High Blood Pressure in Pregnancy.
  2. The National Working Group Consensus Report encourages recording both the muffled sound (K4) and the disappearance sound (K5).
  3. Some experts recommend that both phases be recorded and that the K4 sound be used for diagnosis. This can result in an overdiagnosis of preeclampsia, but this "risk" is acceptable.
- Place the woman in a lateral recumbent or semirecumbent position. This avoids compression of the maternal vena cava and aorta; improves renal function by enhancing cardiac output, renal circulation, and urinary output; and can enhance uterine/placental perfusion, thus benefiting the fetus.
- Continuous fetal monitoring for uteroplacental insufficiency is done even after BP has been controlled because it is unclear whether the underlying pathologic condition has been controlled as well. Electronic fetal monitoring is recommended.
- Record hourly intake and output using a Foley catheter with a urometer. Careful assessment of fluid balance is critical in preventing a hydrostatic and oncotic pressure imbalance that could lead to pulmonary edema.

Oliguria (less than 30 mL/h for 2 hours) can result from intravascular volume depletion, renal vasospasm, or cardiac failure. Oliguria is an ominous sign. Report a trend toward this immediately. Do not wait until fully evolved oliguria has occurred.

- Reduce stimulation from noise and light. Place the woman in the quietest room in the labor and delivery unit and dim the lights.
- Maintain the woman on strict bed rest. Side rails should be padded with a blanket for patients with severe preeclampsia or eclampsia.
- Give intravenous fluids to ensure adequate hydration and electrolyte balance and for drug administration.
  - Crystalloid solutions (e.g., 5% dextrose and water or lactated Ringer's solution) should be used.
  - Limit fluid administration to no more than 150 mL/h. Some authorities suggest a more cautious use of 1 mL/kg per hour.
  - Continuous monitoring is necessary to maintain adequate output.
- Obtain appropriate laboratory workup, which includes the following:
  - Complete blood count (CBC), type and crossmatch, and platelets
  - Liver studies
  - DIC profile
- When testing urine for protein, *use a fresh specimen* from the Foley catheter tubing.
- Assess deep tendon reflexes to determine an early sign of magnesium sulfate toxicity.
- Ask the woman to tell you if she develops a headache, blurred vision, dizziness, or epigastric pain, or if she feels uncomfortable or different.
- Observe the woman for restlessness or apprehension.
- HAVE EMERGENCY EQUIPMENT READY—SEIZURE PRECAUTIONS.
  - Oxygen and suctioning equipment must be immediately available. Check that the equipment is in operating order.
  - Keep an emergency cart nearby.
- Administer magnesium sulfate according to the physician's orders. Magnesium sulfate ($MgSO_4 \cdot 7H_2O$) is currently believed the safest and most effective anticonvulsant drug available. It can be given intramuscularly or intravenously.

Intravenous administration is recommended because it permits more precise control of serum magnesium blood levels in the woman. Also, the pain of an intramuscular injection is avoided.

The woman **with severe preeclampsia or eclampsia** needs intensive monitoring. She should never be left alone!

Management of HELLP Syndrome

Management of the woman with HELLP syndrome is the same as that for the woman with severe preeclampsia.[3,5]

In addition:
- Monitor platelet count for changes indicating worsening thrombocytopenia.
- Assess for clinical signs and symptoms of bleeding:
  - Petechiae
  - Easy bruising
  - Epistaxis
  - Gingival bleeding
  - Hematuria
  - Gastrointestinal bleeding
  - Conjunctival/retinal hemorrhage
  - Oozing from the intravenous site
- Administer blood products per the physician's orders.
- Monitor serial liver function tests.
- Observe and report signs of the following:
  - Malaise
  - Anorexia
  - Nausea and vomiting
  - Right upper quadrant or epigastric pain

- Jaundice
- Hypoglycemia
- Avoid sedatives.

NOTE: Decreased blood glucose can occur as a result of hepatic congestion that is caused by microemboli in the small vessels of the liver.

- Use electronic fetal monitoring to assess for signs of fetal hypoxemia.
- Deliver oxygen at 10 L/min via face mask as indicated.

NOTE: Late decelerations and loss of short-term variability are nonreassuring signs associated with fetal hypoxia.

Intrapartum Pain Management[3,5]

- Vaginal birth is preferable to cesarean delivery, even with the presence of severe disease.
- Regional anesthesia techniques are relatively contraindicated in preeclampsia accompanied by coagulopathy.
- Continuous epidural anesthesia for pain relief during labor in women with severe hypertensive disease does not appear to increase cesarean birth rates, maternal pulmonary edema, or acute renal failure.

Anticonvulsant Therapy

▶ **What is the current recommended treatment schedule for administering magnesium sulfate ($MgSO_4 \cdot 7H_2O$) to the preeclamptic woman?**

Magnesium sulfate is given for anticonvulsant therapy. **It is not given to treat hypertension.**

A number of sound clinical studies provide significant evidence that magnesium sulfate is the anticonvulsant drug of choice. Diazepam (Valium) and phenytoin (Dilantin) are no longer accepted anticonvulsant therapies for preeclampsia.

The following recommendations represent currently accepted therapeutic practices in the treatment of the preeclamptic woman with magnesium sulfate.[3,5]

- If a rapid therapeutic effect is desired, an initial loading dose of 4 to 6 g of magnesium sulfate in 100 mL of IV solution is administered intravenously over 20 to 30 minutes, followed by controlled, continuous infusion of 2 g/h.
- Maintenance therapy is delivered at the rate of 2 g in 100 mL of solution per hour. Some women require infusions of 3 g/h to maintain effective plasma levels of magnesium.

NOTE: Administration of the loading dose at these rates is likely to induce vomiting. Do not speed up the loading dose infusion beyond the stated rate.

The effect of magnesium sulfate is immediate when administered intravenously.

Magnesium sulfate is stable in both 5% dextrose and water and in lactated Ringer's solutions for extended periods. However, attention should be given to maintaining sterilization in a preparation administered over more than 24 hours. A new preparation of the solution is recommended.

▶ **What special monitoring of the patient is required during administration of magnesium sulfate?**

Magnesium is believed to exert a specific anticonvulsant action on the cerebral cortex. In therapeutic ranges, magnesium sulfate slows neuromuscular conduction and depresses central nervous system irritability. The purpose of giving the drug is to reduce muscle excitability and hyperreflexia, thus reducing the possibility of convulsions.

To monitor the woman during magnesium sulfate administration:

- Assess patellar reflexes. Absence of the reflex is the earliest sign of magnesium sulfate toxicity.
- Count respirations; they should not be less than 12 per minute and should be of normal depth. **Discontinue the infusion if signs of respiratory compromise are present.**
- Measure urinary output hourly. Use of a Foley catheter is imperative. Indications of impaired renal function as seen in laboratory tests (e.g., elevated plasma creatinine levels) or diminished urinary output (less than 30 mL/h) necessitate a critical reevaluation of not only fluid therapy but also anticonvulsant therapy. **Because parenterally administered magnesium is cleared almost exclusively by renal excretion, notify the primary care provider immediately if you suspect any renal function compromise.**
- Assess the patient's state of consciousness.

The therapeutic range for magnesium sulfate is between 4 and 7 mEq/L (4.8 and 8.4 mg/dL) of serum magnesium. Concentrations greater than 7 mEq/L (8.4 mg/dL) result in signs of maternal toxicity, including the following:

- Nausea and vomiting
- Respiratory depression
- Disappearance of the patellar reflex
- Respiratory and cardiac arrest if toxicity is not remedied
  Consider the following:
- Extensive experience indicates that intravenous doses of magnesium sulfate at dosages up to 2 g/h are safe in the patient with normal renal function.
- Protocols for nursing supervision of patients with maternal disease, such as severe preeclampsia, should address a 1:1 nurse-to-patient ratio.
- Magnesium sulfate is discontinued 24 hours after birth or with evidence of disease reversal.

TO AVOID TOXICITY:
Make sure the patient has excreted at least 100 mL of urine in the past 4 hours, that respirations are at least 12 per minute, and that patellar reflexes are present. Monitoring of serum magnesium levels is indicated if signs of toxicity are present.

The most common causes of toxicity are:
1. Iatrogenic overdosage
2. Deteriorating renal function, which can be common with severe preeclampsia

---

► **How is a magnesium sulfate overdose managed?[3,5]**

Calcium gluconate is the antidote to magnesium toxicity.

- Administer 1 g of calcium gluconate intravenously slowly over 10 to 20 minutes; for example, use 10 mL of a 10% calcium gluconate solution (each milliliter contains 0.1 g of calcium gluconate).
- Provide airway and ventilatory support as needed.

Calcium gluconate is commonly packaged in 1g ampules containing 10 mL of a 10% solution. Read the label carefully when drawing up the solution.

Antihypertensive Therapy: Current Recommendations[3,5]

Although controversy exists regarding how aggressively hypertension should be treated in pregnancy, there is a consensus that patients with diastolic BP measurements of 110 mmHg or higher should be treated. In some situations, pressures lower than this might warrant antihypertensive treatment. Maternal benefits from this therapy are the prevention of pulmonary edema and cerebral hemorrhage, two severe complications of preeclampsia.[3–5,7,8,11] The major concern in using antihypertensive drugs is that, while maternal BP is reduced, uteroplacental perfusion is also lowered, thus potentially compromising fetal oxygenation. The goal of treatment is aimed at maintaining a diastolic pressure between 90 and 100 mmHg, but not lower.

A review of recent literature indicates a few selective drugs:

Hydralazine (Apresoline) (arteriolar dilator)
- A drug of choice for many in the treatment of severe hypertension near term or during labor
- Administered intravenously and intramuscularly
- See protocol that follows for specific directions

Labetalol (adrenergic blocker)
- Is used as a second-line drug of choice
- May be used in intravenous bolus injections beginning with 20 mg; if not effective within 20 minutes, give 40 mg, then 80 mg every 10 minutes, *but not to exceed 220 mg total dose*
- May be used as a continuous infusion of 1 mg/kg per hour as needed

NOTE: The drug is premixed as a 20-mL vial containing a concentration of 5 mg labetalol per milliliter. Add 40-mL vial of labetalol to 160 mL of intravenous fluid; the resultant 200 mL contains 1 mg labetalol per milliliter.

- Must watch for the delayed effect of sudden maternal hypotension (reactive hypotension); **stop the infusion immediately**
- Use with caution in women with asthma and those with congestive heart failure

Nifedipine (calcium entry blocker)
- Used in preeclamptic hypertensive emergencies
- Start with 10 mg dose orally and repeat in 30 minutes if needed
- Short-acting nifedipine not approved by U.S. Food and Drug Administration for hypertension management

Guidelines for the Use of Hydralazine in Antihypertensive Therapy[3–5,7,8,11]

Hydralazine should be administered using plastic containers or syringes. A significant but unpredictable decrease in effectiveness has been observed when glass containers are used.

NOTE: The patient's response to vasodilators depends on the status of her intravascular blood volume. Severely preeclamptic patients have a depleted volume. WHEN ADMINISTERING HYDRALAZINE, WATCH FOR EARLY SIGNS OF HYPOTENSION. THESE PATIENTS CAN EXPERIENCE SUDDEN AND PROFOUND HYPOTENSION.

- A test dose of 1 mg is given intravenously over 1 minute. BP is checked to determine any idiosyncratic hypotension.
- Administer a 5 mg dose intravenously over 1 to 2 minutes, or give 10 mg intramuscularly.
- Subsequent doses are dictated by the patient's response to the initial dose. For example, another 5 to 10 mg dose may be given intravenously after 20 minutes if the diastolic BP remains higher than 110 mmHg.

The pharmacokinetics of hydralazine involve a peak and maximal effect in 20 minutes, with a 6 to 8 hour duration of action. This is why intermittent bolus injections are appropriate. However, because the time to maximum effect of any given dose can vary, DO NOT ADMINISTER THE 5 MG DOSES TOO CLOSE TOGETHER.

- Recheck BP every 5 minutes.
- Once BP control is achieved, the dose is repeated as needed—usually about every 3 hours.
- Maintain a properly functioning IV line. Monitoring of input and output is critical to prevent hypotensive episodes or overload.
- Do not mix this medication with any other medications in the same intravenous bag.

NOTE: A desired response to hydralazine therapy is defined as a decrease in the diastolic BP to 90 to 100 mmHg, but not any lower because placental perfusion can be compromised. If, after giving 20 mg intravenously or 30 mg intramuscularly total dose, success has not been achieved, another drug should be considered.

COMPREHENSIVE PROTOCOLS THAT ADDRESS NURSING RESPONSIBILITIES FOR ANTICONVULSANT THERAPY OR ANTIHYPERTENSIVE THERAPY (e.g., HYDRALAZINE) SHOULD BE DEVELOPED AT EACH INSTITUTION. THESE PROTOCOLS SHOULD INCLUDE CRITERIA FOR PATIENT SELECTION, RESPONSIBILITY FOR INFORMATION TO BE COVERED IN THE INFORMED CONSENT, DRUG PREPARATION AND ADMINISTRATION, PATIENT MONITORING, POTENTIAL SIDE EFFECTS, AND THERAPEUTIC GOALS.

Special Delivery Preparations

- Maternal corticosteroid administration is strongly recommended to reduce the risk of newborn respiratory distress syndrome if a preterm birth is anticipated. A single course of corticosteroids should be given 24 hours before birth is anticipated. All pregnant women between 24 and 34 weeks' gestation should be considered candidates. See Module 8 for treatment dose.

NOTE: Maternal administration of corticosteroids can give a transient increase in platelet counts and elevate serum glucose.

- If the preeclamptic woman is at a Level I or Level II hospital, is preterm, and does not respond to the conservative management of diet control and bed rest with a decrease in BP, disappearance of proteinuria, and lessening of edema, it is recommended that she be transferred to a high-risk regional center. She may need fetal maturity tests, electronic fetal monitoring, and induction of labor. **PREPARE FOR A HIGH-RISK INFANT.**
- If a preterm or term woman is admitted to the labor and delivery unit of a Level I or Level II hospital with severe preeclampsia, it is recommended that she be transferred to the high-risk regional center as soon as she is stabilized enough for the transfer.
- In the event that the preeclamptic woman delivers at the community hospital because there is no time for transfer to the regional center, **PREPARE FOR A HIGH-RISK INFANT.**
- *The preeclamptic woman maintained on therapeutic levels of magnesium sulfate is at risk for postpartum hemorrhage. This is of great concern because the woman with severe preeclampsia or eclampsia is unable to tolerate a large blood loss at delivery. She is already experiencing reduced blood volume and hemoconcentration. Be prepared for this. Oxytocic drugs and manual uterine stimulation usually control uterine atony.*

Recognize that any significant fall in BP soon after delivery in these women often reflects excessive blood loss and not the disappearance of vasospasm with return to a more normotensive state.

Oliguria soon after delivery may signify blood loss. Hematocrit should be evaluated frequently to detect this. Treatment with careful blood transfusion might be implemented.

- **Whenever anticipating a possible HIGH-RISK INFANT** *have the appropriate personnel on hand—not on call.* Their presence at the birth can make a critical difference to the quality of life for the newborn.
- Epidural anesthesia is considered safe and is the anesthetic of choice in severe preeclampsia, if preceded by volume preloading, to prevent maternal hypotension. Fluid management consists of infusion of normal saline or lactated Ringer's solution at a rate of 100 to 125 mL/h. Intravenous fluids can decrease colloidal osmotic pressure and also result in fluid accumulation in interstitial tissue. Be vigilant in monitoring for hypotension and pulmonary edema. Women who are experiencing severe preeclampsia or eclampsia and develop pulmonary edema most often do so in the postpartum period.

Postpartum Care and Education, Including Long-Term Prognosis[3-5,7,8,11]

- Delivery is the "cure" for preeclampsia.
- Magnesium sulfate should be continued in the severely preeclamptic and eclamptic woman for at least 24 hours after delivery and even longer if the woman complains of persistent headache, blurred vision, or scotomata.
- BP monitoring is continued after magnesium sulfate administration is discontinued.
- Approximately 25% to 30% of eclampsia cases occur within the first few days postpartum.
- Recovery, including resolution of abnormal laboratory values, is not always immediate in women with HELLP syndrome. These women are very ill.
  - Thrombocytopenia worsens for 3 to 4 days after delivery.
  - Patients may appear to worsen initially and then slowly begin to improve.
- Close monitoring within the first 48 hours is critical to detect the development of pulmonary edema, renal failure, or hypertension encephalopathy. Watch for the following:
  - Hemoconcentration
  - Oliguria
  - Respiratory changes, such as pulmonary rales, tachypnea, and dyspnea; chest discomfort; and tachycardia
- Women who are at risk for postpartum complications are those with underlying cardiac disease, chronic renal disease, superimposed preeclampsia, placental abruption complicated with DIC, and hypertension that requires several antihypertensive medications.
- Breastfeeding is encouraged and can be done safely using selected antihypertensive drugs and reduced doses under careful BP supervision. Studies indicate that all antihypertensive agents are excreted into human breast milk. The breastfed infant requires close monitoring for any adverse effects.
- At 3 months postpartum, BP is usually normal and proteinuria disappears. However, in some women hypertension may persist for as long as 3 months.
- The sequelae of underlying renal disease are few.

> The longer hypertension diagnosed during pregnancy persists postpartum, the greater the likelihood that the cause is underlying chronic hypertension.

> The existence of normal BP in a pregnancy subsequent to a hypertension-complicated pregnancy has been found to be predictive of reduced risk for chronic hypertension in the future.[9]

- Approximately 3% to 19% of women with HELLP syndrome experience the disorder in a subsequent pregnancy; 43% experience preeclampsia. When the syndrome does occur, it tends to develop later in the pregnancy and tends to be less severe after two episodes.

NOTE: Preeclampsia does not cause chronic hypertension.

- Oral contraceptives usually can be used safely under medical BP supervision.
- Women with HELLP syndrome should be screened for the presence of antiphospholipid antibodies (APLA testing), which may be indicative at specified levels of a syndrome associated with a variety of medical problems, including arterial and venous thrombosis, autoimmune cytopenia, and fetal loss.

PRACTICE/REVIEW QUESTIONS

After reviewing this module, answer the following questions.

1. Hypertension complicates pregnancy in approximately

   _____ % to _____ % of women.

2. A general term that has been used to describe all new

   onsets of hypertension in pregnancy is _____

   _____ .

3. A general term identifying chronic hypertension wors-

   ened by pregnancy is _____ .

4. A hypertensive state in pregnancy that occurs after the

   20th week and is characterized by convulsions is

   _____ .

5. Pregnancy complicated by hypertension and proteinuria

   is called _____ .

6. Match the terms in Column B with the descriptions given
   in Column A.

   Column A

   _____ 1. Hypertension
   during the last
   20 weeks of
   pregnancy or
   in the first 24
   hours postpartum
   without other signs
   of preeclampsia

   _____ 2. A term sometimes
   used to designate
   expectant women
   who have elevated
   BP after 20 weeks
   but without
   accompanying
   proteinuria

   _____ 3. A subset of
   preeclampsia

   _____ 4. Sometimes seen in
   normotensive women
   within the first hours
   after delivery but with
   a subsequent return to
   baseline BP levels
   in 24 hours

   _____ 5. The development of
   a BP of 140/90 mmHg
   or higher after the 20th
   gestational week and
   accompanied by
   proteinuria

   Column B

   a. Preeclampsia

   b. Transient
   hypertension

   c. Eclampsia

   d. Chronic hyperten-
   sion

   e. HELLP syndrome

   f. Superimposed
   preeclampsia

   g. Gestational hyper-
   tension

   _____ 6. Occurs before the
   20th week in the
   presence of pathologic
   changes in the placenta

   _____ 7. A disorder that can
   begin with implantation,
   but has no overt signs
   or symptoms for weeks
   or even months

   _____ 8. Exists in a severe
   form when BP reaches
   160/110 mmHg or higher

   _____ 9. Can occur in women
   who enter pregnancy
   with preexisting
   hypertension

   _____ 10. Has as its underlying
   pathophysiology arterial
   vasospasm leading to
   microangiopathic
   hemolytic anemia

   _____ 11. Is accompanied by
   convulsions not caused
   by neurologic disease

   _____ 12. Is diagnosed with a history
   of persistent BP elevation
   of at least 140/90 mmHg
   before the 20th gesta-
   tional week

   _____ 13. Convulsions can occur
   in the presence of mildly
   elevated BP or mild
   proteinuria

   _____ 14. The presence of this
   hypertensive disorder,
   together with diabetes,
   renal disease, or a cardiac
   condition, increases the
   mother's risk

7. The following statements elicit your understanding of the
   current thinking about hypertensive states in pregnancy.

   a. Perinatal mortality rates tend to increase as maternal
      BP increases.

      a. True

      b. False

   b. Chronic hypertension and preeclampsia have the same
      etiology.

      a. True

      b. False

   c. Several reliable screening tests can be used to identify
      women at risk for pregnancy-induced hypertensive
      disorders.

a. True

b. False

d. Eclampsia can be mild or severe.

a. True

b. False

e. A diagnostic criterion for hypertension is a BP of 140/90 mmHg.

a. True

b. False

f. Severe hypertension is diagnosed when the BP reaches 150/100 mmHg.

a. True

b. False

g. Gestational hypertension is the same thing as transitional hypertension.

a. True

b. False

h. A BP of 146/100 mmHg in a laboring woman with no previous hypertension history and with no proteinuria can indicate transient hypertension.

a. True

b. False

i. If the laboring woman mentioned above in "h" has transient hypertension, it can be diagnosed only in the postpartum period.

a. True

b. False

8. Name the two principal signs present in the hypertensive states of pregnancy.

a. _____

b. _____

9. Select the hypertensive state that fits the descriptions given in a through j.

T = Transient hypertension

P = Preeclampsia

H = HELLP syndrome

E = Eclampsia

_____ a. Is not accompanied by adverse fetal outcomes

_____ b. Complicates approximately 20% of teenage pregnancies

_____ c. Is characterized by microangiopathic hemolytic anemia, as diagnosed by abnormal red blood cells on a peripheral smear

_____ d. Accompanied by malaise, flulike symptoms, and nausea and vomiting

_____ e. A disorder that can begin with implantation

_____ f. A fairly benign disease that can, however, be predictive of possible future chronic hypertension with aging

_____ g. Proteinuria often a late sign

_____ h. Microvascular damage to the endothelial lining of blood vessels and platelet activation diagnosed in laboratory studies

_____ i. Convulsions that are sometimes not accompanied by dramatic warning signs

_____ j. Associated with poor maternal and perinatal outcomes and its presence is a risk factor for postpartum eclampsia

10. State at least five predisposing risk factors for developing preeclampsia.

a. _____

b. _____

c. _____

d. _____

e. _____

11. "Significant" proteinuria means:

a. 300 mg/L or more in 24 hours

b. 200 mg/L in 24 hours

c. 1+ on dipstick tested twice 4 hours apart

d. The presence of a urinary tract infection

12. When a pregnant woman presents with a BP of 144/96 mmHg, how is a diagnosis of chronic hypertension versus preeclampsia made?

_____

_____

13. Mark with an "X" the statements that characterize what is known about chronic hypertension and pregnancy.

_____ a. Most chronic hypertensive pregnant women have primary or essential hypertension.

_____ b. It occurs more often in white women than in black women.

_____ c. It is not associated with increased risk of IUGR.

_____ d. Mild, uncomplicated chronic hypertension in pregnancy is associated with moderate maternal and fetal morbidity.

_____ e. Preconceptional and antepartal antihypertensive medications are not advised in the moderately chronic hypertensive woman.

_____ f. Sodium restriction is advocated to reduce the potential for edema.

14. Pregnancy-aggravated hypertension exists in two forms: _____ and _____ .

15. State at least five characteristics that are common to the woman presenting with HELLP syndrome.

    a. _____

    b. _____

    c. _____

    d. _____

    e. _____

16. The second leading cause of maternal death in the United States is:

    a. Hemorrhage

    b. Infection

    c. Thromboembolic disease

    d. Preeclampsia

17. The underlying disease process in preeclampsia is:

    a. Not known

    b. Thought to be strictly neurologic in origin

    c. Widespread vasospasms of the arterioles

    d. DIC

18. In preeclampsia, hypertension is the:

    a. Primary clinical feature

    b. Cause of the disease

    c. Earliest symptom

    d. Latest symptom

19. Preeclampsia (choose all that apply):

    a. Can involve one or more organ systems

    b. Is thought to be inherited

    c. Begins late in pregnancy

    d. Never occurs in the older primigravida

20. Pathophysiologic processes related to preeclampsia involve all of the following except:

    a. A balance in two potent vasoactive substances

    b. Increased sensitivity to angiotensin II

    c. Incomplete invasion of the spiral arteries in the endometrium

    d. Microangiopathy

21. Match the terms in Column B with the descriptions given in Column A.

    Column A

    _____ 1. Stimulates platelet aggregation

    _____ 2. Synthesized in the endothelium of blood vessels

    _____ 3. A potent vasodilator

    _____ 4. Inhibits platelet aggregation

    _____ 5. A potent vasoconstrictor

    _____ 6. A precursor in the liver requiring the action of renin

    _____ 7. Affects smooth muscle contractions, stimulates aldosterone production, and sensitizes smooth muscles of the vasculature to norepinephrine

    Column B

    a. Thromboxane

    b. Prostacyclin

    c. Angiotensin II

    d. Angiotensinogen

22. Fill in the blanks from the following list of terms:

    Angiotensin I

    Angiotensin II

    Angiotensinogen

    Endothelin-derived releasing factor

    Prostacyclin

    Renin

    Thromboxane

    Preeclamptic women have increased sensitivity to a chemical substance called _____ . In the liver, _____ converts _____ to an inactive substance called _____ . In turn, this becomes biologically active _____ . Normal pregnant women have a moderate vasoactive response to _____ .

23. Define *microangiopathy*.

    _____

    _____

    _____

24. List the changes that vasospasms can lead to in terms of the following:

    a. Pressure and blood flow through the arteriole

    _____

    _____

    b. Loss of fluid components

    _____

    _____

    c. Blood supply to target organs

    _____

    _____

25. Vasospasm leading to formation of endothelial lesions activates the body's _____ system. _____ accumulate at lesion sites, and a _____ network forms. Blood continues to be forced through the damaged vessels, and consequently, _____ are forced through the fibrin network. The damage sustained by the fragmentation of these cells results in _____.

26. The process described in question 25 results in a disorder called _____ anemia. This is a unique sign of what disease state? _____

27. Ongoing endothelial vessel damage continues to result in more lesions with increasing numbers of platelets used up in laying down fibrin networks. This platelet consumption results in _____.

28. Maternal death resulting from the extreme pathologic processes described in questions 23 through 27 is usually caused be one of four conditions:

    a. _____

    b. _____

    c. _____

    d. _____

29. A significant elevation of BP requiring careful watching is a diastole of _____ mmHg or a systole of _____ mmHg.

30. A BP elevation to 140/90 mmHg seen throughout a morning in a woman in the clinic who is beyond 20 weeks' gestation indicates _____.

31. With preeclampsia, there is a shift of fluids within the circulatory system, resulting in decreased _____. A sign of this can be either _____ or _____.

32. This shift of fluid also results in hemoconcentration within the circulatory system. A sign of this can be seen in a rising _____.

33. Thrombocytopenia is diagnosed with platelets lower than _____. It is severe with a platelet count of less _____.

34. Proteinuria:

    a. Usually develops early in the disease process

    b. Is a result of renal arteriolar vasospasm

    c. Generally indicates integrity of kidney tissue

    d. Is correlated with a mild disease process

35. Patient complaints of what four symptoms may indicate spasms of retinol blood vessels and cerebral edema

    a. _____

    b. _____

    c. _____

    d. _____

36. Vascular spasms occurring in the liver capsule should be suspected when the patient complains of _____.

37. Irritation of the central nervous system is suspected in the presence of _____.

38. Hypertension in pregnancy can compromise blood supply to the placenta and lead to _____.

39. Increases in systolic and diastolic pressures are always pathologic.

    a. True

    b. False

40. Relative gradual increases in BP can be interpreted as "normal."

    a. True

    b. False

41. The diagnosis of preeclampsia requires the presence of proteinuria and edema.

    a. True

    b. False

42. Edema is not a valid diagnostic sign of preeclampsia.

    a. True

    b. False

43. Most pregnant women exhibit some edema.

    a. True

    b. False

44. A 19-year-old gravida 1 is at 37 weeks' gestation; her BP is 150/100 mmHg, and she has no lower extremity edema. A 24-hour urine specimen collected is reported to have 5 g of protein. By definition the diagnosis is

    _____.

45. Significant proteinuria is based on:

    _____

    _____

46. A 17-year-old African American primigravida is admitted to labor and delivery in a Level I hospital at 27 weeks' gestation. Her BP is 170/114 mmHg, and her urine output is 30 mL/h. Stabilization and transport to a high-risk regional center is important because

    _____

    _____.

47. List three diagnostic criteria for HELLP syndrome.

    a. _____

    b. _____

    c. _____

48. Indicate whether the following statements are true (T) or false (F).

    _____ a. Arteriolar vasospasm is the underlying factor in hemolytic anemia that occurs in HELLP syndrome.

    _____ b. In HELLP syndrome, platelets accumulate in small blood vessels, causing those vessels to swell and rupture.

    _____ c. The liver is the primary organ that is damaged as a result of HELLP syndrome.

    _____ d. Hepatic distention can cause subjective symptoms of epigastric and/or right upper quadrant pain.

49. To diagnose the complication of HELLP syndrome, a pregnant woman must show clinical evidence of preeclampsia (i.e., hypertension, proteinuria, and edema).

    a. True

    b. False

50. List at least five areas that you need to address in admission history when screening a woman for HELLP syndrome.

    a. _____

    b. _____

    c. _____

    d. _____

    e. _____

51. State four primary nursing management goals in the care of a preeclamptic woman.

    a. _____

    b. _____

    c. _____

    d. _____

52. What four steps should be taken to ensure that BP readings on the preeclamptic woman are standardized?

    a. _____

    b. _____

    c. _____

    d. _____

53. Match the correct responses. BP readings are:

    Column A

    _____ 1. Lowest

    _____ 2. Highest

    _____ 3. Intermediate

    Column B

    a. Supine, standing

    b. Sitting

    c. Laterally recumbent with a 15- to 30-degree tilt

54. In the severely preeclamptic patient, how often is assessment of the following recommended?

    a. BP: _____

    b. Proteinuria: _____

    c. Hyperreflexia: _____

    d. Urinary output: _____

55. An appropriate nurse:patient ratio with a severely preeclamptic woman is _____.

56. Appropriate laboratory workup for the preeclamptic woman includes:

    a. _____

    b. _____

    c. _____

    d. _____

    e. _____

57. State five precautions to be taken in caring for the severely preeclamptic woman.

    a. _____

    b. _____

    c. _____

    d. _____

    e. _____

58. State the initial steps you would take if an 18-year-old primigravida at 34 weeks' gestation presented in early labor at the labor unit of a Level I hospital and had signs and symptoms of severe preeclampsia.

    _____

    _____

    _____

    _____

59. The woman with HELLP syndrome is at risk for hemorrhage due to a severely low platelet count. Which of the following are clinical signs and symptoms of this condition? (Circle all that apply.)

    a. Hematuria

    b. Epistaxis

    c. Proteinuria

    d. Petechiae

    e. Hypertension

    f. Epigastric pain

    g. Easy bruising

    h. Oozing from the IV site

    i. Bleeding gums

60. When caring for the woman with HELLP syndrome, what two laboratory values should be monitored closely?

    a. _____

    b. _____

61. The recommended fetal monitoring approach for a woman with HELLP syndrome is intermittent, external fetal monitoring throughout her labor.

    a. True

    b. False

62. Epidural blocks can safely be used for pain management during labor and delivery and for anesthesia during cesarean delivery in the woman with HELLP syndrome.

    a. True

    b. False

63. All women with HELLP syndrome should have a cesarean delivery.

    a. True

    b. False

64. To give a woman a loading dose of magnesium sulfate means that:

    _____

    _____

    _____

65. State three signs of magnesium sulfate overdose.

    a. _____

    b. _____

    c. _____

66. The antidote to magnesium sulfate toxicity is the administration of _____.

67. The initial dose of hydralazine (Apresoline) to the severely hypertensive patient is _____ mg intravenously over _____ minutes. BP during hydralazine therapy should be checked every _____ minutes. Another _____ mg may be given intravenously after _____ minutes if the diastolic BP remains above 110 mmHg.

68. Explain why it is critical to observe for any sign of hypotension when administering a vasodilator, such as hydralazine (Apresoline), to the severely hypertensive or eclamptic woman.

    _____

    _____

    _____

    _____

69. A significant drop in BP after delivery in a woman with a severe hypertensive disorder likely reflects _____.

70. When a high-risk baby is anticipated at delivery, it is imperative to prepare by _____.

71. The "cure" for preeclampsia is _____.

72. Eclampsia occurs in almost _____ % to _____ % of cases during the _____ period.

73. Postpartum recovery from HELLP syndrome is:

    a. Gradual

    b. Preceded by worsening of laboratory values and illness

    c. Quite rapid

    d. Uneventful

74. State five signs and symptoms that indicate the development of pulmonary edema.

    a. _____

    b. _____

    c. _____

    d. _____

    e. _____

75. Breastfeeding can be done safely in women taking selected antihypertensive drugs with carefully reduced dosages and BP supervision.

    a. True

    b. False

76. The longer hypertension occurring for the first time during pregnancy persists postpartum, the greater the likelihood that the underlying cause is chronic hypertension.

    a. True

    b. False

77. Most women experiencing HELLP syndrome for the first time have a high risk of reoccurrence in a subsequent pregnancy.

    a. True

    b. False

PRACTICE/REVIEW ANSWER KEY

1. 6; 8%

2. Gestational hypertension

3. Superimposed hypertension

4. Eclampsia

5. Preeclampsia

6.
    1. b
    2. g
    3. e
    4. b
    5. a
    6. a
    7. a
    8. a
    9. f
    10. e
    11. c
    12. d
    13. c
    14. d

7.
    a. a, True
    b. b, False
    c. b, False
    d. b, False
    e. a, True
    f. b, False
    g. a, True
    h. a, True
    i. a, True

8.
    a. Elevated BP: 140/90 mmHg or higher
    b. Proteinuria

9.
    a. T
    b. P
    c. H
    d. H
    e. P
    f. T
    g. P, E, or H
    h. H
    i. E
    j. H

10. Any five of the following:
    a. Young and pregnant for the first time
    b. Young and experiencing a pregnancy with a new father
    c. History of chronic hypertension
    d. Twin pregnancy
    e. Has diabetes
    f. History of preeclampsia
    g. Black race and older than 35 years of age

11. a

12. A diagnosis of chronic hypertension preceding pregnancy is made based on a history of persistent BP elevation before the 20th week of gestation. Preeclampsia is diagnosed with BP elevations after the 20th week of gestation.

13. Mark an "X" by statement a.

14. Superimposed preeclampsia; superimposed eclampsia

15. Any five of the following:
    a. Is remote from term (less than 36 weeks' estimated gestational age)
    b. Is white, multiparous, and 25 years of age or older
    c. Demonstrates excessive weight gain with generalized edema

d. Complains of epigastric or right upper quadrant pain and a history of malaise for a few days

e. Complains of flulike symptoms and nausea and vomiting

f. Complains of hematuria, bleeding gums, jaundice, or diarrhea

16. d

17. c

18. a

19. a and b

20. a

21. 1. a
    2. b
    3. b
    4. b
    5. a
    6. d
    7. c

22. Angiotensin II; renin; angiotensinogen; angiotensin I; angiotensin II

23. A disease of small blood vessels in which the basement membrane of capillaries thickens, or thrombi microangiopathy, in which thrombi form in arterioles or capillaries

24. a. Pressure is increased (hypertension) and blood flow is diminished

    b. Lesions in the vessel wall result in fluid (plasma) loss, leading to changes in oncotic pressures and extracellular fluid accumulation

    c. Perfusion to the target organs is reduced, leading to ischemia and necrosis

25. Immune; platelets; fibrin; red blood cells; hemolysis

26. Microangiopathic hemolytic; HELLP syndrome

27. Thrombocytopenia

28. a. Abruptio placentae
    b. Cerebral hemorrhage
    c. Acute renal or cardiac failure
    d. DIC

29. 30; 15

30. Gestational hypertension

31. Intravascular volume; edema; sudden weight gain

32. Hematocrit

33. 100,000 mm^3; 50,000 mm^3

34. b

35. a. Blurred vision
    b. Dizziness
    c. Scotomata
    d. Headache

36. Epigastric pain in the right upper quadrant of the abdomen

37. Hyperactive reflexes

38. Intrauterine growth restriction

39. b. False

40. b. False

41. b. False

42. a. True

43. a. True

44. Preeclampsia

45. 300 mg/L or more of protein in a 24-hour specimen or protein concentration of 2+ or higher on at least two random urine tests done 6 hours apart

46. She has severe preeclampsia. If delivery is required, a preterm, low-birth-weight infant will require neonatal intensive care.

47. a. Hemolysis
    b. Elevated liver enzymes
    c. Low platelets

48. a. T
    b. F
    c. T
    d. T

49. b. False

50. Any five of the following:
    a. Nausea and vomiting
    b. General sick feeling
    c. Epigastric or right upper quadrant pain
    d. Worsening edema
    e. Diarrhea
    f. Hematuria
    g. Bleeding gums
    h. Abdominal, flank, or shoulder pain

51. a. To prevent convulsions through the use of magnesium sulfate
    b. To ensure adequate kidney function
    c. To monitor fetal status continuously for signs of utero-placental insufficiency
    d. To stabilize the woman so that a vaginal or cesarean birth can be accomplished

52. a. Use the same arm throughout.
    b. Use the arm with the higher reading if pressure readings differ in each arm by more than 10 mmHg.
    c. Fit the appropriate size sphygmomanometer to the patient's arm.
    d. Perform BP readings with the woman in essentially the same position each time, preferably laterally recumbent and at a 15- to 30-degree tilt when on bed rest.

53. 1. c
    2. a
    3. b

54. a. Every 15 to 30 minutes
    b. Every hour
    c. Every hour
    d. Every hour

55. 1:1

56. a. CBC with peripheral smear
    b. Type and crossmatch
    c. Liver enzymes
    d. DIC profile
    e. Serum creatinine

57. a. Control the environment by keeping lights dim, noise level down, and visitors to a minimum.
    b. Pad the sides of the bed.
    c. Have emergency airway equipment immediately available.
    d. Have oxygen and suctioning equipment available.
    e. Check that the equipment is in operating order and have the emergency cart nearby.

58. Notify the primary care provider immediately. Anticipate a maternal transport to a high-risk regional center after the patient is stabilized.

59. a, b, d, g, h, i

60. a. Platelet count
    b. Liver enzymes

61. b. False

62. b. False

63. b. False

64. The woman receives 4 to 6 g of magnesium sulfate in 100 mL of solution administered at a rate that ensures that the entire 4 to 6 g is received over a 15- to 20-minute period. This is done when a rapid therapeutic effect is desired. To reduce the risk of vomiting (the side effect of rapid magnesium sulfate administration), administer the dose over 25 to 30 minutes in nonemergency situations.

65. a. Absence of the patellar reflex
    b. Respirations that are shallow and fewer than 12 per minute
    c. Urinary output less than 25 mL/h

66. Calcium gluconate; using 10 mL of a 10% calcium gluconate solution (each milliliter contains 0.1 g of calcium gluconate)

67. 5 mg; 1 to 2 minutes; 2 to 5 minutes; 5 to 10 mg; 20 minutes

68. Women who are severely hypertensive or eclamptic usually have reduced intravascular blood volume. Giving a potent vasodilator such as hydralazine causes blood vessels to dilate. This can result in poor blood return to vital organs in a patient with an abnormally low blood volume. The woman might experience sudden, severe hypotension.

69. Excessive blood loss

70. Having appropriate personnel present, not on call

71. Delivery

72. 25; 30; postpartum

73. b

74. a. Chest discomfort
    b. Tachycardia
    c. Pulmonary rales
    d. Tachypnea
    e. Dyspnea

75. a. True

76. a. True

77. b. False

REFERENCES

1. Chang, J., Elam-Evans, L., Berg, C., Hendon, J., Flowers, L., Seed, K., & Syverson, C. J. (2003). Pregnancy-related mortality surveillance—United States, 1991–1999. *Surveillance Summaries, Morbidity and Mortality Weekly Report, 52*(SS-2), 1–8.
2. Martin, J. A., Hamilton, B. E., Sutton, P. D., Ventura, S. J., Menacker, F., & Kormeyer, S. (2006). Births: Final data for 2004. *National Vital Statistics Reports, 55*(1), 1–102.

3. Roberts, J. M. (2004). Pregnancy-related hypertension. In: Creasy, R., & Resnik, R., (Eds.), *Maternal-fetal medicine* (5th ed., pp. 859–900). Philadelphia: Saunders.

4. National High Blood Pressure Education Program Working Group on High Blood Pressure in Pregnancy. (2000). Report of the National High Blood Pressure Education Program Working Group on high blood pressure in pregnancy. *American Journal of Obstetrics and Gynecology, 183*(1), S1–S22.

5. National High Blood Pressure Education Program. (2000). *Working group report on high blood pressure in pregnancy*. Bethesda, MD: Heart Lung and Blood Institute.

6. Gifford, R., August, P., Cunningham, G., Green, L., Lindeheimer, M., McNellis, D., et al. (2000). *National High Blood Pressure Education Program Working Group National High Blood Pressure in Pregnancy* [NIH Publication No. 00-3029]. Bethesda, MD: National Institutes of Health, National Heart, Lung, Blood Institute.

7. American College of Obstetricians and Gynecologists. (2002). *Diagnosis and management of preeclampsia and eclampsia* [ACOG Practice Bulletin No. 33]. Washington, DC: Author.

8. August, P. Hypertensive disorders in pregnancy. In: Burrow, G., Duffy, T., & Copel, J. (Eds.), *Medical complications during pregnancy* (6th ed., pp. 43–68). Philadelphia: Elsevier.

9. Cunningham, F. G., Gant, N. F., Leveno, K. J., Gilstrap, L. C., Hauth, J. C., & Wenstrom, K. D. (eds). (2001). Hypertensive disorders in pregnancy. In: *Williams' Obstetrics* (21st ed., pp. 567–618). New York: McGraw-Hill.

10. Norwitz, E. R., & Repke, J. T. (2000). Preeclampsia prevention and management. *Journal of the Society for Gynecologic Investigation, 7*(1), 21–36.

11. Martin, J. M., Thigpen, B., Moore, R., Rose, C., Cushman, J., & May, W. (2005). Stroke and severe preeclampsia and eclampsia: A paradigm shift focusing on systolic blood pressure. *Obstetrics and Gynecology, 105*(2), 246–254.

12. Saphier, C. J., & Repke, J. T. (1998). Hemolysis, elevated liver enzymes, and low platelets (HELLP) syndrome: A review of diagnosis and management. *Seminars in Perinatology, 22*(2), 118–133.

13. Coppage, K., & Sibai, B. M. (2004). Hypertensive emergencies. In Foley, M. T., Strong, J., & Garite, T. (Eds.). *Obstetric intensive care manual* (pp. 51–65). New York: McGraw-Hill.

14. American College of Obstetricians and Gynecologists. (2001). Chronic hypertension in pregnancy. ACOG Committee on Practice Bulletins. *Obstetrics and Gynecology, 98*(1), 177–185.

15. Mulrow, C. D., Chiquette, E., Ferrer, R. L., Sibai, B. M., Stevens, K. R., Harris, M., et al. (2000). *Management of chronic hypertension in pregnancy* [Evidence report/technology assessment no. 14 (Prepared by the San Antonio Evidence-based Practice Center based at the University of Texas Health Science Center at San Antonio under Contract No. 290-97-0012). AHRQ Publication No. 00-E011.]. Rockville, MD: Agency for Healthcare Research and Quality.

16. American College of Obstetricians and Gynecologists. (2001). *Chronic hypertension in pregnancy*. Washington, DC: Author.

17. vonDadelszen, P., Ornstein, M. P., Bull, S. B., Logan, A. G., Koren, G., & Magee, L. A. (2000). Fall in mean arterial pressure and fetal growth restriction in pregnancy hypertension: A meta-analysis. *Lancet, 355,* 87–92.

18. Beevers, G., Lip, G. Y. H., & O'Brien, E. (2001). ABC of hypertension. Blood pressure measurement. Part I—Sphygmomanometry: Factors common to all techniques. *British Medical Journal, 322,* 981–985.

19. Feldman, D. M. (2001). Blood pressure monitoring during pregnancy. *Blood Pressure Monitoring, 6*(1), 1–7.

20. Marx, G. F., Schwalbe, S. S., Cho, E., & Whitty, J. E. (1993). Automated blood pressure measurements in laboring women: Are they reliable? *American Journal of Obstetrics and Gynecology, 158*(3, Pt. 1), 796–798.

21. O'Brien, E., Beevers, G., & Lip, G. Y. H. (2001). ABC of hypertension. Blood pressure measurement. Part III—Automated sphygmomanometry: Ambulatory blood pressure measurement. *British Medical Journal, 322,* 1110–1114.

22. Shennan, A. H., & Halligan, A. W. (1999) Measuring blood pressure in normal and hypertensive pregnancy. *Bailliere's Clinical Obstetrics and Gynecology, 13*(1), 1–26.

23. Bell, S. C., Halligan, A. W., Martin, A., Ashmore, J., Shennan, A. H., Lambert, P. C., et al. (1999). The role of observer error in antenatal dipstick proteinuria analysis. *British Journal of Obstetrics and Gynecology, 106,* 1177–1180.

24. Rinehart, B. K., Terrone, D. A., May, W. L., Magann, E. F., Isler, C. M., & Martin, Jr, J. N. (2001). Change in platelet count predicts eventual maternal outcome with syndrome of hemolysis, elevated liver enzymes and low platelet count. *Journal of Maternal-Fetal Medicine, 10*(1), 28–34.

MODULE

10 Caring for the Laboring Woman With HIV Infection or AIDS

FRANCILLA A. THOMAS ■ KELLY GEE ■
MARY COPELAND MYERS

Objectives

As you complete this module, you will learn:

1. The current status of the HIV/AIDS epidemic
2. Recommendations by the U.S. Public Health Service for HIV screening of pregnant women
3. The pathogenic process of HIV
4. How to correctly diagnose HIV infection
5. Risk factors for HIV infection
6. The current definition of *AIDS* and common opportunistic infections
7. How HIV infection is transmitted horizontally
8. The timing and mechanisms of vertical transmission
9. Methods to prevent vertical transmission
10. The impact of HIV infection on pregnancy
11. The impact of pregnancy on HIV infection
12. Recommendations for delivery of a newborn of an HIV-infected pregnant woman
13. Pharmacotherapeutic treatment recommendations for the HIV-infected pregnant woman
14. Diagnosis of HIV infection in the infant of an HIV-infected mother
15. How to use universal precautions recommended by the U.S. Centers for Disease Control and Prevention
16. Intrapartum and immediate postpartum management of the HIV-infected mother and newborn
17. Psychosocial issues related to the care of the HIV-infected mother
18. Ethical issues related to the care of the HIV-infected mother
19. Educative issues to discuss with the HIV-infected mother

Key Terms

When you have completed this module, you should be able to recall the meaning of the following terms. You should also be able to use the terms when consulting with other health professionals. The terms are defined in this module or in the glossary at the end of this book.

AIDS
antiretroviral therapy
AZT (or ZVD or Retrovir)
CD4$^+$ T cell
confirmatory test
EIA (formerly called the ELISA)
highly active antiretroviral therapy
  (HAART)
HIV DNA PCR test
HIV-1

HIV-2
HIV RNA test (or viral load or RNA)
horizontal transmission
perinatal transmission
sensitivity
specificity
sexually transmitted infection (STI)
SUDS (Single Use Diagnostic System) HIV-1 test
vertical transmission
Western blot test

Epidemiology and Pathophysiology of HIV

▶ What is known about the epidemiology of HIV?

The human immunodeficiency virus (HIV) was first identified in the early 1980s; ever since, it has been the focus of worldwide medical, political, and research efforts. Unfortunately, today it is believed that all cases of AIDS will eventually result in the death of the infected person. Worldwide, based on estimates from the Joint United Nations Programme on HIV/AIDS (UNAIDS), as of December 2006, a total of 39.5 million people are living with HIV or AIDS. Of these, 17.7 million are women and 2.3 million are children (younger than 15 years of age). In 2006, 530,000 children were newly diagnosed with HIV infection.[1]

In the United States, at the end of 2005, the Centers for Disease Control and Prevention (CDC) reported a cumulative number of 988,376 AIDS cases, with 182,822 cases in females and 9,078 cases in children younger than 13.[2] African-American and Hispanic women continue to be disproportionately affected by the epidemic. At the end of 2005, an estimated 8,438 perinatally acquired AIDS cases were reported, with the highest incidence still among African-American and Hispanic children.[2]

More than 90% of all adolescent and adult HIV infections worldwide are a result of heterosexual transmission, and women are particularly susceptible owing to substantial mucosal exposure to seminal fluid. Studies in the United States and abroad have shown that sexually transmitted infections (STIs), especially infections causing ulcerations to the vagina (e.g., genital herpes, syphilis chancroid), greatly increase a woman's risk of becoming infected with HIV. Other factors associated with an increased risk of heterosexual HIV transmission include alcohol use, history of childhood sexual abuse, domestic abuse, and illicit drug use.[3]

From 1985 to 1995, approximately 6,000 to 7,000 HIV-infected women gave birth in the United States. The number of children reported with AIDS attributed to perinatal HIV transmission peaked at 945 in 1992 and declined 95% to 48 in 2004.[4] According to the CDC Revised Recommendation for HIV Testing of Adults, Adolescents, and Pregnant Women in Health-care Settings, the dramatic decrease is attributable mainly to the identification of HIV-infected pregnant women and the effectiveness of antiretroviral prophylaxis in reducing mother-to-child transmission.[4] This decline could be even more dramatic; however, many pregnant women who are HIV positive are not diagnosed during their pregnancy. Therefore, they do not receive the appropriate treatment to reduce the risk of transmission to their babies.

In an effort to confront the growing problem of HIV infection and AIDS in women, the National Institute of Allergy and Infectious Disease (NIAID) has made woman-focused research an important part of the Institute's AIDS research program. The disease is tracked through studies and clinical trials, for example the Women's Interagency HIV Study (WIHS), Adult AIDS Clinical Trials Group (ACTG), and Pediatric AIDS Clinical Trials Group (PACTG).[3]

Risk Factors for HIV Infection

As health care providers evaluate pregnant women, they must be aware of certain factors and behaviors that place women at risk for becoming HIV infected. Assessment is essential throughout pregnancy and on admission for delivery. *A complete history and assessment of risk factors must be accomplished.* It is essential to formulate a plan of care that will provide for the special needs of the woman, her infant, and the hospital staff.

Some of the factors that place women at risk for HIV infection include a history of the following:

- **Intravenous (IV) drug use**—One way HIV is transmitted is through blood. Because drug users often share syringes and needles without adequate cleaning, the virus can be transferred from one person to another in this manner.
- **Multiple sexual partners**—Having multiple sexual partners increases the risk of exposure to HIV.
- **Sex with partners who are infected or at risk for infection**—Partners at risk include people with hemophilia, bisexual men, IV drug users, and partners who have or have had multiple sexual partners.
- **Receiving a blood transfusion before blood was being screened *but after* HIV infection occurred in the United States (1978–1985)**—Before 1986, no tests or heat-treating techniques were available to detect and destroy HIV in donated blood. Consequently,

people who received blood during that period were at increased risk for HIV infection. Today, because of blood screening and heat treatment, the risk of HIV transmission from transfusion is extremely small.

- **Multiple sexually transmitted infections (STIs)**—Infection with multiple STIs is often associated with other risk factors such as multiple sexual partners, IV drug use, and high-risk partners.
- **Currently living in or born in communities or countries where there is a known or suspected high prevalence of HIV infection**—There is more opportunity for exposure to HIV.

▶ What are the recommendations for HIV screening of pregnant women?

In 1995, after studies showed that treatment with ZDV decreased perinatal HIV transmission by 67.5%, the U.S. Public Health Service published guidelines recommending the following:
- Universal HIV counseling of all pregnant women
- Voluntary HIV testing of all pregnant women
- Voluntary treatment of pregnant women infected with HIV

Health care providers rapidly implemented these guidelines. Perinatal AIDS cases declined by 83% in 1999.[4] However, infants are still becoming infected perinatally, with about 100–200 infants in the U.S. infected annually.[2] These numbers emphasize the need for improved strategies to ensure that all pregnant women are offered HIV testing and, if positive, treatment to reduce their transmission risk.

Reasons for not being tested include the following[4]:
- Lack of prenatal care (especially among women who use illicit drugs)
- Lack of strong recommendation by the health care provider
- Perception of low risk by the patient and the provider
- Provider perception of the difficulties and complexity of required counseling
- Misunderstanding of counseling requirements by providers
- Complex logistics of testing

The U.S. Public Health Service published the following *revised* recommended guidelines for HIV screening of pregnant women in the United States[5]:
1. HIV screening should be a routine part of prenatal care for all pregnant women.
2. Recommend simplifying the testing process so that pretest counseling is not a barrier to testing.
3. Increase the flexibility of the consent process to allow for various types of informed consent.
4. Providers need to explore and address reasons for refusal.
5. Emphasize HIV testing and treatment at the time of labor and delivery for women who have not received prenatal testing.

Many nationwide professional and governmental organizations, including the American Academy of Pediatrics, the American College of Obstetricians and Gynecologists, and the U.S. Preventive Services Task Force, have underscored the importance of universal HIV counseling and testing of all pregnant women.[4]

Current recommendations from the CDC urge three approaches to HIV testing during pregnancy:
- An "opt-out" approach to testing, whereby a pregnant woman, unless she specifically declines, is tested.
- Routine testing with a rapid HIV test for women with unknown or undocumented HIV status who present in labor, to offer those testing HIV positive antiretroviral prophylaxis during labor.
- Rapid HIV testing for newborns of mothers of unknown HIV status so that they can receive postexposure antiretroviral prophylaxis, if needed.

Because state laws regarding HIV testing during pregnancy vary widely, health care providers should be familiar with their state and local laws, regulations, and policies concerning HIV screening of pregnant women and infants. The U.S. Public Health Service revised guidelines also provide recommendations on HIV prevention, counseling, education, interpretation of HIV test results, recommendations for HIV-infected pregnant women, and recommendations for postpartum follow-up of HIV-infected women and perinatally exposed infants.[4–6]

Pathophysiology of HIV Infection

▶ What is the human immunodeficiency virus?

The human immunodeficiency virus (HIV-1) is one of five known retroviruses. These viruses store genetic information in the form of RNA. The five known retroviruses are as follows.[7]

1. Human T-cell lymphotrophic virus (HTLV)-I	Causes adult T-cell leukemia/lymphoma
2. HTLV-II	Causes hairy cell leukemia
3. HTLV-III	Causes HIV-1 (previously called human T-cell lymphotrophic virus type III)
4. HTLV-IV	Causes HIV-2
5. HTLV-V	Causes cutaneous T-cell lymphoma/leukemia

HIV-1 was discovered in 1984.
HIV-2 was discovered in 1986.

In the United States, and in most of the world, HIV infection is usually caused by HIV-1. HIV-2 infection is predominantly found in West Africa.

Because of the extremely high replication rate of the viruses, there is substantial genetic variation of HIV. Within HIV-1, the two major groups are group M and group O. HIV-1 group M consists of nine subtypes, which are subtypes A though I.[7]

Findings reported at the Sixth Conference on Retroviruses and Opportunistic Infections in 1999 indicate that HIV-1 originated in nonhuman primates, that is, chimpanzees. The establishment of HIV-1 in humans is likely to have resulted from the cross-species transmission. The origin of HIV-2 has been identified with the sooty mangabey, another monkey species.[8]

Both HIV-1 and HIV-2 have the same modes of transmission, cause similar opportunistic infections, and cause AIDS.

HIV-2 seems to develop more slowly. It is milder and is less infectious early in the course of infection. As disease advances, the duration of increased infectivity is shorter. HIV-2 infection in children is rare. When compared with HIV-1, it seems to be less transmissible from mother to child. ZVD treatment is recommended for HIV-2–infected pregnant women. Because epidemiologic data indicate that the prevalence of HIV-2 is very low in the United States, *the CDC does not recommend routine HIV-2 testing at HIV counseling and test sites or in settings other than blood centers.*[8]

The Pathogenic Processes in HIV Infection

HIV has a great affinity for a protein complex called CD4, which is an antigen on the surface of certain cells.

The following cells have extremely high levels of CD4 surface antigen[9]:

- Lymphocytes (especially CD4$^+$ T cells)
- Monocytes
- Neural cells

Cells with a high surface density of CD4 are most at risk for invasion.

The following cells also have high levels of CD4 surface antigen[9]:

- Macrophages
- Langerhans' cells
- Endothelial cells
- Cells of the placenta

The large number of cell types affected by the virus explains the wide range of organs/systems affected by HIV infection.

Infection occurs when the human immunodeficiency virus envelope glycoprotein attaches itself to the CD4 receptors on the cellular membrane of its target cell. The virus then enters the cell; because the virus carries only RNA, it must invade the nucleus, accessing DNA of a host cell, to replicate. The following outlines the process of HIV replication.

1. After entering the host cell, the virus uses an enzyme called "reverse transcriptase" to convert its RNA to DNA. This process is called *reverse transcription.*
2. The new viral DNA is incorporated into the host cell's chromosomal DNA, where it forms a provirus.
3. Transcription of the viral DNA begins and results in multiple copies of viral RNA. This RNA codes for the production of viral proteins and enzymes.
4. Viral RNA and proteins are packaged as budding viruses. They are released from the host lymphocyte surface. They can now invade other host cells.

New viral particles that leave the infected cell destroy part of the host cell's outer membrane. As a consequence of this viral replication, the host cell dies. **Declining numbers of CD4$^+$ T cells result in the progressive decline of the individual's immune response.** Replication of HIV in macrophages can occur *without cellular destruction.*[10] Because macrophages are widely distributed throughout the body, they may play a critical role in the persistence of HIV infection because they provide reservoirs for chronically infected cells. *Viral replication is active throughout the course of the infection, and replication proceeds at a faster rate than what was predicted before the more sensitive tests were developed to detect viral loads.* Ongoing HIV replication in an active but incompletely effective immune system is probably responsible for secondary manifestations of HIV disease such as wasting and dementia.[11]

The impact of HIV infection is related to its effect on the normal function of the CD4$^+$ T cells. These cells play an essential role in orchestrating the body's immune responses. When CD4$^+$ T cells decline from cellular death or injury, the person becomes more susceptible to opportunistic infections. Progression of HIV infection varies among individuals.

- The average time of progression from the initial infection to AIDS, without antiretroviral therapy or with monotherapy, is approximately 10 to 11 years.
- Approximately 20% of individuals develop AIDS within 5 years.
- Less than 5% have sustained long-term asymptomatic HIV infection without a decline in CD4$^+$ T-cell counts to less than 500 cell/mm.[12,13]

This great variation in disease development depends on several factors, including the following:

- Health of the immune system
- Virulence of the HIV strain
- Viral concentration
- Mode of transmission

With disease advancement, there is increased susceptibility to infection and increased incidence of neoplasms, particularly Kaposi sarcoma, B-cell lymphoma, non-Hodgkin's lymphoma, and some carcinomas.

Diagnosis of HIV Infection and AIDS

▶ How is the diagnosis of HIV infection made?

The standard algorithm (step-by-step procedure) for HIV testing consists of the following:

1. An initial screening with a sensitive FDA-licensed *enzyme immunosorbent assay* (EIA), *followed by*
2. Confirmation with the specific FDA-licensed *Western blot test*

The initial test to screen for HIV antibody status in the adult is the EIA. The EIA detects antibodies produced in response to HIV. The HIV infection causes a reaction in the EIA; therefore, a **positive result is called** *reactive. The EIA is sensitive in that it identifies almost all blood containing antibodies to HIV (true-positive test), but the EIA is not specific. It sometimes produces false-positive results.*

False-positive results with the EIA can be caused by the following conditions[14]:

- Contamination in the laboratory
- Multiple pregnancies
- Cross-reactivity with other retroviruses
- History of injected drug use
- Hemophilia
- Alcoholism with hepatitis
- Hemodialysis

> A **false-positive test** is a positive reading on a blood specimen that *does not* contain antibodies to HIV (the patient does *not* have HIV).

> A **false-negative test** is a negative reading on a blood specimen that *does* contain HIV (the patient does have HIV).

False-negative results are rare with the EIA. False-negative results can occur in the early stage of HIV infection or in the late stage of HIV infection. In early infection, there is an interval in which the test can be negative because the patient has not yet produced antibodies against HIV.

> The average time to develop detectable antibodies is 25 days.[15] At the point in time when antibodies are detectable by testing, it is said that **seroconversion** has occurred.

Although an initial EIA may be reactive, it should not be considered a positive test until another EIA is repeated on the same blood sample. If the two tests are reactive, the test is reported as repeatedly reactive and the results are confirmed using a second, more specific antibody test called the *Western blot*. The Western blot is not used as the initial screening test because it is expensive and time consuming. *The Western blot is an immunoelectrophoresis procedure that identifies antibodies to nine specific viral proteins.* **Western blot test results are reported as unequivocal positive or indeterminate.**

- An *unequivocal positive result* means that HIV antibody–positive serum reacts with all nine viral antigens. This means the patient is infected with HIV.
- An *indeterminate result* means that there are not enough detectable antibodies to the viral antigens. Retesting in 1 month is recommended.[16]
- If the test results are indeterminate, the test can mean that either it is too early to detect HIV antibodies or the blood has produced something to cause a test reaction.
- When the test remains indeterminate for 6 months or longer, it is called a *stable indeterminate*. If the results remain stable indeterminate for 6 months or longer, the patient is considered uninfected *unless* clinical conditions of HIV infection are present.

> When used together, the EIA and Western blot are greater than 99% accurate.[17]

▶ What other tests are available to diagnose HIV?

In addition to blood test for the diagnosis of HIV, the FDA has also approved tests that detect HIV antibodies using oral fluids and urine. These tests were developed because many patients are more willing to have these tests, which are less invasive compared with the blood test.

The *immunofluorescent antibody* (IFA) *test* can be used to confirm the results if an EIA is repeatedly reactive and an indeterminate Western blot is obtained. The IFA is highly sensitive and specific. Although the IFA is less likely than the Western blot to yield indeterminate results, it is rarely used because it is difficult to perform.

Additional tests that are less commonly used to identify HIV infection include the following:

- HIV-1 p24 antigen assays
- Viral load assays
- Viral culture
- Polymerase chain reaction (PCR)

These tests are used most often to clarify an indeterminate Western blot, monitor therapeutic intervention, monitor disease progression, and identify the infected neonate or infant.[16]

Two rapid blood tests, approved by the FDA and increasing in popularity are **the OraQuick HIV-1 Antibody Test** and **the SUDS HIV-1 Test** (*Single Use Diagnostic System*). These tests are particularly useful for women with no prenatal care and those presenting in active labor who are unaware of their HIV status. **These tests are easier to perform when compared with the EIA, and the sensitivity and specificity are higher than 99%.**[5,18] Although the SUDS test costs more than the EIA, research indicates that rapid HIV testing is more cost effective than the current EIA/Western blot testing. The rapid tests have been found to be feasible, accurate, timely, and useful in providing prompt access to intrapartum and neonatal antiretroviral prophylaxis and in reducing perinatal transmission. Results can be obtained within minutes to a few hours[19] as opposed to several days with the EIA. With rapid HIV testing, antepartal patients can learn their results at the initial visit, and because a second visit is not required to obtain results, patients tend to be more compliant.[14,16] *As with the EIA, a negative test does not require a confirmation, yet a positive or reactive test does require a confirmation with the Western blot or IFA.*

▶ Can HIV be accurately diagnosed during pregnancy?

HIV infection during pregnancy can usually be diagnosed using the standard algorithm consisting of the EIA and Western blot. Before the development of more sensitive HIV antibody test, the estimated time between exposure and HIV antibody seroconversion (time delay from infection to positive antibody status) was 2.4 months. Now, with more sensitive tests, detection of HIV antibody is approximately 12 to 22 days.[18]

Individuals at risk for HIV infection should have repeated testing at appropriate intervals. Some individuals do not seroconvert for 3 to 4 weeks, but almost all do so by 6 months. The period between actual infection with HIV until the time when enough antibodies are produced, by the body, to cause a positive HIV test result is called the *window period*. Because of this period, repeated HIV tests may be necessary due to false-negative results, and after additional risky behaviors.[18]

Because some common complaints and problems associated with pregnancy are similar to those seen in the initial phase of HIV infection, accurate differential diagnosis can be difficult and thus delayed. Problems common to both early HIV infection and pregnancy are fatigue, malaise, anemia, and dyspnea. If an individual has a recent history of known or possible exposure to HIV and has a negative HIV-1 test, a false-negative result should be considered. Additional testing should be performed, including testing for HIV-2 and HIV-1 group O infections.

▶ What is AIDS?

AIDS is the result of advanced HIV infection. Studies have suggested that all HIV-positive individuals will *eventually* develop AIDS. At present, AIDS is considered a lethal disease. In January 1993, the CDC expanded the AIDS surveillance case definition to include (a) laboratory evidence of infection, (b) laboratory evidence of severe immunosuppression, and/or (c) 1 or more of the 26 identified clinical conditions for AIDS.[19] Display 10.1 presents an outline of the most current CDC diagnostic criteria (definition) for AIDS in adults and adolescents.

▶ What are opportunistic infections?

Opportunistic infections are caused by organisms that a healthy immune system, under normal situations, could easily destroy on its own or manage to overcome with the assistance of medication. However, with HIV infection, the immune system is compromised, and an opportunistic infection can be deadly. Some of the most common opportunistic infections that often occur early in HIV infection are:

- Thrush
- Shingles
- Herpes simplex
- Pneumococcal pneumonia
- Oral hairy leukoplakia
- Thrombocytopenic purpura

Opportunistic infections that occur late in the course of HIV infection are the following[20]:

- *Pneumocystis carinii* pneumonia (PCP)
- Kaposi sarcoma
- Tuberculosis
- Toxoplasmosis
- Cryptococcosis
- Cryptosporidiosis

DISPLAY 10.1	CURRENT DIAGNOSTIC CRITERIA FOR AIDS IN ADULTS AND ADOLESCENTS[19]

LABORATORY EVIDENCE OF HIV INFECTION

1. Repeatedly reactive EIA
2. Subsequent confirmatory Western blot or immunofluorescence assay

plus
Laboratory evidence of severe immunosuppression
1. Less than 200 CD4$^+$ T lymphocytes
2. CD4$^+$ T lymphocytes <14% of total lymphocytes

and/or
One or more of the following:
1. Candidiasis of the bronchi, trachea, or lungs
2. Candidiasis, esophageal
3. Recurrent pneumonia (bacterial, more than one episode)
4. Invasive cervical cancer (diagnosed by biopsy)
5. Coccidioidomycosis, disseminated or extrapulmonary
6. Cryptococcosis, extrapulmonary
7. Cryptosporidiosis, chronic intestinal (≥1 month's duration)
8. Cytomegalovirus disease (other than liver, spleen, or nodes)
9. Cytomegalovirus, retinitis (with loss of vision)
10. HIV encephalopathy
11. Herpes simplex: chronic ulcer(s) (≥1 month's duration); or bronchitis, pneumonitis, or esophagitis
12. Histoplasmosis, disseminated or extrapulmonary
13. Isosporiasis, chronic intestinal (of at least 1 month's duration)
14. Kaposi's sarcoma
15. Lymphoma, Burkitt's (or equivalent term)
16. Lymphoma, immunoblastic (or equivalent term)
17. Lymphoma, primary, of brain
18. Mycobacterium avium-intracellulare complex or Mycobacterium kansasii, disseminated or extrapulmonary
19. Mycobacterium tuberculosis, disseminated or extrapulmonary
20. Mycobacterium, other species or unidentified species, disseminated or extrapulmonary
21. Pneumocystis carinii pneumonia (PCP)
22. Progressive multifocal leukoencephalopathy
23. Salmonella septicemia, recurrent
24. Toxoplasmosis of the brain
25. Wasting syndrome due to HIV
26. Pulmonary tuberculosis

Methods of HIV Transmission

HIV can be transmitted through the following three routes:
1. Sexual contact
2. Exposure to infected blood or blood products
3. Perinatally from an infected mother to her baby

HIV has been isolated from the following:

- Blood
- Semen
- Vaginal secretions
- Saliva
- Tears
- Breast milk
- Cerebrospinal fluid
- Amniotic fluid
- Urine

However, evidence reveals that it is transmitted only by the following[21]:

- Blood
- Semen
- Vaginal secretions
- Breast milk
- Body fluids such as amniotic fluid and urine *that contain visible blood*

> The two methods of transmission for HIV are:
> 1. Horizontal transmission
> 2. Vertical transmission

Horizontal Transmission of HIV

Horizontal transmission **means that the virus is transmitted from one person to another by direct contact.** Examples of such contact include the following:

- **Intimate sexual contact (oral, anal, or vaginal) with someone infected with the human immunodeficiency virus**—Studies demonstrate that the receptive partner in intercourse has a greater chance of acquiring HIV infection than does the insertive partner. Receptive rectal intercourse has an approximate risk of 0.1% to 3% per episode, whereas receptive vaginal intercourse has an approximate risk of 0.1% to 0.2% per episode. Insertive rectal intercourse has an approximate risk of 0.06% per episode, and insertive vaginal intercourse has an approximate risk of 0.1% per episode.[22,23] Other factors associated with an increased risk of HIV infection are exposure to blood, such as with genital ulcer disease, trauma during sex, menstruation of the HIV-infected woman, and exposure to inflammation of the genital or rectal mucosa, which can occur with STIs.[24] Open-mouth kissing is considered very low risk; however, prolonged open-mouth kissing could damage the mouth or lips and allow HIV transmission through bloody saliva. Therefore, the CDC recommends against open-mouth kissing with an infected partner.[5]
- **Sharing of drug needles and syringes with an infected individual**—Sharing IV drug paraphernalia has an approximate risk of 0.67% per exposure.[25]
- **Receipt of a blood transfusion that contains HIV**—Risk from blood transfusions has been virtually eliminated through careful screening procedures now done on all donated blood and plasma.
- **Inadvertent contamination of mucous membranes or breaks in the skin (e.g., of a nurse or other health care provider) by the blood or body fluid of the infected person**—The overall risk for HIV infection after percutaneous exposure to HIV-infected blood is approximately 0.3% and is 0.09% after mucous membrane exposure.[26] The Public Health Service provides specific management guidelines for postexposure antiretroviral intervention. Every institution should use these guidelines.

Vertical Transmission of HIV

Vertical transmission **of HIV occurs when the virus is passed from the mother to her infant during the perinatal period.** Transmission can occur during the antepartum, intrapartum, or postpartum period. HIV has been isolated from many sources (early gestational embryo, blood, breast milk, amniotic fluid, cord blood, and the placenta), which indicates multiple potential routes of fetal or neonatal transmission. The virus has been isolated in 13- to 20-week-old fetuses, but **transmission is generally believed to occur most often in late pregnancy.**[27,28] In nonbreastfeeding populations, antepartum transmission accounts for 25% to 40% of infections, and intrapartum transmission accounts for 60% to 75% of HIV infections. In breastfeeding populations, antepartum transmission accounts for 20% to 25% of infections, intrapartum transmission accounts for 60% to 70% of infections, and postpartum transmission accounts for 10% to 15% of infections.[5]

The HIV-1 vertical transmission rate *in the absence of antiretroviral use* is approximately 16% to 25% in studies from Europe and North America, 25% to 40% in Africa, and up to 24% in Thailand.[4] In the United States, the extensive implementation of the Public Health Service guidelines for universal counseling and testing, and the use of ZDV sharply reduced transmission risk and the number of mother-to-infant transmission. **Studies have reported transmission rates of 5% to 6% and as low as less than 1% among women with undetectable plasma viral load. ZVD combined with cesarean section or combination antiretroviral drugs taken antenatally have been shown to achieve a rate of 2% or lower transmission rate.**[5]

Mechanisms of Vertical Transmission

Antepartum transmission most likely occurs through transplacental transmission of HIV. An example is when HIV is transmitted after placental disruption, as in placental abruption or during amniocentesis. *Intrapartum transmission* can occur through maternal–fetal transfusion of blood during labor and through contact of the infant with infected blood or other maternal secretions during delivery. *Postpartum transmission* can occur by inoculation, if infant is injected before maternal secretion is removed from its body, or through breastfeeding because of prolonged exposure of the infant's oral and gastrointestinal tracts to infected breast milk. Most studies indicate that transmission by breastfeeding occurs during the early weeks of breastfeeding. Randomized trial of formula versus breastfeeding showed approximately 44% of HIV infection resulted from breastfeeding, and most infections occurred during the first few weeks to months of life.[5,29]

Risk Factors for Vertical Transmission

The following are risk factors for vertical transmission:

- **Clinical**
  - Immunologically or clinically advanced HIV disease in mother
  - Increased plasma viral load
  - Maternal injected drug use during pregnancy
  - Low CD4 lymphocyte count
  - Breastfeeding
  - Nonreceipt of chemoprophylaxis[5,29,30]

NOTE: No link has been established between perinatal transmission and maternal age, race/ethnicity, or history of having a previously infected child.[5]

- **Obstetric**
  - Delivery more than 4 hours after rupture of fetal membranes doubles the risk for transmission
  - Maternal infection with other STIs during pregnancy
  - Invasive procedures; for example, amniocentesis, fetal scalp electrode insertion, fetal scalp sampling, episiotomy
  - Use of forceps and vacuum extractors
  - Chorioamnionitis
  - Preterm delivery[5,29,30]

Prevention of Perinatal HIV Transmission

Every infant that is born HIV infected is a sentinel health event as a result of either a missed prevention opportunity or, rarely, prophylaxis failure.[5]

Strategies to Prevent Transmission
- Early prenatal care
- Offer and acceptance of HIV testing
- Reducing viral load
- Chemoprophylaxis
- Reducing exposure of infant to HIV during the intrapartum period
- Reducing exposure to HIV infection during the postpartum period
- Cesarean delivery performed before onset of labor and rupture of membranes

Prevention strategies incorporating HIV screening can be highly effective in reducing perinatal transmission.

Transmission rate can be reduced to less than 2% with universal screening of women in combination with antiretroviral prophylaxis, scheduled cesarean section, when indicated, and avoidance of breastfeeding.[5]

Reducing the Viral Load

The viral load (also called the HIV-RNA test) is a measurement of the magnitude of active HIV replication. The viral load assesses the relative risk for disease progression and assesses the efficacy of antiretroviral therapies. *The CD4$^+$ T-cell count is an indicator of the extent of immune system damage.* The CD4$^+$ T-cell count assesses the risk of developing specific opportunistic infections and other sequelae of HIV infection. *When the viral load and the CD4$^+$ T-cell count are used together, the risk for disease progression and death can be predicted.*

As in the nonpregnant patient, the viral load should be monitored every 3 months in pregnant women.

The viral load correlates with the risk of perinatal transmission.

At a viral load of less than 1,000 copies per milliliter, the incidence of vertical transmission was about 2%.[31–33] However, *perinatal transmission has occurred in women with viral loads below the level of detection.* This indicates that other factors must play a role in the transmission.[18,34–36]

Current therapeutic intervention goals are as follows[36]:

1. Early initiation of an aggressive combination of antiretroviral regimens to maximally suppress viral replication
2. Preservation of immune function
3. Reduction in the development of resistance to drug therapy

Potent antiretroviral drugs (which can inhibit the protease enzyme of HIV-1) used in combination with nucleoside analog reverse transcriptase inhibitors can reduce viral loads to undetectable levels for prolonged periods. **The current recommended standard treatment for HIV-1–infected women who are *not* pregnant is a combination of two nucleoside analog reverse transcriptase inhibitors and one protease inhibitor. *Although pregnancy should not preclude the use of this standard, considerations must be made for potential dosing changes due to the physiologic changes of pregnancy and for potential short- and long-term effects of drugs on the fetus and newborn.*[36]**

Reducing Exposure of the Fetus to HIV During the Intrapartum Period

Because not all infants born to HIV-positive mothers are infected with HIV, care must be taken to protect and prevent further exposure of these infants to the virus. Avoiding procedures that increase risk for infection is an important element in reducing the risk.

Procedures that increase risk of HIV infection to the infant include invasive procedures and extended exposure to potentially infected body fluids. Invasive procedures include the following:

- **Internal fetal heart monitoring**—The electrode pierces the scalp of the fetus and permits exposure to bloody maternal amniotic fluid. As a result, the risk of contracting HIV is greatly increased.
- **Fetal pH scalp sampling**—Fetal scalp sampling involves breaks in the skin surface of the fetus. It can increase the potential for inoculation with HIV. Unless an urgent medical reason exists for performing this procedure, it is not recommended in the HIV-infected patient.
- **Eye prophylaxis, the giving of injections, or drawing of blood from the newborn before removal of maternal body fluids and blood**—Before these procedures are done, the newborn must be bathed with soap and water. Alcohol should be used afterward to prepare the injection site. The alcohol should be allowed to dry completely before the puncture is made to prevent possible skin contamination and body fluids from being transmitted into the tissues.
- **Cutting the cord with contaminated instruments**—Use sterile instruments to cut and clamp the cord after delivery. This reduces the risk of cross-contamination from instruments that have been in contact with maternal tissues and body fluids. After cutting the cord, apply an antimicrobial agent to the cord.

Newborns can also be infected during the birth process by exposure to the mother's infected body fluids. The following guidelines should be used to reduce the length of neonatal exposure to these fluids.

- Avoid cutting an episiotomy.
- Avoid using forceps or vacuum extraction.
- Dry the infant immediately after the delivery to remove all maternal blood and amniotic fluid.
- Gently remove excess fluid and blood from the nares and oropharynx with a bulb syringe, mucus extractor, or meconium aspirator with wall suction set on low setting. Because of the operator's risk of exposure to body fluids, do not use a suction device that requires the operator to provide suction by placing one end of the device in his or her mouth.
- Bathe the newborn under a radiant warmer as soon as the newborn is stable. Thorough cleansing with a mild, nonmedicated soap removes amniotic fluid and blood from the body surface, which is essential in reducing the chance of infection.
- Thoroughly clean the eye area before applying antibiotic prophylaxis. Failure to remove the maternal fluids from the ocular area before prophylaxis placement can result in exposure of the mucous membranes to the virus.
- Instruct the mother to avoid breastfeeding.

- Cesarean delivery for women with a high viral load. Pregnant women with HIV should be counseled with the following information:
  - Without ZDV therapy, the risk of vertical transmission is approximately 25%.
  - With ZDV therapy, the risk is reduced to 5% to 8%.
  - **With both ZDV therapy and a scheduled cesarean delivery (delivery before the onset of labor and before rupture of membranes), the risk is approximately 2%.**
  - With a viral load of fewer than 1,000 copies per milliliter, a vaginal delivery has a risk of 2% or less.
  - If a cesarean delivery is planned, delivery is recommended at 38 completed weeks of gestation rather than the usual 39 weeks, to minimize the chance of ruptured membranes or the woman going into labor. For women receiving ZDV therapy, adequate levels of the drug in the blood should be obtained *by starting the IV infusion 3 hours preoperatively.* Because morbidity is increased, prophylactic antibiotics should be considered. The risk of maternal morbidity associated with cesarean delivery should also be discussed with the woman. Her decision regarding the method of delivery should be respected.[37,38]

Reducing Risk of Infection if Exposed to HIV

In some cases, antiretroviral therapy given during or after an infant's exposure to HIV during labor and delivery blocks infection. For example, if HIV-infected women are treated only with ZDV within 24 hours of birth, only 8% of infants are infected, as opposed to 20% to 28% of infants who are infected if no treatment is given.[5,18] With highly active antiretroviral therapy (HAART), the transmission rate dropped 1% to 2%.[18,39] In Africa, the effectiveness of neonatal antiretroviral prophylaxis in infants who received either ZDV-3TC or nevirapine during labor and delivery and during the first week of life was demonstrated.[30]

Reducing Exposure to HIV During the Postpartum Period

Infants are at risk for HIV infection if they are breastfed by HIV-infected mothers. Most infection from breastfeeding occurs during the first few weeks to the first few months of life.[40] **In the United States and other developed countries where safe alternative sources of nutrition are available, breastfeeding is contraindicated in mothers with HIV infection.**[5,18,41]

A worldwide policy statement was issued in May 1997 by UNAIDS and cosponsored by the World Health Organization (WHO) and the United Nations Children's Fund (UNICEF). The guidelines state the following[42]:

- HIV infection can be transmitted though breastfeeding.
- Appropriate and affordable alternatives to breastfeeding should be available to HIV-infected women.
- HIV-positive women should be assisted in making fully informed decisions about the best way to feed their infants. This includes weighing the risk of (a) illness/death from infectious diseases and (b) the availability of safe alternatives to breastfeeding to reduce the risk of HIV transmission through breastfeeding.
- Women need to know and accept their HIV status.
- More voluntary and confidential counseling and testing needs to be available to women and their partners.
- Primary prevention of HIV infection is an essential priority for all adults of reproductive age and young people.

To counter the negative effects of the introduction of breast milk substitutes in developing countries, the International Code of Marketing of Breastmilk Substitutes was developed by the WHO in 1981.[42,43]

Management of the HIV-Infected Pregnant Woman

▶ **What is the effect of pregnancy on HIV infection?**

Even though pregnancy is accompanied by a mildly immunosuppressive state, **no conclusive evidence exists that pregnancy aggravates the health of the expectant woman who has**

early HIV infection.[10] During pregnancy, a decline in absolute CD4 cell counts is seen in both HIV-positive and HIV-negative women. It is thought to be secondary to hemodilution of pregnancy. Therefore, the use of a percentage of CD4 cells, rather than an absolute number of CD4 cells, is the most accurate method to measure immune function. Pregnancy does not accelerate a decline in CD4 cells, and HIV RNA levels remain relatively stable during pregnancy.[24]

▶ What is the effect of HIV infection on pregnancy?

HIV-infected women often have multiple coexisting problems that negatively affect pregnancy, including STIs, malnutrition, poverty, substance abuse, domestic violence, and inadequate or no prenatal care. These problems are often difficult to separate from problems stemming from the HIV infection.

Adverse pregnancy outcomes may occur not only because of secondary disease processes, but also because of antiretroviral therapy side effects and complications.

In regard to fertility with HIV, recent studies in Africa, as well as developed countries, suggest that HIV may have an adverse effect on fertility in both symptomatic as well as asymptomatic women. Prospective studies show lower pregnancy rates and losses more common in HIV-infected women. Longer intervals between births in HIV-positive women and longer times to achieve pregnancy in those with high viral loads was also noted.[24] The United States and developing countries have reported fetal loss associated with HIV infection. In West Africa, higher rates of both spontaneous abortion and stillbirths are found in women infected with HIV-1 or HIV-2.[44]

Many studies have revealed no increased risk of adverse outcome of asymptomatic or mildly symptomatic HIV-infected women. Reports regarding infant outcomes in developing countries indicate reduced birth weight for infants exposed to or infected with HIV-1. In the United States, mean birth weight was reported as 0.28 kg lighter and length was 1.64 cm shorter in HIV-infected infants. However, two confounding factors were maternal drug use and limited maternal antiretroviral therapy.[45]

Contradicting data exist on the impact of HIV infection on preterm delivery. In the United States, the incidence of pregnancy ending prematurely is 10%, and preterm birth is the leading cause of perinatal morbidity and mortality.[24] However, developing nations report an incidence of preterm labor as high as 26%, and an increased risk in infant mortality among HIV-infected women. Many coexisting medical problems contribute to the mortality.[46] HIV infection may predispose pregnant women to a variety of poor outcomes, such as preterm labor, prematurity, low birthweight infants, and postpartum endometritis. However, these poor obstetric outcomes occur mostly in women who are severely immunocompromised.[47]

In addition, some common infections often seen in HIV-negative women are more prevalent and often more severe in HIV-positive pregnant women. These infections include:

- Genital herpes simplex
- Human papillomavirus
- Syphilis
- Cytomegalovirus
- Hepatitis B
- Hepatitis A
- Vulvovaginal candidiasis

In conclusion, the effect of HIV infection on pregnancy is difficult to measure because of many confounding factors. The risk varies depending on the following factors:

- Population location (developed or developing countries)
- Clinical stage of HIV
- Availability of antiretroviral treatment
- Availability of obstetric care

Assessment and Monitoring of HIV-Infected Pregnant Women and Their Infants

Along with an initial social, emotional, and nutritional assessment, the initial medical assessment of the HIV-infected woman should include the following:

- CD4+ T-cell count to evaluate the degree of existing immunodeficiency
- Viral load to evaluate the risk for disease progression
- History of prior and current antiretroviral medications

The decision to initiate therapy or alternative therapy should be the same for women who are not receiving antiretroviral therapy and who are not pregnant. The discussion should include the following:

- Potential impact of therapy on the fetus and infant
- Ability to adhere to the prescribed regimen
- Long-term treatment plans for the mother

The final decision regarding treatment is the responsibility of the woman.

> The standard of care is the simultaneous use of multiple antiretroviral drugs to suppress the viral load below detectable limits.

Although the standard of care is the simultaneous use of multiple antiretroviral drugs to suppress the viral load below detectable limits, the decision to use any antiretroviral drug should be made by the woman after discussing with her health care provider the known and unknown benefits and risks to her and her fetus.[24,36]

A decision by the woman (a) to refuse treatment of ZDV, (b) to only use ZDV, or (c) to refuse other antiretroviral drugs should not result in denial of care or punitive action.

Also included in the initial medical assessment is a review of the woman's current immunization status. *Immunizations should be given as early as possible in the course of HIV infection because the ability to form specific antibodies after immunizations becomes progressively impaired as the disease advances. (Remember that immune system function declines as the disease advances.)* Live pathogen vaccines, such as the MMR (measles-mumps-rubella), are contraindicated, but killed or inactivated vaccines are considered safe.[24]

Recommended vaccines include the following[24]:
- Pneumococcal vaccine
- Hepatitis B immunization series (in the presence of a negative screen)
- Influenza vaccine
- *Haemophilus influenzae* type B (Hib) vaccine
- Tetanus-diphtheria vaccine
- Hepatitis A vaccine
- Polio vaccine
- Immune globulins

In addition to the aforementioned assessments and a physical examination, the following laboratory data should be evaluated:
- All routine prenatal laboratory tests, including blood type and Rh, antibody screen, rubella, urine culture, gonorrhea/chlamydia screening, Pap smear, syphilis serology, and hemoglobin electrophoresis (as indicated)
- Complete blood count (CBC) every 3 months
- Hepatitis serology to screen for vaccine candidates
- Serum chemistry panel to screen for adverse effects of some drug therapies
- Purified protein derivative (PPD) skin test for tuberculosis
- Cytomegalovirus immunoglobulin G (IgG)
- Toxoplasmosis IgG if with a low CD4 count
- Maternal serum α-fetoprotein if patient desires
- Glucose challenge test at 24 to 28 weeks (remember that protease inhibitors are diabetogenic, so repeat if indicated)
- Group B streptococcal culture

During pregnancy, **continued monitoring should include measurement of CD4$^+$ T-cell counts and an HIV-RNA test approximately every 3 months** to determine whether:
- Antiretroviral therapy is needed
- Current therapy needs to be altered
- Prophylaxis against *P. carinii* pneumonia should be started

Although ZDV is not associated with an increased risk for fetal complications, less is known about the effect of combination antiretroviral therapy on the fetus. **More intensive fetal surveillance is recommended with the use of combination antiretroviral therapy,** including the following[36]:
- Assessment of fetal anatomy with a level II ultrasound
- Assessment of fetal growth
- Assessment of fetal well-being during the third trimester, with fetal kick counts, nonstress tests, or biophysical profiles

For the postpartum woman, comprehensive care and support services are required to optimize the woman's own medical care and to provide proper family planning assistance. Services must be coordinated between the obstetrician and the HIV specialist. It must be determined whether continuing antiretroviral treatment is required for the woman's health. If continuing antiretroviral treatment is best for the woman, compliance with drug therapy is essential.

The following guidelines should be used for initial assessment and for follow-up monitoring of newborns of HIV-infected women[36]:

- A baseline CBC and differential should be determined before the initial administration of ZDV.
- Hemoglobin measurements are required (at a minimum) after the completion of the 6-week ZDV regimen and again at 12 weeks of age. *ZDV can cause anemia complications in the newborn.*
- Newborns who are anemic at birth or who are born premature need more intensive hemoglobin monitoring.
- If the infant's mother used combination antiretroviral therapy, more intensive monitoring of hematologic and serum chemistry values are advised.
- To prevent *P. carinii* pneumonia, all infants should begin prophylaxis at 6 weeks of age after the completion of ZDV therapy.
- Infants with negative virologic tests during the first 6 weeks of life should have the evaluation repeated after the completion of neonatal antiretroviral prophylaxis therapy. The effect of combination therapy on the sensitivity of infant virologic diagnostic testing is not known.[24,36]

Pharmacotherapeutic Treatment for HIV Infection

> In 1994, during the PACTG 076 study, the use of zidovudine (ZDV, Retrovir, AZT) therapy in pregnant women who were HIV positive, resulted in a 70% reduction in the risk of HIV perinatal transmission. The estimated risk of perinatal transmission without ZDV therapy was 25.5% compared with an 8.3% risk of transmission with ZDV therapy.[6,36]

ZDV is an antiretroviral drug that attacks the HIV virus. It is a nucleoside analog reverse transcriptase inhibitor (NRTIs) whose action inhibits viral replication in the cells by targeting the HIV reverse transcriptase enzyme. Since 1994, major advances in the understanding of the pathogenesis of HIV-1 infection, the treatment, and monitoring of the disease have been made. Given that the mean half-life of plasma virions (a complete virus particle) is estimated at only 6 hours, the focus of intervention is to initiate aggressive combination antiretroviral regimens quickly to maximally suppress viral replication, preserve immune function, and reduce the development of drug resistance.[24,36] *Maximal suppression of viral replication is now recommended.*

Protease inhibitors (PIs) prevent maturation of virus protein by competitively inhibiting HIV protease (an enzyme essential for viral protein cleavage). Blockage of this enzyme leads to immature, noninfectious virus particles being produced.[24]

PIs along with NRTIs can reduce plasma HIV-1–RNA to undetectable levels for prolonged periods.

In making decisions regarding treatment in a pregnant patient, the following must be considered:

- The treatment of HIV infection
- Reduction of the risk of perinatal transmission
- The known and unknown benefits and risks of therapy

> Although unique considerations associated with pregnancy should be discussed, pregnancy is not a reason to defer antiretroviral treatment.

Antiretroviral monotherapy is now considered suboptimal treatment for pregnant women with HIV infection.[36] Along with ZDV chemoprophylaxis, standard antiretroviral therapy should be offered to HIV-infected pregnant women.

Combination antiretroviral therapy is often called *highly active antiretroviral therapy* **(HAART).**

The current HAART standard of care for HIV-1–infected adults who are not pregnant consists of two nucleoside analog reverse transcriptase inhibitors and one protease inhibitor.

Guidelines for initiation and optimal antiretroviral therapy for pregnant women should be the same as guidelines for nonpregnant adults. The primary issues to consider in guiding treatment decisions are the woman's clinical, virologic, and immunologic status. However, the potential effect on the fetus must also be considered.

In the first trimester of pregnancy, women who have not begun antiretroviral therapy may wish to delay initiation of therapy until after 10 to 12 weeks' gestation. This is the period of organogenesis, when major organs are developing. Some women who are already receiving antiretroviral therapy may consider temporarily stopping therapy until after the first trimester; however, most experts recommend continuation of maximally suppressive therapy.

If antiretroviral therapy is discontinued for any reason, all agents should be stopped and restarted simultaneously to prevent the development of drug resistance.[36]

Currently, minimal data exist on the pharmacokinetics and safety of antiretroviral agents used during pregnancy. Drug choice needs to be individualized based on the patient's status. **The combination of medications that seems to work best in many people and is strongly recommended consists of a choice of one protease inhibitor** *plus* **a choice of two nucleoside analog reverse transcriptase inhibitors**[48] (Table 10.1). Alternative recommendations are available, for instance through ATIS.[48]

TABLE 10.1 RECOMMENDED HAART REGIMENS

PROTEASE INHIBITORS	NUCLEOSIDE ANALOG REVERSE TRANSCRIPTASE INHIBITORS
Efavirenz	Stavudine + lamivudine
Indinavir	Stavudine + didanosine
Nelfinavir	Zidovudine + lamivudine
Ritonavir + saquinavir	Zidovudine + didanosine

There are currently six approved nucleoside analog reverse transcriptase inhibitors (Table 10.2). ZDV and d4T *should not* be used together.[48]

TABLE 10.2 NUCLEOSIDE ANALOG REVERSE TRANSCRIPTASE INHIBITORS

NAME OF DRUG	FDA PREGNANCY CATEGORY
Zidovudine (Retrovir)	C
Didanosine (Videx, ddi)	B
Lamivudine (Epivir, 3TC)	C
Stavudine (Zerit, d4T)	C
Zalcitabine (HIVID, ddc)	C
Abacavir (Ziagen, ABC)	C

There are three non-nucleoside analog reverse transcriptase inhibitors (Table 10.3).[48] Nevirapine has been evaluated, and to date, no adverse effects have been seen in women or infants. Because of teratogenic effects seen in primate studies with efavirenz, pregnancy should be avoided in women receiving this drug. No studies are currently planned with efavirenz in pregnant women.

TABLE 10.3 NON-NUCLEOSIDE ANALOG REVERSE TRANSCRIPTASE INHIBITORS	
NAME OF DRUG	**FDA PREGNANCY CATEGORY**
Delavirdine (Rescriptor)	C
Efavirenz (Sustiva)	C
Nevirapine (Viramune)	C

There are five approved protease inhibitors (Table 10.4). In the United States, the use of four protease inhibitors is currently being studied in pregnant women and their infants. No data are available at this time. Amprenavir has not been studied in pregnant women.[48]

TABLE 10.4 PROTEASE INHIBITORS	
NAME OF DRUG	**FDA PREGNANCY CATEGORY**
Indinavir (Crixivan)	C
Nelfinavir (Viracept)	B
Ritonavir (Norvir)	B
Saquinavir (Fortovase)	B
Amprenavir (Agenerase)	C

At present, if combination antiretroviral drugs are going to be used during the antepartum period, *whenever possible,* ZDV should be included as a component of the antenatal therapeutic regimen. During the intrapartum and neonatal period, ZDV should be used to reduce the risk of perinatal transmission.

The current standard ZDV dosing regimen for the antenatal period is 200 mg three times daily or 300 mg twice daily. This is a change from the regimen used in the PACTG 076 study, which used 100 mg five times a day. The current regimen has shown comparable clinical responses and is expected to enhance maternal adherence.[36]

Recommendations for the Use of Antiretroviral Drugs to Reduce Perinatal HIV Transmission

The Public Health Service Task Force has made the following recommendations regarding the use of antiretroviral drugs to reduce perinatal transmission[36]:

1. *If an HIV-infected pregnant woman has not received prior antiretroviral therapy, the three-part ZDV chemoprophylaxis regimen should be recommended.* The three-part ZDV regimen consists of the following:
   - **An antepartum regimen**—The dosage is zidovudine 200 mg three times daily or 300 mg twice daily.
   - **An intrapartum regimen**—The dosage is an initial loading dose of zidovudine 2 mg/kg intravenously followed by a continuous infusion of 1 mg/kg per hour until delivery.
   - **A neonatal regimen**—The dosage is zidovudine syrup 2 mg/kg orally four times a day for 6 weeks. Treatment of the newborn must begin as soon as possible after delivery. Optimally, treatment should begin within 12 to 24 hours after birth.
   - The combination of additional antiretroviral drugs should be discussed and recommended based on the woman's clinical, immunologic, and virologic status. A woman in the first trimester may consider delaying initiation of treatment until after 10 to 12 weeks' gestation.

2. *If an HIV-infected pregnant woman has already been receiving antiretroviral therapy during the current pregnancy, the recommendations are as follows:*
   • If past the first trimester, the woman should continue with her therapy.
   • If in the first trimester, the woman should be counseled on the risks versus the benefits of antiretroviral therapy during this period. Continuation of therapy should be considered. If therapy is discontinued, all drugs should be stopped simultaneously and restarted simultaneously to prevent the development of drug resistance.
   • If the current regimen does not contain ZDV, the addition of ZDV (or substitution of another nucleoside analog reverse transcriptase inhibitor) is recommended after 14 weeks' gestation. Also, ZDV administration is recommended during the intrapartum period and for the newborn.

3. *If an HIV-infected pregnant woman presents in labor with no prior therapy, the recommendations are as follows:*
   • A single dose of nevirapine at the onset of labor, followed by a single dose of nevirapine for the newborn at 48 hours of age **OR**
   • Oral ZDV and 3TC during labor, followed by 1 week of oral ZDV-3TC for the newborn **OR**
   • Intrapartum IV ZDV, followed by 6 weeks of ZDV for the newborn **OR**
   • The single-dose maternal/infant nevirapine regimen combined with intrapartum IV ZDV and 6 weeks of ZDV for the newborn
   • If single-dose nevirapine is given to the mother, alone or in combination with ZVD, adding ZVD/3TC may be considered to be given intrapartum or immediately postpartum for 3 to 7 days to aid in reducing nevirapine resistance.
   • The woman should be assessed in the immediate postpartum period to determine whether antiretroviral therapy is necessary for her health.

4. *If an infant is born to a mother who has received no antiretroviral therapy during her pregnancy or intrapartum period, the recommendations are as follows:*
   • A 6-week course of ZDV therapy for the infant should be offered and discussed with the mother.
   • ZDV should be initiated as soon as possible after delivery, preferably within 6 to 12 hours of birth.
   • The appropriate dosing for premature infants is currently being studied in infants less than 34 weeks' gestation. The regimen being studied is 1.5 mg/kg body weight orally or intravenously every 12 hours for the first 2 weeks of life, then increased to 2 mg/kg body weight every 8 hours for infants 2 to 6 weeks of age.

5. *The woman should be assessed in the immediate postpartum period to determine whether antiretroviral therapy is recommended for her health.*[36]

Serious Side Effects of Antiretroviral Therapy

ZDV has been associated with hematologic toxicity, including granulocytopenia and severe anemia (especially in patients with advanced HIV disease). Prolonged use has also been associated with symptomatic myopathy. Rare occurrences of potentially fatal lactic acidosis and severe hepatomegaly with steatosis have been reported. Nucleoside analog drugs are also known to cause mitochondrial dysfunction. Toxicity related to mitochondrial dysfunction has been reported in patients who have received long-term treatment. It resolved with discontinuation of the drugs.[48]

Protease inhibitors have been reported to cause hyperglycemia, new-onset diabetes mellitus, exacerbation of existing diabetes mellitus, and diabetic ketoacidosis. Because pregnancy can also cause hyperglycemia (as seen with gestational diabetes), pregnant women receiving protease inhibitor drugs should be monitored closely for hyperglycemia.[48]

▶ Does zidovudine present any threat to the fetus?

Studies of ZDV use at recommended dosages during pregnancy indicate that it is well tolerated by adults and term infants. Long-term data are not available, but short-term data are reassuring. Infants who were exposed to ZDV in utero have been followed for up to 6 years. They show no significant findings in immunologic, neurologic, or growth parameters. In the PACTG 076 study, the only significant side effect observed with ZDV use in infants was the presence of anemia. The anemia was mild and resolved spontaneously without transfusions.[48]

> Providers who are treating HIV-infected pregnant women and their infants are advised to report cases of prenatal exposure to antiretroviral drugs to the Antiretroviral Pregnancy Registry.

The Antiretroviral Pregnancy Registry[49]

The Antiretroviral Pregnancy Registry is an epidemiologic project to collect observational, non-experimental data on the use of antiretroviral drugs during pregnancy and their potential teratogenicity. The registry is a collaborative project among pharmaceutical companies, the CDC, the National Institutes of Health, and obstetric and pediatric practitioners.

The registry data will be used to supplement animal studies and assist providers in evaluating the risks and benefits of treatment for their patients. *The registry does not use patient names.* Information is obtained from reporting providers who call the project office at 800-258-4263, fax the enrollment form to 800-800-1052, or mail the form to Antiretroviral Pregnancy Registry, Research Park, 1011 Ashes Drive, Wilmington, NC 28405.

Current Recommendations Regarding Delivery in the Woman With HIV Infection

Baseline rate of perinatal HIV transmission without prophylaxis is 25%, timing of transmission is therefore critical to the development of preventive interventions. Evidence has shown that transmission can occur during the antenatal period, the intrapartum period or postpartum through breastfeeding; however, two thirds to three quarters of transmission appears to occur during or close to the intrapartum period, particularly in the non-breastfeeding populations.[24]

Because of these findings, studies that examine the delivery method and transmission have been conducted. **A significant relationship has been noted between the mode of delivery and vertical transmission.**

Research indicates that cesarean delivery (scheduled or elective) performed before the onset of labor and or membrane rupture, is associated with a 55% to 80% decrease in mother-to-child transmission with the use of ZVD alone.[24]

When making a decision about mode of delivery, potential maternal risks with cesarean section should be considered. Maternal morbidity is increased with cesarean delivery compared with vaginal delivery. The postpartum morbidity is greatest among HIV-infected women with low CD4$^+$ T-cell counts.[24,37]

Current recommendations by the Perinatal HIV Guidelines Working Group and The American College of Obstetricians and Gynecologists include[24,36,37]:

- Counsel all HIV-infected pregnant women about benefits and risks of scheduled cesarean section. The woman's freedom to make an informed decision regarding route of delivery should be respected and honored.
- Scheduled cesarean section should be recommended in the following situations:
  - HIV-RNA less than 1,000 copies/mL (regardless of ARV therapy).
  - Women with unknown HIV-RNA level, not on ARV therapy or receiving ZDV alone.
- Cesarean section is unlikely to add additional benefit in reduction of maternal-to-child transmission with HIV-RNA below 1,000 copies/mL in ARV-treated mothers.
- Plasma viral load should be evaluated every 3 months or after changes in therapy. The most recently determined HIV-RNA level should be used when counseling about mode of delivery.
- Women who have scheduled cesarean section but present in early labor or shortly after membranes rupture should be counseled and managed on an individual basis, based on most recent HIV-RNA level, ARV therapy, and projected length of labor.
- Other ARV medications taken during pregnancy should be given on schedule.
- The patient should receive antiretroviral chemotherapy during pregnancy according to the current guidelines. Adequate ZDV levels should be achieved if the IV infusion is begun 3 hours preoperatively.
- Prophylactic antibiotics should be considered during all cesarean deliveries.

- Cesarean delivery is recommended at 38 completed weeks of gestation to reduce the likelihood of onset of labor or rupture of membranes.
- Amniocentesis to determine fetal lung maturity should be avoided. The expected date of confinement should be made based on clinical and ultrasonographic estimates.

NO THERAPIES GUARANTEE A 0% RISK OF VERTICAL TRANSMISSION. THE HIGHEST RISK FOR VERTICAL TRANSMISSION IS AMONG WOMEN WITH RELATIVELY HIGH PLASMA VIRAL LOADS.

▶ How is HIV infection diagnosed in the newborn?

The presence of maternal HIV antibodies is a normal finding in babies born to HIV-infected mothers, regardless of whether the newborn is infected. These passively acquired maternal antibodies may persist for up to 15 to 18 months of age because of transplacental passage. Because these antibodies form the basis for standard HIV testing with the EIA and Western blot, these tests are invalid in the determination of whether the newborn has contracted HIV. **Using viral diagnostic assays, HIV infection can be diagnosed in most infants by 1 month of age and in virtually all infants by 6 months of age.**

Diagnostic testing in infants with known perinatal HIV exposure is recommended[50]:

- At birth to 14 days of life.
- 1 to 2 months of age
- 3 to 6 months of age

The following tests are available for the diagnosis of HIV infection in infants[50]:

- **HIV-DNA PCR is the *preferred* virologic method for diagnosing HIV infection in infants.** It is both sensitive and specific; it detects proviral HIV DNA in patient's peripheral blood mononuclear cells (PBMCs).
- **HIV-RNA assays** may also be useful in the diagnosis of HIV infection in infants; it detects extracellular viral RNA in the plasma.
- **HIV viral culture** has a similar sensitivity compared with HIV-DNA PCR. However, the culture is more complex and expensive to perform, and has a longer turn around time (2 to 4 weeks) for definitive results.
- **The p24 antigen** test is another highly specific test for HIV infection, but is not recommended for infant diagnosis in the United Stated because the sensitivity and specificity of the assay in the first months of life is lower than that of other HIV virologic tests.

Initial testing is recommended between birth and 14 days of age. Thirty percent to 40% of HIV infected infants can be identified by 48 hours of life. Infants with positive virologic tests at or before 48 hours are considered to have *intrauterine* or *antepartum infection.* Infants with negative virologic tests during the first week of life and subsequent positive tests are considered to have *intrapartum infection.*[50] Infants with an initially negative test should be retested at 1 to 2 months of age. Most HIV-exposed infants receive 6 weeks of antiretroviral prophylaxis to prevent mother-to-child transmission. HIV-exposed infants who have had repeatedly negative virologic assays at birth and 1 to 2 months of age should be retested at 3 to 6 months of age.

> HIV infection in the infant is diagnosed with two positive HIV virologic tests performed on separate blood samples.

HIV infection in the infant can be reasonably excluded in the following situations:

- A non-breastfed infant who has two or more negative virologic tests performed at 1 month of age or older, with one performed at 4 months of age or older.
- An infant has two or more negative HIV IgG antibody tests performed after 6 months of age with an interval of at least 1 month between tests, *and* the infant has no clinical evidence of HIV infection.

HIV infection in the infant can be *definitely* excluded in the following situations[50]:

- HIV IgG antibody is negative in the absence of hypogammaglobulinemia at 18 months of age, AND
- The infant has no clinical symptoms of HIV infection, AND
- HIV virologic assays are negative.

Special Issues to Consider in the Intrapartum and the Immediate Postpartum Management of HIV-Infected Women

The following factors must be addressed so that an effective, individualized plan of care can be developed and implemented:

- Infection control
- Pharmacotherapeutic options (as previously outlined)
- Psychosocial needs
- Ethical issues
- Patient education

Infection Control

Infection control measures must be a primary concern when providing care for the pregnant HIV-positive patient. The potential for infection of hospital personnel is certainly important; however, it is not the only consideration in the labor management of these patients. Obvious concerns are for fetal infection with HIV and for maternal infection because of potential immunocompromise and anemia. The following procedures are meant to help protect the HIV-positive woman from infection:

- **Reduce exposure to opportunistic organisms**—Limit vaginal examinations, avoid invasive procedures, avoid episiotomies and lacerations, attend to aseptic and sterile technique when performing procedures, and use the proper suturing techniques when episiotomy or laceration repair is necessary.
- **Monitor the patient closely for signs of infection**—Check vital signs and be especially alert for increasing temperature and pulse. Perform respiratory auscultation at regular intervals. Closely review laboratory results.
- **Review the patient's chart for history of infection**—especially a history of recent infections and evidence of cure.
- **Be alert for signs of chorioamnionitis**—The higher incidence of STIs combined with the potential for immunocompromise in HIV-positive women place the woman at risk for ascending infection. These infections have been implicated as possible causes of premature rupture of the membranes. These women require close monitoring of maternal vital signs (especially elevations of temperature and pulse), antibiotic usage when chorioamnionitis occurs, and continuous external intensive fetal surveillance to detect any signs of infection (e.g., increasing baseline rate, tachycardia, or decreasing variability).
- **Screen for colonization of group B streptococcus at 35 to 36 weeks' gestation**—If cultures are positive, provide chemoprophylaxis during labor.

Additional guidelines for the delivery of a mother at high risk or infected with HIV include the following:

- Follow universal precautions carefully to protect *yourself* from accidental needlesticks, splatter, or contact with body fluids.
- Carefully maintain patient hygiene. Keep the skin and perineum as clean and dry as possible. Change disposable underpads frequently. Closely follow institutional guidelines for care of urinary catheters and intravenous lines.
- Review the woman's chart for evidence of normal or abnormal fetal growth (ultrasound reports, maternal weight gain, and fundal height measurements). Palpate the mother's abdomen to obtain an estimation of the fetal weight. Many factors associated with HIV infection, such as drug use, poverty, and inadequate prenatal care, have an impact on the weight and condition of the baby at birth.
- Carefully monitor for blood loss, contraction pattern, and fetal heart rate pattern during labor.
- Observe the patient and laboratory values for signs of thrombocytopenia and anemia (common side effects of ZDV therapy).
- Handle blood– and body fluid–stained linen according to institutional infection control guidelines. Dispose of soiled linens promptly after use to reduce the chance of accidental contact with personnel.
- Precisely follow the recommended guidelines of the institution for sterilization, disinfection, and housekeeping.
- Inform the nursery staff of the mother's HIV status.
- Use universal precautions when caring for the newborn.

Psychosocial Needs

For most people, the birth of a baby is a time of happiness, joy, and celebration. **However, the HIV-positive mother *might* have ambivalent feelings about the whole process.** She might feel happy about motherhood, *but* at the same time be worried about her health and her baby's health. This can interfere with bonding and can contribute to the development of postpartum blues or depression. The following actions can help promote maternal–infant bonding.

- Encourage the new mother to hold her baby as soon as possible after delivery.
- Personalize the baby. Reinforce positive qualities of the newborn (e.g., pretty eyes, hair; has all her fingers and toes) and call the newborn by name.
- Encourage maternal–infant interaction. Encourage the mother to touch, talk to, and examine the baby.
- Promote family involvement in the birth process by allowing family attendance. Encourage participation in the labor, delivery, and postpartum period.

Many emotional and psychological adjustments are also occurring during this critical time. The following actions can help to promote psychological adjustment.

- If a psychiatric professional or a social worker has followed the mother, with her permission, notify that person of her status.
- Allow the mother to verbalize her feelings. Listening to her concerns will often help to reduce her anxiety and assist her in coming to terms with issues she must face.
- Do not avoid the mother because of her HIV status. Your time with her is therapeutic because women like her often feel isolated and are commonly ostracized by others.
- Avoid judgmental behavior and attitudes when providing care.
- Keep the new mother informed of both her status and that of her baby (before and after delivery). Counsel the mother regarding necessary health screenings for her newborn and herself.

> Remember that HIV is a family disease. It affects every family member, regardless of whether they are infected.

Ethical Issues

The care of the HIV-positive patient includes many emotionally charged issues for both patients and staff. These issues demand recognition and consideration to ensure that optimal care is provided to patients. The following are some of the key issues that affect both the patient and staff in the care of HIV-positive patients.

- **Confidentiality**—It is a central issue in the treatment of HIV/AIDS patients. Unauthorized disclosure of a patient's HIV status by health care workers is not only unethical but can cause irreparable damage to the patient by affecting social, occupational, and personal relationships. Fear of disclosure can keep patients from seeking early prenatal care, receiving any prenatal care, and consenting to testing for HIV. Organizations must have well-established policies and procedures for handling and maintaining HIV-related confidential information that conform to state and federal laws. **If a breach of confidentiality occurs, it can serve as grounds for legal action.**
- **Advance directives**—They provide the patient with an opportunity to direct her own care in advance. All health care facilities that receive federal money must follow guidelines set by the Federal Patient Self-Determination Act of 1991. This act requires institutions to make information accessible to all patients regarding options open to them for care if they become incapable of making their own decisions. Staff members should be aware of these options and should respect the patient's plans, values, and beliefs.
- **Right to medical care**—This means that each individual has a right to expect the best possible health care regardless of his or her disease state.
- **Consent and coercion issues**—These include the fact that each patient has the right to full information regarding treatment options available. Decisions made by HIV-positive patients about their care should be with the full knowledge of the potential benefits, risks, indications, and side effects for both her and her unborn or newborn baby. Threat, coercion, and incomplete information have no place in patient care. Health care professionals have the opportunity and responsibility to help the woman to understand options for and implications of treatment.

Patient Education

The HIV-positive woman, in labor, might not be able to fully concentrate on complex or lengthy explanations; therefore, effective patient education during this period can be difficult. In addition to information related to the labor and delivery process, the following should be presented in a thorough, but concise, manner.
- Risks and benefits of drug therapy
- Contraindications to breastfeeding
- Immediate care of the newborn
- Immediate care of the mother after delivery

As long as the mother and baby are stable, the primary focus in the immediate post-partum period should be on the promotion of bonding. Extensive information concerning self-care, baby care, contraception, lifestyle, nutrition, and transmission of HIV should be covered later.

Universal Precautions Recommended by the CDC

Because most people with blood-borne viral infection (HIV, HBV) do not have symptoms, nor can they be visibly recognized as being infected, Standard Precautions are designed to care for **all** persons (patients, clients, staff) regardless of whether or not they are infected.

Standard precautions should be used by *all* health care workers in *all* situations involving the care of patients or contact with the environment.

This approach was recommended by the CDC in 1996 for isolation precaution in hospitals. **Standard precautions recommend that you consider all patients as potentially infected with HIV, hepatitis B virus, or other blood-borne pathogens.** These precautions are standards of practice for all health care personnel and must be used with every patient. In addition, *hepatitis B vaccine is recommended as an important adjunct to universal precautions for all health care workers who are exposed to blood.*[51,52]

Nursing, medical, and housekeeping personnel on an obstetrics unit are exposed on a daily basis to a variety of body fluids. The following precautions should be followed rigorously to minimize the risk of exposure to blood and body fluids of all patients.
- Universal precautions apply to blood and other body fluids containing visible blood.
- Universal precautions apply to semen, vaginal secretions, tissue, cerebrospinal fluid, synovial fluid, pleural fluid, peritoneal fluid, and amniotic fluid.
- Universal precautions do *not* apply to feces, nasal secretions, sputum, sweat, tears, urine, and vomitus, unless they contain visible blood. The risk of transmission of HIV and hepatitis B virus from these fluids and materials is extremely low.
- Although universal precautions do not apply to human breast milk, gloves may be worn in situations in which exposures to breast milk might be frequent, such as with breast milk banking.
- Use protective barriers such as gloves, gowns, masks, and protective eyewear to reduce the risk of exposure of skin or mucous membranes to these fluids. The type of barrier should be appropriate for the procedure and type of exposure anticipated.
- Be careful when using needles, scalpels, and other sharp instruments. Use caution when handling or cleaning sharp instruments. Do not recap, bend, or break needles after use. In addition, do not recap Vacutainer devices. Dispose of used syringes immediately after use in a designated waste container designed for sharp hazardous waste materials. These special containers should be readily accessible to the staff to prevent accidental punctures during transport. They should be available in every patient room, examination room, treatment room, and delivery area. They should be emptied often to prevent accidental sticks when trying to push needles into an overflowing container.
- Immediately and thoroughly wash hands and other skin surfaces that are contaminated.
- Wear gloves during phlebotomy. Gloves should be made of latex or vinyl. Never wash or disinfect surgical or examination gloves for reuse.

Additional considerations include the following:
- Wear vinyl or latex gloves when contact with blood, amniotic fluid, mucous membranes, broken skin, or other body fluids is anticipated. To reduce the chance of exposure caused by tears or imperfections in the gloves, some institutions recommend double gloving when exposure to these substances will be prolonged or intense. Examples of intense

exposure include surgery, delivery, episiotomy repair, and placement of internal monitoring devices. Gloves should also be worn when changing dressings, underpads, perineal pads, and diapers and when giving perineal care.

- Remove gloves and wash hands immediately after giving care to one patient and before giving care to another patient. A single pair of gloves should not be repeatedly used because potential defects could render the gloves useless as a protective barrier.
- Always wear protective coverings such as gloves, impervious gowns/aprons, masks, and eye/face shields when doing invasive procedures that can contaminate you. This includes births (both vaginal and cesarean) and cleaning procedures that can cause splashing of blood and body fluids.
- Use protective eyeglasses or a face shield during any procedure that could result in contamination of the eyes. Providing goggles for employees is the responsibility of the employing institution.
- Refrain from all direct patient contact and from handling potentially contaminated equipment if you have exudative lesions, weeping dermatitis, or breaks in the skin that cannot be adequately covered.
- Wear gloves when inserting or discontinuing an IV catheter.
- Remove a glove torn by a needlestick or other injury and cleanse the area immediately. Report all accidents and follow institutional protocol.
- Place all specimens of blood and body fluids in containers with secure lids or sealed plastic bags to prevent leaking during transport. Care should be taken when collecting each specimen to prevent contamination of the outside of the container and the laboratory form.
- Blood, body fluids, soiled linen, and other potentially contaminated articles from all patients should be handled according to the infection control measures recommended by your institution.
- If you are pregnant, there are no special guidelines to follow. You should use the same universal precautions for patient care as other staff members.

Conclusion

HIV infection continues to rise in women of childbearing age with many learning of their HIV status when they become pregnant. Recent advances in both antiretroviral and obstetric interventions can aid in reducing perinatal transmission; this involves comprehensive planning of care for the woman who is planning on becoming pregnant or who is already pregnant. Health care providers can have a major positive influence on these women and their ability to access and maintain care.

Resources for Current HIV Information

AIDS Education Global Information System (AGEiS)
A comprehensive website of HIV information and resources.
www.aegis.com

AIDS Treatment Information Service (ATIS)
Provides all the Public Health Service treatment guidelines and up-to-date information.
New data is reviewed by the Perinatal HIV Guidelines Working Group and regular updates
    to the guidelines are made.
www.hivatis.org
Phone: 800-HIV-0440

Association of Nurses in AIDS Care (ANAC)
Professional association that provides information and advises members about clinical and
    policy issues related to nursing and HIV care.
www.anacnet.org
Phone: 800-260-6780

The Body
A comprehensive website of HIV information and resources.
www.thebody.com

Centers for Disease Control and Prevention National Prevention Information Network
Offers up-to-date epidemiologic information, daily updates on HIV/AIDS, and patient-
oriented information.
www.cdcnpin.org

HIV Medication Guide
A website providing drug information.
www.hivmedicationguide.com

International Association of Physicians in AIDS Care (IAPAC)
This organization provides a website with policy information about ongoing efforts to
expand access to health care services and lifesaving drugs and technologies.
www.iapac.org
Phone: 312-795-4930

Important Phone Numbers
AIDS Clinical Trials Information Services (ACTIS): 800-874-2572
CDC National Prevention Information Network: 800-458-5231
HIV/AIDS Treatment Information Service (ATIS): 800-448-0440
National AIDS Hotline: 800-342-2437
STD Hotline: 800-227-8922

PRACTICE/REVIEW QUESTIONS
After reviewing this module, answer the following questions.

1. What three parameters does the CDC use in its definition of AIDS?

   a. _____

   b. _____

   c. _____

2. What is the difference between AIDS and HIV infection?

   _____

   _____

   _____

3. State five ways in which HIV can be transmitted.

   a. _____

   b. _____

   c. _____

   d. _____

   e. _____

4. The standard algorithm for HIV testing consists of which two tests?

   a. _____

   b. _____

5. Having a sexually transmitted disease increases a person's chance of getting HIV infection.

   a. True

   b. False

6. Give two reasons why HIV in pregnant women can go undetected.

   a. _____

   b. _____

7. According to the PACTG 076 study, the rate of HIV transmission from an infected mother to her infant without ZDV treatment is estimated to be _____%. The rate of HIV transmission from an infected mother to her infant with ZDV treatment is estimated to be _____%.

8. What is meant by the *window period?*

   _____

   _____

9. A negative HIV antibody testing may need to be repeated in 3 to 6 months after a high-risk exposure.

   a. True

   b. False

10. State three ways in which newborns can acquire HIV from their mothers.

    a. _____

    b. _____

    c. _____

11. Breastfeeding should be encouraged for all women in the United States.

    a. True

    b. False

12. What is the primary means of postpartum vertical transmission of HIV?

_____

13. What is the World Health Organization position on breastfeeding and HIV infection?

_____

_____

14. What does practicing "standard precautions" as recommended by the CDC mean?

_____

_____

15. What are five characteristics or factors in a woman's history that increase her risk for contracting HIV?

a. _____

b. _____

c. _____

d. _____

e. _____

16. Which body fluid has the highest concentration of the human immunodeficiency virus?

_____

17. The concept of universal precautions presumes that

_____.

18. List those body fluids to which universal precautions apply. _____

_____

_____

_____

19. Regarding universal precautions:

a. When will you wear gloves? _____

_____

b. How often should gloves be changed? _____

_____

c. What rule will guide you in handwashing? _____

_____

d. When should protective coverings such as gloves, impervious gowns/aprons, masks, and eye/face shields be used? _____

_____

e. How should one dispose of used needles? _____

_____

f. How should specimens of blood and body fluids be handled? _____

_____

g. What specimens require special infection warning labels? _____

_____

20. Pregnant health care workers are at greater risk of contracting HIV infection than nonpregnant health care workers.

a. True

b. False

21. The CDC recommends routine HIV antibody testing of all health care workers.

a. True

b. False

22. Explain why invasive procedures on the fetus during labor should be avoided if possible.

_____

_____

23. List six steps you need to take in caring for the delivering woman who has HIV.

a. _____

b. _____

c. _____

d. _____

e. _____

f. _____

24. List six steps you should take while caring for the newly delivered baby that can reduce the risk of HIV transmission to the newborn.

a. _____

b. _____

c. _____

d. _____

e. _____

f. _____

25. Isolation is not necessary for the HIV-infected mother or mother with AIDS.

a. True

b. False

PRACTICE/REVIEW ANSWER KEY

1. a. Laboratory evidence of infection, plus
    b. Laboratory evidence of severe immunosuppression, and/or
    c. One or more of the 26 identified clinical conditions for AIDS

2. HIV infection occurs when an individual is infected with the human immunodeficiency virus. This individual has no clinical signs or symptoms of the disease. *AIDS* is the term used to denote the disease stage when individuals develop a severely weakened immune system and opportunistic infections occur.

3. a. Intimate sexual contact (oral, anal, or vaginal) with someone infected with HIV
    b. Sharing of drug needles and syringes with an infected person
    c. Receipt of a blood transfusion that contains HIV
    d. Inadvertent contamination of either mucous membranes or breaks in the skin with the blood or bodily fluids of an infected person
    e. Vertical transmission from a mother who transfers the virus to the fetus during the perinatal period

4. a. Enzyme immunosorbent assay (EIA)
    b. Western blot

5. a. True

6. a. Testing too soon, before the antibodies develop, results in a false-negative test.
    b. Some signs and symptoms of pregnancy (e.g., anemia, fatigue, dyspnea) are similar to symptoms of progressing HIV infection and AIDS and can mask or delay the diagnosis.

7. a. 25.5
    b. 8.3

8. The "window period" is the period between actual infection with the virus through the time when enough antibodies are produced by the body to cause a positive HIV test result.

9. a. True

10. a. Vertical transmission during pregnancy
    b. Through contact with infected blood and bodily fluids during delivery
    c. Breastfeeding

11. b. False

12. Breastfeeding

13. Women at risk for HIV infection should feed their babies infant formula if it is easily accessible. In areas where accessibility of formula is a problem, it is recommended that women, even those at risk for HIV infection, breastfeed their infants.

14. All health care workers should use precautions when dealing with blood and body fluids on all patients. All patients should be considered as potentially infected with HIV, hepatitis B virus, or other blood-borne pathogens.

15. Any five of the following:

    a. Is an IV drug user
    b. Has had multiple sexual partners
    c. Has had sexual partners who are infected or at risk for infection because they are hemophiliacs, bisexual, or IV users, or they have had multiple sexual partners
    d. Had a blood transfusion received before blood was being screened but after HIV infection occurred in the United States
    e. Had or has multiple STIs
    f. Currently living in or born in communities or countries where there is a known or suspected high prevalence of HIV infection

16. Blood

17. All patients are considered potentially infected with a blood-borne pathogen such as HIV or hepatitis B virus. No distinction is made among patients as needing precautionary care by the health care worker.

18. Blood and other body fluids containing visible blood, semen, vaginal secretions, tissues, cerebrospinal fluid, synovial fluid, pleural fluid, peritoneal fluid, pericardial fluid, or amniotic fluid

19. a. Wear gloves when contact with blood, amniotic fluids, mucous membranes, broken skin, or other body fluids is anticipated or when giving baths if your hands are cut, are chapped, or have abrasions.
    b. Gloves should be changed after giving care to one patient and before providing care to another. A single pair of gloves should *not* be used repeatedly in giving care to a single patient because defects can occur.
    c. Handwashing occurs after gloves are removed and after care is rendered to each patient.
    d. Protective coverings should be used when carrying out or assisting with invasive procedures that might contaminate an individual with droplets or splashing of body fluids or tissue.
    e. Never recap, bend, or break needles. Dispose of needles immediately in a designated container. Keep needle disposal containers in each patient's room. Avoid overfilled containers. Also, do not recap Vacutainer devices. Either remove the needles with a hemostat or dispose of the unit according to your institution's protocol.
    f. Place specimens in containers with secure lids or sealed plastic bags to prevent leaking during transport. Avoid contaminating the outside of the container.

g. None. Blood and body fluids from all patients should be considered infective.

20. b. False

21. b. False

22. Some infants can be infected with HIV by inoculation during an invasive procedure.

23. a. Follow universal precautions to protect yourself from splatter or contact with body fluids.
    b. Maintain patient hygiene carefully.
    c. Promote maternal–infant bonding by all possible means as you would in any birthing situation.
    d. Handle blood– and body fluid–stained linen as you would for any infection control measure.
    e. Follow institutional recommended sterilization, disinfection, or housekeeping guidelines.
    f. Alert nursery staff to expect the newborn and of the HIV infection status of the mother.

24. a. Assign one nurse to attend to the newborn after delivery.
    b. Dry the infant immediately after the delivery to remove all maternal blood and amniotic fluid.
    c. Gently remove excess fluid and blood from the nares and oropharynx.
    d. Aspirate stomach contents using a bulb syringe, mucus extractor, or meconium aspirator with wall suction on a low setting.
    e. Delay administration of vitamin K until after the infant is bathed.
    f. Bathe the newborn early and thoroughly with a mild, nonmedicated soap under radiant heat as soon as the infant is stable.

25. a. True

REFERENCES

1. UNAIDS. (2006, December). *AIDS epidemic update: December 2006* [On-line]. Available at: www.unaids.org/en/hiv_data/epi2006.
2. Centers for Disease Control and Prevention. (2005). *HIV/AIDS surveillance report, Vol. 17.* Available at: www.cdc.gov/hiv/topics/surveillance/resources/reports.
3. National Institute of Allergy and Infectious Disease. (2006). *HIV infection in women.* Available at: www.niaid.nih.gov/factsheets/womenhiv.htm.
4. Centers for Disease Control and Prevention. (2006). Revised recommendations for HIV testing of adults, adolescents, and pregnant women in health-care setting. *Morbidity and Mortality Weekly Report, 55*(RR14), 1–17 [On-line]. Available at: www.cdc.gov/mmwr/preview/mmwrhtml.
5. Centers for Disease Control and Prevention. (2001). Revised recommendations for HIV screening of pregnant women. *Morbidity and Mortality Weekly Report, 50*(RR19), 59–86. Available at: www.cdc.gov/mmwr/preview/mmwrhtml.
6. AIDS Education and Training Centers. (2006). *Clinical manual for management of the HIV-infected adult. Reducing maternal-infant HIV transmission.* Available at: www.aids-ed.org.
7. Minkoff, H. (1994). Human immunodeficiency virus. In Resnick, R. & Creasy, R. K. (Eds.), *Maternal-fetal medicine principles and practice* (3rd ed., Rev., pp. 1310–1312). Philadelphia: WB Saunders.
8. Centers for Disease Control and Prevention. (1999, January). *CDC statement in response to presentation on origin of HIV-1 at 6th conference on retroviruses and opportunistic infections* [On-line]. Available at: www.cdcnpin.org/hiv/faq/virus.htm.
9. Centers for Disease Control and Prevention. (1998). *Human immunodeficiency virus type 2* [On-line]. Available at: www.cdc.gov/hiv/pubs/facts/hiv2.htm.
10. Watts, D. H. (2002). Management of human immunodeficiency virus infection in pregnancy. *New England Journal of Medicine, 346*(24), 1879–1891.
11. Green, W. (1991). The molecular biology of the human immunodeficiency virus type-1 infection. *New England Journal of Medicine, 324*(5), 308–317.
12. Centers for Disease Control and Prevention. (1998). Report of the NIH panel to define principles of therapy of HIV infection. *Morbidity and Mortality Weekly Report, 47*(RR-5), 1–41. Available at: www.epo.cdc.gov/wonder/prevguid/.
13. Enger, C., Graham, N., Peng, Y., Chmiel, J. S., Kingsley, L. A., Detels, R., & Munoz, A. (1996). Survival from early, intermediate, and late stages of HIV infection. *Journal of the American Medical Association, 275*, 1329–1334.
14. Haynes, B., Panteleo, G., & Fauci, A. (1996). Toward an understanding of the correlates of protective immunity to HIV infection. *Science, 271*, 324–328.
15. Centers for Disease Control and Prevention. (1997). *Gateway to AIDS knowledge: Accuracy of tests.* Available at: http://hivinsite.ucsf.edu/topics/testing/2098.3075.html.
16. Centers for Disease Control and Prevention. (1998). *Frequently asked questions about HIV and AIDS—HIV testing* [On-line]. Available at: www.cdcnpin.org/hiv/faq.
17. Centers for Disease Control and Prevention National AIDS Clearinghouse. (1997). *Guide to information and resources on HIV testing.* Atlanta: Author.
18. Lachat, M., Scott, C., & Relf, M. (2006). *HIV and pregnancy: Consideration for nursing practice. American Journal of Maternal and Child Nursing, 31*(4), 233–240.
19. Centers for Disease Control and Prevention. (1992). 1993 revised classification system for HIV infection and expanded surveillance case definition for AIDS among adolescents and adults. *Morbidity and Mortality Weekly Report, 41*(RR-17), 1–11.
20. COHIS. (2000, May). *AIDS/HIV opportunistic infections* [On-line]. Available at: www.medvalet.com/index.html.
21. Centers for Disease Control and Prevention. (1987). Recommendations for prevention of HIV transmission in health-care settings. *Morbidity and Mortality Weekly Report, 36*(SU02), 1–19.
22. Mastro, T., & de Vinceni, I. (1996). Probabilities of sexual HIV-1 transmission. *AIDS, 10*(Suppl. A), S75–S82.
23. Vittinghoff, E., Douglas, J., Judson, F., McKirnan, D., MacQueen, K., & Buchbinder, S. P. (1999). Per-contact risk of human immunodeficiency virus transmission between male sexual partners. *American Journal of Epidemiology, 150*(3), 306–311.
24. Anderson, J. (Ed.). (2006). *A guide to the clinical care of women with HIV: 2005 edition* [On-line]. Available at: http://www.hab.hrsa.gov.

25. Kaplan, E., & Heimer, R. (1992). A model-based estimate of HIV infectivity via needle sharing. *Journal of Acquired Immune Deficiency Syndromes, 5,* 1116–1118.

26. Centers for Disease Control and Prevention. (2001). Public health service guidelines for the management of occupational exposures to HBV, HCV, HIV and recommendations for post-exposure prophylaxis. *Morbidity and Morality Weekly Report, 50*(RR-11), 1–42.

27. Chin, J. (1994). The growing impact of HIV/AIDS pandemic on children born to HIV-infected women. *Clinics in Perinatology, 21*(1), 111–114.

28. Barkowsky, W., Krasinski, K., Pollack, H., Hoover, W., Kaul, A., & Ilmet-Moore, T. (1992). Early diagnosis of human immunodeficiency virus infection in children less than 6 months of age: Comparison of polymerase chain reaction, culture, and plasma antigen captive techniques. *Journal of Infectious Diseases, 166*(3), 616–619.

29. Fowler, M., Simonds, R., & Roongpisuthipong, A. (2000). HIV/AIDS in infants, children, and adolescents: Update on perinatal transmission. *Pediatric Clinics of North America, 47*(1), 21–38.

30. Northwestern Territories HIV/AIDS. (2006). *Manual for healthcare professionals* [On-line]. Available at: www.hlthss.gov.nt.ca.

31. Mofenson, L., Lambert, J. S., Stiehm, E. R., Bethel, J., Meyer, W. A., 3rd, Whitehouse, J., Moye, J. Jr., Reichelderfer, P., Harris, D. R., Fowler, M. G., Mathieson, B. J., & Nemo, G. J. (1999). Risk factors for perinatal transmission of human immunodeficiency virus type 1 in women treated with zidovudine. Pediatric AIDS clinical trials study 185 team. *New England Journal of Medicine, 341*(6), 385–393.

32. Garcia, P., Kalish, L. A., Pitt, J., Minkoff, H., Quinn, T. C., Burchett, S. K., Kornegay, J., Jackson, B., Moye, J., Hanson, C., Zorrilla, C., & Lew, J. F. (1999). Maternal levels of plasma human immunodeficiency virus type 1 RNA and the risk of perinatal transmission. Women and Infants Transmission Study Group. *New England Journal of Medicine, 341*(6), 394–402.

33. Maternal viral load and vertical transmission of HIV-1: An important factor but not the only one: The European collaborative study. (1999). *AIDS, 13,* 1377–1385.

34. Mock, P., Shaffer, N., Bhadrakom, C., Siriwasin, W., Chotpitayasunondh, T., Chearskul, S., Young, N. L., Roongpisuthipong, A., Chinayon, P., Kalish, M. L., Parekh, B., & Mastro, T. D. (1999). Maternal viral load and timing of mother-to-child transmission. *AIDS, 13,* 407–414.

35. Shaffer, N., Roongpisuthipong, A., Siriwasin, W., Chotpitayasunondh, T., Chearskul, S., Young, N. L., Parekh, B., Mock, P. A., Bhadrakom, C., Chinayon, P., Kalish, M. L., Phillips, S. K., Granade, T. C., Subbarao, S., Weniger, B. G., & Mastro, T. D. (1999). Maternal virus load and perinatal human immunodeficiency virus subtype E transmission, Thailand. *Journal of Infectious Disease, 179,* 590–599.

36. Public Health Service Task Force. (2006, October). *Public Health Service Task Force recommendations for the use of antiretroviral drugs in pregnant HIV-1 infected women for maternal health and interventions to reduce perinatal HIV-1 transmission in the United States* [On-line]. Available at: http://hivatis.org/guidelines/perinatal/.

37. American College of Obstetricians and Gynecologist. (2000, May). *ACOG committee opinion: Scheduled cesarean delivery and the prevention of vertical transmission of HIV infection* [On-line]. Available at: www.acog.com/publications/committee.

38. Aidsinfo. (2006). Delivery options for HIV positive pregnant women. Available at: http://aidsinfo.nih.gov.

39. Saba, J. (1999, February). *Interim analysis of early efficacy of three short ZVD/3TC combination regimens to prevent mother-to-child transmissions of HIV-1: The PETRA trial* [6th Conference on Retroviruses and Opportunistic Infections]. Chicago.

40. Nduati, R., John, G., Mbori-Ngacha, D., Richardson, B., Overbaugh, J., Mwatha, A., Ndinya-Achola, J., Bwayo, J., Onyango, F. E., Hughes, J., & Kreiss, J. (2000). Effect of breastfeeding and formula feeding on transmission of HIV-1: A randomized clinical trial. *Journal of the American Medical Association, 283,* 1167–1174.

41. American College of Obstetricians and Gynecologist. (2000, July). *ACOG news release: ACOG issues guidelines on breastfeeding* [On-line]. Available at: www.acog.org/from_home/publications/press_releases/.

42. WHO, UNAIDS, & UNICEF. (1998). *Technical consultation on HIV and infant feedings, Geneva* [On-line]. Available at: www.unaids.org/publications/documents/mtct/meetrev.html.

43. The Linkages Project. (1998). *Frequently asked questions on breastfeeding and HIV/AIDS* [On-line]. Available at: http://linkagesproject.org/FAQ_Html/FAQ_HIV.htm.

44. De Cock, K. M., Zadi, F., Adjorlolo, G., Diallo, M. O., Sassan-Morokro, M., Ekpini, E., Sibailly, T., Doorly, R., Batter, V., Brattegaard, K., & Gayle, H. (1994). Retrospective study of maternal HIV-1 and HIV-2 infection and child survival in Abidjan, Cote d'Ivoire. *British Medical Journal, 308,* 441–443.

45. Moye, J., Jr., Rich, K. C., Kalish, L. A., Sheon, A. R., Diaz, C., Cooper, E. R., Pitt, J., & Handelsman, E. (1996). Natural history of somatic growth in infants born to women infected by human immunodeficiency virus: Women and infants transmission study group. *Journal of Pediatrics, 128*(58), 58–69.

46. Hanson, C. (1998). HIV and women and pregnancy: Effect of HIV infection on pregnancy outcome. *Immunology and Allergy Clinics of North America, 18*(2), 345–353.

47. Landers, D., Martinez de Tejada, B., & Coye, B. (1997). HIV disease in pregnancy. Immunology of HIV in pregnancy: The effect of each on the other. *Obstetrics and Gynecology Clinics, 24*(4), 821–831.

48. ATIS. (2006). *Guidelines for the use of antiretroviral agents in HIV-infected adults and adolescents* [On-line]. Available at: www.thebody.com/hivatis/.

49. Glaxo Wellcome Inc. (2000). *Antiretroviral pregnancy registry* [On-line]. Available at: www.glaxowellcome.com/preg_reg/antiretroviral.html.

50. The Working Group. (2000). *Guidelines for the use of antiretroviral agents in pediatric HIV infection* [On-line]. Available at: www.thebody.com/hivatis/pediatric/ped1.html.

51. Centers for Disease Control and Prevention. (1996 update). Perspectives in disease prevention and health promotion update: Universal precautions for prevention of transmission of human immunodeficiency virus, hepatitis B virus, and other bloodborne pathogens in health-care settings. *Morbidity and Mortality Weekly Report, 37*(24), 377–388.

52. Garner, J. S.; The Hospital Infection Control Practices Advisory Committee (HICPAC). (1996). Guideline for isolation precautions in hospitals. Infection control hospital epidemiology. *American Journal of Infection Control, 24*(1), 24–52. Available at: www.cdc.gov/ncidod/hip/isolat.htm.

MODULE

11

Hepatitis Infections

E. JEAN MARTIN ■ DONNA JEAN RUTH

A word to the reader:

This topic is extremely complex. Understanding the concepts presented might take several thoughtful readings. DO NOT become discouraged if on the first read through you feel a bit overwhelmed. This will probably be the experience for many. Regarding the diagnostic markers, keep relating the antigens to the schematic drawing of the virus. Try to see them in the context of being pieces of the virus. Appreciate that each antigen is capable of inducing a physiologic immune response in an individual, which gives rise to a unique antibody. The antigens and/or antibodies are referred to as serologic markers because most of them can be identified by laboratory analysis of an exposed individual's blood. Some readers might not feel the need to master the diagnostic interpretation of the serologic markers. Knowing the risk factors, clinical features, and implications for care in various settings may suffice. However, if your level of practice requires an interpretation of laboratory reports, you do need to understand the significance of serologic markers in the report or in the patient's history.

The sad truth is that this disease will be with us for a while, so it behooves health care professionals to stay informed.

Objectives

As you complete this module, you will learn:

1. The distinctions between major forms of viral hepatitis (hepatitis A, B, C, D, and E), that is, how to distinguish each form according to infecting organism, mode of transmission, diagnostic workup, and risks during pregnancy
2. To identify forms of viral hepatitis that can confer a carrier state
3. Immunization recommendations for hepatitis A viral infection, including implications for pregnant women
4. Important information about hepatitis C: epidemiology, pathophysiology, causes of the disease, risk factors, diagnosis, treatments, and implications for pregnant women
5. How hepatitis B antigens and antibodies are used in laboratory tests to identify individuals who are acutely infected, immune, or carriers
6. Facts about the course of hepatitis B disease, including the timing and sequence of serologic titers beginning with exposure
7. The epidemiology of the hepatitis B carrier state
8. Diagnostic markers for the carrier state
9. Transmission risks for the fetus and newborn when the pregnant woman has acute hepatitis B or is a carrier
10. To identify those women who are at high risk of being hepatitis B carriers
11. Clinical implications for mother and fetus during the antepartum period
12. About products for active and/or passive immunization: hepatitis B vaccines and hepatitis B immune globulin
13. Facts about hepatitis B vaccine and recommendations by the Centers for Disease Control and Prevention (CDC) for preexposure immunization

14. CDC recommendations for appropriate hepatitis B status screening in pregnant women
15. Recommendations for hepatitis B screening in women being admitted to the labor unit
16. Risk of hepatitis B transmission to health care personnel and precautions that medical and nursing personnel need to take while caring for the hepatitis B carrier woman in the perinatal setting
17. Nursing care of the mother and newborn during labor, during delivery, and postpartum
18. Treatments and precautions to use in reducing hepatitis B transmission to the newborn
19. Current breastfeeding recommendations for the hepatitis B-infected mother
20. CDC recommendations for immunization treatment of individuals needing preexposure or postexposure immunization for hepatitis A and hepatitis B

Key Terms

When you have completed this module, you should be able to recall the meaning of the following terms. You should also be able to use the terms when consulting with other health professionals. An understanding of the terms will be important in interpreting prenatal and neonatal laboratory results. The terms are defined in this module or in the glossary at the end of this book.

alanine aminotransferase (ALT)	inoculate
antibody	lochia
antigen	nosocomial infections
aspartate aminotransferase (AST)	plasma-derived vaccine
carrier	prevalence
Engerix-B (Engerix-B, Pediatric/Adolescent)	Recombivax HB (Recombivax HB, Pediatric)
Havrix	seronegative
hepatitis B immune globulin (HBIG)	seroprotective
hepatocellular carcinoma	serous exudates
horizontal transmission	serum
immune serum globulin (ISG)	Vaqta
immunization	vertical transmission

Hepatitis infection, its various forms, and how it can affect pregnancy outcomes is a very complex topic. Terms needed for a clear understanding of this module's content are defined here. You may want to refer to these definitions throughout this module until you become familiar with them.

Terms to Know

- **Antigen**—a substance that, when introduced in a host, is capable of inducing the production of antibodies. An antigen can be introduced into the host, or it can be formed within the body. Bacteria and viruses are examples of antigens.
- **Antibody**—protein substances developed by the body in response to the presence of an antigen. Antibodies are produced to inhibit or destroy the antigen and are a defense against foreign substances such as bacteria and viruses.
- **Carrier**—an individual who harbors a pathogen and is capable of transmitting a disease caused by this pathogen to another person. Often, carriers do not experience any significant illness and have no idea that they are capable of spreading the disease.
- **Plasma**—the fluid part of blood.
- **Serum**—that fluid part of blood that remains after clotting has occurred.
- **Inoculate**—to introduce a substance (the inoculum) into the body, which can produce a disease or an immunity to the disease, depending on the circumstances and the substance. The inoculate is sometimes a cultured substance.

Facts About the Major Hepatitis Infections

▶ **What is viral hepatitis?**

Viral hepatitis has the following characteristics:
- It is an infection that occurs in the liver.
- The clinical features in each type of viral hepatitis are similar and are uniquely derived from the consequences of liver cell injury.
- Jaundice, low-grade fever, abdominal pain, or "flulike" symptoms may or may not accompany hepatitis infection. Most people do not develop clinically apparent disease.
- It can exist as an acute or a chronic disease.
- Viral hepatitis is a major cause of death and morbidity in third-world countries.
- Infection can occur any time during pregnancy.
- Hepatitis A, B, and D viral infections can be prevented by immunization in most cases.
- Vaccines do not exist for hepatitis C or E.
- Hepatitis is a major public health problem.
- Chronic liver disease is the tenth leading cause of death among adults in the United States.

Viral hepatic diseases differ with regard to mode of transmission, diagnostic criteria, pathophysiology, infectivity states, and in disease outcome. Five major forms of hepatitis exist, all of which are caused by a virus or "viruslike" particle. They are:
- Hepatitis A virus (HAV), formerly known as "infectious hepatitis"
- Hepatitis B virus (HBV), formerly known as "serum hepatitis"
- Hepatitis C virus (HCV), formerly known as "non-A, non-B"
- Hepatitis D virus (HDV), known as "delta hepatitis"
- Hepatitis E virus (HEV)

> **NOTE:** *Other viral agents such as the herpes simplex virus (HSV), cytomegalovirus (CMV), and Epstein-Barr virus (EBV) can cause acute liver disease but are not included in this module.*

HAV and HEV initially enter the body by way of the gut, where they begin to multiply. HBV, HCV, and HDV enter the body via the bloodstream, eventually passing to the liver, where they replicate (reproduce). The body's immune response to any of these viruses residing in the liver is inflammation, thereby setting up the potential for either mild or severe liver damage.

With HBV infection, the liver is usually able to repair itself readily. However, with HCV infection, resolution of liver damage may not occur. Over many years, unresolved damage may lead to severe liver pathology. Therefore, the quality of life resulting from these two viral infections is usually very different.

Although this module is especially concerned with the impact of HBV on pregnant women and newborns, considerable content on HAV and HCV is included.

Hepatitis A, C, D, and E

Hepatitis A (HAV) Infection[1-4]

- In the United States, about one third of acute hepatitis cases are caused by HAV.
- In the United States, the incidence of acute HAV infection in pregnancy is approximately 1 per 1,000. Pregnant women at greatest risk are those who have recently traveled to or emigrated from developing nations such as Southeast Asia, Africa, Central America, Mexico, and the Middle East, where HAV infection is endemic.[5]
- This disease is spread through the fecal–oral route, usually by person-to-person contact (*horizontal transmission*) or ingestion of contaminated food or water.
- Outbreaks are common in winter and spring.
- The incubation period averages 28 days (15 to 50 days).
- Transmission by blood transfusion or injection is rare.

- Risk factors for HAV infection include personal contact with infected individuals (26%), employment in a day care center (14%), intravenous drug use (11%), travel to an area where HAV infection is prevalent (4%), and consumption of food or water contaminated with feces (3%).[2]
- Acute infection is diagnosed by the identification of antibody immunoglobulin (Ig)M anti-HAV in the individual's blood (serum). This is always present at the first sign of the disease and remains present for several months to a year.
- IgG anti-HAV develops during convalescence. This antibody persists and is responsible for the individual's subsequent immunity to HAV infection.
- There is no chronic carrier state that can transmit HAV to others after recovery from acute infection.
- HAV infection in pregnant women is generally no more severe than in nonpregnant women.
- There is no evidence that this viral infection is teratogenic in pregnancy.
- Pregnancy can be complicated by poor outcomes from this disease in vulnerable populations in third-world countries. Perinatal and maternal morbidity can be increased.
- Pregnant women exposed to HAV should be given human serum immunoglobulin containing antibodies to the virus (confers passive immunization).
- Hepatitis A vaccines contain formalin-inactivated virus and *are safe for use in pregnant women* (active immunization). Two vaccines, called Havrix and Vaqta, were released in 1995. They both require two doses. A single dose provides immunity for 1 year. A booster dose administered 6 to 12 months after the initial injection provides protection for approximately 15 years. A third vaccine TWINRIX is a combined hepatitis A and hepatitis B vaccine. Primary immunization requires three doses of this vaccine.

Immunization Recommendations

Current recommendations include routine hepatitis A vaccination of all children age 1 year or older in the United States. Vaccinations should be integrated into the routine childhood vaccination schedule. This represents a change from the previous recommendations, and in areas that did not have an existing hepatitis A vaccination program, catch-up vaccination of unvaccinated children age 2 to 18 years should be considered.[1]

Recommendations for vaccinating individuals in groups known to be at high risk for HAV infection remain a focus and are intended to further reduce hepatitis A in the United States. This list includes travelers to countries with high or intermediate infections incidence, men who have sex with men, users of injection and noninjection illicit drugs, persons with occupational risk exposure (e.g., persons who work with HAV infected primates or with HAV in a research laboratory setting), persons with clotting disorders, and persons with chronic liver disease.

Hepatitis C (HCV) Infection[4,6-8]

HCV infection is a major cause of acute and chronic hepatitis, both of which are asymptomatic in most individuals.

Epidemiology

Worldwide, it is estimated that 170 million people are infected (3% of the world's population), many of whom have no idea they are infected. In some endemic regions of the world (e.g., Egypt), prevalence rates range from 10% to 30%. The CDC reports a seroprevalence rate in the United States of 4 million chronically infected Americans.[7] The incidence rate in the United States is 200,000 new infections each year; about 30% of these are symptomatic. Approximately 8,000 to 10,000 deaths from chronic HCV infection occur yearly.[7]

Pregnancy

The prevalence of prenatal infection varies with the population studied. Risk factors include intravenous drug use, sexually transmitted disease, increased age and parity, multiple sex partners, and sex partners who used intravenous drugs.[4] Reported incidence ranges from 5% at a public clinic to 1.5% in private patients. The concern is that the hepatitis C infection will be transmitted vertically (pregnant mother to infant). The rate of transmission varies between 3%

and 6%.[4] However, the risk of transmission seems to be greatest if the mother is co-infected with HIV. Investigators find significantly higher rates of transmission (14% to 17%) in women coinfected with HIV. This is thought to be due to higher maternal hepatitis C viremia.[7]

NOTE: Maternal antibodies to HCV (anti-HCV) are not protective!

Perinatal outcomes appear to be no different than among mothers who do not have the infection. Universal screening is not recommended.

Breastfeeding

The average rate of HCV infection in both bottle-fed and breastfed infants is 5%. It appears that breastfeeding does not appreciably increase transmission risk to the newborn.[7,8]

Transmission

Transmission modes appear to be the same as for HBV infections, that is, parenteral; contact with infected blood (as in intravenous drug blood use); and use of contaminated needles, razors, tattoo equipment, acupuncture needles, and shared straw use among cocaine users. It is not nearly as easily spread through sexual contact as is HBV infection. Health care workers are at risk through needlesticks and other exposures.

Blood transfusion was a significant source of HCV transmission before 1992, at which time routine screening of blood donors was initiated. Blood transfusion from an anti–HCV-positive donor results in very high infectivity for recipients (more than 80%). Since the advent of rigorous screening procedures, transfusion transmission in the United States is very low. However, the risk is not 0%.

Infection

There are 10 or more types and numerous subtypes of this virus, some of which appear uniquely in different geographic regions of the world. Most infected individuals are not symptomatic, and most do not know they are infected. Symptoms are the same as with HBV infection. Sequelae are very serious in that 75% to 85% of infected persons develop chronic infection and a very high percentage (about 70%) develop chronic liver disease, eventually leading to the need for transplantation or to death. The likelihood of developing chronic HCV infection is a function of the following:

- Viral genotype (certain types are correlated with high chronicity rates)
- Mode of acquisition (e.g., a transfusion with HCV-contaminated blood is associated with a greater risk of chronic infection versus a lower risk with a small amount of inoculate involved in illicit drug use)
- Host immune response (the more vigorous the antibody and T-cell responses to severe acute infections, the more likely there will be a spontaneous resolution of the infection)[6]

Serologic Markers

Infection with HCV results in the presence of unique serologic markers to indicate the virus presence. Two major markers are actual viral material called HCV RNA and the antibody anti-HCV, produced by the host immunologic response. *Research indicates that a large percentage of anti–HCV-positive individuals do not clear HCV RNA; in other words, they are HCV RNA positive and can transmit the infection to others.*

Diagnosis

Diagnosis is made by detecting the antibody to hepatitis C through enzyme immunoassay (EIA). All positive EIA results are verified with a supplemental assay called the recombinant immunoblot assay (RIBA). Sensitivity is 97% or greater.[7] *This test does not distinguish between acute, chronic, or resolved infection.*

Another diagnostic test can be done to quantify or qualify the amount of HCV RNA by using gene amplification techniques (e.g., polymerase chain reaction [PCR]). The PCR process takes a very small amount of viral or bacterial content not detectable in usual laboratory analysis and multiplies the content to detectable levels. HCV RNA analysis measures a part of the hepatitis C virus.

The gold standard in diagnostic workup for individuals with HCV infection is a liver biopsy, especially when treatment is being considered for a person with suspected chronic hepatitis C.

Recommendations for routine testing for HCV are shown in Display 11.1. Postexposure follow-up recommendations are given in Display 11.2.

DISPLAY 11.1 TESTING FOR HEPATITIS C VIRUS

PERSONS WHO SHOULD BE TESTED ROUTINELY FOR HEPATITIS C VIRUS (HCV) INFECTION BASED ON THEIR RISK FOR INFECTION

- Persons who ever injected illegal drugs, including those who injected once or a few times many years ago and do not consider themselves drug users
- Persons with selected medical conditions, including the following:
  - Persons who received clotting factor concentrates produced before 1987
  - Persons who were ever on chronic (long-term) hemodialysis
  - Persons with persistently abnormal alanine aminotransferase levels
- Prior recipients of transfusions or organ transplants, including the following:
  - Persons who were notified that they received blood from a donor who later tested positive for HCV infection
  - Persons who received a transfusion of blood or blood components before July 1992
  - Persons who received an organ transplant before July 1992

PERSONS WHO SHOULD BE TESTED ROUTINELY FOR HCV INFECTION BASED ON A RECOGNIZED EXPOSURE

- Health care, emergency medical, and public safety workers after needlesticks, sharps, or mucosal exposures to HCV-positive blood
- Children born to HCV-positive women

PERSONS FOR WHOM ROUTINE HCV TESTING IS NOT RECOMMENDED

- Health care, emergency medical, and public safety workers
- Pregnant women
- Household (nonsexual) contacts of HCV-positive persons
- The general population

Reprinted with permission from Centers for Disease Control and Prevention (1998). Recommendations for prevention and control of hepatitis C virus (HCV) infection and HCV-related chronic disease. *MMWR Morbidity and Mortality Weekly Report, 47*(RR-19), 21, 24.

DISPLAY 11.2 POSTEXPOSURE FOLLOW-UP

POSTEXPOSURE FOLLOW-UP OF HEALTH CARE, EMERGENCY MEDICAL, AND PUBLIC SAFETY WORKERS FOR HEPATITIS C VIRUS (HCV) INFECTION

- For the source, baseline testing for anti-HCV
- For the person exposed to an HCV-positive source, baseline and follow-up testing, including the following:
  - Baseline testing for anti-HCV and ALT activity
  - Follow-up testing for anti-HCV (e.g., at 4 to 6 months) and ALT activity (if earlier diagnosis of HCV infection is desired, testing for HCV RNA may be performed at 4 to 6 weeks.)
- Confirmation by supplemental anti-HCV testing of all anti-HCV results reported as positive by enzyme immunoassay

Reprinted with permission from Centers for Disease Control and Prevention (1998). Recommendations for prevention and control of hepatitis C virus (HCV) infection and HCV-related chronic disease. *MMWR Morbidity and Mortality Weekly Report, 47*(RR-19), 24.

Treatment

Current treatments with interferon–ribavirin combinations are having encouraging success. However, therapies are fairly toxic and accompanied by severe side effects. "Cure" is currently defined as a loss of detectable HCV RNA in serum using a sensitive PCR assay at least 6 months after cessation of therapy.

Currently, there are insufficient data to recommend treatment of acute HCV infection. HCV-positive persons should be referred for ongoing evaluation to detect the presence or development of chronic disease and treatment according to current practice guidelines. Counseling is needed to prevent further liver damage. Counseling for reducing the risks of HCV transmission to others is critical.[7]

Immunization

No vaccine exists for hepatitis C. Development of a vaccine is complicated by the fact that antibodies to HCV are not protective against the infection. In addition, the virus has a rapid mutation rate, especially when under efforts to eradicate it (i.e., during treatment).

Hepatitis D (HDV) Infection (Delta Hepatitis)[2,4]

The virus was named "delta" virus, hence hepatitis D. This infection is caused by a defective virus that can replicate and cause infection only in the presence of an active HBV infection; therefore, it never outlasts HBV infection. HDV infection occurs worldwide, but is most common in nations bordering the Mediterranean Sea and is less common in the United States. It exists as an acute coinfection acquired simultaneously with hepatitis B, or it can be a superinfection in a chronic hepatitis B carrier and can produce more severe disease.

HDV is diagnosed in the following ways:
- By detecting the antibody to the delta virus antigen (anti-HDV) in blood
- By liver biopsy, which identifies the delta antigen
- By identifying the IgM antibody to the hepatitis D virus in blood

HDV is transmitted by exposure to blood and blood products and by sexual contact (similar to HBV transmission). It is most prevalent in intravenous drug users, patients with hemophilia, and patients who have received multiple blood transfusions. It is highly infectious and associated with serious illness.

Hepatitis B vaccination usually protects against hepatitis D. Neonatal transmission is rare because neonatal hepatitis B vaccination prevents hepatitis D.[4] There is no cure for or prevention of HDV infection in hepatitis B carriers.

Hepatitis E (HEV) Infection[2,4,5]

Hepatitis E is an enteric disease associated with large epidemics from sewage-contaminated food and water. It is widespread in developing countries, such as India, Southeast Asia, Africa, and South America. The disease is characterized by acute infection similar to that of hepatitis A and affects primarily persons of childbearing age (ages 15 to 40). Hepatitis E does not exist as a chronic infection. The development of antibodies to the hepatitis E antigen (IgG anti-HEV) confers immunity.

Although the disease is usually characterized by a mild illness, there is a high mortality rate for fulminant hepatic failure in pregnant women. The reason for this is unknown. Infection in the third trimester of pregnancy is associated with an increased incidence of fetal complications. Neonates die from HEV infection much more than from any other type of viral hepatitis. Vertical transmission of HEV has been reported.[5]

Acute infection can be diagnosed by a positive serum test for IgM anti-HEV antibody, but this test is not available in most laboratories, especially in developing countries. Diagnosis is made by the signs and symptoms of liver disease, excluding other causes such as HAV, HBV, cytomegalovirus, and Epstein-Barr virus.

Hepatitis B (HBV) Infection

Hepatitis B infection is caused by the hepatitis B virus. It is found in liver cells (hepatocytes), where it replicates (reproduces itself). The virus also travels to the bloodstream. Infection often goes unrecognized.

Prevalence[9,10]

More than 1.25 million people are chronically infected with HBV in the United States.[9] In 2005, a total of 5,494 acute, symptomatic cases were reported; the overall incidence of acute hepatitis

B was 1.8/100,000. This was the lowest ever recorded and represented an 80% decline since the national strategy to eliminate HVB transmission was implemented in 1991.[10] Some differences in prevalence still remain with regard to region, age, gender, and racial/ethnic groups. Rates remain the highest in non-Hispanic blacks with the rate of 2.9/100,00 being twice the rate of any other racial or ethnic group.[10] The long-term consequences of hepatitis B may include cirrhosis of the liver, liver cancer, liver failure, and death.

Clinical Features[9]

Clinical features of HBV infection include the following:
- The virus has been found in body fluids such as saliva, menstrual, and vaginal discharge, semen, colostrum, breast milk, and serous exudates. These fluids have been implicated as vehicles of infection transmission.[9]
- The incubation period ranges from 14 to 180 days.
- Most patients have no symptoms.
- One third of patients with symptoms have jaundice (evident in the skin and eyes).
- Some individuals experience fatigue, lassitude, loss of appetite, nausea, vomiting, and/or abdominal pain.
- Occasionally, joint pain (arthralgia), and a rash can be present.
- The symptoms are often misdiagnosed as "the flu," especially if no jaundice is present.
- Liver enzymes, **alanine aminotransferase** (ALT) and **aspartate aminotransferase** (AST), are elevated (e.g., above 1,000 U/mL in the acute phase of viral hepatitis).
- Acute infection generally runs its course over a 3- to 4-week period, but symptoms can remain for as long as 6 months.
- For pregnant women, the disease generally does not assume any greater virulence, but there are serious implications if the virus is transmitted to the newborn.
- In vulnerable populations, such as third-world countries, fulminant hepatitis B results in increased perinatal and maternal mortality.
- When individuals develop the disease whether symptomatic or not, there are only two possible outcomes: they experience complete resolution or they might retain the virus in their bodies in a chronic state. Individuals who retain the virus in a chronic state are at risk for two potential situations:
  1. Becoming a chronic active hepatitis carrier who can transmit the disease to others under certain conditions.
  2. They are at risk for developing cirrhosis and/or *hepatocellular carcinoma* (cancer of the liver).

> Mothers who develop the disease (symptomatic or not) might recover completely, or they might retain the virus in their bodies in a chronic state. These hepatitis B carriers can transmit the disease to others, including the newborn.

Diagnosis

▶ What laboratory tests are used to diagnose hepatitis B active disease or carrier status?

Identifying the antigens and antibodies for HBV that are found in the blood of infected individuals confirms that the individual is either:
- In the active disease state

OR
- A carrier

OR
- Immune

HBV contains three antigens. These antigens are protein particles that derive from the virus, as shown in Figure 11.1. When found in blood, they are called *serologic markers*. As you study the following antigen names and characteristics, refer to Figure 11.1 to identify from where they derive.

Hepatitis B Virus

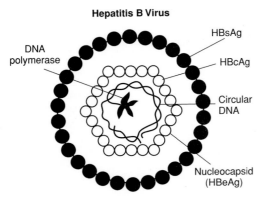

FIGURE 11.1 Hepatitis B virus and serologic markers. (Source unknown)

HBV Antigen Serologic Markers

Hepatitis B surface antigen (**HBsAg**)—protein coat
Hepatitis B core antigen (**HBcAg**)—core of the virus
Hepatitis B e antigen (**HBeAg**)—part of the core

> Study these abbreviations so that you know exactly what each stands for as you read on.

Hepatitis B Antigens

Hepatitis B Surface Antigen (HBsAg)

- Is the protein coat of the virus
- Is detectable in large quantities in serum because more HBsAg is produced than is needed to cover the core
- Can be present even in the absence of any symptoms of the disease
- Has several subtypes detectable only in research laboratories
- Is associated with chronic hepatitis B and denotes a carrier state when its presence persists in blood

> *Laboratory studies of blood serum can identify the presence of HBsAg in infected persons. This is one of the earliest indications of HBV infection.*

> *The persistent presence of HBsAg in serum is associated with chronic hepatitis B.*

Hepatitis B Core Antigen (HBcAg)

- Comes from the center, or core, of the virus
- Is not found in the blood, and therefore, no commercial test is available to detect this antigen in infected persons; is located in the nuclei of liver cells (hepatocytes)
- Can be detected by a liver biopsy

> HBcAg cannot be found in the blood serum of infected persons.

Hepatitis B e Antigen (HBeAg)

- Is found only in association with the surface antigen HBsAg in the blood
- Evidence suggests that it is derived from the core antigen or is a breakdown product of the core antigen
- Its presence is correlated with high titers of hepatitis B viral DNA and an increased infectivity state

> *Laboratory studies of blood serum can identify the presence of HBeAg in infected persons.*

> *HBeAg is found in serum during the early part of the acute phase of the infection and then disappears. This antigen is never found alone. It always occurs after HBsAg is present and the infection state has begun.*

If a pregnant woman has HBsAg in her blood at the time of birth, she has HBV infection. She may not have symptoms. If the mother is positive for only HBsAg, the rate of transmission to the baby who is not immunized is about 10% to 20%.[5]

If a pregnant woman has both HBsAg and HBeAg at the time of birthing, the risk of perinatal transmission of HBV to her infant, if not immunized, is approximately 90%.[5,9]

> MORE THAN 90% OF WOMEN FOUND TO BE HBsAg POSITIVE ON ROUTINE SCREENING WILL BE HEPATITIS B CARRIERS.[11]

Antigen levels tend to be higher in early and midstages of the disease process and then fall to levels so low that they cannot be detected by laboratory examination. During the recovery phase of HBV infection, HBsAg is cleared and not detectable.

Hepatitis B Antibodies

Most individuals infected with HBV are capable of producing antibodies against the viral antigens. Because three **antigens** have been identified, it is not surprising to learn that there are three **antibodies** that the human body can produce against the antigens. These antibodies also can be detected in blood and are referred to as *serologic markers.*

Combinations of antigen and antibodies tell us whether an individual is:
• Infectious (in an active disease state)

OR
• A carrier

OR
• Immune

HBV Antibody Serologic Markers

Antibody to HBsAg (**anti-HBs**)
Antibody to HBcAg (**anti-HBc**)
Antibody to HBeAg (**anti-HBe**)

> Study these abbreviations so that you know exactly what each stands for as you read on.

Antibody to the Surface Antigen (Anti-HBs)

Anti-HBs can be present 2 to 6 weeks after the disappearance of HBsAg. The surface antigen (HBsAg) and surface antibody (anti-HBs) do NOT exist together. Study Figure 11.2 to see the timing and rise and fall of titers for these two markers.

NOTE: An exception to this diagram (and laboratory findings) occur in the presence of both a subtype HBsAg and an anti-HBs produced from a different subtype. In such occasional situations, both markers could exist together.

> When anti-HBs is found alone without HBsAg, the individual:
> • Has developed immunity to the disease
> • Is not infectious
> • Is not a carrier

Antibody to the Core Antigen (Anti-HBc)[12]

• Can be easily detected in blood
• Appears in blood around the time of onset of symptoms or when liver tests abnormalities appear and persists for life
• Refers to one or both immunoglobulins (i.e., IgM and IgG)
• Acute or recently acquired infection can be detected by the presence of IgM, which may persist for up to 6 months if the disease resolves
• In persons who have chronic HBV infections, IgM anti-HBc can persist during viral replication at low levels that are not detectable by assays commonly used in the United States

Sometimes, neither the hepatitis B surface antigen (HBsAg), the hepatitis B e antigen (HBeAg), nor the antibodies for these are found in blood serum. However, if the hepatitis B core antibody is found, it is evidence that the individual has encountered the hepatitis B virus. The antibody to hepatitis B core antigen is the only factor that is detectable by laboratory studies during all phases of the infection.

The presence of the antibody to hepatitis B core antigen (anti-HBc)
- Can remain for an individual's lifetime
- Can indicate a carrier state postinfection if the hepatitis B surface antigen (HBsAg) is also present
- Can indicate the possibility of passing the infection on to the baby at birth if the surface antigen (HBsAg) is present

Antibody to the Hepatitis B e Antigen (Anti-HBe)

- Appearance of this antibody occurs as levels of HBsAg are diminishing and the disease is resolving.
- This antibody develops in most hepatitis B infections.
- It can persist along with HBsAg in the carrier state.
- The presence of anti-HBe correlates with low levels of hepatitis viral DNA.

Timing and Titers in Hepatitis B Virus Infection

Figure 11.2 demonstrates the timing and sequence of titers in the majority of patients with acute HBV infection who go on to resolution with resulting immunity. Immunity is indicated by the sustained rise in the antibody to the surface antigen (anti-HBs) and/or core antibody (anti-HBc). Study the graph carefully and, as you do, try to relate the following facts correlating with the graph.

- The incubation period is long, varying from 14 to 180 days and averaging about 120 days.
- Symptoms do not appear for at least 1 to 3 months after exposure.
- Symptoms, if present, can last for several weeks.
- HBsAg can be identified in blood anywhere from 1 to 2 months after exposure.
- HBeAg appears after HBsAg *and never exists without the presence of HBsAg.*

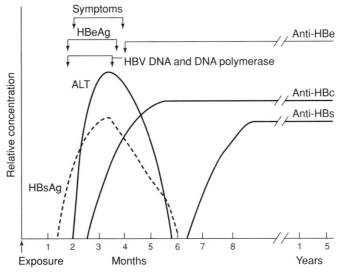

FIGURE 11.2 Course of hepatitis B disease. (Adapted with permission from Cohen, M., & Cohen, H. [1990]. Current recommendations for viral hepatitis. *Contemporary OB/GYN, 35*[11], 65.)

- The presence of HBeAg is associated with high levels of circulating HBsAg. This indicates a highly infectious state.
- By the time symptoms appear, it is usually possible to detect HBsAg and HBeAg in blood.
- Detectable levels of HBsAg generally disappear by 6 months after exposure.
- The antibody to the core antigen, anti-HBc, begins to appear during the acute viremic phase (high virus levels), can be detected easily, and can persist for an individual's lifetime.
- The antibody to the e antigen, anti-HBe, appears before the production of the surface antibody, anti-HBs, but after production of anti-HBc; it can persist indefinitely.
- The appearance of anti-HBs does not occur until many weeks or months after the appearance and eventual disappearance of HBsAg. Titers for the surface antigen and antibody do not exist together. This antibody (anti-HBs) indicates that the individual has developed an immunity to hepatitis B infection. The antibody can persist for a lifetime.
- Diminishing of anti-HBs after a resolved infection to below-detectable levels can occur over many years, but immunity is believed to be retained ("immune memory").
- HBV is associated with several serologic subtypes and is now known to have mutations associated with its replication. This may be related to recurrent disease, failure to clear the virus, or altered response to therapy in chronic infection.[3]

Carrier State

▶ How serious is the carrier state, and what impact does it have on pregnancy?

Carriers have the potential of transmitting the disease to others under certain circumstances. Carriers have a 12 to 30 times higher risk of developing primary liver cancer than noncarriers. Carriers also have increased risk of cirrhosis of the liver, liver cancer, liver failure, and death.[12]

The global prevalence of HBsAg varies greatly. In areas where the disease is highly prevalent, perinatal transmission is the primary transmission route. In low endemic areas, sexual contact in the high-risk adult population is the predominant route. The disease is highly endemic in China, Southeast Asia, most of Africa, most Pacific Islands, the Middle East, and the Amazon Basin. The risk of developing chronic HBV infection after acute exposure ranges from 90% in newborns of HbeAg positive mothers to 25% to 30% in infants and children under age 5 and to less than 5% in adults in endemic areas.[13]

Hepatitis B Carriers[14,15]

- Hepatitis B carriers are unable to clear HBsAg from their blood, and they harbor the virus in a chronic state.
- They can have an intermittent but chronic symptomatic infection. These individuals have serologic evidence of HBsAg, constant or intermittent elevations of liver enzymes, and evidence of liver inflammation. Symptoms come and go, but liver biopsies reveal a chronic form of hepatitis.
- Carriers can be asymptomatic. This state is characterized by a "healthy" carrier who has no symptoms and usually has normal liver studies but continues to be HBsAg positive serologically. Liver biopsies show evidence of viral infection.
- These patients are frequently also immunocompromised (e.g., HIV-infected individuals).
- Can include infants infected at birth who have a high likelihood of becoming carriers.
- Typically, carriers have high titers of anti-HBc and *do not have anti-HBs.*
- Carriers who demonstrate the presence of HBeAg are considered to have a high degree of infectivity.

▶ How is the carrier state diagnosed?

When detectable levels of HBsAg are found in an individual on at least two occasions, at least 6 months apart, that individual probably is a carrier. This means the individual will indefinitely be capable of transmitting the disease to others through blood and other body fluids and through sexual contact.

Certain immunoglobulins serve as serologic markers, which also denote infectiousness and the carrier state. Immunoglobulins are unique types of antibodies. Different antigens are capable of stimulating the body's production of immunoglobulins in response to foreign antigenic substances. These immunoglobulins or antibodies inactivate the foreign antigen as part of the body's defense system. Currently, five classes of antibodies (immunoglobulins) have been identified.

The two classes of immunoglobulins relevant to hepatitis B are called IgG and IgM.

NOTE: When a laboratory report identifies the presence of the antibody to the core antigen, anti-HBc, it refers to the "total" amount of anti-HBc. Depending on the individual's disease state, the "total" anti-HBc may contain either IgG or IgM antibodies or both. This is an important concept to understand as you read on about these two unique and different immunoglobulins, which serve as important diagnostic markers for the hepatitis B carrier state.

IgG Immunoglobulins

- These are the major immunoglobulins in the blood, comprising approximately 75% to 80% of the total antibodies in a normal individual. Because of relatively small molecular size, these are the only immunoglobulins capable of crossing the placenta.
- IgG immunoglobulins are protein complements specific to the antigen responsible for their production. Numerous IgG immunoglobulins exist for different diseases, including one for hepatitis B. It is referred to as **IgG anti-HBc. IgG blood levels of individuals exposed to a given antigen may remain present for years or a lifetime.** The presence of IgG to a specific antigen simply means that the individual has been exposed to that antigen (e.g., bacteria, virus).
- Because IgG is usually produced as a response to a disease, it is associated with resolving or postinfectious states and in many diseases signals postinfection immunity.

IgM Immunoglobulins

- These are the *first immunoglobulins produced during the body's immune response.*
- There are specific IgM complements for individual antigens, including one for hepatitis B, called **IgM anti-HBc**.
- IgM levels rise, peak, and fall within a few weeks or months of contracting a disease.
- IgM immunoglobulins serve as important markers for the acute phase of a disease.

Figure 11.3 represents a chronic carrier state with persisting HBsAg, HBeAg, and anti-HBc titers.

The following additional serologic markers play a role in diagnosing the hepatitis B carrier state:

- IgM class of anti-HBc
- IgG class of anti-HBc

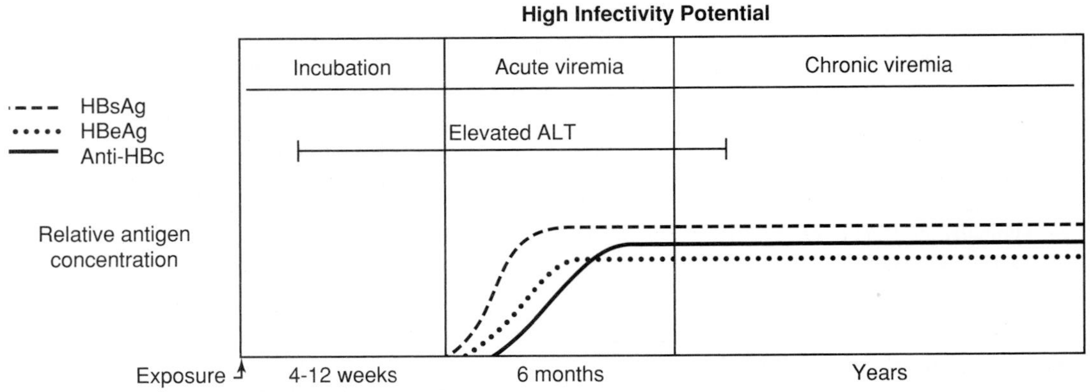

High Infectivity Potential

	Incubation	Acute viremia	Chronic viremia

- - - HBsAg
······ HBeAg
—— Anti-HBc

Elevated ALT

Relative antigen concentration

Exposure   4-12 weeks   6 months   Years

FACTS

*All three serologic markers persist: HBsAg, HBeAg, and Anti-HBc.

*It is the continued presence of HBeAg along with HBsAg that indicates high blood levels of HBsAg and therefore an elevated degree of infectivity.

*Liver enzymes (e.g., ALT) will be elevated in the chronic, active, and highly infectious carrier.

FIGURE 11.3   Hepatitis B titers of a chronic carrier.

When patients have an *acute* or *recent* HBV infection, *the IgM class of anti-HBc is present* in the blood. However, if patients have the *chronic* form of the disease or have recovered from the acute disease, the IgM anti-HBc is absent and the *IgG class of anti-HBc is present.*

REMEMBER: *When a report identifies "anti-HBc," it refers to "total" anti-HBc. Depending on the patient's disease state (active or chronic), this "total" may include both IgM anti-HBc and IgG anti-HBc. The distinction is made by a laboratory order to identify the IgM anti-HBc marker.*

IgM Anti-HBc

- Is an immunoglobulin produced by the body's defense system early in the disease
- Is an immunoglobulin or antibody to the core antigen HBcAg
- Indicates recent infection with HBV
- Is detectable for several weeks to months after infection

NOTE: *Absence of the IgM class antibody means there is no acute infectious process present.*

To summarize, a carrier is a person who is either HBsAg positive on at least two occasions at least 6 months apart or **who is anti-HBc positive and IgM anti-HBc negative when only a single blood serum specimen is tested.**[14]

CAUTION: *Chronic active carriers who are having an exacerbation of the disease will test positive for IgM anti-HBc.*

Care must be exercised when labeling an individual a carrier. Occasionally, 6 to 8 months may be required to clear the system of HBsAg. HBsAg-positive individuals should be tested after 6 months to establish chronicity.

▶ **If the pregnant woman has had hepatitis B, will she necessarily be a carrier?**

Fortunately, no. Sometimes individuals completely recover from the disease, and when tested, HBsAg and HBeAg are not present. These individuals are not carriers and will not transmit the disease.

▶ **How common is the infection in pregnant women?**

There are an estimated 1.2 million carriers in the United States and 350 million carriers worldwide.[4] Approximately 22,000 women with chronic hepatitis B deliver infants in the United States. However, increased migrations to the United States of high-carrier populations, such as Vietnamese, Haitians, and Africans, may lead to an increased frequency of maternal hepatitis B encountered in perinatal units in the United States.

Hepatitis B is also a sexually transmitted disease. Epidemiologic studies indicate that males having sex with males, intravenous drug use, and heterosexual exposure with a hepatitis B carrier or sex with multiple partners account for the major modes of transmission in individuals.

One of the major risk factors for hepatitis B currently is intravenous drug abuse.	The proportion of individuals whose risk factor for hepatitis B is heterosexual exposure has increased.

▶ **Can pregnant women who have acute hepatitis B or who are carriers give the disease to the newborn?**

Yes, these mothers can transmit this disease to the newborn. This mother-to-infant transmission process is known as ***vertical transmission.*** Transmission of HBV by carrier mothers to their babies occurs during the perinatal period. This appears to be the single most important factor in the prevalence of the infection in many regions of the world including Southeast Asia and China.

Vertical Transmission Most Likely Occurs in the Following Ways

- Transplacental infection is not as common as was once thought[14]
- Infant ingestion of infected maternal fluids (blood, amniotic fluid, or breast milk) during the process of birth and postpartum

Risk of Transmission Is Most Likely in the Following Circumstances [2,5,9]

- When infection occurs during the third trimester
- When the mother is in an especially acute infectious state, with her blood testing positive for both HBsAg and HBeAg serologic markers

The acute infectious state occurs when the mother's blood has two serologic markers:

HBsAg positive and HBeAg positive   =   90% to 95% risk of perinatal transmission
HBsAg positive and HBeAg negative   =   10% risk of perinatal transmission

---

▶ Which women are at high risk of being hepatitis B carriers?

Women in any of the following categories are at high risk for being hepatitis B carriers[4,13]

- Women who have ever injected drugs (needles can be contaminated)
- Women who are partners of intravenous drug abusers
- Women with multiple sexual partners
- Women who have had household or sexual contact with HBsAg-positive partners
- Health care workers such as nurses, physicians, medical technologists, dentists, and dental hygienists (because of exposure to blood or to blood-tinged saliva)
- Women from the following areas: South Asia (except Sri Lanka), Africa, South Pacific Islanders, Middle East (except Cyprus), European Mediterranean (Greece, Italy, Malta, Portugal and Spain), the Arctic, South America (Argentina, Bolivia, Ecuador, Guyana, Suriname, Venezuela, and the Amazon regions of Peru and Columbia), independent states of the former Soviet Union, Eastern Europe (including Russia but excluding Hungary), the Caribbean (Haiti, Antigua, Barbados, Dominican Republic, Granada, Jamaica, Puerto Rico, St. Kitts, St. Lucia, St. Vincent, Grenadines, Trinidad and Tobago, and Turks and Caicos) owing to epidemic/endemic exposure in their mother country or refugee camps
- Women with active disease or a history of hepatitis (can be a chronic carrier)
- Women with a history of sexually transmitted disease
- Women are undergoing dialysis. This also includes partners of men who are receiving dialysis treatment as a result of frequent exposure to blood and semen
- Inmates of correctional facilities
- Women infected with hepatitis C or HIV
- Women who have received many blood transfusions (as a result of receiving donated blood)
- Women with acute and chronic liver disease or chronically elevated ALT or AST

NOTE: *The CDC Immunization Practices Advisory Committee recommends routine screening of all pregnant women as the only strategy that will provide control of perinatal transmission of HBV infection in the United States.*[14,16]

Antepartum Care

▶ What are the maternal complications and clinical implications during the antepartum period?

Maternal complications from hepatitis B are not common. The following facts are known about the course of HBV infection during pregnancy[2,11]:

- Pregnancy is *not* thought to aggravate the course of the disease in developed countries.
- Most infections go unrecognized.
- Fifty percent or fewer of HBV infections are accompanied by clinical signs and symptoms.
- Usual *clinical signs* are jaundice, hepatic tenderness, and weight loss.
- Most symptoms appear 45 to 180 days after exposure. These symptoms include anorexia, nausea, malaise, weakness, and abdominal pain.
- Acute infection lasts 3 to 4 weeks.
- Mothers rarely need hospitalization unless dehydration or marked liver damage has occurred.
- No special dietary prescriptions are needed.

- In the event of severe symptoms of anorexia, nausea, vomiting, and diarrhea, hospitalization is recommended and the goals of treatment are to:
  - Correct fluid and electrolyte imbalance
  - Assess for liver damage
  - Conserve energy
  - Minimize infection transmission

> Fulminant hepatitis with encephalopathy is a rare complication of hepatitis B but one that has high rates of morbidity and mortality.

Screening

During pregnancy, every woman should be screened for hepatitis B. This is done by testing for the surface antigen, HBsAg. The presence of HBsAg in serum identifies any infected person in either an acute or carrier state. *The test does not differentiate members of the two groups.*

If HBsAg is present, additional tests need to be carried out to identify the following:
- The degree of infectivity
- Whether the mother is in the acute or chronic carrier state

The hepatitis B laboratory panel for disease identification includes the following serologic markers:
- HBsAg
- anti-HBs
- anti-HBc

NOTE: HBeAg and anti-HBe are looked for only when HBsAg is found. They are prognostic indicators of degree of infectivity.

Although the presence of the marker IgM anti-HBc would identify acute or recent (within the last 4 to 6 months) infection, this is not routinely included in initial laboratory panels.

If a mother tests positive for HBsAg, her liver biochemistry should be analyzed to determine whether any liver damage has occurred. If the results are abnormal or if her liver is enlarged, she should be further evaluated to assess whether the disease is acute or chronic.

Hepatitis B is a sexually transmitted disease. The presence of a sexually transmitted disease in an individual indicates the possibility of others. HBsAg-positive mothers should be screened for gonorrhea, syphilis, chlamydial infection, HIV, herpes, and human papillomavirus. An additional disease, group B streptococcus, has strikingly increased in incidence among young sexually active persons over the last decade. It can be sexually transmitted. Because this organism is currently the most common cause of sepsis and meningitis in the neonate and young infant, GBS screening in pregnancy is recommended.[17] (See Appendix A and E.)

Women who are HBsAg negative but at high risk of contracting HBV infection need to be counseled that vaccination is recommended during pregnancy. Health care providers need to be aware that recent findings indicate that maternal obesity, advancing age, and smoking tend to reduce the efficacy of HBV vaccination in pregnant women.[18]

Screening mothers also means that families of infected or carrier patients can then be tested and immunized. This is an important component in the strategy to prevent hepatitis B transmission.

Counseling and testing are recommended in all prenatal settings, where women who are at risk for hepatitis B are encountered. In addition, women should be educated about the following:
- A description of the infection
- Risk behaviors associated with contracting or transmitting the infection
- Potential social and familial implications (carrier transmission risks in home and employment settings)
- Testing and immunization benefits for family members and sexual contacts

Immunization

Products for Active and/or Passive Immunization

Two types of immunizing products are available for prophylaxis against hepatitis B. These are *vaccines, which confer active immunization, and hepatitis B immune globulin, which confers passive immunization.*

Hepatitis B Vaccines

Recombinant vaccines are produced by inserting the HBsAg gene into *Saccharomyces cerevisiae*, common baker's yeast cells, which are capable of synthesizing large quantities of HBsAg in the host cell. Purified HBsAg is obtained by lysing the yeast cell and extracting the surface antigen particles. Hepatitis B vaccines are packaged to contain 10 to 40 mg of HBsAg protein per milliliter. The HBsAg is absorbed by aluminum hydroxide and preserved through the addition of thimerosal. Currently licensed recombinant vaccines are Recombivax HB (Merck & Co., West Point, PA) and Engerix-B (SmithKline Beecham, Philadelphia, PA).[19]

Plasma-derived vaccines are produced from pooled serum of hepatitis B-infected individuals. There are 15.[20]

> Both plasma-derived vaccine and recombinant vaccine are used throughout the world; 80% of hepatitis B vaccine production is plasma derived. Both vaccines confer equal and long-term protection.[3]

> Clinical trials have established that the achievement of a level of 10 mIU/mL of anti-HBs in a vaccinated individual is associated with protection against clinical infection.[3]

> A series of three IM doses of hepatitis B vaccine induces a protective antibody response (anti-HBs in ≥95% or more of infants, children, and adolescents).[3]

NOTE: Viruses that use RNA and reverse transcriptase for replication are capable of multiple mutations. There is concern about HBV mutants that may develop vaccine and treatment resistance. Preliminary data on enhancing hepatitis B vaccine immune-producing capabilities against one or more of these mutants has been established, but no such vaccines are as yet licensed in the United States.[3]

Hepatitis B Immune Globulin

Hepatitis B immune globulin (HBIG) is prepared from the plasma of donors known to contain a high titer of antibody against HBsAg. This human plasma is carefully screened for antibodies to HIV and HCV. In addition, the process used to prepare HBIG actually inactivates and eliminates HIV from the final globulin product. The final product is also free of HCV RNA. Since 1999, all products available in the United States have been manufactured by methods that inactivate HCV and other viruses.[21] No evidence exists that HIV can be transmitted by HBIG. Because administration of HBIG confers antibodies to the recipient directly, immediate passive protection is received that is temporary (3 to 6 months) and is usually recommended prophylactically in the case of newborn exposure risk or health care personnel parental exposure (e.g., needlestick) or within hours after exposure in certain postexposure situations. This serves as an intermediate and transient step while the individual begins to develop his or her own antibodies after immunization with hepatitis B vaccine.

CDC Recommendations for Prevention of Hepatitis B Infection and Management of Pregnant Women[18]

- All pregnant women should be routinely tested for HBsAg during an early prenatal visit
- Women who were not screened prenatally, those who engage in behaviors that put them at risk for infection, and those with clinical signs should be tested on admission to the hospital for delivery
- Women who are HBsAg positive should be referred to an appropriate case management program to ensure that their contacts receive timely postexposure prophylaxis and follow-up
- Women who are HBsAg positive should be provided with or referred for appropriate counseling and medical management. HBsAg-positive women should receive information concerning hepatitis B that discusses the following:
  - Mode of transmission
  - Perinatal concerns (e.g., infants born to HBsAb-positive mothers may breastfeed)
  - Prevention of HBV transmission to contacts

- Substance abuse treatment, if appropriate
- Medical evaluation and treatment for chronic hepatitis B
- When HBsAg testing of pregnant women is not feasible, all infants should receive hepatitis B vaccine within 12 hours of birth and should complete vaccine series according to schedule for infants born to hepatitis B-positive mothers

Intrapartum Care

▶ **How is the disease transmitted to others, including health care personnel?**

HBV is viable in blood and in secretions containing serum or those derived from serum. Transmission of the virus can be by one of five routes[21]:

1. Direct inoculation through the skin (percutaneous) of infected serum or plasma or by transfusion of infected blood or blood products
2. Indirect inoculation through the skin of infected serum or plasma through abrasions or small skin cuts
3. Absorption of infected serum or plasma through mucosal surfaces (e.g., eye, mouth)
4. Absorption of infective secretions (e.g., saliva, semen) through mucosal surfaces (could occur during vaginal, anal, or oral sexual contact)
5. Transfer of infected serum or plasma by way of inanimate surfaces or possibly vectors

Besides blood, body fluids include the following:

Serous fluid (e.g., cerebrospinal fluid, synovial fluid, pleural fluid, peritoneal fluid)	Breast milk
	Vaginal secretions
	Semen
Amniotic fluid	Urine
Saliva	Sweat
Tears	Feces

Universal precautions involve a mindset that incorporates practices performed every hour of the professional day to be used consistently to reduce transmission of blood-borne pathogens, whether that be from patients to health care workers, from health care workers to patients, or from patient to patient. Precautions include appropriate use of personal protective equipment such as gloves, gowns, face shields, and goggles, as well as proper instrument/equipment cleaning, disinfection, or sterilization procedures.

Precautions Recommended for Hospital Personnel[21,22]

Nursing, medical, and housekeeping personnel are exposed to a variety of body fluids on an obstetrics unit during an average workday.

HBV has been isolated from blood, semen, urine, breast milk, saliva, tears, and brain tissue of infected individuals. However, research to date indicates that the virus is not transmitted to individuals through saliva, sweat, tears, urine, or stool.

> The concentration of HBV in bodily fluids is proportional to the number of white blood cells in the fluid. Blood has the highest concentration of HBV, whereas saliva and tears have much lower concentrations.

Precautions do not apply to feces, nasal secretions, sputum, sweat, tears, urine, and vomitus *unless they contain gross, visible blood.*

> The risk of HBV transmission from these fluids and material is low or nonexistent.

Pregnant health care workers have additional motivation for adhering to universal precautions because of the risk of perinatal transmission to the fetus.

> The CDC strongly recommends hepatitis B vaccination for all at-risk health care workers.

> Pregnant women who are considered at high risk of becoming infected with HBV should be considered for HBV immunization. Pregnancy is not a contraindication to the use of hepatitis B vaccine.[14,16]

A major aim of appropriate intrapartum care is the prevention of nosocomial infection in patients and health care workers. *Nosocomial infections* are those acquired while in the hospital and as a result of being in a hospital, as opposed to community-acquired infections. The infection is neither present nor in the incubation stage at the time the patient is admitted to the hospital. Symptoms of a nosocomial infection are not necessarily present during hospitalization, but may become evident after discharge.

Basic guidelines are as follows:
- Universal precautions should be followed by all staff, medical, nursing, allied health workers, and housekeeping personnel.
- Focusing only on patients known to be infected puts the health care provider at risk from patients who are infected but not yet identified and, therefore, are not being properly treated.
- Hospital personnel who are at high risk of exposure to blood and other body fluids should have hepatitis B screening and immunization made available to them.

Hospital Admission Screening

▶ **Which women require hepatitis B screening on admission?**

- All pregnant women should have prenatal screening for hepatitis B infection.
- Women who present with no prenatal care or without documentation of prenatal care and laboratory testing results should have a hepatitis B screen done immediately.
- Women who have incomplete documentation of their hepatitis B status should have the remaining serologic markers evaluated to determine their infectious and/or carrier state. (For example, an HBsAg-positive marker documented from a screening examination always needs further evaluation. Is HBeAg present? Has the HBsAg marker cleared and is anti-HBs present, denoting immune status? Has the HBsAg marker persisted for more than 6 months, indicating a carrier state?)

REMEMBER: Many persons clear their systems of HBsAg over a 6-month period and go on to develop an immune state.

Therefore, when admitting a pregnant woman who is at increased risk for being a hepatitis B carrier, the following should be done:
- Review her prenatal record to determine the results of her hepatitis screen.
- If no record is available, contact the primary care provider immediately.
- If no documentation can be obtained for her hepatitis B status, HBsAg testing on the mother should be done immediately.
- After an initial positive test for HBsAg on a laboring woman, treatment of the infant should begin within 24 hours of birth.
- **If a hospital does not possess the capacity to do the hepatitis B screen and the mother has no documentation of her status, the infant should be presumed to be at risk. Treatment with both HBIG and hepatitis B vaccine should begin within 12 hours of birth.**[19]

Prevention of Perinatal Transmission

▶ **How can the risk of transmission of hepatitis B to the newborn be reduced?**

In 1991 and 1995, the CDC Immunization Practices Advisory Committee[19,23] recommended strategies to eliminate HBV transmission in infancy and childhood, as well as in adolescence and adulthood. Immunization of all susceptible persons will prevent new infections. **Therefore, routine vaccination of children born to HBsAg-negative mothers is now recommended.** Infants and children should receive the vaccine during routine visits to clinical or private practices.

THE PRIMARY GOAL IN TREATING THE NEWBORN IS PREVENTION OF THE INFANT BECOMING A CARRIER OF HEPATITIS B. NINETY PERCENT OF INFECTED INFANTS BECOME CHRONIC CARRIERS OF HBsAg. APPROXIMATELY 25% OF THESE INFANTS WILL DIE FROM CIRRHOSIS OF THE LIVER OR LIVER CANCER.

> **The best newborn treatment to prevent acute or chronic hepatitis B infection is timely immunization using a combination of HBIG and hepatitis B vaccine.**

CAUTION: *Currently the American Academy of Pediatrics and the CDC recommend delaying the initiation of hepatitis B immunization beyond the first week of life for premature infants at low risk for hepatitis B infection, especially those weighing less than 1,700 g at birth. Studies indicate an inadequate immune response in these infants. Vaccination can be considered once the infants reach 2,200 g of weight or until 2 months of age.[24]*

Because newborns are most often infected by exposure to the mother's infected secretions during the birthing process, *the following guidelines are intended to reduce that risk in infants of carrier mothers.* Remember that blood and amniotic fluid are the predominant contaminants in this situation.

Precautions aimed at preventing the spread of infection from the mother to the newborn during the intrapartum period include the following:

- Consider the intact fetal skin as a protective barrier. *Maintain the integrity of the skin when possible.*
- Avoid invasive procedures. These should be performed only after careful assessment of risks versus benefits. Examples include the following:
  - Internal scalp electrode monitoring
  - Fetal scalp blood sampling
  - Internal uterine pressure monitoring
  - Vaginal examination after rupture of membranes
  - Vacuum extraction
  - Forceps delivery
- Studies do not demonstrate that cesarean section lowers the risk of neonatal hepatitis B infection. Therefore, this route of delivery should be reserved for obstetric indications only.
- Women admitted for delivery who have no record of prenatal HBsAg testing should have blood drawn for testing. While awaiting the test results and within the first 12 hours of birth, the infant should receive hepatitis B vaccine.
  - If the mother is found to be HBsAg positive, the infant should also receive HBIG as soon as possible and within 7 days of birth. If for some reason HBIG is not given, it is important that the infant be given the second vaccination treatment at 1 month and no later than 2 months of age because the risk of infection is somewhat greater when HBIG has not been given at birth.
  - Even if the mother tests negative for HBsAg, the infant should continue with the vaccination schedule.
- In populations where pregnant women are not routinely screened for HBsAg, all newborns should receive the first dose of hepatitis B vaccine and HBIG within 12 hours of birth, the second dose at 1 to 2 months of age, and the third dose at 6 months of age.

Guidelines for Delivery of At-Risk Newborns

- Obtain informed consent for treatment of the infant before delivery.
- Assign one nurse to attend to the newborn after delivery when possible.
- Dry the infant immediately after the delivery to remove maternal blood and amniotic fluid.
- Mucous membrane exposure should be reduced by careful suctioning of the nares and oropharynx. Gently remove excess fluid and blood from the nares and oropharynx.
- Aspirate stomach contents.

> Take care to avoid traumatizing the mucous membranes.
>
> Always use low wall suction or newly devised mucus extractors, which prevent potentially contaminating fluids from coming in contact with the mouth.

- **Delay administration of vitamin K until after the infant is bathed.**
- Bathe the newborn early and thoroughly with a mild, nonmedicated soap under radiant heat as soon as possible.

> Prompt removal of infectious fluids reduces the chance of exposing both the infant and caregivers to infection. Attention should also be given to cleansing around the eyes.

- Remove potentially infectious maternal blood and secretions before any application of eye medications.
- Begin immunization treatment immediately on infants of hepatitis B-infected or carrier mothers.
- If the infant is born with additional problems, any life-threatening situation takes priority.

> In performing invasive procedures, avoid introducing the mother's blood or amniotic fluid into the baby.

- If the baby must be transported:
  - Inform the receiving physician/flight nurse/hospital that the baby's mother is infected with hepatitis B or is a carrier.
  - Label the maternal blood as HBsAg positive before transport.
  - Inform the transport team of what has been done for the baby regarding the prevention of transmission of the infection.
  - Document all steps taken in the newborn's chart.

Guidelines for At-Risk Newborn Vaccine Administration[18]

> STUDIES DEMONSTRATE THE HIGHEST EFFICACY (85% TO 95%) OF COMBINED HBIG AND HEPATITIS B VACCINE PROPHYLAXIS WHEN HBIG IS ADMINISTRATED WITHIN 1 TO 12 HOURS AFTER BIRTH.[19]

Newborns at risk should receive a three-dose series of Recombivax HB, Pediatric, or Engerix-B, Pediatric/Adolescent. The first dose, which is given at birth, should be combined with a single dose of HBIG given intramuscularly at another site. The second dose of Recombivax HB, Pediatric, or Engerix-B, Pediatric/Adolescent, is administered at 1 to 2 months of age and the third dose at 6 months of age.[19] There is a four-dose series with Engerix-B, Pediatric/Adolescent.[23]

Treatment

One dose at birth: HBIG 0.5 mL intramuscularly; use the anterolateral thigh muscle in the newborn

Passive immunity is developed with the dose of HBIG. This gives babies the antibodies needed immediately to protect them from infection with HBV through maternal blood and body fluids.

Treatment

Dose: Recombivax HB, Pediatric, 5 μg/dose, 0.5 mL intramuscularly
OR
Engerix-B, Pediatric/Adolescent, 10 μg/dose, 0.5 mL intramuscularly
Use the *other* anterolateral thigh muscle.

Active immunity is developed by the administration of hepatitis B vaccine. This simulates the baby's immune system to begin producing its own hepatitis B antibody protection.

NOTE: Infants born to HBsAg-negative mothers should receive 2.5 μg of Recombivax-HB, Pediatric, or 10 μg of Engerix-B, Pediatric/Adolescent, ideally at birth or before discharge. The second dose should be administered at least 1 month after the first dose. The third dose should be at least 2 months after the first dose but not before 6 months of age.

Failures of immunization for some newborns are believed to occur because a small percentage of these babies probably acquired the infection transplacentally before birth. Testing for efficacy of immunization in the infant is usually done at 9 months of age.

REMEMBER:
- *These medications should be administered within 12 hours after delivery. Recent studies indicate that administration of the first does of hepatitis B vaccine at birth*

is associated with increased likelihood of completion of the hepatitis B vaccination series.[25]

- *Different sites for each injection should be used. In the newborn, only the anterolateral thigh muscles should be used.*
- *Be sure the baby has been bathed thoroughly before the injections are given.*
- *The baby will require two additional immunizations: one at 1 month of age and one at 6 months of age.*

Communication with private physicians and community health departments is important. Arrangements can be made for babies to receive their second and third doses of the vaccine at the public health immunizations clinic or at the private physician office.

▶ Can hepatitis B be diagnosed in the newborn?

Currently, there are no available methods for prenatal diagnosis of fetal HBV infection. It is generally believed that vertical transmission occurs primarily at birth.[5] Although transplacental passage of viral particles can occur, it is rare. Hepatitis B viral particles, including the surface antigen, are too large to pass through the placenta easily.

Obtaining a definite diagnosis of HBV infection in the newborn is also a problem. Infected infants cannot be distinguished from noninfected infants through testing. Laboratory testing of newborns in the first few months of life is not conclusive because transplacentally acquired maternal HBsAg or anti-HBs in the infant's blood complicates the diagnosis. Basically, all infants born to mothers who are positive for hepatitis B antigens or antibodies will be seropositive for those markers at birth. The exception to this will be IgM markers, whose large molecular size does not permit transplacental passage. IgG immunoglobulins are of smaller size and are passed from mother to newborn.

Postpartum Care

▶ What are the important aspects of postpartum care?

There is no reason to separate the mother and infant after the infant has been bathed.

NOTE: *Mothers should be permitted to hold their infants immediately after birth, even though the baby has not been bathed.*

Until a complete bath is given, strict isolation procedures for the infant should be instituted. Before the baby is bathed, health care personnel should do the following:

- Wear gown and gloves when handling the baby.
- Wear masks and goggles or large-size glasses if there is a possibility of blood being spattered during a particular procedure.
- Consider all linens and other articles that come in contact with the baby to be sources of contaminated blood and/or amniotic fluid.

Once the infant has been thoroughly bathed with a detergent soap and water, there is no need to isolate the baby.

Although there is no urgent need to place the mother in a private room, it might be reasonable and prudent to do so when possible because a shared bathroom is probably the most

---

Only infants who are stable and able to tolerate the heat loss that occurs with bathing should be given a bath.

REMEMBER: *The reason for isolation procedures is to prevent transmission of the infection to staff or other patients through contact with the mother's infected blood or amniotic fluid.*

Handle these linens and other discarded articles according to infection control guidelines.

likely source of contamination. Heavy lochia can contaminate the toilet, her hands, and anything that she might touch before washing her hands. If she is sharing a bathroom, she should be taught to report any contamination with blood immediately.

After the infant has been bathed, teach the mother the following:
- To wash her hands before handling the baby
- Precautions for blood spills, lochia, and perineal pads
- To avoid letting the baby come in contact with soiled linen
- Why it is important to delay breastfeeding for 48 hours after administration of HBIG to the baby
- To inspect her breasts and nipples for infection or breaks in the skin if she is breastfeeding (the nurse should make this inspection with the mother once a day)

Education is a critical part of the mother's care after delivery. Be sure that the mother and her family members understand the following:
- Her hepatitis carrier status
- How the infant is infected and the importance of proper handwashing after handling blood-soiled materials (e.g., in changing her perineal pads before handling the baby)
- The potential for transmission via saliva
- The risks her hepatitis carrier status poses for the infant
- The risks and benefits of immunization for the infant
- The need for complete immunization plans for the baby over the next 6 months

Breastfeeding

▶ **What are the breastfeeding recommendations for the infant of a carrier mother?**

The CDC states that the infant of a hepatitis B-infected or carrier mother is not likely to be at risk for contracting the disease through breastfeeding. The infant has already received intense exposure to the virus during the birth process.[11]

> However, it is recommended that breastfeeding be delayed for 48 hours after HBIG treatment of the infant. This precaution ensures the conferring of passive immunity to the infant.

Breastfeeding is not contraindicated unless the mother develops any of the following:
- Cracked nipples
- Mastitis
- Other breast lesions

Feeding from the breast with any of these problems must be stopped because highly infectious discharge from the lesions can mix with breast milk.

Teach the breastfeeding mother the following:
- Nipple care
- Good breastfeeding techniques to prevent nipple trauma
- To stop breastfeeding the baby on the breast that develops a cracked nipple, mastitis, or other lesions and to express milk from that breast to prevent engorgement; to feed the infant from the unaffected breast (*The mother does not have to stop breastfeeding.*)

> Engorgement slows the healing in breasts affected with these problems.

Discharge Planning

▶ **What unique components need to be incorporated in discharge planning?**

Essential discharge preparation for the postpartum hepatitis B-positive mother and her infant include the following:
- Education about self-care
- Guidance to reduce transmission risks for household members
- Screening needs of household members, including sexual partner

- Scheduling the newborn for HBV immunization
- Counseling about safe sexual practices and contraceptive methods

Education About Self-Care

In addition to instructions concerning self-care, additional emphasis should be placed on a discussion of likely sources of contamination, such as body fluids, especially blood. Proper handling and use of sanitary pads, razor blades, toothbrushes, and bathroom facilities need to be reviewed. Handwashing practices related to handling objects that could be sources of contamination (e.g., a sanitary pad) should be explained. At the same time, it should be made clear that urine, tears, and stool are not sources of contamination. Giving the mother and family balanced perspective for a reasonable and responsible lifestyle is important.

The mother should be encouraged to seek regular, ongoing medical follow-up for herself. If she is in the acute infectious stage, periodic screening will eventually reveal seroconversion to an immune or carrier state. She needs to know her postinfection status when the acute stage passes so that appropriate medical interventions can be instituted. If she is a carrier, periodic medical follow-up is imperative. She is at risk for long-term sequelae including cirrhosis of the liver and/or hepatocellular carcinoma.

Guidance to Reduce Transmission Risks for Household Members

Teach the hepatitis B-positive mother that her hands and other skin surfaces should be washed immediately and thoroughly if contaminated with her blood. Warm water and soap suffice. Waterless antiseptic hand cleaners are appropriate if handwashing facilities are not available. Household surfaces should be cleaned with an Environmental Protection Agency (EPA)-approved germicide solution or a 1:100 solution of a household bleach when any blood is spilled. Blood-soiled linen can be contaminated with HBV, but the risk of actual disease transmission is negligible. The linen should be handled as little as possible and washed quickly. Normal laundry cycles and detergent can be used.

EVERY HOSPITAL CARING FOR OBSTETRIC PATIENTS SHOULD HAVE UNIVERSAL PRECAUTIONS GUIDELINES READILY AVAILABLE FOR NURSES, PHYSICIANS, ALLIED HEALTH WORKERS, AND HOUSEKEEPING PERSONNEL TO FOLLOW WHEN CARING FOR MOTHERS AND THEIR INFANTS ON INTRAPARTUM AND POSTPARTUM UNITS.

Postexposure Management

Management of Employees in Exposure-Prone Occupations

In June 2001, the CDC released updated guidelines for the management of occupational exposures to HBV, HCV, and HIV, as well as recommendations for postexposure prophylaxis.[26] The following comments reflect these recommendations and report.

The CDC defines *health care personnel* as those persons whose activities involve contact with patients or with blood or other body fluids from patients in a health care setting or a laboratory or public safety setting. This includes employees, students, contractors, attending clinicians, public safety workers, or volunteers in any of these settings.

Occupational exposure is defined as exposure that could reasonably be anticipated from skin, eye, mucous membranes, or parenteral contact with blood or other potentially infectious materials resulting from the performance of an employee's duties. Exposures placing a worker at risk for HBV, HCV, or HIV infection could be a percutaneous injury such as a needlestick or contact of mucous membranes or nonintact skin (chapped, abraded, or affected with dermatitis) with potentially infectious blood, tissue, or other body fluids.

Facts About Occupational Exposure[26]

- Blood contains the highest HBV titers of all body fluids.
- Semen and vaginal secretions are considered potentially infectious.
- Other potentially infectious fluids are cerebrospinal fluid, synovial fluid, pleural fluid, peritoneal fluid, pericardial fluid, and amniotic fluid. *The risk for transmission of HBV, HCV, or HIV infection from these fluids is unknown.*

- Feces, nasal secretions, saliva, sputum, sweat, tears, urine, and vomitus *are not considered potentially infectious unless they contain visible blood.* Transmission risk from these fluids and materials is extremely low. It appears that the risk of acquiring HBV infection is higher than for acquiring HIV or HCV. Also, the risk of acquiring HCV is greater than that the risk of contracting HIV.[27]
- Occupational exposure should be considered an urgent medical concern with the appreciation for the need of timely postexposure management.

HBV infection is the major infectious risk for health care personnel. There is no doubt that regulations issued under the Occupational Safety and Health Act,[28,29] making HBV vaccine available to all occupationally exposed health care personnel, have been instrumental in marked improvement. Studies indicate that 5% to 10% of HBV-infected workers become chronically infected. These individuals are at risk for chronic liver disease (e.g., cirrhosis, primary hepatocellular carcinoma) and are potentially infectious for their lifetime. Current estimates indicate that 100 to 200 health care personnel have died each year during the past decade owing to consequences of HBV infection, yet vaccines exist that could have prevented most of those deaths.[29]

Important Data Cited by the CDC[26]

- The risk of HBV infection is primarily related to the degree of contact with blood in the workplace.
- In needlestick injuries, the risk of developing *clinical* HBV infection (with signs and symptoms) from a contaminated needle was 22% to 31% if the blood contained both HBsAg and HBeAg.
- The risk of developing serologic evidence of HBV infection (i.e., the laboratory markers such as HBsAg, etc., can be identified) was 37% to 62%.
- When the surface antigen was present (HBsAg positive) without the e antigen (HBeAg negative), the risk was considerably lower: *Clinical* evidence of infection is 1% to 6%, and *serologic* evidence of infection is 23% to 37%. Considering that 5% to 10% of those infected will become chronically infected, these numbers are sobering and should motivate all "at-risk" personnel to seek vaccination.
- Having hepatitis B-vaccinated personnel reduces the risk of infection transmission to patients.
- HBV has been demonstrated to survive in dried blood at room temperature on surfaces for as long as 1 week and is seen as a potential for infection transmission.
- HCV is not efficiently transmitted through *occupational exposure* to blood, including blood on environmental surfaces. One study indicated that percutaneous transmission occurred only with hollow-bore needles as compared with other sharps.

Postexposure Recommendations

Since 1992, with the Occupation Safety and Health Administration's (OSHA) blood-borne pathogen standard, employers have been required to establish a control plan for cases of exposure that includes postexposure follow-up for employees. This includes the following:

- Availability of postexposure care during all working hours, including nights and weekends
- Provision of HBIG, HBV vaccine, and antiretroviral agents for HIV postexposure treatment *for timely administration* (Table 11.1)

NOTE:

- *Prescreening is not required as a condition for receiving the vaccine.*
- *Employees must sign a form stating that they decline the vaccine if they choose not to be vaccinated.*
- *If booster doses are later recommended by the U.S. Public Health Service, employees must be offered them.*

The control plan, among many stipulations, requires the following:

- That employers identify tasks, procedures, and job classifications where occupational exposure to blood occurs
- That evaluation plans be developed for postexposure circumstances
- The use of universal precautions in all exposure-prone work settings
- That engineering and work practice controls be implemented (e.g., procedures to minimize needlesticks and splashing and spraying of blood)
- Appropriate packaging and labeling of specimens and waste

▶ Who should have postvaccination testing?[19,26]

- **Health care personnel who are in contact with patients and/or blood and are at ongoing risk for percutaneous injuries should be tested for anti-HBs 1 to 2 months after they have completed the three-dose vaccination series; includes surgeons and dentists**
- Infants born to HBsAg-positive mothers (Knowledge of their immune status dictates subsequent clinical management.)
- Dialysis patients and staff
- HIV-infected individuals

TABLE 11.1 RECOMMENDED POSTEXPOSURE PROPHYLAXIS FOR EXPOSURE TO HEPATITIS B VIRUS

VACCINATION AND ANTIBODY RESPONSE STATUS OF EXPOSED WORKERS[a]	TREATMENT		
	Source HBsAG Positive	Source HBsAG Negative	Source Unknown or Not Available for Testing
Unvaccinated	HBIG[b] ×1 and initiate HB vaccine series[c]	Initiate HB vaccine series	Initiate HB vaccine series
Previously vaccinated			
Known responder[d]	No treatment	No treatment	No treatment
Known nonresponder[e]	HBIG ×1 and initiate revaccination or HBIG ×2[f]	No treatment	If known high-risk source, treat as if source were HBsAg positive
Antibody response unknown	Test exposed person for anti-HBs 1. If adequate,[d] no treatment is necessary 2. If inadequate,[e] administer HBIG ×1 and vaccine booster	No treatment	Test exposed person for anti-HBs 1. If adequate,[d] no treatment is necessary 2. If inadequate,[e] administer vaccine booster and recheck titer in 1–2 months

[a]Persons who have previously been infected with HBV are immune to reinfection and do not require postexposure prophylaxis.
[b]Dose is 0.06 mL/kg intramuscularly.
[c]Hepatitis B vaccine.
[d]A responder is a person with adequate levels of serum antibody to HBsAg (i.e., anti-HBs ≥10 mIU/mL).
[e]A nonresponder is a person with inadequate response to vaccination (i.e., serum anti-HBs <10 mIU/mL).
[f]The option of giving one dose of HBIG and reinitiating the vaccine series is preferred for nonresponders who have not completed a second three-dose vaccine series. For persons who previously completed a second vaccine series but failed to respond, two doses of HBIG are preferred.
Reprinted with permission from Centers for Disease Control and Prevention. (2001). Updated U.S. Public Health Service guidelines for the management of occupational exposures to HBV, HCV, and HIV and recommendations for postexposure prophylaxis. *MMWR Morbidity and Mortality Weekly Report, 50*(RR-11), 22.

Management of Nonresponders[26]

Important information:

    Nonresponders to the primary hepatitis B vaccination series are those who do not develop an antibody titer (anti-HBs) at a level equal to or above 10 mIU/mL. A second three-dose vaccine series should be given, or the nonresponder should be evaluated to determine whether he or she is HBsAg positive. See Table 11.1 for options with known nonresponders.

A second vaccine series for nonresponders has a 30% to 50% chance of producing appropriate antibody levels.

Nonresponders who are determined to be HBsAg positive need to be counseled regarding further medical evaluation and how to prevent transmission to others.

Nonresponders who are determined to be HBsAg negative are at risk for contracting HBV and need to be counseled regarding precautions and the need to obtain HBIG prophylaxis in the event of any parenteral exposure to HBsAg-positive blood.

For any occupational exposure, the infectious status of the source should be determined for the presence of the following:
- HBsAg
- HCV antibody
- HIV antibody

Hepatitis B Virus Exposure Treatment

- Prophylactic treatment to prevent infection after exposure should be considered in situations involving the following:
  - Percutaneous (e.g., needlestick, lacerations, bites) or perimucosal (ocular or mucosal) exposure to HBsAg-positive blood
  - Perinatal exposure of an infant born to an HBsAg-positive mother
  - Sexual exposure to an HBsAg-positive person
  - Household exposure of an infant younger than 12 months to a primary caretaker who has acute HBV infection
- In situations of perinatal exposure to an HBsAg-positive, HBeAg-positive mother, treating the newborn with HBIG and initiation of hepatitis B vaccine at birth is 85% to 95% effective in preventing infection.
- Regimens of either multiple doses of HBIG alone or the hepatitis B vaccine series alone are 70% to 75% effective in preventing infection.
- In occupational settings, the combination HBIG plus hepatitis B vaccine is recommended, as cited in Table 11.1, with the following guidelines:
  - Administer HBIG as soon as possible after exposure (preferably within 24 hours). Effectiveness is unknown when HBIG is administered later than 7 days.
  - Administer hepatitis B vaccine as soon as possible after exposure (preferably within 24 hours); it can be administered simultaneously with HBIG at a separate site.
  - Administer the vaccine only in the deltoid muscle using a 1- to 1.5-inch-long needle.
  - Persons exposed to HBsAg-positive blood or body fluids who are nonresponders to a primary vaccine series should receive a single dose of HBIG and the three-dose vaccine series initiated.

Booster Recommendations

A booster dose constitutes the amount of vaccine used in the vaccine dose for the three-dose series.[19]

Under current guidelines, the CDC states that booster doses of hepatitis B vaccine are not necessary and that periodic serologic testing to monitor antibody concentrations after completion of the vaccine series is not recommended.[26]

Occupational exposure–prone individuals need to know their hepatitis B serologic status. Postvaccination serologic testing for anti-HBs is strongly recommended by some authors. Nonresponse rates have been demonstrated in several studies. One study cites a 29% nonresponse rate among health care workers who were vaccinated against hepatitis B. Booster vaccination response in six of six subjects in this study suggests immunity. These authors recommend the following[30]:

- Postvaccination testing within 1 to 2 months to document immunity
- Periodic anti-HBs monitoring
- Booster vaccination to maintain protective titer levels

Hepatitis C Virus Exposure Treatment[26]

- After accidental percutaneous exposure from a hepatitis C-positive source, an average of 1.8% persons demonstrate anti-HCV seroconversion. Transmission rarely occurs from mucous membrane exposure to blood; no transmission has been documented from intact or nonintact skin exposures to blood.
- Immune globulin and antiviral agents such as interferon with or without ribavirin *are not recommended for postexposure treatment.*
- The HCV infection status of the source and the person exposed should be evaluated. If the source tests positive for anti-HCV, follow-up testing of the exposed person should be performed to determine whether infection develops. This is intended to identify chronic hepatitis C infection early so that referral for treatment can be made. Currently, data are insufficient to recommend treatment of acute HCV infection; that is, HCV RNA is first detected, but no evidence of liver disease is seen (normal ALT levels).
- Review Display 11.2 for CDC recommendations on postexposure follow-up.

PRACTICE/REVIEW QUESTIONS

After reviewing this module, answer the following questions.

1. List the five major forms of hepatitis:

   a. _____

   b. _____

   c. _____

   d. _____

   e. _____

2. All forms of hepatitis are caused by a(n) _____ or _____.

3. The five major forms of hepatitis differ in which of the following factors? Select all that apply.

   a. Mode of transmission
   b. How they affect people
   c. How they are diagnosed
   d. All of these
   e. None of these

4. Which of the following statements about hepatitis A reflect current knowledge? Select all that apply.

   a. The disease is spread by the fecal–oral route or ingestion of contaminated food or water.
   b. The disease is commonly contracted through contaminated blood.

   c. About one third of acute hepatitis cases in the United States are caused by HAV.
   d. The infection is much more severe when contracted by pregnant women.
   e. No vaccine exists for this disease.
   f. Viral infection in pregnancy is not associated with teratogenicity.
   g. Persistent antibody after infection (IgG anti-HAV) means the individual is immune.
   h. Absence of the IgG anti-HAV antibody after infection indicates a carrier state.

5. HCV is estimated to have infected about _____ people worldwide or _____ % of the world's population.

6. In the United States, the CDC reports that about _____ people are chronically infected with HCV.

7. Annually, approximately _____ deaths occur from chronic HCV infection.

8. Most hepatitis C-infected individuals are:

   a. Symptomatic
   b. Not symptomatic

9. Of hepatitis C-infected persons, _____ % to _____ % develop chronic liver disease, leading to the need for a liver transplant or resulting in death.

10. Hepatitis C postinfected persons who test positive for anti-HCV are:

    a. Infectious

    b. Immune

11. Hepatitis _____ exists as an acute coinfection acquired simultaneously with hepatitis B or as a superinfection in a chronic hepatitis B carrier.

12. Hepatitis _____ has a high mortality rate for fulminant hepatic failure in pregnant women, is associated with serious neonatal mortality, and does not exist as a chronic infection.

13. An *antigen* is defined as:

    _____

    _____.

14. An *antibody* is defined as: _____

    _____.

15. Match the symbols in Column B with the appropriate hepatitis B antigen or antibody term listed in Column A.

    Column A

    _____ 1. Surface antigen

    _____ 2. Core antigen

    _____ 3. e antigen

    _____ 4. Antibodies to the surface antigen

    _____ 5. Antibodies to the core antigen

    _____ 6. Antibodies to the e antigen

    Column B

    a. HBcAg

    b. anti-HBe

    c. HBeAg

    d. HBsAg

    e. anti-HBs

    f. anti-HBc

16. Match the terms in Column B with the appropriate characteristic or definition in Column A.

    Column A

    _____ 1. The protein coat of the virus can be found in infected persons.

    _____ 2. This antigen cannot be found in the blood of infected persons.

    _____ 3. The presence of this antigen in serum indicates that hepatitis B infection is one of the earliest indicators of the infection.

    _____ 4. This antigen is never found alone. It always occurs after HBsAg is present and the infection state has begun.

    _____ 5. When this antibody is found alone with HBsAg, the individual has developed an immunity to the disease and is neither infectious nor a carrier.

    Column B

    a. HBcAg

    b. anti-HBe

    c. HBeAg

    d. HBsAg

    e. anti-HBs

    f. anti-HBc

_____ 6. The detection of this antibody indicates that the core antigen is or was present in the body at one time (i.e., the individual has had hepatitis B).

_____ 7. This antibody is the only one that is detectable by the laboratory studies during all phases of a hepatitis B infection.

_____ 8. Whenever this antibody is found together with the HBsAg surface antigen, the individual is a carrier of hepatitis B infection but is of decreased infectiousness.

_____ 9. The presence of this antibody can remain for an individual's lifetime, can indicate a carrier state after infection, and in a pregnant woman, can indicate the possibility of passing the infection to the baby if the HBsAg surface antigen is also present.

_____ 10. The persistent presence of this antigen occurs in chronic hepatitis B.

17. Mark an "X" beside those statements that accurately reflect what Figure 11.4 depicts about the course of hepatitis B infection.

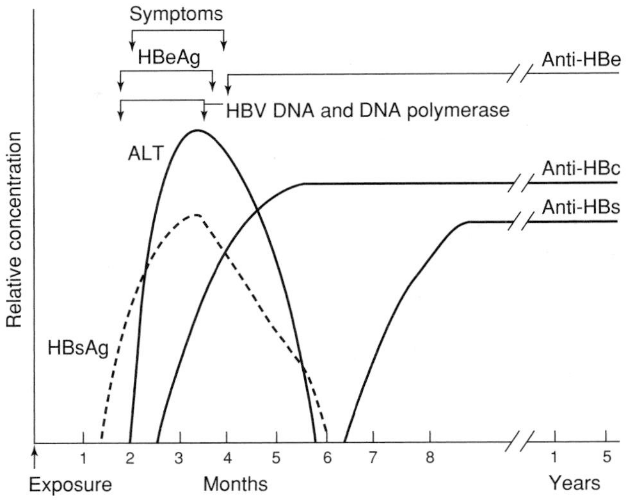

FIGURE 11.4

_____ a. Symptoms appear approximately 1 to 3 weeks after exposure.

_____ b. The appearance of symptoms (if any) usually correlates with the ability to detect HBsAg and HBeAg in blood.

_____ c. HBcAg is not detectable in blood.

_____ d. Detectable levels of HBsAg generally disappear after 6 months.

_____ e. The antibody to the core antigen begins to appear during the symptom phase and can be detected easily. It can persist for a lifetime.

_____ f. HBsAg and anti-HBs do not exist together.

18. Complete the statement. Select all that apply. Carrier states

    a. Are a key factor in the spread of hepatitis B worldwide

    b. Pose minimal problems for individual carriers themselves

    c. Are associated with high prevalence rates in most populations worldwide

    d. Are easily identified through symptoms of the disease

19. A child's best chances of avoiding the hepatitis B carrier state would be if he or she were born in which of the following areas? Select all that apply.

    a. The Philippines

    b. East Africa

    c. Hong Kong

    d. Canada

20. Which of the following statements is true about children in endemic areas of hepatitis B carriers, such as in the Pacific Islands or Southeast Asia? Select all that apply.

    a. They develop an immunity to the disease in the majority of cases.

    b. They have the greatest risk of contracting the infection at birth.

    c. They have the greatest risk of contracting the infection as adults.

    d. They can contract the infection but rarely become carriers.

21. The major influences on the increase of hepatitis B in the United States are _____ and _____.

22. List eight groups of women who are at high risk for hepatitis B carrier status during pregnancy.

    a. _____

    b. _____

    c. _____

    d. _____

    e. _____

    f. _____

    g. _____

    h. _____

Select from the following list the serologic marker to complete the statement(s) in questions 23 through 25:

HBsAg   anti-HBs

HBeAg   anti-HBe

HBcAg   anti-HBc

23. A highly infectious carrier has HBsAg and _____ in his or her blood.

24. A carrier of diminished infectivity has HBsAg and _____ in his or her blood.

25. An immune state exists when _____ is found in the blood.

26. Which of the following statements is true about mothers who have had hepatitis B?

    a. They will always be carriers.

    b. They can recover completely from the disease and not be carriers.

27. There is no evidence that hepatitis B is transmitted to the fetus through the placenta during pregnancy.

    a. True

    b. False

28. Transmission from an infected or carrier mother to the baby is most likely to occur as the baby comes into contact with infected amniotic fluid or blood during the birth process.

    a. True

    b. False

29. In the United States, hepatitis B is contracted most often during adulthood.

    a. True

    b. False

30. Infants who contract hepatitis B are less likely to become chronic carriers than are adults who contract the disease.

    a. True

    b. False

31. Carriers are the predominant vehicle by which the hepatitis B virus is passed on from person to person.

    a. True

    b. False

32. Many carriers are asymptomatic and do not know that they have been exposed to the virus.

    a. True

    b. False

33. A patient's hepatitis B screen shows the presence of HBsAg. Which of the following serologic markers should be ordered to identify whether the patient might be a carrier? Select all that apply.

    a. anti-HBc

    b. IgM anti-HBc

    c. HBeAg

    d. anti-HBe

34. IgM anti-HBc and IgG anti-HBc serologic markers are requested on the patient referred to in question 33. The report reads as follows: *IgG anti-HBc = positive; IgM anti-HBc = negative*. Which of the following are the correct diagnostic interpretations? Select all that apply.

    a. Carrier state

    b. Immune

    c. Infectious

    d. Recently infected

35. A patient's laboratory report reads as follows: *Anti-HBs = present; IgG anti-HBc = present*. Which of the following is the appropriate interpretation? Select all that apply.

    a. Carrier state

    b. Immune state

    c. Minimally infectious

    d. Recent infection

36. Betty Lou's hepatitis B screen reads as follows: *HBsAg = positive*. Which of the following is a correct conclusion? Select all that apply.

    a. She is infected.

    b. She is a carrier.

    c. She is immune.

    d. She is susceptible.

37. In a follow-up test on Betty Lou (the patient referred to in question 36), the following report is sent: *HBsAg = positive; HBeAg = positive; IgM anti-HBc = positive*. What can you correctly conclude about this patient? Select all that apply.

    a. That she is acutely infected.

    b. That she is chronically infected.

    c. That she is of a lower infectivity level.

    d. That she is not infectious at all.

38. Despite the 1988 universal screening guidelines for pregnant women, transmission during the perinatal period still occurs in the United States. Which of the following is a reason for this? Select all that apply.

    a. A relatively high percentage of women do not receive prenatal care.

    b. Hepatitis B immunization is not 100% effective.

    c. There is a high rate of viral transmission across the placenta.

    d. There is a high viral transmission rate to newborns from infected health care personnel.

39. Which of the following pregnant women should be screened for hepatitis B? Select all that apply.

    a. 35-year-old mother of four children, married to the same man for 16 years

    b. 29-year-old lawyer in a monogamous relationship

    c. 20-year-old college graduate who tested negative for HBsAg 1 year ago

    d. 25-year-old nurse who tested anti-HBs positive 1 month ago

40. Which of the following women need liver function tests? Select all that apply.

    a. 16-year-old at 16 weeks' gestation with a palpable liver and who is positive for HBsAg, IgG anti-HBc, and anti-HBe

    b. 18-year-old at 39 weeks' gestation who is positive for anti-HBs

    c. 30-year-old at 18 weeks' gestation who is negative for HBsAg and positive for anti-HBc

    d. 21-year-old at 6 weeks' gestation who tests positive for HBsAg on her hepatitis screen

41. Jane Rupp is a 20-year-old woman, gravida 1, at 7 weeks' gestation. Her hepatitis B screen reads as follows: *HBsAg = negative*. You interpret this to mean that she is:

    a. Highly infectious

    b. Immune

    c. Needs no further workup

    d. Infectious but not acutely so

42. Mandy Soffit is a 26-year-old woman, gravida 1, who is at 9 weeks' gestation. Her hepatitis B screen is reported as: *HBsAg = positive*. You interpret this to mean that (select all that apply):

    a. She is infectious

    b. Further workup is needed

    c. She is immune

    d. A risk of perinatal transmission exists

43. Hettie Swan is a 30-year-old woman, gravida 3, who is 32 weeks pregnant. Late entry to prenatal care leads to her hepatitis workup being received today. The report reads as follows: *HBsAg = positive; HBeAg = negative; anti-HBe = positive.* You interpret this to mean that:

    a. There is a 10% risk of perinatal transmission

    b. She has a history of hepatitis B but is now immune

    c. There is a 90% risk of perinatal transmission

    d. There is no risk of perinatal transmission

44. Ida Plano is the mother of a 3-year-old and is approximately 34 weeks pregnant. Her hepatitis B screen at 12 weeks' gestation was negative. Owing to a recent exposure through a new sexual partner, she is tested again. Today, the results read as follows: *HBsAg = positive; HBeAg = positive.* What can you conclude about perinatal transmission risk?

    a. It is *low* because maternal infectiousness is occurring during the third trimester

    b. It is *low* because of the presence of HBeAg

    c. It is *high* because maternal infectiousness is occurring during the third trimester

    d. It is *high* because of the presence of HBeAg

45. What is the appropriate follow-up to Ida Plano's test result?

    a. Test her 3-year-old immediately if never immunized with hepatitis B vaccine

    b. Immunize Ida immediately

    c. Arrange for hepatitis B testing for Ida's recent sexual partner and other intimate household contacts

    d. Order liver tests for Ida

46. When caring for infants of hepatitis B carrier mothers, what is your primary goal?

    _____

47. State seven steps, other than the immunization treatment, that are aimed at reducing the risk of transmission of the disease to the infant of a carrier mother or a mother of unknown HBV status.

    a. _____

    b. _____

    c. _____

    d. _____

    e. _____

    f. _____

    g. _____

48. The immunization treatment for the newborn of a carrier mother includes administering both _____ and _____ within _____ after delivery.

49. _____ is given at birth only and ideally within 12 hours of delivery.

50. The correct dose of HBIG for the newborn given at birth is _____.

51. HBIG and Recombivax HB, Pediatric (or Engerix-B, Pediatric/Adolescent), should always be administered to the newborn in the same site.

    a. True

    b. False

52. Should the baby be bathed before or after the injections of HBIG and Recombivax HB, Pediatric, or Engerix-B, Pediatric/Adolescent? _____

53. The appropriate injection sites to use for administration of HBIG and Recombivax HB, Pediatric, or Engerix-B, Pediatric/Adolescent, are in the _____ muscles.

54. HBIG confers _____ immunity in the newborn, whereas Recombivax HB, Pediatric, or Engerix-B, Pediatric/Adolescent, confers _____ immunity in the newborn.

55. There are never any justifiable reasons for waiving risk reduction measures for hepatitis B transmission in the newborn.

    a. True

    b. False

56. If the baby must be transported, besides preparing the infant for transport, what additional steps would you take with the infant of a carrier mother?

    a. _____

    b. _____

    c. _____

57. If an infant is born to a mother who has not been screened for hepatitis B but belongs to one of the risk groups, what is the recommendation? Select all that apply.

    a. Obtain a blood specimen from the mother for a hepatitis B screen

    b. Obtain a blood specimen from the baby for a hepatitis B screen

    c. Give the baby HBIG 0.5 mL intramuscularly within 12 hours of birth

d. Give Recombivax HB, Pediatric, or Engerix-B, Pediatric/Adolescent, to the newborn within 12 hours of birth

58. Which of the following statements reflects what is known about newborn testing for HBV? Select all that apply.

   a. Accurate methods exist for testing the newborn within the first month of life.

   b. Transplancentally acquired maternal HBsAg or anti-HBs in the newborn's blood complicates the diagnosis.

   c. All infants born to mothers who are positive for hepatitis B antigens or antibodies will be seropositive for these markers at birth.

   d. The maternal IgM marker can be identified in the newborn's blood.

59. Active immunization can be conferred in most newborns through the administration of which of the following? Select all that apply.

   a. Hepatitis B immune globulin (HBIG)

   b. Recombivax HB, Pediatric

   c. Engerix-B, Pediatric/Adolescent

   d. Vitamin K

60. A Vietnamese patient who has no record of having a hepatitis B screening delivers a healthy 7-pound infant. While awaiting the results from the mother's hepatitis B test, what is the recommendation for care of this infant? Select all that apply.

   a. No special care is required

   b. Isolation should be maintained after bathing the infant

   c. 0.5 mL of Recombivax HB, Pediatric, should be administered intramuscularly within 12 hours of birth

   d. 0.5 mL of HBIG should be administered intramuscularly within 12 hours of birth

61. An analysis of a newborn's cord blood for hepatitis B markers reveals the following results: *HBsAg = negative; anti-HBc = positive; anti-HBs = positive.* Which of the following conclusions can be drawn? Select all that apply.

   a. The mother is an HBV carrier.

   b. The baby is immune.

   c. The mother is immune.

   d. The baby is infected with HBV.

62. Which of the following practices correctly reflect universal precautions? Select all that apply.

   a. Gloves are worn when bathing newly delivered babies.

   b. Gown, face shields, and goggles are worn while performing an amniotomy.

   c. Full-size eye glasses are used for eye protection during a vaginal birth.

   d. Double gloving is done when discontinuing a woman's IV line.

   e. Gloves are worn while giving an HBsAg-positive laboring woman a bedpan.

63. A registered nurse works in a labor and delivery unit in a busy metropolitan area. Which of the following activities are likely to put her at risk of contracting HBV infection? Select all that apply.

   a. Screening high-risk patient charts to identify patients most at risk for being infected with HBV

   b. Recapping all needles carefully after use

   c. Choosing to wear gloves only while bathing babies who have been born of intravenous drug users or of women who are partners of intravenous drug users

   d. Hugging a hepatitis B carrier mother after the birth of her child

64. You are going to bathe a newly delivered hepatitis B carrier mother. After the bath, you need to begin an IV line. Which sequence of steps is recommended in the universal precautions guidelines?

   a. Wash hands, put on gloves, remove gloves after the bath, immediately put on another pair of gloves before starting the IV line.

   b. Continue to use the same pair of gloves without interrupting for handwashing.

   c. Wash hands, put on gloves for the bath, remove gloves, wash hands, and put on the same pair of gloves if you see no tears.

   d. Remove gloves after the bath, wash hands immediately, and put on another pair of gloves before starting the IV line.

65. A pregnant nurse working on a labor and delivery, nursery, or postpartum unit should do which of the following? Select all that apply.

   a. Request a change to another hospital unit

   b. Be assigned to low-risk patients on those units

   c. Know her hepatitis B status

   d. Use universal precautions

66. List five areas of education that should be addressed with the newly delivered hepatitis B carrier mother and her family.

   a. _____

   b. _____

   c. _____

d. _____

e. _____

67. Indicate whether the following statements are true (T) or false (F):

_____ a. Infants who are not bathed need to be kept isolated from their hepatitis B carrier mothers in the delivery or birthing room.

_____ b. An unstable newborn who has not been able to be bathed should be kept in isolation after being brought from the delivery or birthing room.

_____ c. Nursing and medical staff to the nursery should use gowns and gloves when handling a baby who has not been bathed.

_____ d. The reason for any isolation procedure used with the baby is to prevent transmission of hepatitis B to the baby.

_____ e. Even if a baby has been infected with HBV, the baby will not be infectious to nurses and medical personnel after a thorough bathing.

_____ f. Hepatitis B carrier mothers need not be placed in a private room.

68. Explain why a baby of a hepatitis B carrier mother, after being thoroughly bathed, need not be kept isolated from other mothers or babies in the nursery or on the postpartum unit.

_____

69. List four areas of self-care and precautions about which you need to instruct the newly delivered hepatitis B carrier mother.

a. _____

b. _____

c. _____

d. _____

70. Which of the following mothers have contraindications to any breastfeeding throughout the postpartum course? Select all that apply.

a. Angie is a known hepatitis B carrier mother who has just delivered her third child this morning. The baby received HBIG after birth.

b. Mary Beth is an intravenous drug abuser who tested positive for both HBV and HIV. Her newborn is doing well at 2 hours of age and has received HBIG.

c. Claire has recently tested positive for HBsAg and HBeAg but has no clinical signs or symptoms of infection. She delivered a healthy newborn yesterday. The baby received HBIG after birth.

d. Isun is a nurse who works on a labor and delivery unit. Because she was found to be susceptible (no history of immunization and no anti-HBs), she received the full course of hepatitis B immunization during the last 6 months of her pregnancy. She delivered a healthy baby today.

e. Teryl, a carrier mother, delivered by cesarean birth 4 days ago. The baby was given HBIG after birth. Today both of Teryl's nipples are cracked, with a slight serosanguinous discharge.

71. Which of the following statements best applies to recombinant vaccines? Select all that apply.

a. Production involves HBsAg gene manipulation in a yeast host cell.

b. They confer short-term, passive immunity.

c. They are no longer being produced in the United States.

d. Production involves using the plasma of chronically infected persons.

72. Studies indicate that approximately 5% to 10% of infected health care workers become carriers.

a. True

b. False

73. An unvaccinated health care worker could potentially infect susceptible patients with the hepatitis B virus.

a. True

b. False

74. The gluteal muscle is not recommended for HBV vaccination in children or adults.

a. True

b. False

75. Which of the following statements accurately profile the recommended use of HBIG in postexposure treatment?

a. When HBIG is given in conjunction with hepatitis B vaccine, efficacy of the immune response is improved.

b. An exposed health care worker's immune response is improved if given HBIG 2 weeks after a documented percutaneous exposure to HBsAg-positive blood.

c. HBIG is administered in postexposure situations in calculated amounts based on the body weight of the individual at risk.

d. HBIG may be given in two doses, 1 month apart, to a vaccinated individual who shows inadequate anti-HBs levels (a nonresponder) and who suffers an inadvertent exposure to HBsAg-positive blood.

76. When a health care worker accidentally receives a needlestick from a needle used on an individual with

unknown serologic status, which of the following is an appropriate action? Select all that apply.

a. Obtaining an immediate hepatitis B blood (and HIV) workup of the health care worker to assess immune status

b. Beginning hepatitis B immune globulin injections only after the health care worker's and the patient's status are known

c. Evaluating the patient's hepatitis B status immediately

d. Giving the health care worker HBIG immediately and beginning immunization within 7 days if the patient is a carrier and the worker is nonimmune

PRACTICE/REVIEW ANSWER KEY

1. a. Hepatitis A virus (HAV)
   b. Hepatitis B virus (HBV)
   c. Hepatitis C virus (HCV)
   d. Hepatitis D virus (HDV)
   e. Hepatitis E virus (HEV)

2. virus; virus-like particles

3. d. All of these

4. a, c, f, and g

5. 170 million; 3

6. 4 million

7. 8,000 to 10,000

8. b

9. 75; 85

10. a

11. D

12. C

13. A substance that, when introduced into a host, is capable of producing antibodies; bacteria and viruses are examples of antigens.

14. A protein substance developed in response to the presence of an antigen; they are part of the body's defense against foreign substances such as bacteria and viruses.

15. 1. d
    2. a
    3. c
    4. e
    5. f
    6. b

16. 1. d
    2. a
    3. d
    4. c
    5. e
    6. f
    7. f
    8. b
    9. f
    10. d

17. X at b, c, d, e, and f

18. a and c

19. d

20. b

21. Drug abuse; migration of high-carrier populations, such as Vietnamese, Haitians, and Africans, to the United States

22. a. Drug abusers who inject drugs under the skin or into veins
    b. Women who are partners of intravenous drug abusers or bisexual men or those who have multiple partners
    c. Health care workers such as nurses, physicians, medical technologists, dentists, dental hygienists
    d. Southeast Asians, Native Alaskans, Pacific Islanders, and Haitians
    e. Those with active disease or a history of hepatitis
    f. Those with a history of venereal disease
    g. Those rejected as blood donors—these individuals might have had the hepatitis surface antigen (HBsAg) detected
    h. Those who work in a renal dialysis unit (this also includes wives of men who are receiving dialysis)

23. HBeAg

24. Anti-HBe

25. Anti-HBs

26. b

27. b, False

28. a, True

29. a, True

30. b, False

31. a, True

32. a, True

33. a

34. a and c

35. b

36. a

37. a

38. a and b

39. a, b, and c

40. a and d

41. c

42. a, b, and d

43. a

44. c and d

45. a, c, and d

46. Prevention of the infants from becoming carriers of hepatitis B

47. Any seven of the following:
    a. Obtaining informed consent for treatment of the infant before delivery
    b. Avoiding invasive procedures on the fetus during the labor and birth period if possible
    c. Assigning one nurse to attend to the newborn after delivery
    d. Drying the infant immediately after the delivery to remove all maternal blood and amniotic fluid
    e. Gently removing excess fluid and blood from the nares and oropharynx
    f. Aspirating stomach contents using a mucus extractor or meconium aspirator with wall suction on a low setting
    g. Delaying the administration of vitamin K until after the infant is bathed
    h. Bathing the newborn early and thoroughly with a mild, nonmedicated soap under radiant heat as soon as the infant is stable
    i. Treating the infant of a hepatitis B infectious or carrier mother immediately

48. HBIG; Recombivax HB, Pediatric, or Engerix-B, Pediatric/Adolescent; 12 hours

49. HBIG

50. 0.5 mL

51. b, False

52. Before

53. Anterolateral thigh

54. Passive; active

55. b, False (life-threatening situations take priority)

56. a. Inform the receiving physician/flight nurse/hospital that the baby's mother is infected with hepatitis B or a carrier.
    b. Label the maternal blood as HBsAg positive before making the transport.
    c. Inform the transport team of what has been done for the baby regarding the prevention of transmission of the infection.

57. a, c, and d

58. b and c

59. b and c

60. c and d

61. c

62. a, b, and c

63. a and c. These activities represent selective identification of some women and not others for the practice of universal precautions. Treat all patients as if they were potentially infected with a blood-borne pathogen.

64. d

65. c and d

66. a. How hepatitis B could be transmitted to the infant and the importance of proper handwashing after handling blood-soiled materials (e.g., in changing the mother's perineal pads before handling the baby)
    b. The potential for saliva causing transmission of the infection
    c. The risks the mother's hepatitis carrier status poses for the infant
    d. The risks and benefits of immunization for the infant
    e. The need for complete immunization plans for the baby over the next 6 months

67. a. F
    b. T
    c. T
    d. F
    e. T
    f. T

68. Because the production of viruses in an infant who is infected with hepatitis B does not occur for several weeks

69. Any four of the following:
    a. To wash her hands before handling the baby
    b. Precautions for blood spills, lochia, and perineal pads
    c. To avoid letting the baby come in contact with soiled linen
    d. Why it is important to delay breastfeeding for 48 hours after administration of HBIG to the baby
    e. To inspect her breasts and nipples for infection or breaks in the skin if she is breastfeeding (maternal HIV infection is a contraindication to breastfeeding)

70. b and e

71. a

72. a. True

73. a, True

74. a, True

75. a and c

76. a, c, and d

REFERENCES

1. Centers for Disease Control and Prevention. (2005). Prevention of hepatitis A through active or passive immunization: Recommendations of the Advisory Committee on Immunization Practices (ACIP). *MMWR Morbidity and Mortality Weekly Report, 55*(RR-12), 1–29.

2. Reinus, J. F., & Leiken, E. L. (1999). Viral hepatitis in pregnancy. *Clinics in Liver Disease, 3*(1), 115–130.

3. Regev, A., & Schiff, E. R. (2000). Viral hepatitis A, B, and C. *Clinics in Liver Disease, 4*(1), 47–71.

4. Cunningham, F. G., Gant, N. F., Leveno, K. J., Gilstrap, L. C., Hauth, J. C., & Wenstrom, K.D. (2005). *Williams obstetrics* (22nd ed., pp. 1129–1133). New York: McGraw-Hill.

5. American College of Obstetricians and Gynecologists. (1998). ACOG educational bulletin: Viral hepatitis in pregnancy. No. 248. *International Journal of Gynaecology and Obstetrics, 63*(2), 195–202.

6. Strader, D. B., Wright, T., Thomas, D. L., Seeff, & L. B.; American Association for the Study of Liver Disease. (2004). AASLD practice guideline: Diagnosis, management and treatment of hepatitis C. *Hepatology, 39*, 1147–1171.

7. Centers for Disease Control and Prevention. (1998). Recommendations for prevention and control of hepatitis C virus (HCV) infection and HCV-related chronic disease. *MMWR Morbidity and Mortality Weekly Report, 47*(RR-19), 1–39.

8. American College of Obstetricians and Gynecologists. (1998). ACOG committee opinion: Breastfeeding and the risk of hepatitis C virus transmission. No. 220. *International Journal of Gynaecology and Obstetrics, 66*(3), 307–308.

9. Zuckerman, J. N., & Zuckerman, A. J. (1999). The epidemiology of hepatitis B. *Clinics in Liver Disease, 3*(2), 179–187.

10. Center for Disease Control and Prevention. (2007). Surveillance for acute viral hepatitis—United States, 2005. *MMWR Surveillance Summaries, 56*(SS03), 1–24.

11. Centers for Disease Control and Prevention. (1988). Recommendations of the Immunization Practices Advisory Committee: Prevention of perinatal transmission of hepatitis B virus—Prenatal screening of all pregnant women for hepatitis B surface antigen. *MMWR Morbidity and Mortality Weekly Report, 37*(22), 341–346, 351.

12. Centers for Disease Control and Prevention. (2006). A comprehensive strategy to eliminate transmission of hepatitis B virus infection in the United States: Recommendations of the Advisory Committee on Immunization Practices (ACIP) Part II: Immunization of adults. *MMWR Morbidity and Mortality Weekly Report, 55*(RR16), 1–25.

13. Lok, A. S., & McMahon, B. J.; American Association for the Study of Liver Disease. (2007). AASLD practice guideline: Chronic hepatitis B. *Hepatology, 45*, 507–539.

14. Centers for Disease Control and Prevention. (1990). Protection against viral hepatitis: Recommendations of Immunization Practices Advisory Committee (ACIP). *MMWR Morbidity and Mortality Weekly Report, 39*(RR-2), 1–26.

15. Towers, C. V., Asrat, T., & Rumney, P. (2001). The presence of hepatitis B surface antigen and deoxyribonucleic acid in amniotic fluid and cord blood. *American Journal of Obstetrics and Gynecology, 184*, 1514–1520.

16. Committee on Obstetrics: Maternal and Fetal Medicine. (1992, March). *Guidelines for hepatitis B virus screening and vaccination during pregnancy* [ACOG Committee Opinion No. 103]. Washington, DC: American College of Obstetricians and Gynecologists.

17. Centers for Disease Control and Prevention. (1996). Prevention of perinatal group B streptococcal disease: A public health perspective. *MMWR Morbidity and Mortality Weekly Report, 45*(RR-7), 1–24.

18. Ingardia, C. J. (1999). Hepatitis B vaccination in pregnancy: Factors influencing efficacy. *Obstetrics and Gynecology, 93*(6), 983–986.

19. Centers for Disease Control and Prevention. (2005). A comprehensive strategy to eliminate transmission of hepatitis B virus infection in the United States: Recommendations of the Advisory Committee on Immunization Practices (ACIP) Part 1: Immunizations in infants, children and adolescents. *MMWR Morbidity and Mortality Weekly Report, 54*(RR16), 1–23.

20. Jefferson, T., Demicheli, V., Deeks, J., MacMillan, A., Sassi, F., & Pratt, M. (2000). Vaccines for preventing hepatitis B in health-care workers. *Cochrane Database System Review, (2)*, CD000100.

21. Centers for Disease Control and Prevention. (1989). Guidelines for the prevention of transmission of human immunodeficiency virus and hepatitis B virus to healthcare and public safety workers. *MMWR Morbidity and Mortality Weekly Report, 38*(S-6), 177.

22. Department of Labor, Occupational Safety and Health Administration. (1991). OSHA blood-borne pathogens final rule. *Federal Register, 56*(235, Pt II, excerpts), 64175–64182.

23. Centers for Disease Control and Prevention. (1995). Recommended childhood immunization schedule—United States. *MMWR Morbidity and Mortality Weekly Report, 44*(RR-5), 1–9.

24. Losonsky, G. A., Wasserman, S. S., Stephens, I., Mahoney, F., Armstrong, P., Gumpper, K., Dulkerian, S., West, D. J., & Gewolb, I. H. (1999). Hepatitis B vaccination of premature infants: A reassessment of current recommendations for delayed immunizations. *Pediatrics Electronic Pages, 103*(2), E14.

25. Yusuf, H. R., Daniels, D., Smith, P., Coronado, V., & Rodewald, L. (2000). Association between administration of

hepatitis B vaccine at birth and completion of the hepatitis B and 4: 3: 1: 3 vaccine series. *Journal of the American Medical Association, 284*(8), 978–983.

26. Centers for Disease Control and Prevention. (2001, June 29). Updated U.S. Public Health Service guidelines for the management of occupational exposures to HBV, HCV, and HIV and recommendations for postexposure prophylaxis. *MMWR Morbidity and Mortality Weekly Report, 50*(RR-11), 1–52.

27. American College of Obstetricians and Gynecologists. (1998). Hepatitis virus infections in obstetricians-gynecologists. ACOG committee opinion. *International Journal of Obstetrics and Gynecology, 63*, 203–204.

28. Department of Labor, Occupational Safety and Health Administration. (1991). (29 CFR Part 1910. 1030.) Occupational exposure to bloodborne pathogens: Final rule. *Federal Register, 56*, 64004–64182.

29. Centers for Disease Control and Prevention. (1997). Immunization of health-care workers: Recommendations of the Advisory Committee on Immunization Practices (ACIP) and the Hospital Infection Control Practices Advisory Committee (HICPAC). *MMWR Morbidity and Mortality Weekly Report, 46*(RR-18), 1–42.

30. Barash, C., Conn, M. I., DiMarino, A. J., Jr., Marzano, J., & Allen, M. L. (1999). Serologic hepatitis B immunity in vaccinated health care workers. *Archives of Internal Medicine, 159*(13), 1481–1483.

M O D U L E

12 Caring for the Pregnant Woman With Diabetes

MARY COPELAND MYERS

Objectives

As you complete this module, you will learn:

1. The epidemiology of diabetes mellitus and gestational diabetes
2. Perinatal consequences for women with preexisting diabetes and gestational diabetes
3. Preconception health care issues for diabetic women
4. Current classification and diagnostic criteria for diabetes mellitus
5. Characteristics of type 1 diabetes
6. Characteristics of type 2 diabetes
7. Characteristics of secondary diabetes
8. Characteristics of gestational diabetes
9. Physiology of normal glucose metabolism
10. Physiology of glucose metabolism during pregnancy
11. Pathophysiology of type 1, type 2, and gestational diabetes
12. Effect of pregnancy on preexisting diabetes
13. Effect of preexisting diabetes on pregnancy
14. Antepartum management goals for women with preexisting diabetes
15. Intrapartum management for women with preexisting diabetes
16. Postpartum management for women with preexisting diabetes
17. The pathophysiology of gestational diabetes
18. Diagnostic criteria for gestational diabetes
19. Antepartum management of pregnancy complicated by gestational diabetes
20. Intrapartum management of pregnancy complicated by gestational diabetes
21. Postpartum management of pregnancy complicated by gestational diabetes
22. Blood glucose goals during pregnancy
23. Signs and symptoms of hypoglycemia and proper treatment
24. Medical nutritional therapy requirements for diabetes during pregnancy
25. Exercise guidelines for women with diabetes during pregnancy
26. Insulin types and treatment regimens

diabetic ketoacidosis (DKA)
diabetogenic
endogenous insulin
euglycemia
exogenous insulin
hemoglobin A_{1c} (HbA_{1c})
hyperglycemic hyperosmolar nonketotic syndrome (HHNS)
hyperpnea
maturity-onset diabetes of youth (MODY)
nephropathy

neuropathy
organogenesis
polydipsia
polyphagia
polyuria
postprandial
preexisting diabetes or pregestational diabetes
proliferative retinopathy
retinopathy
tumor necrosis factor alpha (TNF-α)
leptin

Epidemiology of Diabetes

Diabetes is a significant public health challenge for the United States. In the United States, 20.8 million people (7% of the population) have diabetes. Of these people, 14.6 million are diagnosed and 6.2 million are undiagnosed. In addition, 54 million have prediabetes. Approximately 9.7 million or 8.8% of all women age 20 or older have diabetes. Each year, approximately 1.5 million people are diagnosed with new cases of diabetes.[1] Diabetes is becoming more common, with an increase in both prevalence and incidence. Currently, it is a chronic disease that has no cure and is the sixth leading cause of death in the United States.

Age, gender, and race affect the prevalence of diabetes. Prevalence increases with age (Table 12.1). In women age 20 and older, the prevalence increases to 9.7 million, compared with 10.9 million men. Diabetes is increased in non-Hispanic blacks, Hispanic/Latino Americans, American Indians, Alaska Natives, Asian Americans, and Native Hawaiian and Pacific Islanders (Table 12.2).[1]

TABLE 12.1 AGE AND PREVALENCE OF DIABETES

AGE (Y)	PERCENTAGE OF PEOPLE WITH DIABETES	NUMBER OF PEOPLE WITH DIABETES
$\leq$20	0.22	176,500
20–59	9.6	20.6 million
$\geq$60	20.9	10.3 million

TABLE 12.2 RACE/ETHNICITY AND PREVALENCE OF DIABETES AMONG PEOPLE AGED $\geq$20 YEARS

RACE/ETHNICITY	PERCENTAGE WITH DIABETES	INCREASED RISK OVER WHITES
Whites	8.7	—
African Americans	13.3	1.8
Hispanic/Latino Americans	9.5	1.7
American Indians and Alaska Natives	12.8	2.2
Asian Americans and Native Hawaiian or other Pacific Islanders	Not available	1.5–2.0

During pregnancy, 90% of all cases of diabetes are women with gestational diabetes mellitus (GDM). Approximately 7% of women in the United States are diagnosed with gestational diabetes.

Depending on race and ethnicity of the population, the prevalence may range from 1% to 14%.[2] Women with type 1 and type 2 diabetes have the most risk for perinatal consequences. Risks to the fetus depend on maternal glucose control during the time of conception and throughout the pregnancy.

Perinatal Consequences of Diabetes

Perinatal consequences depend on blood glucose control. In addition, the consequences differ depending on the gestational age when glycemic control is poor. If glycemic control is poor during conception and in the first trimester during *organogenesis* (first 8 weeks of gestation, when major organs are developing), congenital anomalies or miscarriage can occur. If glycemic control is poor during the second and third trimesters, metabolic consequences occur. The metabolic problems are attributable to increased insulin production by the fetus in response to the elevated blood glucose of the mother. However, in gestational diabetes, which usually develops and is diagnosed after 24 weeks' gestation, congenital anomalies are not a consequence. However, metabolic problems can be encountered if glycemic control is not optimal.

> If blood glucose is controlled during conception and throughout the pregnancy, perinatal consequences can be minimal.

Preconception health is an integral component of care for all women contemplating pregnancy. The March of Dimes Birth Defects Foundation recommends that preconception (prepregnancy planning) visits become a standard component of care.[3] *Unfortunately, preconception health care has not become a standard of care.* Unplanned pregnancies occur in about two thirds of women with diabetes.[4] In addition, fewer than one third of all diabetic women seek preconception counseling.[5] New goals aim at establishing preconception health screening as a part of routine care for all women of reproductive age.[6]

> Preconception care is recommended as a standard of care for all women of childbearing age.

> All women of childbearing age should be placed on a daily multivitamin with 0.4 mg of folic acid. Folic acid helps to reduce the risk of neural tube defects.

Preconception health care management for diabetic women should include the following:
- Patient education about the interaction of diabetes and pregnancy
- Education about diabetes self-management skills
- Medical care and laboratory testing
- Counseling by a mental health professional, as necessary, to reduce stress and improve adherence to the treatment plan

The specific goal is to lower HbA$_{1c}$ before conception to a level that is associated with optimal development during organogenesis. Organogenesis is the time of organ development and occurs 17 to 56 days after conception. The target goal is to have the HbA$_{1c}$ value at a level that is less than 1% above the normal range.[5] Normal values are 4% to 6%. See page 384

The following assessment should be completed:
- **Complete history and physical examination.**
- **Laboratory testing**—This should include Pap smear, complete blood count (CBC), HbA$_{1c}$, serum creatinine, thyroid studies, and 24-hour urine evaluation for total protein, creatine clearance, and microalbumin.
- **Medication usage**—All medications should be evaluated regarding their safety during pregnancy. For example, statins are pregnancy category X and should be discontinued before conception. In addition, angiotensin-converting enzyme (ACE) inhibitors and angiotension receptor blockers (ARBs) should be discontinued. Women taking these hypertensive medications should be assessed to determine whether the drug should be stopped or switched to another hypertensive medication.[7]
- **Current insulin regimen**—The blood glucose log should be reviewed and insulin adjustments made for optimal control. If oral diabetic agents are being used, the woman should be switched to insulin therapy. The FDA has not approved glyburide or metformin

for use during pregnancy. Both have been studied during pregnancy and currently we know the following:

- Glyburide does not cross the placenta and has been used successfully to treat gestational diabetes.
- Metformin, which is a category B drug, has been primarily used in patients with polycystic ovary syndrome (PCOS).

Although glyburide, which does not cross the placenta, has been used to treat gestational diabetes, and metformin, which is category B, has been used primarily in patients with PCOS, the use of oral agents to control type 2 diabetes should be limited until data regarding the safety and efficacy can be established.[4,5]

- **Dilated retinal examination**—Before pregnancy, evaluation should be performed by an ophthalmologist to assess for retinopathy.
- **Screening test for coronary artery disease if cardiac or vascular diseases are present**—Testing includes a lipid panel (cholesterol, high-density lipoprotein, low-density lipoprotein, very-low-density lipoprotein, and triglycerides), electrocardiogram (ECG), and blood pressure. This evaluates whether the patient can tolerate the increased cardiac demands of pregnancy.
- **Neurologic examination**—Assess for signs of peripheral and autonomic neuropathy.
- **Referral to a diabetes educator and a registered dietitian**—They will assist the woman with her diet, exercise, and self-management skills.
- **Counseling regarding risks associated with the effects of diabetes on the pregnancy and the effects of pregnancy on diabetes.**
- **Counseling regarding lifestyle changes to enhance health**—Examples include daily exercise, smoking cessation, cessation of alcoholic beverage intake, and adequate rest.
- **Contraception**—Stress the importance of using effective contraception while obtaining optimal glycemic control. If without vasculopathy and a nonsmoker, there are no specific contraceptive methods that are contraindicated in women with diabetes.[5] The woman's support system must be explored. She should be seen every 1 to 2 months after the initial visit to determine whether goals are being achieved and to assess for the presence of other coexisting medical complications. *Once goals are achieved, contraception may be discontinued.* Once conception has been achieved, the woman should be evaluated as early as possible to confirm her pregnancy and reinforce goals and management plans. She and her partner need to understand that even with *euglycemia* (normal blood glucose levels), it is not possible to reduce the incidence of congenital anomalies to zero. There remains the 2% to 3% incidence of congenital malformations found in the general population.[8]

Classification and Physiology of Diabetes

▶ **How is diabetes diagnosed?**

In 1997, the Expert Committee on the Diagnosis and Classification of Diabetes Mellitus updated the classification and diagnostic criteria for diabetes and impaired glucose homeostasis (Display 12.1). The committee also recommended eliminating the old categories of insulin-dependent diabetes mellitus (IDDM) and non–insulin-dependent diabetes mellitus (NIDDM). The new recommendations use the Arabic 1 and 2 (type 1 and type 2) instead of the Roman numerals I and II. In 2003, modifications were made regarding the diagnosis of impaired fasting glucose (IFG).[9]

DISPLAY 12.1 DIAGNOSTIC CRITERIA FOR DIABETES MELLITUS[4]

Diabetes can be diagnosed using any of the following three methods and **must** be confirmed on a subsequent day unless unequivocal symptoms of hyperglycemia are present.

1. Acute symptoms of diabetes (polyuria, polydipsia, and unexplained weight loss) plus a random plasma glucose 200 mg/dL or higher
2. Fasting (no calorie intake for 8 hours) plasma glucose 126 mg/dL or higher
3. 2-Hour plasma glucose 200 mg/dL or higher during an oral glucose tolerance test (OGTT); the OGTT should be performed according to the World Health Organization using a glucose load containing 75 g anhydrous glucose dissolved in water

The committee recognized two categories that indicate prediabetic conditions in which glucose metabolism is impaired: impaired fasting glucose (IFG) and impaired glucose tolerance (IGT; Display 12.2). IFG and IGT are risk factors for future diabetes and cardiovascular disease. Providers who care for pregnant women with these laboratory findings need to be aware of their relationship to a prediabetic condition.

DISPLAY 12.2 DIAGNOSTIC CRITERIA FOR IMPAIRED GLUCOSE[4]

1. IFG is diagnosed when the fasting glucose levels are 100 mg/dL to 125 mg/dL.
2. Impaired glucose tolerance (IGT) is diagnosed when the 2-hour oral glucose tolerance values are 140 mg/dL to 199 mg/dL.

NOTE: Impaired fasting glucose and impaired glucose tolerance are officially termed "prediabetes."[10]

▶ **What are the classifications of diabetes?**

The four etiologic classifications of diabetes are: type 1 diabetes, type 2 diabetes, other specific types of diabetes, and gestational diabetes.[10]

Type 1 diabetes is defined by the following characteristics:
- It accounts for 5% to 10% of all cases of diabetes in the United States.
- It develops at any age, but two thirds of all cases are diagnosed before age 18, and results from cellular-mediated autoimmune destruction of β cells in the pancreas. It usually leads to absolute insulin deficiency.
- Symptoms include significant weight loss, polyuria, and polydipsia with significant hyperglycemia.
- It has strong HLA associations with linkage to the DQA and B genes, and it is influenced by the DRB genes.
- The patient is dependent on **exogenous insulin** to prevent ketoacidosis and sustain life.
- **Diabetic ketoacidosis** (DKA) can occur. Coma and death can result if diagnosis and/or treatment are delayed.

Type 2 diabetes is defined by the following characteristics:
- It accounts for 90% to 95% of all cases of diabetes among people in the United States.
- It is usually diagnosed after the age of 30 but can occur at any age. Results from insulin resistance that progresses to an insulin secretory defect.
- Often, patients are asymptomatic at the time of diagnosis. Because type 2 diabetes frequently goes undiagnosed for years, many patients have end-organ complications such as retinopathy, neuropathy, or nephropathy at the time of diagnosis.
- Endogenous insulin levels may be increased, normal, or decreased. The need for exogenous insulin is variable.
- Insulin resistance with impaired glucose tolerance is usually seen in the first stages.
- Seldom does ketosis occur unless associated with a stressor such as another illness or an infection.
- Hyperglycemic hyperosmolar nonketotic syndrome (HHNS) may develop.
- Most patients are obese or have an increased percentage of body fat distributed mainly in the abdominal region.
- Risk of developing type 2 diabetes increases with age, obesity, and lack of physical activity.
- It has a strong genetic predisposition.

Other specific types of diabetes are diagnosed when diabetes occurs as the result of other disorders or the treatment of disorders (Display 12.3). The following are classified as other specific types of diabetes:
- Genetic defects of the pancreatic β cell
- Genetic defects in insulin action
- Diseases of the exocrine pancreas
- Endocrinopathies
- Drug- or chemical-induced diabetes
- Infections
- Uncommon forms of immune-mediated diabetes
- Other genetic syndromes sometimes associated with diabetes

| **DISPLAY 12.3** | ETIOLOGIC CLASSIFICATIONS OF DIABETES MELLITUS—OTHER SPECIFIC TYPES[10] |

A. Genetic defects of β-cell function
  1. Chromosome 12, HNF-1alpha (MODY3)
  2. Chromosome 7, glucokinase (MODY2)
  3. Chromosome 20, HNF-4alpha (MODY1)
  4. Chromosome 13, insulin promoter factor-1 (IPF-1: MODY4)
  5. Chromosome 17, HNF-1beta (MODY5)
  6. Chromosome 2, *NeuroD1* (MODY6)
  7. Mitochondrial DNA
  8. Others

B. Genetic defects in insulin action
  1. Type A insulin resistance
  2. Leprechaunism
  3. Rabson-Mendenhall syndrome
  4. Lipoatrophic diabetes
  5. Others

C. Diseases of the exocrine pancreas
  1. Pancreatitis
  2. Trauma/pancreatectomy
  3. Neoplasia
  4. Cystic fibrosis
  5. Hemochromatosis
  6. Fibrocalculous pancreatopathy
  7. Others

D. Endocrinopathies
  1. Acromegaly
  2. Cushing syndrome
  3. Glucogonoma
  4. Pheochromocytoma
  5. Hyperthyroidism
  6. Somatostatinoma
  7. Aldosteronoma
  8. Others

E. Drug or chemical induced
  1. Vacor
  2. Pentamidine
  3. Nicotinic acid
  4. Glucocorticoids
  5. Thyroid hormone
  6. Diazoxide
  7. β-Adrenergic agonists
  8. Thiazides
  9. Dilantin
  10. α-Interferon
  11. Others

F. Infections
  1. Congenital rubella
  2. Cytomegalovirus
  3. Others

G. Uncommon forms of immune-mediated diabetes
  1. "Stiff-man" syndrome
  2. Anti-insulin receptor antibodies
  3. Others

H. Other genetic syndromes sometimes associated with diabetes
  1. Down syndrome
  2. Klinefelter syndrome
  3. Turner syndrome
  4. Wolfram syndrome
  5. Friedreich ataxia
  6. Huntington chorea
  7. Laurence-Moon-Biedl syndrome
  8. Myotonic dystrophy
  9. Porphyria
  10. Prader-Willi syndrome
  11. Others

Adapted with permission: American Diabetes Association (2007). Diagnosis and classification of diabetes mellitus. *Diabetes Care*, 30,S42–S47.

Gestational diabetes has the following characteristics:
- Glucose intolerance develops or is first discovered during pregnancy. Definition does not exclude the possibility that the patient may have had previously undiagnosed type 2 diabetes.
- After pregnancy, the diagnostic classification may be changed to type 1, type 2, IFG, IGT, or normoglycemic.
- The occurrence of gestational diabetes increases the future risk for progression to type 2 diabetes.

Many classification systems have been developed to assist the health care provider in identifying risk factors. Priscilla White first published one commonly used classification system in 1932. It classifies patients on the basis of age at onset of diabetes, duration of disease, and secondary vascular and other end-organ complications, and it predicts perinatal risk according to these parameters (Table 12.3).

Normal Glucose Metabolism

Normal glucose metabolism involves the following pathways[11]:
1. After eating, carbohydrates are broken down into glucose.
2. The glucose is absorbed into the blood.
3. The glucose in the blood stimulates the pancreas to release insulin.

TABLE 12.3	WHITE'S CLASSIFICATIONS OF DIABETES			
CLASS	**DIABETES ONSET AGE (y)**			**DURATION (y)**
Gestational diabetes				
A1	Any			Any
A2	Any			Any
Pregestational diabetes				
B	>20		*or*	<10
C	10–19		*or*	10–19
D	<10		*or*	>20
F	Any			Any
R	Any			Any
T	Any			Any
H	Any			Any

From White, P. (1949). Pregnancy complicating diabetes. *American Journal of Medicine, 7,* 609–616.

4. The insulin is released from the β cells in the islets of Langerhans. Insulin is released in two phases:
   - A bolus release is the immediate rapid spike insulin response owing to hyperglycemia caused by the meal.
   - A basal release is the gradual release of insulin and is under the feedback control of the blood glucose. As glucose increases, the insulin release is increased. As glucose decreases, the insulin release is decreased.
5. Insulin causes the following actions:
   - Stimulates entry of glucose into cells for utilization as energy
   - Promotes the storage of glucose as glycogen in muscles and liver cells
   - Inhibits release of glucose from the liver or muscle glycogen
   - Stimulates entry of amino acids into cells
   - Enhances fat storage and prevents the mobilization of fat for energy
   - Inhibits the formation of glucose from non-carbohydrates (e.g., amino acids)

Normal Glucose Metabolism During Pregnancy

Many metabolic changes occur during pregnancy to optimize the growth of the fetus. Because the fetus depends entirely on the mother for its supply of energy, maternal adaptations must occur to increase glucose supply to the fetus.

Early in pregnancy, glucose homeostasis is altered by the increases in estrogen and progesterone that cause pancreatic β-cell hyperplasia (the cells multiply), with subsequent increased insulin secretion.

At the end of the first trimester, women with preexisting diabetes often experience hypoglycemia as a result of the following factors:
   - Increased glucose utilization (results in approximately a 10% reduction of maternal glucose)
   - Increased insulin secretion (results in increased glycogen stores and decreased hepatic glucose production)

In the second and third trimesters, levels of human placental lactogen (HPL), progesterone, estrogen, prolactin, placental growth hormone, and cortisol increase progressively and cause increasing tissue resistance to insulin action. Recent studies found that tumor necrosis factor alpha (TNF-α) and leptin also contribute to insulin resistance.[5] Insulin resistance is caused by a defect in the insulin receptor sites on cells. The defect does not allow the insulin to transport glucose into the cell. This causes a decrease in insulin function or sensitivity. If a patient has preexisting borderline β-cell reserve, hyperglycemia results. The following changes are seen:
   - Increased basal insulin level requirements owing to insulin resistance
   - Increased bolus insulin level requirements owing to insulin resistance
   - Increased infant glucose utilization

Throughout pregnancy, there is an increased risk for DKA and fasting ketosis due to the following factors:

- Decreased levels of alanine (a gluconeogenetic amino acid that is able to form glucose from substances other than carbohydrates such as fats and protein)
- Increased levels of fatty acids
- Increased triglycerides
- Increased ketones

These metabolic factors cause increased fat catabolism (breakdown), and decreased maternal glucose production in the fasting state. This allows for increased utilization of fat stores for energy, therefore protecting muscle mass breakdown.

Pathophysiology of Type 1, Type 2, and Gestational Diabetes

Type 1 diabetes is a result of an autoimmune attack on the β cells in the pancreas in individuals who carry a genetic marker identified on chromosomes 6 and 11, and possibly 10 other genes.[12] The stages of development involve a genetic predisposition, an environmental trigger, active autoimmunity directed against the β cells, progressive β-cell dysfunction, and then the clinical onset of diabetes.

Type 2 diabetes is a result of abnormal insulin secretion and resistance to insulin action in target tissue. There is not a genetic marker, but there is a genetic susceptibility. The following three phases occur before overt diabetes presents[13]:

1. In phase one, insulin resistance begins but plasma glucose remains normal because of an elevated insulin level.
2. In phase two, insulin resistance increases and *postprandial* (following a meal) hyperglycemia develops.
3. In phase three, insulin resistance remains the same but declining insulin secretion causes fasting hyperglycemia and overt diabetes.

Gestational diabetes is a result of the combination of insulin resistance and a diminished insulin secretion. *Pregnancy hormones such as HPL, estrogen, progesterone, prolactin, and cortisol are responsible for the increase in insulin resistance that is found later in pregnancy as the fetal–placental unit grows.* HPL is a hormone produced by the placenta. It is found in increasing levels as the pregnancy progresses and the placenta grows. Most recently, TNF-α and leptin have been identified as contributors to insulin resistance.[5] The diagnosis of gestational diabetes applies even if unrecognized glucose intolerance began before the onset of pregnancy.

▶ **What is the effect of pregnancy on preexisting diabetes?**

NOTE: Preexisting (type 1 and type 2) diabetes and pregnancy cause multiple effects on each other. Pregnancy affects insulin requirements, retinopathy, nephropathy, coronary artery disease, neuropathy, and DKA. In addition, diabetes can cause both maternal and fetal complications. (See Appendix B.)

Insulin requirements undergo many changes throughout pregnancy (Table 12.4). During the first trimester, the effect of morning sickness on nutritional intake may cause necessary changes in insulin requirements. By the end of the first trimester (10 to 16 weeks), because of metabolic changes, insulin needs may slightly decrease; however, from that point onward, insulin requirements steadily increase. During the third trimester, a two- to threefold increase in insulin requirements may be seen.[14] After delivery, insulin requirements dramatically decrease because the insulin resistance caused by HPL, progesterone, estrogen, prolactin, and cortisol is decreased.

TABLE 12.4	INSULIN REQUIREMENTS DURING PREGNANCY
GESTATIONAL PERIOD	**INSULIN REQUIREMENTS**
First trimester	Same or may be decreased (because of decreased nutritional intake from nausea and vomiting)
End of first trimester	Decreased
Second trimester	Increased
Third trimester	Increased
Postpartum	Decreased

Retinopathy (damage to the retina of the eye caused by microvascular deterioration from elevated blood glucose levels) is the leading cause of blindness in patients 24 to 64 years of age. Poor glycemic control contributes to the presence and severity of retinopathy. A woman with background retinopathy at the beginning of her pregnancy is at risk for progression. In most situations, background retinopathy regresses after delivery. Studies show that although pregnancy may accelerate the short-term progression of retinopathy, it has no long-term effect. One main contributor to this progression is the rapid change in glycemic control. *A rapid change in glycemic control of the blood glucose can cause short-term progression of retinopathy.* This is often the situation encountered when the patient begins pregnancy in poor control, and because of the risks of congenital anomalies, she is encouraged to obtain quick glycemic control.[15] Also, hypertensive patients are more likely to have progression of retinopathy.[16] Women with untreated **proliferative** retinopathy should undergo laser photocoagulation to stabilize their eyes before pregnancy. During pregnancy, close surveillance must be maintained by an ophthalmologist. Recommendations include an eye examination in the first trimester with close follow-up throughout pregnancy and for 1 year postpartum.[4]

> Because of the increased pressure in the eyes caused by pushing during the second stage of labor, Valsalva pushing in a vaginal delivery is **contraindicated** in a woman with untreated proliferative retinopathy. This, however, does not prevent a vaginal delivery. Delivery can be accomplished with open glottis and/or passive descent in the second stage of labor.

Diabetic nephropathy occurs in 5% to 10% of pregnancies. *Nephropathy* is disease of the kidneys caused by microvascular changes. Although progression to end-stage renal disease has been reported in women with serum creatinine levels greater than 1.5 mg/dL or severe proteinuria, most studies indicated that women with mild to moderate diabetic nephropathy do not have permanent deterioration in renal function.[5] The most serious consequences of diabetic nephropathy during pregnancy are maternal hypertensive complications including preeclampsia, preterm birth secondary to worsening maternal disease, and fetal growth restrictions secondary to uteroplacental insufficiency. *The incidence of preeclampsia is 15% to 20% among women with type 1 diabetes without nephropathy. However, if nephropathy is present, approximately 50% will develop preeclampsia.*[17] *Renal function should be assessed initially and every trimester.* Proteinuria progresses during gestation, but studies have failed to demonstrate a permanent worsening to advanced renal disease or end-stage renal disease.[18,19]

In regard to chronic hypertension, ACE inhibitors are contraindicated in pregnancy. They cause fetal hypotension and oligohydramnios. Methyldopa and hydralazine have been proven safe for use in pregnancy. **Perinatal complications encountered with hypertension associated with nephropathy include intrauterine growth restriction (IUGR), preeclampsia, and abruptio placentae.**[20]

Coronary artery disease is commonly seen in women with long-standing diabetes along with nephropathy and hypertension. Myocardial stress may occur due to pregnancy associated hemodynamic changes and may result in myocardial infarction and death.[21]

> Coronary heart disease during a pregnancy complicated with diabetes is a serious situation. It is a potential contraindication to pregnancy.

Diabetic *neuropathy* is a disease of the nervous system that involves peripheral nerve dysfunction. Potential complications from diabetic neuropathy in the pregnant woman may involve the following:
- Nausea and vomiting secondary to gastroparesis
- Urinary retention
- Hypoglycemia unawareness
- Orthostatic hypotension
- Carpal tunnel syndrome

Metoclopramide (Reglan) can be used for women with gastroparesis. This drug may aid in improving nutritional status and glucose control. Both family and patient education regarding safety must be provided for those with hypoglycemia unawareness, orthostatic hypotension, and carpal tunnel syndrome. Hand braces may provide some relief for patients with carpal tunnel syndrome. Foot care should be discussed with all patients.

DKA is a life-threatening emergency seen in 5% to 10% of pregnancies complicated by diabetes. Maternal mortality is rare, but fetal mortality ranges from 10% to 35%.[5] A higher incidence is seen during pregnancy because DKA develops more rapidly and at less severe levels of hyperglycemia. Most cases of DKA are in patients with undiagnosed new-onset diabetes. **The most common cause of DKA is infection.** Additional risk factors unique to pregnancy are the use of β-sympathomimetic tocolytic drugs and antenatal corticosteroids.[22] *The hallmarks of DKA treatment consist of fluid replacement and insulin therapy.*

► What is the effect of preexisting diabetes on pregnancy?

The effect of diabetes on pregnancy impacts both the mother and the fetus. The following risks are increased:

Maternal Consequences
- Preeclampsia
- Bacterial infections
- Polyhydramnios
- Birth trauma from macrosomic infants
- Preterm labor
- Cesarean delivery
- Postpartum hemorrhage
- DKA

Fetal Consequences
- Congenital anomalies
- Spontaneous abortion
- Macrosomia
- Intrauterine fetal death (IUFD)
- Delayed pulmonary maturity
- Hypoglycemia at birth
- Hyperbilirubinemia and polycythemia
- Hypocalcemia
- Decreased magnesium serum levels
- Intrauterine growth restriction
- Delayed lung maturity
- Learning disabilities
- Childhood obesity and type 2 diabetes later in life

> Congenital anomalies and spontaneous abortion are the two major fetal complications seen in women who have poor glycemic control during the period of fetal organogenesis.

Hyperglycemia in the first trimester can result in numerous complications. Organogenesis is the development of the major organs of the fetus and occurs during the first 8 weeks of gestation. The average risk of congenital anomalies among diabetics is 6% to 12%. This is four times more frequent than the general population.[5] Structural anomalies *mainly* involve the following:
- Central nervous system (neural tube defects)
- Cardiovascular system
- Skeletal system (sacral agenesis)

Glycosylated hemoglobin levels correlate directly to the rate of fetal anomalies. If the level is less than 7%, fetal anomalies are not increased. At less than 7%, the risk is close to the general population risk of 2% to 3%. If the level of the glycosylated hemoglobin is close to 10%, the risk of fetal anomalies is 20% to 25%.[23]

In regard to spontaneous abortion, rates also correlate with blood glucose control at the time of conception. Ensuring normal blood glucose values at the time of conception and during the first trimester, when organ development occurs, can reduce the risk of both spontaneous abortion and congenital anomalies.

Hyperglycemia in the second and third trimesters results in metabolic complications. If maternal physiologic glucose control is lacking, maternal hyperglycemia occurs. Pathologic elevated glucose levels lead to higher amounts of glucose transfer across the placenta to the fetus. Because the fetal pancreas begins to function at approximately 13 weeks' gestation, the fetal pancreas responds to the elevated fetal glucose levels. Fetal hyperglycemia results in increased fetal insulin output or fetal hyperinsulinism. The outcome of the fetal response is accelerated fetal growth, resulting in large-for-gestational-age (LGA) infants and macrosomia. *Macrosomia is generally defined as an infant weight above the 90th percentile or greater than 4,000 g.* Macrosomic infants and LGA infants have increased requirements for oxygen. If the increased demand for oxygen exceeds the supply available, fetal distress or IUFD may occur. Hyperglycemia also causes an increase in fetal erythropoietin production, which leads to polycythemia and hyperbilirubinemia. In addition, severe prolonged hyperinsulinemia interferes with the transport of oxygen and carbon dioxide, which leads to a decrease in fetal pH, increased P_{CO_2}, lactate, and erythropoietin incompatible with life.[24]

An additional risk for diabetic women is **preterm labor**. Management includes nifedipine, magnesium sulfate, or indomethacin. β-Sympathomimetics are not recommended because they can cause severe hyperglycemia. In addition, corticosteroids should be used only under close observation of blood glucose values and intensive insulin therapy to avoid the potential risk of hyperglycemia.

When delivery plans are being made, the **pulmonary maturity of the infant** must be ensured. *Among preexisting diabetic women, the risk of pulmonary immaturity is not passed until after 39 weeks' gestation.* In the nondiabetic patient, by 37 weeks' gestation more than 99% of infants have mature pulmonary profiles. However, with diabetic mothers, hyperglycemia and hyperinsulinemia cause a delay in fetal maturity due to an interference with the production of phosphatidyl glycerol.[24]

Lung maturity must be assessed through amniocentesis in all preexisting diabetic women if delivery is planned before 39 weeks' gestation.

In addition, **at the time of delivery, the infant must be assessed carefully for signs of hypoglycemia.** *Hypoglycemia is a plasma glucose level of less than 35 mg/dL in the term infant* and less than 25 mg/dL in the premature infant. Hypoglycemia is caused by the elimination of excess maternal blood glucose when the cord is cut and the continued excess production of insulin by the infant. *The peak incidence of neonatal hypoglycemia is 6 to 12 hours after birth.*[14] *The incidence of neonatal hypoglycemia is 64.1% and occurs in both macrosomic and non-macrosomic infants.*[25] In regard to future implications for infants of diabetic mothers, both an increased risk for glucose intolerance and obesity have been noted. If the mother has type 2 diabetes, the risk for her child to develop type 2 diabetes later in life is 70%. Due to the islet cell injury that occurs in utero secondary to the exposure to hyperglycemia, the risk of childhood obesity and childhood type 2 diabetes is higher.[26]

Management of Diabetes in the Pregnant Woman

Preexisting Diabetes

Antepartum Management for Mothers with Preexisting Diabetes

The three hallmarks in the treatment of diabetes during pregnancy include the following:
1. Medical nutritional therapy (MNT)
2. Exercise
3. Insulin therapy

Careful attention to each component is essential for optimal glucose control.

Antepartum management includes the evaluation, education, and/or treatment for the following factors:
- MNT
- Exercise

- Self-management of blood glucose (SMBG)
  - Preprandial capillary blood glucose goals are below 95 mg/dL.
  - One-hour postprandial glucose values are more predictive of macrosomia than fasting values. The goal for the one hour postprandial glucose value is less than 130 to 140 mg/dL.
  - Two-hour postprandial glucose goals are below 120 mg/dL.[27]
- Insulin regimen
- Medications
  - All women should continue a prenatal vitamin, which contains 0.4 mg of folic acid.
  - All medications should be assessed for their safety during pregnancy.
- Prenatal laboratory tests
  - In addition to routine prenatal laboratory tests, an HbA_{1c}, thyroid panel, serum creatinine, 24-hour urine for total protein, microalbumin, and creatinine should be obtained.
- ECG
  - A baseline ECG should be obtained to rule out a preexisting cardiac problem.
- Ophthalmologic examination
  - A thorough baseline examination is needed to determine the existence or extent of retinopathy.
  - Recommendations include an eye examination in the first trimester with close follow-up throughout pregnancy and for 1 year postpartum.[4]
- Maternal serum α-fetoprotein (MSAFP)
  - MSAFP should be offered to all diabetic women between 14 and 22 weeks gestation because of the increased risk of neural tube defects.
- HbA_{1c}
  - Repeat every 4 to 6 weeks to monitor glucose control.
- Ultrasound
  - An ultrasound should be done initially to confirm viability. It should be repeated at approximately 18 to 20 weeks for anatomic survey. A screening fetal echocardiogram is indicated. Cardiac views are best imaged near 20 to 22 weeks of pregnancy.
  - Growth should be assessed every 4 weeks as clinically indicated.
- Fetal kick counts
  - Fetal kick counts should be taught to women and should begin daily at 28 weeks' gestation.
- Antepartum fetal monitoring
  - Includes nonstress test (NST), the biophysical profile, and the contraction stress test (CST).
  - Initial testing should begin at 32 to 34 weeks. The NST is most commonly used. Twice weekly testing has been adopted because of the risk of stillbirth. With poor glycemic control, NSTs may begin as early as 28 weeks' gestation. If the test is nonreactive, a biophysical profile should be obtained. In women with vascular complications, Doppler velocimetry of the umbilical artery may be used.[5]
- Delivery plan
  - The timing of delivery should be based on maternal glucose control, maternal health, and fetal status.
  - As a general rule, diabetic women should be delivered between 39 and 40 weeks. If delivery is planned electively before 39 weeks, an amniocentesis must be performed to confirm lung maturity.
  - A cesarean delivery is recommended if the estimated fetal weight is greater than 4,500 g.[18]

Intrapartum Management for Mothers With Preexisting Diabetes

Timing of delivery and the route of delivery should be based on clinical judgment. Indications for delivery include the following:

- Nonreassuring fetal status
- Arrest or decline in fetal growth rate owing to vasculopathy
- Macrosomia with fetal lung maturity
- Severe preeclampsia
- Nephropathy
- Decreased maternal renal function

- Poor glucose control
- Preterm labor with failure of tocolysis
- Fetal maturity greater than 38.5 weeks
- History of stillbirth

> Intrapartum management goals include providing adequate carbohydrate intake for energy requirements and maintaining maternal glucose control.

In patients with excellent glucose control, delivery may be delayed; **however, after 40 weeks' gestation, the benefits of delivery outweigh the benefits of conservative management because of the danger of fetal compromise.**

A protocol for insulin infusion to maintain glycemic control includes the following algorithm[28]:

- At bedtime, give usual dose of intermediate acting insulin.
- Withhold the morning insulin.
- Begin and maintain a glucose infusion of D_5W at 100 to 150 cc/hr once active labor begins or glucose levels decrease to less than 70 mg/dL.
- Goal is to maintain blood glucose level at approximately 100 mg/dL.
- Monitor maternal blood glucose every hour.
- Administer regular insulin by IV infusion at a rate of 1.25 U/hr if glucose levels exceed 100 mg/dL.

In addition to using an intravenous insulin drip, the insulin pump may also be used to maintain euglycemia during labor and delivery. For type 2 diabetic patients in excellent control, blood glucose control may be achieved by avoiding dextrose intravenous fluids. Blood glucose must be monitored hourly. At delivery, the newborn must be assessed for hypoglycemia. Preventing intrapartum hyperglycemia reduces the chance of neonatal hypoglycemia.[29]

Continuous fetal monitoring should be used during labor to monitor the infant closely for signs of distress. **The provider must watch carefully for indications of shoulder dystocia because many infants are macrosomic.** Indications of shoulder dystocia include an estimated fetal weight of more than 4,000 g, a dysfunctional labor curve, a prolonged second stage, and the "turtle" sign occurring with the delivery of the head (the head is extremely tight against the perineum). Early induction of labor for macrosomia is not endorsed by ACOG. However, among diabetic women, a cesarean delivery should be considered if the estimated fetal weight is greater than 4,500 g.[5]

Postpartum Management for Mothers With Preexisting Diabetes

The management issues during the postpartum period include insulin adjustment, care of the newborn, breastfeeding, and balancing of self-care needs of the mother with the needs of her newborn.

> **After the delivery, insulin requirements decrease dramatically. Often, very little or no insulin is required for the first 24 to 72 hours. If required, the insulin dose should be recalculated based on one half of the predelivery dose.**

Breastfeeding should be encouraged. *Oral hyperglycemic agents cannot be used while lactating.* Breastfeeding patients should also be informed that hypoglycemia may occur during a nursing session. Postpartum caloric requirements are increased. Breastfeeding women need an additional caloric intake of 500 kcal/d.[30]

At the postpartum visit, a complete physical examination should be performed, and education on contraceptive methods, diet, exercise, insulin regimen, glucose control, and HbA_{1c} should be assessed. Counseling regarding future pregnancies is important. Last, assurance must be made that the woman has a health care provider to monitor and assist her with diabetes care between pregnancies.

Gestational Diabetes

Gestational diabetes is defined as carbohydrate intolerance and consists of both insulin resistance and diminished insulin secretion during pregnancy. It has implications for both the mother and the baby. The mother has an increased risk for the following:

- Preeclampsia and hypertensive disorders
- Polyhydramnios
- Cesarean section because of fetal macrosomia
- Excessive weight gain

Of great significance is the risk for the mother to develop type 2 diabetes or glucose intolerance later in life. Estimates vary on the risks of type 2 diabetes after gestational diabetes. Estimates range from 17% to 63% within 5 to 16 years after pregnancy.[31] A recent study revealed the 8th-year cumulative risk of postpartum diabetes was 52.7%.[32] Insulin use, ethnicity, elevated body mass index, detection of islet autoantibodies and age at delivery are all predictors for the long-term development of type 2 diabetes; however, insulin use during pregnancy is the strongest predictor.[33]

The fetus has an increased risk for the following:
- Macrosomia
- Birth trauma
- Shoulder dystocia
- Hypoglycemia
- Hypocalcemia
- Hyperbilirubinemia
- Respiratory distress syndrome
- Polycythemia

Long-term implications for the offspring are an increased risk for obesity and impaired glucose tolerance or diabetes later in life.[34] Of importance is that in the presence of fasting hyperglycemia greater than 105 mg/dL is associated with an increased risk of intrauterine fetal death in the last 4 to 8 weeks of gestation.[2]

▶ **How is gestational diabetes diagnosed?**

The diagnosis of gestational diabetes is a two-step process[35]

1. An initial screening test—1-hour glucose challenge test (GCT; Table 12.5)

TABLE 12.5	IMPLICATIONS OF 1-HOUR GLUCOSE CHALLENGE TEST (GCT)
GCT RESULTS (mg/dL)	**IMPLICATION**
>140–199	Requires 3-hour GTT
≥200	Treat for gestational diabetes; do not perform a 3-hour GTT

2. A diagnostic test—3-hour glucose tolerance test (GTT; for those who fail the screening test; Table 12.6)

TABLE 12.6	CUT-OFF VALUES FOR THE 3-HOUR GLUCOSE TOLERANCE TEST (GTT)	
TIME	**NATIONAL DIABETES DATA GROUP (mg/dL)**	**CARPENTER AND COUSTAN (mg/dL)**
Fasting	105	95
1 hour	190	180
2 hour	165	155
3 hour	145	140

All women should be screened by their history, clinical risk factors, or laboratory screening. The optimal method of screening is controversial; therefore, many providers elect to screen all their patients by laboratory testing. However, if a woman is low risk, laboratory testing may be omitted. Women are considered low risk if they meet the following criteria:

1. Younger than 25 years of age
2. Body mass index of 25 or less
3. No first-degree relatives with diabetes mellitus

4. Not of an ethnic group that is at increased risk of type 2 diabetes mellitus (including Latinos, Native Americans, Asians, Africans, African Americans, Pacific Islanders, indigenous Australians, and women from the Indian subcontinent)
5. No previous history of abnormal glucose tolerance
6. No previous history of adverse obstetric outcomes usually associated with gestational diabetes[18,35]

Some women are considered at high risk for developing gestational diabetes and should be screened earlier at the initial visit. If she passes the initial early screen, she should be rescreened at 24 to 28 weeks' gestation. In addition, in the situation where a high-risk woman passes the laboratory screening at 24 to 28 weeks, if clinically indicated, additional laboratory screening should be done at a later date. High-risk factors include[2]:

- Positive family history for diabetes in parents or siblings
- Poor obstetric history, including unexplained stillbirth, fetal anomaly, or recurrent spontaneous abortions
- History of delivery of infant with birth weight of 9 pounds or more
- Obesity
- Multiple gestation
- Polycystic ovary syndrome
- Hypertensive disorder
- Recurrent monilial vaginitis
- Polyhydramnios without fetal anomalies
- Glycosuria on two consecutive visits
- High-risk ethnic descent: Native American, Hispanic American, Asian American, African American, or Pacific Islander

The initial screening with a 1-hour GCT is recommended between 24 and 28 weeks' gestation. The screening 1-hour Glucola test consists of having the woman drink a 50-g glucose solution and drawing a venous plasma glucose measurement in 1 hour. The screening test can be done at any time of the day. The woman does not need to be fasting before the test. She must be sitting during the test and smoking is contraindicated. A value of 140 mg/dL or lower is considered normal. A value greater than 140 to 199 requires a 3-hour GTT. If the test is 200 mg/dL or higher, the 3-hour GTT is contraindicated and the patient is diagnosed and treated for gestational diabetes.[18]

The 3-hour GTT is the diagnostic test and should be performed fasting but after the women has consumed at least 3 days of an unrestricted diet of at least 150 g of carbohydrates. It consists of obtaining a fasting (at least 8 hours but no more than 14 hours) blood glucose level followed by having the patient drink 100 g of glucose. The venous blood glucose is drawn at 1 hour, 2 hours, and 3 hours. The diagnosis of gestational diabetes can be made with the diagnostic criteria of the National Diabetes Data Group (NDDG) *or* the diagnostic criteria of Carpenter and Coustan. The diagnostic criteria of Carpenter and Coustan have been endorsed by the American Diabetes Association. **If two or more values are met or exceeded, the patient is diagnosed with gestational diabetes.**[18] If only one abnormal value is obtained on the 3-hour GTT, it is recommended that the test be repeated in 4 weeks. Women with only one elevated value have an increased risk of macrosomia.[36] Another method for diagnosing gestational diabetes is based on the results of a 75-g GTT based on the World Health Organization (WHO) criteria. It is most commonly used outside of the United States and is not as well validated.

Antepartum Management for Mothers With Gestational Diabetes

Treatment of gestational diabetes includes the following:

- MNT
- SMBG
- Exercise
- Pharmacologic therapy if indicated
- Fetal surveillance

MNT, exercise, and SMBG are usually the first line of therapy. Exercise, if not medically contraindicated, does improve insulin sensitivity. Women should be encouraged to exercise daily for 20 to 30 minutes.

MNT based on maternal weight and height is recommended. For women with ideal prepregnancy body weight, the caloric prescription is 30 kcal/kg. If underweight, the caloric prescription is 35 kcal/kg. For obese women, 25 kcal/kg is recommended. **Among obese**

women, a reduction of carbohydrates to 35% to 40% of calories has been shown to decrease maternal glucose levels and improve maternal and fetal outcomes.[37] Recommended blood glucose goals are as follows: fasting levels below 95 mg/dL, 1-hour postprandial values below 130 to 140 mg/dL, and 2-hour postprandial below 140 mg/dL.[18,35]

Women should check their fasting and 1- or 2-hour postprandial glucose values each day. If more than one half of blood glucose values are repeatedly above the desired goal even with diet and exercise, pharmacologic treatment should be initiated. Approximately 30% to 40% of women require pharmacologic treatment.[38] Either insulin therapy or glyburide therapy are acceptable.

The choice of insulin type and regimen should be based on the patient's glucose profile and lifestyle. *The same calculations used in calculating insulin requirements for type 1 and type 2 diabetes are used to calculate insulin requirements for gestational diabetes.* The recommended dose of insulin is based on the women's weight and gestational age. During the first trimester, it is 0.8 U/kg per day. During the second trimester it is 1.0 U/kg per day, and during the third trimester it is 1.2 U/kg per day.[39,40] If with type 2 diabetes, higher doses of 1 to 2 U/kg may be necessary due to insulin resistance plus the requirements of pregnancy. In regard to achieving optimal glucose control and reducing the risk of fetal macrosomia, the insulin analogs LiPro and Aspart have been proven more effective than regular insulin.[41] Throughout pregnancy, due to the increasing placental diabetogenic hormones, adjustments to insulin therapy must be made every 7 to 14 days. Changes of approximately 10% of the total dosage can be made to achieve SMBG goals.

In the past several years, glyburide has become an alternative to insulin therapy. As with insulin, the main risk is hypoglycemia. It is contraindicated in women with an allergy to sulfa. The starting dose is 2.5 mg twice a day and can be increased to a maximum dose of 10 mg twice a day.[18] Although research has been done to compare the use of glyburide (an oral diabetogenic medication) with insulin use among women with gestational diabetes, its use during pregnancy has *not* been approved by the U.S. Food and Drug Administration.

In addition, metformin has been studied in the first trimester for women with polycystic ovary syndrome, but at this time, it is not approved for use in gestational diabetes. Initial studies indicate that metformin may be safe and reduce the risk of miscarriage and development of gestational diabetes when used the entire pregnancy.[42]

Much controversy remains regarding the criteria for initiation and timing of fetal testing. All GDM patients should begin daily fetal movement counts at 28 weeks' gestation. Patients with well-controlled diabetes are at low risk for intrauterine fetal death. Fetal surveillance for patients with diet-only therapy usually consists of NSTs twice a week beginning at 40 weeks. *Fetal surveillance for patients receiving pharmacologic therapy, have a history of stillbirth, or have hypertension, is managed in a manner similar to the management in preexisting diabetes.* Initial testing with a NST is performed each week from 32 weeks until 36 weeks and then twice a week until delivery.

Fetal movement counts are taught to all patients and should begin on a daily basis at 28 weeks' gestation until delivery. The most common technique is the "count to 10" technique, which involves the mother monitoring the time it takes to feel 10 fetal movements. If 10 movements are not felt within a 2-hour limit, the patient is to call her provider. In addition to the NSTs and fetal movement counts, an ultrasound examination is often completed to evaluate fetal growth. Frequency of performing ultrasound is based on clinical judgment. If estimated fetal weight is 4,500 grams or more, a cesarean delivery should be considered to decrease the risk of shoulder dystocia.[18]

Delivery plans are based on glucose control and cervical evaluation. If well controlled, patients may progress to their due dates. If poorly controlled, elective delivery may be considered at 38 to 39 weeks' gestation. If delivery is scheduled before 39 weeks gestation, fetal lung maturity must be assessed.[18] Elective delivery at term should be considered if the following conditions are true:

- Glycemic control is suboptimal.
- The patient requires pharmacologic therapy.
- Fetal monitoring is not reassuring.
- The patient has a history of stillbirth.
- Other complications exist (e.g., hypertension, preeclampsia).

> If delivery is planned before the 39th week of gestation, lung maturity should first be assessed.[18]

If expectant management is used, fetal growth must be monitored carefully because of the risk of macrosomia with advancing gestational age. Induction should not be based only on suspected fetal macrosomia. Evidence from multiple studies does not support a policy of early induction of labor for suspected fetal macrosomia.[43]

Intrapartum Management for Mothers With Gestational Diabetes

The goals of glucose management during labor are the same as those for preexisting diabetes. The blood glucose should be monitored and, if necessary, an insulin drip initiated. With diet-controlled gestational diabetes, rarely is glucose control a problem during labor. **A major risk factor during delivery for all diabetic patients is shoulder dystocia.** Risk factors for shoulder dystocia are multifactorial and include the following:

- Fetal macrosomia
- Maternal diabetes
- Maternal obesity
- Excessive maternal weight gain
- Multiparity
- Advanced gestational age
- Prolonged second stage of labor
- Midpelvic delivery
- Postdate pregnancy
- Previous macrosomia
- Previous shoulder dystocia

Infants of mothers with either gestational or preexisting diabetes usually weigh more than infants of nondiabetic mothers. These infants often display asymmetric growth in which there is a disproportionate increase in chest and shoulder size related to the head circumference. **Although the occurrence of shoulder dystocia is often difficult to predict, health providers should always be aware of its potential effect on the delivery and know the proper techniques to manage it.**

Postpartum Management for Mothers With Gestational Diabetes

With the delivery of the fetal–placental unit, the diabetogenic (diabetic-causing) effect of placental hormones are diminished. Therefore, women with gestational diabetes usually regain glycemic control. To ensure that this occurs, blood glucose values should be assessed in the immediate postpartum period by checking fasting and postprandial glucose values. Assessment of maternal glycemic status should be reevaluated at approximately 6 weeks.

> **All women with gestational diabetes should receive a 2-hour oral glucose tolerance test with 75 g of glucose during the postpartum period.**

Because breastfeeding can cause a lower blood glucose reading, the 2-hour GTT should be performed after the patient has stopped breastfeeding. Upon testing, the woman should be reclassified as diabetic, IFG, impaired glucose tolerance (IGT), or normoglycemic (normal blood glucose). After delivery, approximately 15% of patients will have the diagnosis of IFG, IGT, or diabetes.[18] All patients should also be educated regarding lifestyle modifications such as exercise and diet. Exercise, proper diet, and breastfeeding help the mother to maintain normal body weight, which helps to decrease insulin resistance. Symptoms of hyperglycemia should be reviewed with her. If these symptoms occur later in life, medical attention should be obtained. Assessment of glucose control should be recommended at a minimum of 3-year intervals.[2] Future pregnancy plans and contraceptive methods should also be discussed. Future pregnancy plans should be reviewed, with emphasis on ensuring optimal glycemic control before the next conception. A comprehensive literature review from 1965 to 2006 revealed a recurrence rate of GDM between 30% to 84%.[44]

▶ What are blood glucose goals during pregnancy?

SMBG is an *essential* element in the treatment plan of patients with diabetes. It provides the patient with immediate feedback. It assists her in achieving and maintaining her blood glucose goals, preventing and detecting hypoglycemia, and determining necessary adjustments in pharmacologic therapy, diet, and exercise. Remember, however, that the accuracy of the values obtained depends on the accuracy of the blood glucose meter. All patients should be taught how to properly do the following:

- Use the meter
- Check the meter calibration
- Use control solutions
- Store reagent strips
- Perform proper fingerstick technique
- Clean the meter
- Dispose of lancets
- Interpret data

Maternal glucose goals during pregnancy are shown in Table 12.7.

The frequency and timing of SMBG must be individualized. The best method of SMBG requires obtaining both premeal, postprandial glucose levels, and bedtime levels; however, few patients are willing to collect all of these samples. Most patients taking insulin prefer to obtain

TABLE 12.7 MATERNAL GLUCOSE GOALS DURING PREGNANCY[18]

TIME	BLOOD GLUCOSE GOALS: ACOG RECOMMENDATIONS (mg/dL)[18,35]	BLOOD GLUCOSE GOALS: ADA RECOMMENDATIONS (mg/dL)[27]
Preprandial plasma glucose	<95	<105
1-Hour postprandial plasma glucose	<130–140	<155
2-Hour postprandial plasma glucose	<120	<130

premeal blood glucose values because it is the most convenient and because this is the time they administer their insulin. A premeal blood glucose reading allows them to adjust their insulin according to their current blood glucose. However, patients following dietary therapy or taking oral medications should obtain postprandial blood glucose values. This value allows them to observe how their blood glucose responded to the carbohydrate content of the meal. During pregnancy, a 1-hour postprandial glucose value is more predictive of macrosomia than fasting values.

Many glucose meters are available to patients. Basic teaching should include the demonstration of proper technique and allow time for return demonstration by the patient. The accuracy of the results depends mainly on three factors: the quality of the meter, the quality of the test strips, and the proper training of the patient. Additional factors include hematocrit, altitude, temperature, humidity, and other substances. High hematocrit values test lower for blood glucose and low hematocrit values test higher for blood glucose than patients with a normal hematocrit. Altitude, room temperature, and humidity can cause unpredictable results. Substances such as uric acid, glutathione, and ascorbic acid also may interfere with testing results.[45]

Alternative site testing in the upper arm, forearm, base of the thumb, and thigh are allowed by some glucose meters. Although desirable, limitations exist. The common fingertip samples show changes in glucose more quickly than blood samples from other parts of the body. Therefore values may differ due to the actual glucose concentration in the body part. The FDA endorses further research due to the impact on patients.

In addition to standard glucose meters, the FDA has approved one minimally invasive meter and one noninvasive glucose meter. They are not meant to replace standard testing, but to obtain additional values between fingerstick values. The minimally invasive meter is from MiniMed. The MiniMed Continuous Glucose Monitoring System uses a catheter inserted subcutaneously into the abdomen to collect small amounts of liquid that passes through a "biosensor" to measure the amount of glucose present. It collects values over a 72-hour period and must be downloaded to a computer. It is intended to reveal trends in glucose levels. The noninvasive glucose meter is the Cygnus GlucoWatch Biographer. It is worn on the arm like a wristwatch and pulls tiny amounts of fluid from the skin. It can provide up to three glucose measurements per hour for 12 hours. The results can be immediately read by the patient. It is useful in detecting and treating episodes of hypoglycemia. The results are to show trends and not replace finger stick glucose values.[45]

An additional method used to monitor glucose control over an extended period is the **glycosylated hemoglobin (HbA$_{1c}$)**. The HbA$_{1c}$ measures the percentage of glycosylation that occurs in red blood cells (RBCs). Glycosylation is the linkage of hemoglobin to glucose.

Most of the hemoglobin in adults is hemoglobin A. Glycosylated hemoglobin can be separated from hemoglobin A by a laboratory technique called "electrophoresis." The three separated factions of hemoglobin A are HbA$_{1a}$, HbA$_{1b}$, and HbA$_{1c}$. Normally, only HbA$_{1c}$ is measured.

Glycosylation of hemoglobin is a slow, continuous process throughout the replenishing of RBCs during their 120-day life span. The more RBCs are exposed to glucose, the higher the percentage of glycosylated hemoglobin. Because the RBC has a life span of approximately 120 days, the test is able to reflect the blood glucose control during this time (Table 12.8).

Although this test is useful to providers and patients as a method to measure overall blood glucose control, it is not useful in adjusting insulin levels on a daily basis. SMBG must be performed daily. Of importance, several factors can alter the results and cause false values. These factors include[45]:

- Diseases affecting hemoglobin such as anemia or sickle cell disease.
- Vitamins C and E
- High levels of lipids
- Diseases of the liver and kidneys

TABLE 12.8	BLOOD GLUCOSE AND HbA₁c CORRELATION
HbA₁c (%)	**BLOOD GLUCOSE WEIGHTED MEAN (mg/dL)**
10.0	275
9.0	240
8.0	205
7.0	170
6.0	135

> The HbA₁c reflects the weighted mean of blood glucose over the previous 4 to 6 weeks. A normal HbA₁c is 4% to 6%.

Signs and Symptoms of Hyperglycemia and Hypoglycemia

Hyperglycemia, or **high blood glucose,** can be caused by either too much food, too little insulin, illness, or stress. Symptoms of hyperglycemia include the following:

- Polydipsia (extreme thirst)
- Polyuria (frequent urination)
- Polyphagia (hunger)
- Blurred vision
- Headache
- Drowsiness
- Hyperpnea (deep respirations)
- Nausea

> If not treated, prolonged hyperglycemia can lead to diabetic ketoacidosis or hyperglycemic hyperosmolar nonketotic syndrome.

DKA is most common with type 1 diabetes and is characterized by hyperglycemia, ketosis, acidosis, and dehydration. DKA is caused by insulin deficiency and often occurs as a result of illness or infection. Because of the insulin deficiency, the body uses stored fat for energy. The use of stored fat causes ketone buildup. Polyuria, nausea, and vomiting can cause dehydration and electrolyte imbalance. DKA is a medical emergency. If not properly treated, ketoacidosis can lead to coma and eventually death. Treatment of DKA includes correction of fluid and electrolyte imbalances, initiation of insulin to restore normal glucose metabolism and correct acidosis, and prevention of further complications.

Hyperglycemic hyperosmolar nonketotic syndrome (HHNS) occurs in type 2 diabetes and is characterized by extreme hyperglycemia, absence of ketosis, severe dehydration, and decreased consciousness. The hyperglycemia causes polyuria, nausea, and vomiting, which lead to extreme dehydration. HHNS is usually caused by infection, illness, or medications that cause impaired glucose tolerance or increased fluid loss. It is also seen in noncompliant patients or undiagnosed diabetic patients. Prompt medical attention is needed to prevent these adverse outcomes.

Hypoglycemia, or **low blood glucose,** is a blood glucose level of 70 mg/dL or lower. It can be caused by too little food, too much insulin or diabetic medication, or extra exercise. The initial symptoms are as follows:

- Shakiness
- Sweating
- Tachycardia
- Hunger
- Irritability
- Light-headedness

As the blood glucose continues to drop, confusion, inability to concentrate, slurred speech, irrational behavior, blurred vision, or extreme fatigue may be exhibited. If left untreated, a continued drop in blood glucose can lead to seizures or loss of consciousness.

Hypoglycemia treatment must be initiated quickly. If the patient is alert, hypoglycemia should be treated by having the patient eat a simple, fast-acting source of carbohydrate. The lower the drop in blood glucose, the greater the amount of carbohydrate needed to raise the blood glucose. Foods with a high fat content should be avoided because fat slows the absorption of glucose, which slows the rise in blood glucose. General guidelines for hypoglycemia treatment are as follows:

1. Check the blood glucose.
2. If the blood glucose is 70 mg/dL or less, treat with a simple, fast-acting carbohydrate. The amount of carbohydrate depends on the blood glucose value. Approximately 15 g of carbohydrate will raise the blood glucose by 20 mg/dL. Examples of 15 g of glucose include 4 ounces of fruit juice, four Dex-4 tablets, or five LifeSavers.
3. Wait 10 to 15 minutes, then check the blood glucose. If the blood glucose is not above 70 mg/dL, re-treat with carbohydrates.
4. Repeat the previous step. Continue the treatment until the blood glucose is above 70 mg/dL.

During severe hypoglycemia, the patient may become uncooperative, combative, unresponsive, unconscious, or seize. If it is not possible to give the patient a carbohydrate source by mouth, the patient should be given an intramuscular injection of glucagon and emergency services called.

Glucagon is a hormone that stimulates hepatic glucose production. To administer, mix the solution and inject 1.0 mg (all the solution) in the arm, thigh, or buttock. If there is no response, the injection may be repeated in 15 minutes. When awake and alert, treat the patient with 15 g of carbohydrates. Continue to check the blood glucose and treat appropriately until the blood glucose is above 70 mg/dL.[47]

See Appendix B for details on treatment of diabetes during pregnancy.

PRACTICE/REVIEW QUESTIONS

After reviewing this module, answer the following questions.

1. How is diabetes diagnosed?

   a. _____

   b. _____

   c. _____

2. What are the characteristics of type 1 diabetes?

   a. _____

   b. _____

   c. _____

   d. _____

   e. _____

3. What are the characteristics of type 2 diabetes?

   a. _____

   b. _____

   c. _____

   d. _____

   e. _____

   f. _____

   g. _____

   h. _____

4. What is *gestational diabetes?* _____
   _____

5. At what gestational age should laboratory screening for gestational diabetes be performed?_____

6. What are premeal blood glucose goals during pregnancy?
   _____

7. What are 1-hour postprandial blood glucose goals during pregnancy? _____

8. What does the HbA_{1c} measure? _____

9. What is *hypoglycemia?*_____

10. What are the calorie requirements for a type 2 diabetic pregnant woman who is 5 feet, 2 inches tall and weighs 258 pounds? _____

11. What are the general guidelines that should be followed during exercise in pregnancy?

    a. _____

    b. _____

    c. _____

    d. _____

    e. _____

    f. _____

    g. _____

    h. _____

    i. _____

12. What is the major complication of insulin therapy?

    _____

13. Can oral diabetic medications be used during pregnancy in type 2 diabetic women? _____

14. What changes in insulin requirements occur during the first, second, and third trimesters?

    _____

    _____

15. What conditions of diabetes are affected by pregnancy?

    a. _____

    b. _____

    c. _____

    d. _____

    e. _____

    f. _____

16. When does the fetal pancreas begin to function? _____

    _____

17. When and how often should NSTs begin in pregestational diabetes?

    _____

18. Can oral diabetic medications be used while breastfeeding? _____

19. How is gestational diabetes diagnosed? _____

    _____

    _____

    _____

20. Who should be offered preconception health care?

    _____

21. Who should be placed on 0.4 mg of folic acid?

    _____

PRACTICE/REVIEW ANSWER KEY

1. Diabetes can be diagnosed using any of the following three methods and must be confirmed on a subsequent day:
   a. Acute symptoms of diabetes plus a casual plasma glucose concentration that is greater than or equal to 200 mg/dL
   b. Fasting plasma glucose that is greater than or equal to 126 mg/dL
   c. 2-Hour plasma glucose that is greater than or equal to 200 mg/dL during an oral GTT

2. a. It develops at any age, but two thirds of all cases are diagnosed before age 18.
   b. Symptoms include significant weight loss, polyuria, and polydipsia with hyperglycemia.
   c. DKA is possible.
   d. The patient is dependent on exogenous insulin.
   e. Coma and death can result if diagnosis and/or treatment are delayed.

3. a. It accounts for 90% to 95% of all diabetes in the United States.
   b. It is usually diagnosed after the age of 30, but can occur at any age.
   c. Often, patients are asymptomatic at the time of diagnosis. Because type 2 diabetes frequently goes undiagnosed for years, many patients have end-organ complications such as retinopathy, neuropathy, or nephropathy at the time of diagnosis.
   d. Endogenous insulin levels may be increased, normal, or decreased. The need for exogenous insulin is variable.
   e. Insulin resistance with impaired glucose tolerance is usually seen in the first stages.
   f. Risks of developing type 2 diabetes increases with age, obesity, and lack of physical activity.
   g. HHNS may develop.
   h. Most patients are obese or have an increased percentage of body fat distributed mainly in the abdominal region.

4. Glucose intolerance develops or is first discovered during pregnancy; insulin resistance and diminished insulin secretion is usually seen.

5. 24 to 28 weeks gestation

6. 60 to 95 mg/dL

7. <130 to 140 mg/dL

8. The HbA$_{1c}$ reflects the weighted mean of blood glucose over the past 4 to 6 weeks.

9. Blood glucose level of 70 mg/dL or lower

10. 258 pounds = 117 kg

    117 × 25 kcal/kg per day = 2,925

    Her requirements are 2,925 calories each day.

11. a. Before initiating an exercise program, all patients should have a medical evaluation, be educated on benefits and risks of exercise, and understand the potential effects of exercise on glucose levels.
    b. Obtain metabolic control before exercising. Exercise is safe when glucose levels are between 90 and 140 mg/dL. If blood glucose is above 250 mg/dL, the urine should be checked for ketones. If positive for ketones, exercise should be delayed until glycemic control is obtained and ketones are resolved. If ketones are negative but blood glucose is above 300 mg/dL, be cautious with exercise.
    c. Exercise programs should last less than 45 minutes.
    d. Meals should be consumed 1 to 3 hours before the exercise program.
    e. Insulin should be given in the abdomen and not injected into active muscles. Decrease the bolus insulin if its peak coincides with the exercise period.
    f. Monitor blood glucose before and after exercise. Identify when changes in the insulin regimen or diet are necessary. Learn the way the body responds to different types of exercise.
    g. Monitor necessary food intake. Eat extra carbohydrates as needed to prevent hypoglycemia and always have carbohydrates available during and after exercise.
    h. Include a warm-up an cool-down period with each exercise session.
    i. Avoid exercising in the supine position after the first trimester to prevent aortocaval compression and hypotension.

12. Hypoglycemia

13. No. Although research has been done to compare the use of glyburide with insulin use among women with gestational diabetes, its use during pregnancy has *not* been approved by the U.S. Food and Drug Administration.

14. Usually in the first trimester, insulin requirements are slightly decreased, but they increase in the second and third trimesters. They again decrease during the immediate postpartum period.

15. a. Insulin requirements
    b. Retinopathy
    c. Nephropathy
    d. Coronary artery disease
    e. Neuropathy
    f. DKA

16. Approximately 13 weeks

17. Usually begin NSTs at 32 weeks' gestation on a weekly basis and increase to twice a week at 36 weeks' gestation

18. No. The oral medications are secreted through the breast milk and may affect the infant.

19. Gestational diabetes is diagnosed by an elevated 1-hour screening glucose challenge test of 140 mg/dL or greater, which is followed by a diagnostic 3-hour glucose challenge test. The patient is diagnosed with gestational diabetes if two or more values exceed the following: NDDG criteria: fasting, 105 mg/dL; 1 hour, 190 mg/dL; 2 hour, 165 mg/dL; and 3 hour, 145 mg/dL; Carpenter and Coustan criteria: fasting, 95 mg/dL; 1 hour, 180 mg/dL; 2 hour, 155 mg/dL; and 3 hour, 140 mg/dL.

20. All women of childbearing age who are planning a pregnancy

21. All women of childbearing age

REFERENCES

1. U.S. Department of Health and Human Services, National Institute of Health. (2005). *National Diabetes Statistics fact sheet: general information and national estimates on diabetes in the United States, 2005* [On-line]. Available at: http://diabetes.niddk.nih.gov/dm/pubs/statistics/. Retrieved May 20, 2007.
2. American Diabetes Association. (2004). Position statement gestational diabetes. *Diabetes Care, 27*, S88–S90.
3. March of Dimes Birth Defects Foundation. (1993). *Towards improving the outcome of pregnancy—The 90s and beyond.* White Plains, NY: Author.
4. American Diabetes Association. (2007). Standards of medical care in diabetes-2007. *Diabetes Care, 30*, S4–S41.
5. American College of Obstetrics and Gynecology. (2005, March). *Pregestational diabetes mellitus* [ACOG Practice Bulletin No. 60.]. Washington, DC: Author.
6. Department of Health and Human Services Center for Disease Control and Prevention. (2006). *Recommendations to improve preconception health and health care—United States. Morbidity and Mortality Weekly Reports, 55*(RR-6), 1–23.

7. Cooper, W. P., Hernandez-Diaz, S., Arbogast, P. G., Dudley, J. A., Dyer, S., Gideon, P. S., et al. (2006). Major congential malformations after first-trimester exposure to ACE inhibitors. *New England Journal of Medicine, 354,* 2441–2443.

8. Cefalo, R., & Moos, M. (1995). *Preconceptional health care: A practical guide* (2nd ed.). St. Louis: Mosby.

9. American Diabetes Association. (2003). Expert Committee on the diagnosis and classification of diabetes mellitus. Follow-up report on the diagnosis of diabetes mellitus. *Diabetes Care, 26,* 3160–3167.

10. American Diabetes Association. (2007). Diagnosis and classification of diabetes mellitus. *Diabetes Care, 30,* S42–S47.

11. White, J., Campbell, R., & Yarborough, P. (1998). Therapies: Pharmacologic therapies. In Funnell M., Hunt C., Kulkarni K., Rubin R., & Yarborough P., (Eds.), *A core curriculum for diabetes education* (3rd ed., pp. 295–360). Chicago: American Association of Diabetes Educators.

12. American Diabetes Association. (2005). Position statement: Diagnosis and classification of diabetes. *Diabetes Care, 28,* S72–S79.

13. Monnier, L., Colette, C., Dunseath, G. J., & Owens, D. R. (2007). The loss of postprandial glycemic control precedes stepwise deterioration of fasting with worsening diabetes. *Diabetes Care, 30,* 263–269.

14. Jornsay, D. (1998). Pregnancy: Preconception to postpartum. In Funnell M., Hunt C., Kulkarni K., Rubin R., & Yarborough P., (Eds.), *A core curriculum for diabetes education* (3rd ed., pp. 570–629). Chicago: American Association of Diabetes Education.

15. American Diabetes Association. (2005). National standards for diabetes self-management education. *Diabetes Care, 28,* S4–S36.

16. Rosenn, B., Miodovnik, M., Khoury, J., Combs , C. A., Mimouni , F., et al. (1992). Progression of diabetic retinopathy in pregnancy associated with hypertension in pregnancy. *American Journal of Obstetrics and Gynecology, 166,* 1214–1218.

17. Reece, E. A., Sivan, E., Francis, G., & Homko, C. J. (1998). Pregnancy outcomes among women with and without microvascular disease verses non-diabetic controls. *American Journal of Perinatology, 15,* 549–555.

18. Gabbe, S. G., & Graves, C. R. (2007). Management of diabetes mellitus complicating pregnancy. In J. Queenan (Ed.), *High-risk pregnancy* (pp. 98–109). Washington, DC: American College of Obstetrics and Gynecology.

19. Gordon, M. C., Landon, M. B., Samuels, P., Hissrich, S., & Gabbe, S. G. (1996). Perinatal outcome and long-term follow-up associated with modern management of diabetic nephropathy. *Obstetrics and Gynecology, 87,* 401–409.

20. Simpson, L. L. (2002). Maternal medical disease: Risk of antepartum fetal death. *Seminars in Perinatology, 26,* 42–50.

21. American Diabetes Association. (2000). Prepregnancy counseling and management of women with preexisting diabetes or previous gestational diabetes. *Medical management of pregnancy complicated by diabetes* (3rd ed., pp. 4–19). Alexandria, VA: Author.

22. Montoro, M. N. (2004). Diabetic ketoacidosis during pregnancy. In Coustan D., & Gabbe S., (Eds.), *Diabetes in women: Adolescence, pregnancy, and menopause* (3rd ed., pp. 345–350). Philadelphia: Lippincott Williams & Wilkins.

23. Kitzmiller, J. L., Buchanan, T. A., Kjos, S., Combs, C. A., & Ratner, R. E. (1996). Pre-conception care of diabetes, congenital malformation, and spontaneous abortions. *Diabetes Care, 19,* 514–541.

24. Walkinshaw, S. (2004). Type 1 and type 2 diabetes and pregnancy. *Current Opinion in Obstetrics and Gynecology, 14,* 375.

25. Evers, I. M., deValk, H. W., & Visser, G. H. (2004). Risk of complications of pregnancy in women with type 1 diabetes: Nationwide prospective study in the Netherlands. *British Medical Journal, 328,* 915.

26. Dabelea, D., Knowler, W., & Pettitt, D. (2000). Effect of diabetes in pregnancy on offspring: Follow-up research in Pima Indians. *Journal of Maternal Fetal Medicine, 9*(1), 83–88.

27. Metzger, B. E., & Coustan, D. R.; Organizing Committee. (1998). Summary and recommendations of the 4th International Workshop Conference on gestational diabetes. *Diabetes Care, 21*(Suppl. 2), B161.

28. Coustan, D. R. (2004). Delivery, timing, mode, and management. In Reece E., Coustan D., Gabbe S. (Eds.), *Diabetes in women: Adolescence, pregnancy, and menopause* (3rd ed., pp. 63–68). Philadelphia: Lippincott Williams & Wilkins.

29. Oh, W. (2004). Neonatal outcomes and care. In Reece E., Coustan D., Gabbe S. (Eds.), *Diabetes in women: Adolescence, pregnancy, and menopause* (3rd ed., pp. 451–459). Philadelphia: Lippincott Williams & Wilkins.

30. Reader, D., & Franz, M. J. (2004). Lactation, diabetes, and nutritional recommendations. *Current Diabetes Report, 5,* 370–376.

31. Ben-Haroush, A., Yogev, Y., & Hod, M. (2004). Epidemiology of gestational diabetes mellitus and its association with type 2 diabetes. *Diabetes Medicine, 21,* 103–113.

32. Lobner, K., Knopff, A., Baumgarten, A., Mollenhauer, U., Marinfeld, S., Garrido-Franco, M., et al. (2006). Predictors of postpartum diabetes in women with gestational diabetes mellitus. *Diabetes, 55,* 792–797.

33. Lee, A. J., Hiscock, R. J., Wein, P., Walker, S. P., & Permezel, M. (2007). Gestational diabetes mellitus: Clinical predictors and long-term risk of developing type 2 diabetes. *Diabetes Care, 30,* 878–883.

34. Perkins, J. M., Dunn, J. P., & Jagasia, S. M. (2007). Perspectives in gestational diabetes mellitus: A review of screening, diagnosis, and treatment. *Clinical Diabetes, 25,* 57–62.

35. American College of Obstetrics and Gynecology. (2001, September). *ACOG Practice bulletin: Gestational diabetes* (No. 30). Washington, DC: Author.

36. Ergin, T., Lembet, A., Duran, H., Kuscu, E., Bagis, T., Saygili, E., et al. (2002). Does insulin secretion in patients with one abnormal glucose tolerance test value mimic gestational diabetes mellitus. *American Journal of Obstetrics and Gynecology, 186,* 204–209.

37. Major, C., Henry, M., De Veciana, M., & Morgan, M. (1998). The effects of carbohydrate restriction in patients with diet-controlled gestational diabetes. *Obstetrics and Gynecology, 91*(4), 600–604.

38. Durwald, C., & Landon, M. B. (2005). Glyburide: The new alternative for treating gestational diabetes? *American Journal of Obstetrics and Gynecology, 193,* 1–2.

39. Langer, O., Anyaebunam, A., & Brustman, L. (1988). Pregestational diabetes: Insulin requirements throughout pregnancy. *American Journal of Obstetrics and Gynecology, 159,* 616–662.

40. Harris, G. D., & White, R. D. (2005). Diabetes management and exercise in pregnant patients with diabetes. *Clinical Diabetes, 23,* 165–168.

41. Petitt, D. J., Ospina, P., Kolaczynski, J. W., & Jovanovic, L. (2003). Comparison of an insulin analog, insulin Aspart, and regular human insulin with no insulin in gestational diabetes mellitus. *Diabetes Care, 26*, 183–186.

42. Glueck, C. J., Goldenburg, N., Wang, P., Loftspring, M., & Sherman, A. (2004). Metformin during pregnancy reduces insulin, insulin resistance, insulin secretion, weight, testosterone, and development of GDM: Prospective longitudinal assessment of women with polycystic ovary syndrome from preconception throughout pregnancy. *Human Reproduction, 19*, 510–521.

43. American College of Obstetrics and Gynecology. (2000). *ACOG practice bulletin: Fetal macrosomia* (No. 22). Danvers, MA: ACOG Committee on Practice Bulletins.

44. Kim, C., Berger, D. K., & Chamany, S. (2007). Recurrence of gestational diabetes mellitus. *Diabetes Care, 30*, 1314–1319.

45. U.S. Food and Drug Administration. (2005, July 6). Factors that affect glucose meter performance. Available at: www.fda.gov/diabetes/insulin/html. Retrieved May 2, 2007.

46. Rohlfing, C. L., Wiedmeyer, H. M., Little, R.R. England, J.D., Tennill, A., Goldstein, D.E. (2002.) Defining the relationship between plasma glucose and HbAlc: analysis of glucose profiles and HbAlc in the Diabetes Control and Complications Trial. *Diabetes Care*, 25,275–278.

47. Wilson, B.A., Shannon, M.T., Shields, K.M., Stang, C.L. (2008) *Prentice Hall Nurse's Drug Guide 2008*. New Jersey: Prentice Hall.

MODULE

13 Delivery in the Absence of a Primary Care Provider

MARCELLA T. HICKEY ■ ELISABETH D. HOWARD

Skill Unit 1

Managing an Unexpected Delivery

As you complete this module, you will learn:

1. Those situations that can result in an emergency delivery
2. Signs of an impending birth
3. What equipment should always be ready and available for an emergency delivery (emergency delivery pack)
4. How to deliver the baby
5. Precautions taken for the safety of the mother and baby
6. What to do when there is meconium-stained amniotic fluid, difficulty delivering the baby's shoulders, excessive maternal bleeding, hidden maternal bleeding (hematoma), or a newborn with difficulty breathing
7. What should alert the nurse to the possibility of excessive maternal bleeding
8. What to do if the emergency delivery is a breech
9. Dangers of an improperly conducted delivery
10. Immediate care of the newborn
11. Immediate care of the mother
12. Information that must be charted on the hospital record

Key Terms

When you have completed this module, you should be able to recall the meaning of the following terms. You should also be able to use the terms when consulting with other health professionals. The terms are defined in this module or in the glossary at the end of this book.

hematoma	restitute
lochia	shoulder dystocia
nasopharynx	thermoregulation
nuchal cord	uterine atony
oropharynx	

▶ **Why is it important for you to be able to deliver a baby in the absence of a primary care provider?**

The maternity nurse has a responsibility to provide safe care for the mother and baby. If the nurse makes the assessment that a woman will give birth before her primary care provider arrives, the nurse must be prepared to instruct and assist the woman as well as care for the newborn.

> Comprehensive protocols addressing emergency delivery in the absence of the primary care provider should be developed by each institution.

DO NOT WAIT TO PREPARE for the delivery in the hope that the primary care provider will arrive momentarily. Prepare the woman, the place of delivery, yourself, and an assistant.

▶ **Which women are at risk for delivery before the arrival of their primary care provider?**

Women who are at risk include those who:
- Have had at least one vaginal birth
- Are preterm
- Have a history of rapid labors
- Have made rapid progress during the current labor
- Are in active labor and must travel a great distance to the hospital
- Have an unexpectedly small baby

The Delivery Process

Signs of an Impending Delivery

- Nausea and retching as the cervix reaches full dilatation
- Increased bloody show
- Strong urge to "push" or to bear down with contractions
- Feelings expressed by the mother that "the baby is coming!"
- Separation or parting of the labia (Fig. 13.1)

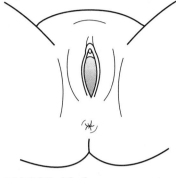

FIGURE 13.1

- Increased fullness and pressure against the perineum (bulging perineum; Fig. 13.2)

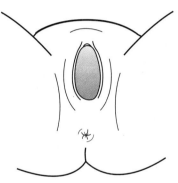

FIGURE 13.2

- Relaxation and bulging of the anus, with or without loss of stool (Fig. 13.3)

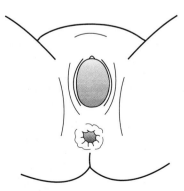

FIGURE 13.3

The Nurse's Role

▶ What must you do to assist with the delivery?

If the primary care provider is not yet present, you should do the following:
- Stay calm.
- Call for assistance. Have another staff member in the room to help with the care of mother and newborn.
- If chart information is not yet available, obtain the most pertinent information from the woman with a 30-second history:
  1. What number baby is this?
  2. When is the due date?
  3. Did you have prenatal care?
  4. Have you had any problems with the pregnancy?
  5. Do you have any health problems?
- Inform the woman and her support person that the birth is about to take place.
- Reassure the woman that she will be assisted and will not be left unattended.
- Instruct the woman to "feather blow" with each contraction, *unless* told to push.
- Open the emergency delivery pack at the bedside. It should contain the following:
  - A package of 4″ × 4″ gauze sponges
  - Two absorbent towels
  - A soft bulb syringe
  - A small drape or sterile field barrier
  - Two clamps, such as Kelly or Rochester
  - A cord clamp or umbilical tape
  - Scissors
  - Baby blanket
  - Gloves
  - Bulb syringe
- Put on sterile gloves, place the sterile barrier under the woman's hips, and prepare to control the delivery of the baby.

> Remember to observe universal precautions.

▶ Why should you instruct the laboring woman to feather blow rather than push with some contractions?

When a woman pushes, she uses abdominal muscles and increases intraabdominal pressure. This enhances the expulsive action of the contracting uterus. Feather blowing helps the woman to control the urge to push. Because you want to protect maternal tissue and the baby from trauma, a controlled delivery with gradual stretching of perineal tissue is desired.

▶ What aseptic techniques should be done in preparation before delivery?

- Wash your hands and forearms thoroughly before putting on sterile gloves.
- Perform perineal and vulvar cleansing. Institutional guidelines and provider preference for cleansing may vary, however the area should be thoroughly washed with an appropriate solution.

▶ Why is control of the head so important?

If the head is delivered too rapidly or with too much force, it can tear the mother's tissues. Remembering the mechanisms of labor will guide your hand maneuvers:
- Flexion
- Extension
- Restitution
- External rotation
- Lateral flexion
- Expulsion

Hand maneuvers:
- Maintain flexion of the fetal head with your left hand
- Allow slow, controlled extension of the head
- Provide perineal support with your right hand
- Suction the nares and oropharynx with a bulb syringe
- Check for a nuchal cord
- Deliver the anterior and then the posterior shoulder
- Support birth of the body by expulsion
- Place baby skin-to-skin on mother

► **Why is it important not to hold back the delivery of the baby's head by pushing against it or crossing the mother's thighs?**

Once it is clear that birth is about to occur, preparation must be made toward a safe and satisfying delivery experience. Pushing back on the head to prevent its delivery can seriously traumatize the baby and maternal tissues.

The nurse should use the pads of the thumb, index, and middle fingers (Fig. 13.4) OR the cupped palm of the hand (Fig. 13.5) to maintain flexion of the head and to provide control as the head delivers.

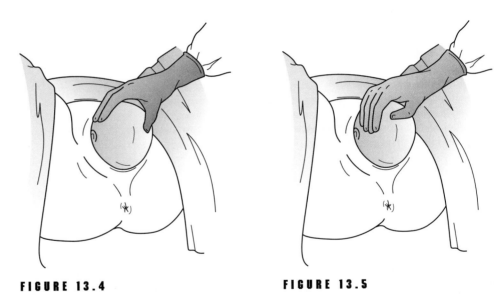

FIGURE 13.4   **FIGURE 13.5**

Never try to hold the head back from delivering!

► **What other safety measures must you take to protect the mother during an emergency delivery?**

Position the mother comfortably so that the perineum, to which you must have access, can easily be viewed. Most often this will be:
- **In the labor bed,** on her back, with her head elevated to a semisitting position (45-degree angle; Fig. 13.6).
  OR
- **In the delivery room.** If the mother has been moved to the delivery room table, the nurse should not "break the table" completely unless skilled in conducting a delivery in this position. Rather, the leg extension should remain partly out to provide safety for the baby with the mother's legs supported by the table stirrups (Fig. 13.7).

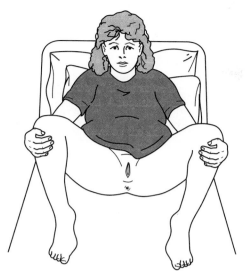

FIGURE 13.6 Position in the labor bed.

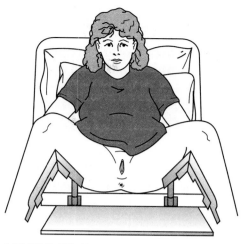

FIGURE 13.7 Position on the delivery room table. The bottom part of the delivery table is left partially extended.

Some women may select alternate positions such as side-lying or squatting. The side-lying position is usually comfortable for the mother and helps to reduce stress on the stretching perineum.

Maintain asepsis (clean technique). Careful handwashing and the use of a sterile emergency pack and sterile gloves will help reduce the possibility of maternal infection.

Allow delivery of the placenta without manipulation. Do not tug on the cord or massage the uterus.

> REMEMBER: If the nurse is observing the progress of the mother's labor and watching closely for signs of an impending birth, the emergency delivery can:
> - Be well planned and conducted in such a way to eliminate last-minute rushing about
> - Provide a safe, satisfying experience for the woman

▶ What safety measures should be taken to protect the newborn?

In addition to careful control of the delivery of the head, you should do the following:
- Inspect the baby for any cord around the neck as the head emerges.
- Wipe off the baby's face and head as soon as possible after delivery. Remove any mucus coming from the nose and mouth.
- Suction the oropharynx and nasopharynx with a bulb syringe to ensure the airway is clear.
- Prevent body heat loss by drying the baby thoroughly, placing the dry baby in the heated crib or directly on the skin of the mother's chest or abdomen, and covering them both well (**thermoregulation**).

Managing Problems

Meconium-Stained Amniotic Fluid[1]

- Occurs more often in high-risk pregnancies
- May be found in the presence of uterine hyperstimulation
- May be associated with maternal hypertension
- Is seen more often when the woman has a biophysical profile (BPP) of less than 6
- Occurs more often in postdate pregnancies
- May be associated with fetal hypoxic episodes
- May also be found with decreased variability in fetal heart rate baseline; late declerations do not have to be present

- May be a physiologic indicator of a mature gastrointestinal tract
- Is not absolutely associated with fetal acidosis

Critical Interventions When Meconium-Stained Amniotic Fluid Is Noted

> Recent research has indicated that routine intrapartum suctioning of the oropharynx and nasopharynx does not always prevent meconium aspiration syndrome in infants.[2]

As soon as the baby's head is delivered and before the shoulders deliver, the baby's oropharynx and then the nasopharynx must be well suctioned with a *bulb syringe*. Have the woman feather blow to avoid pushing. Request for pediatric support to assist with newborn as needed.

Shoulder Dystocia[3]

For a detailed discussion of the nursing responsibilities in the event of a shoulder dystocia, refer to Module 19. These interventions relate specifically to delivery of the fetus when a primary care provider is not present.

A review of the woman's prenatal history may identify antepartum risk factors associated with shoulder dystocia. Risk factors for shoulder dystocia are presented in Module 19.

▶ **What should you do if the baby's shoulders become "stuck" (*shoulder dystocia*)?**

Important steps to take include the following:
- **Be calm and prepared. Call for assistance.**
- Identify which maternal side the fetal back is facing.
- Position a stool on the side of the mother where the fetal back is lying.
- Ensure that the bladder is empty by catheterization.
- Lower the maternal head (i.e., avoid a full Fowler's position).
- Have two nurses assist the mother to sharply flex her knees and hips (McRoberts maneuver) by pulling back on her legs. This action flattens the lumbosacral spine and rotates the symphysis pubis anteriorly. This may dislodge the fetal anterior shoulder (Fig. 13.8).

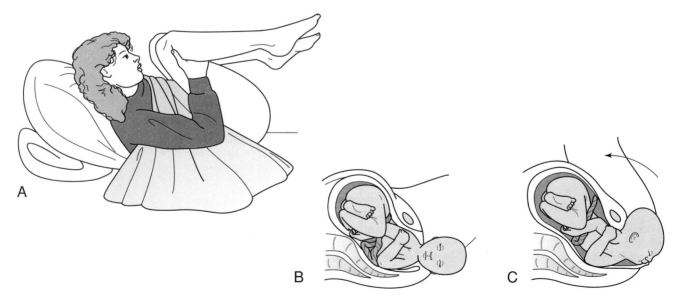

FIGURE 13.8 McRoberts maneuver. **A.** McRoberts maneuver position. **B.** Normal position of the symphysis pubis and the sacrum. **C.** The symphysis pubis rotates and the sacrum flattens. (Adapted with permission from Naef, R. W., & Martin, J. N. (1995). Emergent management of shoulder dystocia. *Obstetrics and Gynecology Clinics of North America, 22*[2], 252.)

- Suprapubic pressure is applied by the nurse who is on the side of the mother where the fetal back lies. This is done while standing on a stool. Using the palmar surface of the hands placed above the pubic bone, apply reasonable pressure straight down (Fig. 13.9). This pressure causes flexion of the shoulder toward the fetal chest, decreasing the diameter of the shoulders. This may aid in the delivery of the shoulder.

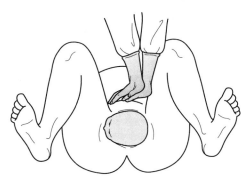

FIGURE 13.9 Pressure is applied by pushing down just above the pubic bone onto the fetal shoulder.

- Consider not suctioning the baby's mouth after the head delivers, but instead take advantage of the baby's rotating shoulders moving to the anteroposterior (AP) position. Do not let the shoulders become directly AP. Shoulders should be delivered in the oblique position.

> Suprapubic pressure is most effective when the person applying it is positioned higher than the maternal body. NEVER USE FUNDAL PRESSURE.

Bleeding

▶ **If the postpartum mother bleeds excessively, what should you do while waiting for the primary care provider to arrive?**

Attempt to identify the source of the bleeding and perform the corresponding nursing interventions (Table 13.1). For a detailed discussion of postpartum hemorrhage, see Module 19. These actions are described for situations in which the primary care provider is not present.

TABLE 13.1	SIGNS AND SYMPTOMS OF AND INTERVENTIONS FOR ACTIVE MATERNAL BLEEDING	
SOURCE	**SIGNS AND SYMPTOMS**	**NURSING INTERVENTION**
Uterine atony OR Retained pieces of placenta	1. Soft and poorly contracting uterus 2. Dark red vaginal bleeding 3. Clots	1. Massage the top of the uterus to stimulate a contraction and express clots 2. Give oxygen if needed 3. Increase rate of intravenous fluids 4. Take and record blood pressure and pulse
Laceration of cervix or vagina	1. Firm uterus 2. Bright red vaginal bleeding	1. Place woman flat or in Trendelenburg position 2. Give oxygen if needed 3. Increase rate of administration of intravenous fluids
Laceration of perineum or labia	1. Firm uterus 2. Obvious tear of tissue 3. Bright red bleeding from tear	1. Apply pressure using a sterile pad 2. Place woman flat or in Trendelenburg position 3. Increase rate of administration of intravenous fluid

Hematoma (Hidden Bleeding)

It is possible for some bleeding to occur under the surface of the tissues (hematoma of the perineum or vagina). The woman might complain of increasing pelvic pain or rectal pressure. A reddish blue mass might be seen in the vagina or at the perineum. This must be noted and observed over several hours.

Additional actions to take include the following:

- Send another person to find a physician or midwife.
- Increase administration of intravenous fluids to more than 125 mL per hour.
- Take and record the woman's blood pressure and pulse.
- Note on the chart the amount, color, and type of blood loss.

To treat a decreasing blood volume caused by excessive bleeding, lactated Ringer's solution should be administered for immediate fluid replacement and prevention of shock. Extreme caution should be used if a large volume of physiologic normal saline is used because it can increase the risk for electrolyte imbalance, coagulation problems, and renal failure.

▶ **Which women are at greatest risk to bleed excessively after the birth?**

Women at greatest risk for excessive bleeding include those women who have had the following:

- A large baby, multiple pregnancy, or hydramnios
- A long labor
- A rapid labor
- Oxytocin induction/augmentation
- A history of many pregnancies (grand multiparity)
- A history of excessive postpartum bleeding

Breech Delivery

▶ **If the emergency delivery is a breech, what should you do to assist it?**

- Avoid excessive handling of the delivering breech.
- Prevent stress on the cord (gently pull a loop free).
- After the breech is delivered, keep the exposed baby warm by carefully applying a warm towel.
- Lift the body, using the towel, to deliver the shoulders. To avoid abdominal trauma, do not grasp the baby's abdomen.
- Lower the body after delivery of the shoulders.

The towel is used to support the infant's lower body *without* grasping the infant's abdomen (Fig. 13.10).

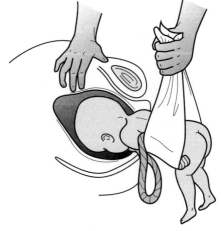

FIGURE 13.10 Use a warm towel and lift the body.

- Keep the head flexed using suprapubic pressure. Another nurse may apply this pressure.
- Using the towel, **raise the body once the hairline is visible;** deliver the chin, mouth, nose, forehead, and top of the head.
- A second nurse may clear the airway as soon as the mouth and nose are visible.

Review

Immediate Care of the Newborn

Immediate care of the newborn involves safety measures discussed previously:
- Maintain a clear airway.
- Maintain body heat (*thermoregulation*).
- Assess general health status (i.e., inspect for any birth injuries or abnormalities).
- Observe vital signs.
- Assess 1- and 5-minute Apgar scores.

In addition, the following must be done:
- Clamp and cut the umbilical cord with sterile scissors.
- Note the number of vessels in the cord (two arteries and one vein).
- Identify the mother/baby unit (mother's fingerprints and baby's footprints, as well as matching name bands for each).

Postpartum Care of the Mother

- Assess firmness and position of the uterus.
- Note the color and quantity of the lochia.
- Note any lacerations.
- Observe and record vital signs every 15 minutes.
- Assess the status of the bladder.
- Provide warmth and rest.

The birth of a baby is a powerful emotional as well as physical experience. Studies indicate a most sensitive period exists immediately after the infant's birth. It is during this time that the parents are most likely to develop strong emotional ties ("bond") with their child. Touching, skin-to-skin contact, holding, nursing, and eye contact all help to develop this tie.

An emergency birth can often be so rushed and hectic that parents miss the opportunity to bond with their baby. The nurse's attitude toward every family's birth should be one of concern for health and safety and a commitment to promote family bonding.

Documentation

Information you should note in the legal record of the birth includes the following:
- Presentation and position of the baby
- Date and time of the birth
- Gender of the baby
- Apgar scores at 1 and 5 minutes
- Presence of cord around the baby's body and the number of times the cord encircles the part (e.g., neck, shoulder, leg)
- Any lacerations to the maternal tissue
- The presence of birth injuries or abnormalities in the baby
- Time of delivery of the placenta
- Appearance of the placenta and membranes (intact, color, abnormalities)
- Appearance of the cord (number of vessels, abnormalities)
- Estimated blood loss
- Any drugs administered to the mother or baby
- Anything unusual about the birth
- First stooling or voiding by the baby
- Vital signs of the mother and the baby
- Name of the person conducting the birth

PRACTICE/REVIEW QUESTIONS

After reviewing this module, answer the following questions.

1. Which of the following situations could result in delivery of the baby before the arrival of the primary care provider? Select all that apply.

   a. An unexpectedly small baby

   b. Rapid progress during labor

   c. Multigravida

   d. History of rapid labors

2. List six signs of impending delivery.

   a. _____

   b. _____

   c. _____

   d. _____

   e. _____

   f. _____

3. List the supplies and equipment that should be available in the sterile emergency delivery pack.

   _____

   _____

   _____

   _____

4. Feather blowing may help the laboring woman control the urge to push.

   a. True

   b. False

5. The woman's thighs and perineal and rectal areas should be cleansed in all situations.

   a. True

   b. False

6. If the baby's head is delivering too fast, you should hold it back.

   a. True

   b. False

7. List at least six things you should do once the baby is delivered to ensure its safety.

   a. _____

   b. _____

   c. _____

   d. _____

   e. _____

   f. _____

8. Meconium-stained amniotic fluid may be associated with which of the following? Select all that apply.

   a. Exercise

   b. Abnormal glucose tolerance test results

   c. Postdated pregnancies

   d. Decreased variability in fetal heart rate baseline

9. What should you do to the baby if the amniotic fluid is stained with meconium?

   _____

   _____

   _____

10. Shoulder dystocia should be a concern when caring for a woman with which of the following? Select all that apply.

    a. History of shoulder dystocia

    b. Height less than 5 feet

    c. Glucose intolerance this pregnancy

    d. Meconium-stained fluid

11. What should you do if the baby's shoulders become stuck?

    _____

    _____

    _____

12. Match the signs and symptoms in Column B with the source in Column A.

    Column A

    _____ 1. Retained placenta

    _____ 2. Lacerations of cervix or vagina

    _____ 3. Laceration of perineum or labia

    Column B

    a. Uterus feels firm but bleeding easily seen from torn tissue

    b. Bright red vaginal bleeding

    c. Soft uterus and dark red bleeding and/or clots

    d. Watery discharge

13. If the source of excessive postpartum bleeding is retained pieces of placenta, what should you do?

    a. _____

    b. _____

    c. _____

    d. _____

14. Which of the following situations place the woman at risk for excessive bleeding after the birth?

    a. Grand multiparity

    b. Short, rapid labor

c. Small baby

d. Oxytocin induction/augmentation

15. What should you do to assist a breech delivery?

a. _____

b. _____

c. _____

d. _____

PRACTICE/REVIEW ANSWER KEY

1. a, b, and d

2. Any six of the following:
   a. Nausea and retching
   b. Increased bloody show
   c. Strong urge to push
   d. Separation of the labia
   e. Increased pressure against the perineum
   f. Bulging of the anus
   g. Mother's feelings

3. 4″ × 4″ gauze sponges, two absorbent towels, soft bulb syringe, small drape, two clamps, scissors, baby blanket, gloves, mucus extractor and trap (e.g., DeLee mucus trap)

4. a. True

5. b. False

6. b. False

7. Any six of the following:
   a. Wipe the baby's face and head.
   b. Inspect the baby's neck for the cord.
   c. Suction the baby's oropharynx and nasopharynx.
   d. Check the airway.
   e. Dry the baby.
   f. Cut the umbilical cord.
   g. Prevent heat loss.

8. c and d

9. Use the bulb syringe to suction the baby's oropharynx and nasopharynx before the shoulders deliver.

10. a, b, and c

11. Have the mother sharply flex her knees and hips, bringing the thighs alongside her abdomen. Occasionally, it may also be necessary to ask another staff member to apply suprapubic pressure.

12. 1. c
    2. b
    3. a

13. a. Massage the top of the uterus.
    b. Administer oxygen, if needed.
    c. Increase the rate of administration of intravenous fluid.
    d. Take and record blood pressure and pulse.

14. a and d

15. a. Avoid excessive handling of the baby.
    b. Prevent stress on the cord.
    c. Lift the baby's body using a towel to help deliver the shoulders and head.
    d. Perform other safety measures, as with a normal delivery.

SKILL UNIT 1 | MANAGING AN UNEXPECTED DELIVERY

The birth of a baby should be planned and conducted to ensure safety for the mother and child and to promote bonding for the family. A birth conducted by the primary care provider who has cared for the woman throughout her pregnancy is ideal. Sometimes, however, circumstances prevent this, and it is then the nurse in the labor and delivery unit who often assists the mother. The labor and delivery nurse must be prepared and have the necessary skills to provide the woman and her baby with the safest and most satisfying experience possible.

The section details how to use the necessary equipment and control the delivery itself. The preceptor will demonstrate the use of hand maneuvers and equipment. You will then be expected to demonstrate *your* skill using a doll.

ACTIONS	REMARKS
Assemble Equipment	
Sterile skin prep kit Sterile emergency delivery pack	It is important to maintain asepsis and prevent infection for both mother and child. USE UNIVERSAL PRECAUTIONS.
Prepare for the Delivery	
1. Call for assistance.	A second person can help care for the newborn, assist the nurse conducting the delivery, and help with any unexpected events.

2. Position the woman.

Position the woman on her back with her head elevated, with or without her legs in stirrups—whichever provides the greatest safety and comfort for the woman.

3. Wash hands

Controlling the delivery of the baby's head is most important

4. Open the sterile emergency delivery pack wherever the birth will take place.

You need to have the pack within easy reach. It is important to maintain sterile technique. This will help to decrease the chances of infection.

5. Put on the sterile gloves. Place the sterile barrier under the buttocks and use the available sterile drapes.

Be sure you know the presentation of the baby. If you are uncertain about the presentation, a vaginal examination should be done to see whether the baby is vertex or breech.

Conduct the Emergency Delivery

6. As the head crowns, break the bag of waters if it does not break by itself.

The bag of waters will usually break by itself, but if not, it must be cut or torn to prevent aspiration of fluid at birth.

7. Use the nondominant hand to support the perineum with a sterile towel or 4″ × 4″ gauze squares.

This protects the sterile glove while supporting the stretching perineum.

8. In the groin area adjacent to the perineum, place the thumb on one side and fingers on the opposite (Fig. 13.11). Exert pressure by drawing the thumb and fingers together. This action is aimed at trying to create a pouch of the perineum.

This relieves pressure on the stretching perineal body.

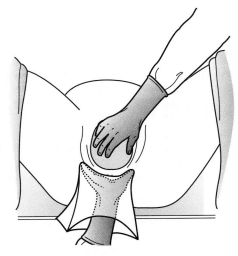

FIGURE 13.11

9. Instruct the woman when to feather blow and when to push.

This helps to prevent uncontrolled, rapid delivery of the head.

10. Gently maintain pressure on the fetal head, using a cupped hand or the pads of the fingers until most of the head is delivered. Then gently assist the head to extend and deliver the forehead, face, and chin.

Keep the head flexed by slowly allowing it to rise under your palm or fingers. Assist extension by raising the head as the forehead comes over the perineum. It is sometimes helpful to have the woman push or bear down after the contraction is over.

Be clear when telling the woman what to do. Make your instructions short and easy to understand.

---

11. Slide your fingers down around the baby's neck to inspect for a cord as soon as the head has delivered (Fig. 13.12).

Need to determine whether cord is present.

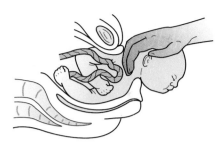

FIGURE 13.12

If loose cord is felt around the baby's neck, gently pull a loop down over the head (Fig. 13.13).

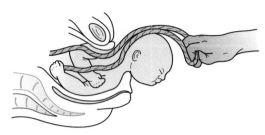

FIGURE 13.13

If a tight cord is felt, try to reduce over baby's shoulders. Put two clamps on the cord (approximately 1 inch apart) and then cut between the clamps (Fig. 13.14). Quickly loosen the cord from around the neck.

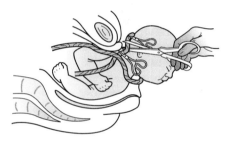

FIGURE 13.14

12. Wipe the head and face dry, paying special attention to mucus coming from the nose and mouth.

Mucus is forced out of the nose and mouth as the baby squeezes through the birth canal. If the mucus is not wiped away, the baby can aspirate it when the baby begins to breathe. At this point, use a bulb syringe to suction out the mouth and nose.

13. Allow the head to **restitute.** Place the hand palm-side up and with the fingers toward the face, under the head for support (Fig. 13.15).

Head and shoulders are resuming normal alignment. The baby's head will turn slightly.

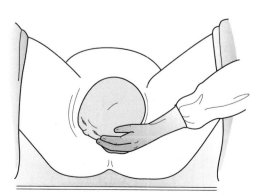

FIGURE 13.15

Allow the shoulders to rotate *externally* (Fig. 13.16).

As the shoulders move into position for birth, you will observe another slight turn of the baby's head. The shoulders are now in the AP diameter of the maternal pelvis.

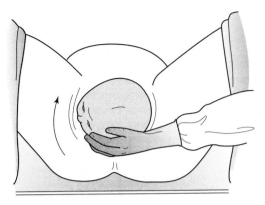

FIGURE 13.16

14. Place the second hand on the other side of the baby's head and, with downward, outward traction on the head, deliver the anterior shoulder (Fig. 13.17).

Keep your fingers flat on the sides of the head. *Do not* grab the baby around the neck.

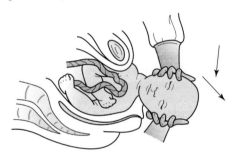

FIGURE 13.17

15. As soon as the anterior shoulder delivers, provide upward, outward traction to the head to deliver the posterior shoulder (Fig. 13.18).

Keep fingers away from eyes and neck.

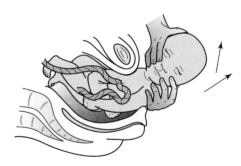

FIGURE 13.18

16. As the shoulder clears the perineum, support the head with the heel of your hand and thumb. Using the fingers of this hand, grasp the baby's arm to the chest wall (Fig. 13.19). Support the baby in your lower hand.

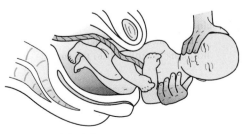

FIGURE 13.19

17. As the body delivers, slide the upper hand down the baby's back to grasp the feet (Fig. 13.20).

Holding the arm to the chest helps to prevent laceration of the perineum by the elbow.

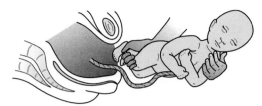

FIGURE 13.20

18. As the feet deliver, turn the baby in an arm hold, with the head turned slightly and the head slightly lower than the feet (Fig. 13.21).

This helps to drain the airway. The nose and mouth can be suctioned with a bulb syringe. Keep the baby close to the perineum to prevent excess pulling on the cord. Avoid grasping the baby's neck and compressing carotid arteries.

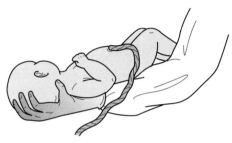

FIGURE 13.21

19. Double clamp the umbilical cord. Cut the cord between the two clamps (Fig. 13.22).

Take care to avoid wide spraying of the blood.

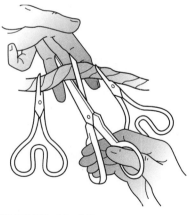

FIGURE 13.22

Care of the Newborn

20. Place the baby directly on the mother's warm chest or abdomen.
21. With skin-to-skin contact, cover the newborn and mother with warm towels or a blanket.
22. Dry the baby thoroughly.

23. Collect blood from the cord attached to the placenta.

This assists in maintaining the baby's body heat with skin-to-skin contact (or a heated crib).
This helps to prevent heat loss in the newborn.

Wet babies lose a great deal of heat. It is important to replace wet towels immediately.
Because the amount of cord blood drawn will depend on the tests needed, check the mother's chart and your hospital's guidelines.

Delivery of the Placenta

24. Check for uterine size, shape, and firmness.	The uterus must contract to expel the placenta and to control bleeding. Signs of placental separation are as follows: • A gush of blood • Lengthening of the cord • A change in the shape of the uterus from oval to globular
25. Control the delivery of the placenta by keeping a gentle, steady, downward traction on the cord as the other hand supports the uterine fundus. The mother can assist by bearing down when she feels a contraction.	Tugging on the cord or vigorous rubbing of the uterus can cause problems and must not be done. Carefully inspect the placenta for signs of missing pieces or abnormalities. Count the number of vessels in the cord: There should be three (two arteries and one vein).
26. Observe the amount and color of the bleeding and the tone of the uterus.	If the uterus feels soft, it can be stimulated to contract by massaging the fundus (the top of the uterus) or by having the baby breastfeed.
27. Inspect for lacerations.	Gently inspect the perineum and labia for bleeding or tears in need of repair by the primary care provider. A sterile pad can be applied to provide pressure to control bleeding of a perineal or labial laceration.
28. Facilitate bonding.	Families need time to inspect, hold, and "take in" the newborn. Immediately after birth, as soon as the mother and baby have settled down, the family must be provided private time to begin to "attach."

You will need to attend a skill session(s) to practice this skill with the help of your preceptor. Mastery of the skill is achieved when you can demonstrate techniques of delivering a baby, including the following:
- Taking preparatory steps
- Positioning the woman
- Using sterile gloves and drapes
- Flexing and controlling the delivery of the head
- Guiding the delivery of the baby's body
- Checking for a nuchal cord
- Cutting the umbilical cord
- Delivering the placenta
- Inspecting the placenta and cord

REFERENCES

1. Creasy, R., K., & Resnik, R. (2004). *Maternal-fetal medicine* (5th ed.) Philadelphia: WB Saunders.
2. Vain, N. E., Szyld, E. G., Prudent, L. M., Wiswell, T. E., Aguilar, A. M., & Vivas, N. I. (2004). Oropharyngeal and nasopharyngeal suctioning of meconium stained neonates before delivery of their shoulders: Multicentre, randomized controlled trial. *Lancet, 364,* 597–602.
3. American College of Obstetricians and Gynecologists. (2002). *Shoulder dystocia* [Practice Bulletin No. 40]. Washington, DC: Author.

SUGGESTED READINGS

Cunningham, G., Leveno, K. J., Bloom, S. L., Hauth, J. C., Gilstrap, L. C., & Wenstrom, K. D. (2005). *Williams obstetrics* (22nd ed.). New York: McGraw-Hill.
Gabbe, S. G., Niebyl, J. L., & Simpson, J. L. (2005*). Obstetrics: Normal and problem pregnancies*. New York: Churchill Livingstone.
Jennings, B. (1979). Emergency delivery: How to attend to one safely. *American Journal of Maternal-Child Nursing, 4*(3), 148–153.
Oxorn, H. (1986). *Oxorn-Foote human labor & birth* (5th ed.). New York: Appleton-Century-Crofts.

MODULE

14

Assessment of the Newborn and Newly Delivered Mother

ANN MOGABGAB WEATHERSBY
■ PENNY WAUGH ■ ERIN RODGERS

1

Initial Assessment of the Newborn

As you complete Part 1 of this module, you will learn:

1. Normal signs of newborn adaptation to extrauterine life
2. Methods to assist the newborn in normal adaptation
3. Methods to evaluate newborn adaptation: Apgar scoring and umbilical cord blood analysis
4. The limitations of these evaluation methods
5. Preparations to be made before delivery of an infant requiring assistance with adaptation
6. Actions that must be taken when an infant requires resuscitation
7. Proper techniques for use when obtaining specimens for cord blood analysis

When you have completed Part 1 of this module, you should be able to recall the meaning of the following terms. You should also be able to use the terms when consulting with other health professionals. The terms are defined in this module or in the glossary at the end of this book.

Apgar score   neonatal resuscitation
asphyxia   newly born
hypopharynx   vagal stimulation

The birth of a baby is a life-changing event for a family, a change that has been anticipated for months or years. The dreams for this new life become reality as parents and family greet the baby and start the process of welcoming a new family member. Family roles shift: A mother becomes a grandmother; the baby becomes the young brother. Two families now have a bond in this new life. Families make this transition in many different ways, sometimes due to cultural conventions, family traditions, or personal decisions. It is a special joy for perinatal nurses to be able to witness this birth of family.

The physical care of the mother is an important part of the role of the perinatal nurse. This chapter contains information to guide the nurse in safe and appropriate care of the newborn and mother. However, it is also important for the nurse to recognize that much more is occurring than these physical changes. Being sensitive to the needs of the woman and her family during the early hours after birth is as important as providing physical care. The nurse has the opportunity to provide care to the whole woman, care that includes the physical and psychosocial, care that considers all aspects of the miracle of birth.

Assessment of the Newborn

▶ What are the normal responses of the newborn to extrauterine life?[1–5]

With birth and the clamping of the umbilical cord, a sequence of events occurs that begins the adaptation of the newborn infant to life outside the womb. The term *newly born* is sometimes used to refer to the infant during this brief period of the first minutes to hours after birth. As the newborn takes the first breaths, the lungs change from fluid filled to air filled. It is thought that newborn respirations are triggered by a combination of factors. After the baby passes through the birth canal, the pressure on the newborn thorax is released and a passive recoil of the chest allows intake of air. Other factors that affect these first respirations include lowered oxygenation of the fetus as a result of occlusion of the cord during birth, clamping of the cord after delivery, and the drop in temperature from the warm uterine environment to the cooler birth room. Circulation begins the transition from the blood flow patterns of the fetus to the blood flow of the newborn. The newborn also begins to regulate temperature. These changes begin in the immediate newborn period, although not without obvious effort on the part of the infant.

An infant responding normally to extrauterine life takes initial breaths and has a lusty cry, maintains heart rate in the normal (greater than 100 bpm) range, and shows good tone and normal reflexes. With adequate respirations and circulation, color gradually changes from dusky blue/pink immediately after birth to the overall pink of body and extremities.

▶ How can the nurse assist the infant in adaptation to the extrauterine environment?[3–5]

Infants showing a normal response to the extrauterine environment can remain with their mother to receive routine care. Care of the mother–infant couple in the first hours after birth is best provided by the mother/baby nurse. The initial status and needs of both the mother and the newborn can be evaluated by this specially trained nurse.

Assisting the newborn with transition to life outside the womb begins with preventing heat loss. The infant is thoroughly dried with warm blankets, placed skin to skin with the mother, and covered with another warm, dry blanket. Covering the head with a cap can also decrease heat loss because the head is a major source of heat loss. This drying of the infant also stimulates the infant to establish spontaneous respirations.

The newborn may need assistance with clearing secretions from the airway. Positioning him or her in a side-lying position may help. Secretions can be wiped from the mouth and nose. If suctioning is necessary, the mouth should be suctioned first, then the nose, with a bulb syringe or suction catheter. Vigorous suctioning must be avoided because this can lead to laryngeal spasms and vagal bradycardia.

▶ What are the methods used to evaluate the adaptation of the newly born?

The newly born infant is initially evaluated for physiologic signs of adaptation to extrauterine life, including heart rate, cry or respirations, movement of extremities, and color. The *Apgar score*, devised in 1952 by Virginia Apgar, allows for an initial rapid assessment of the newly born and is frequently used to identify the infant in need of assistance with adaptation to extrauterine stressors. Five areas are scored, including heart rate, respiratory effort, muscle tone, reflex irritability (grimace), and color. Using this system, scores are determined as follows: heart rate is based on the rate being absent or above or below 100 bpm, and respirations are evaluated as absent, slow, or good. Crying, as a reflection of respiratory effort, can also be measured from absent, or no cry, to weak, or lusty cry. The muscle tone of the infant is evaluated and is rated from flaccid to active motion. Reflexes can be evaluated by a tap on the sole of the foot or by the infant response to a catheter in the nostril, and the infant response can range from no response to cry, cough, or sneeze. The infant color is assessed and can range from blue or pale to completely pink. The components of the score are listed in Table 14.1 and are evaluated at 1 and 5 minutes after birth.

TABLE 14.1	CRITERIA FOR APGAR SCORING		
SIGN	**SCORE 0**	**SCORE 1**	**SCORE 2**
Heart rate	Not detectable	<100	>100
Respiratory rate	Absent	Slow, irregular	Good, crying
Muscle tone	Flaccid	Some extremity flexion	Active motion
Reflex irritability			
Response to tap on sole of foot	No response	Grimace	Grimace
Response to catheter in nostril (after oropharynx is cleared)	No response	Cry	Cough or sneeze
Color	Blue, pale	Body pink, blue extremities	Completely pink

Reprinted with permission from Apgar, V., (1953). A proposal for a new method of evaluation of the newborn infant. *Current Researches in Anesthesia and Analgesia, 32*(4), 260–267.

Umbilical cord blood gas analysis is another method that may be used to evaluate the newborn's need for assistance with adaptation.

Apgar Score

▶ What is the significance of an Apgar score?[1,3-8]

It can be argued that the Apgar scoring system is no longer of clinical significance. Practitioners of newborn care are trained in neonatal resuscitation following the American Academy of Pediatrics (AAP) guidelines. These guidelines recommend assessment of the infant at birth and institution of any needed resuscitation. The delay of resuscitation until a 1-minute Apgar score is obtained is not an appropriate use of the scoring system.

However, the Apgar score continues to be used and can be helpful in the initial evaluation of the newborn's need for further assistance with adaptation and in the evaluation of the newborn's response to resuscitation. Apgar scores may also be useful in resuscitations if continued at 5-minute intervals until the infant has stabilized.

Broad categories of scores that may indicate infant adaptation have been considered:
- **7 to 10**—May indicate adequate adaptation; no assistance is usually needed
- **4 to 6**—May indicate need for some resuscitation
- **0 to 3**—Usually indicates that resuscitation is needed immediately

Even with the guidance of these categories, it is important to consider each infant's condition and needs for assistance with adaptation.

Apgar scoring is most reliable when done by trained personnel and by someone who is giving complete attention to the newborn.

> REMEMBER: The Apgar score is a clinical evaluation of the need for newborn resuscitation. It does not determine newborn hypoxia, acidosis, or neurologic impairment, nor does it predict long-term outcome.

▶ What are some factors that can cause variations in Apgar scores?[2,3,5-7]

Several factors can cause variations in Apgar scores and may not indicate a need for resuscitation. An overall clinical evaluation is important in these situations when considering the care of the infant. Some of these factors include the following:
- **Gestational age**—The standard Apgar goal of 10 points might not be an appropriate gauge of fetal well-being for babies of less than 31 to 34 weeks' gestation. These infants often lack the tone of a term infant and the ability to respond appropriately when reflex irritability is tested.
- **Intubation and cord visualization**—Meconium-stained amniotic fluid may indicate the need for immediate intubation and suctioning of the hypopharynx and trachea. Intubation often produces stimulation of the vagus nerve and subsequent temporary lowering of the heart rate. Babies usually recover from this intervention spontaneously, but this temporary slowing of the heart rate can affect Apgar scoring.
- **Congenital defects**—Babies with congenital defects of the heart or neuromuscular or cerebral malformations may have Apgar scores that do not reflect a need for resuscitation. These infants need further evaluation.
- **Infection**—Infection in the newborn may affect tone, color, and reflexes.

Umbilical Cord Gas Values

▶ How are newborn umbilical cord gas values used to evaluate the newborn?[9,10]

Umbilical cord blood sampling is a useful addition to Apgar scoring in the evaluation of the fetus' condition at the time of birth. Umbilical cord blood gas sampling is a method used to determine the oxygenation and acid–base status of the fetus at birth and the functioning of the placenta. *The arterial values reflect fetal conditions; venous values reflect placental function.*

> REMEMBER: Umbilical arteries carry blood from the fetus to the placenta, and the umbilical vein carries oxygenated blood to the fetus.

The pH value is normal or abnormal. A low pH value indicates acidemia of the fetus, and this acidemia is then further evaluated. Gases are evaluated for the cause of the acidemia and can be classified as respiratory, metabolic, or mixed in origin.

▶ Can Apgar scores and cord blood gases identify a newborn with perinatal asphyxia?[8-11]

Fetal *asphyxia* is a condition of impaired blood gas exchange leading to progressive hypoxemia and hypercapnia with a significant metabolic acidosis. The diagnosis of intrapartum fetal asphyxia requires a blood gas and acid–base assessment. At this time, an exact pH value indicative of arterial acidemia associated with perinatal asphyxia is unknown. However, a reasonable threshold of pH 7.00 or lower has been identified as having an association with significant or pathologic fetal acidemia. Correct umbilical cord gas interpretation requires that other measurements of the blood gas be analyzed. For example, both the pH and the base deficit should be measured. The base deficit is a more precise measurement of a metabolic acidosis. Moderate and severe newborn encephalopathy, respiratory, and other composite complications increase as the arterial base deficit reaches and rises above 12 mmol/L. The AAP and the American College of Obstetricians and Gynecologists (ACOG) have recommended that the term *asphyxia* be applied only to infants who have all of the following conditions:
- Metabolic or mixed acidemia with a pH value below 7.0
- An Apgar score of 0 to 3 for longer than 5 minutes
- Neonatal neurologic manifestations such as seizures, coma, or poor tone and multisystem organ dysfunction

▶ Are cord gas values obtained for all infants?[10]

Some physicians and midwives sample cord blood gases at every delivery. For the normal healthy newborn, little information of clinical value is obtained with this practice. Other practitioners clamp and reserve a segment of cord at every delivery and obtain gas analysis if the infant has low Apgar scores or any signs of distress. Many practitioners routinely obtain gases in high-risk pregnancies or complicated deliveries. ACOG recommends both venous and arterial cord blood samples be obtained in the following situations:
- Cesarean deliveries performed secondary to fetal compromise
- Low 5-minute Apgar score
- Severe intrauterine growth restriction (IUGR)
- Abnormal fetal heart rate tracings
- Maternal thyroid disease
- Intrapartum fever
- Multiple gestation

It is important to understand the expectations of the birth attendant before delivery to prepare for cord gas testing. The Skill Unit at the end of this section will help you to learn the technique for cord blood sampling.

▶ What are normal blood gas values for healthy term babies?[9,10]

Table 14.2 shows a range for normal cord blood gas values for healthy term babies. Other investigators have found a wide range of values to be normal. In general, an umbilical artery pH of 7.10 or higher can be considered normal and is associated with normal Apgar scores and vigorous newborns.

TABLE 14.2	NORMAL UMBILICAL CORD BLOOD pH AND BLOOD GAS VALUES IN TERM NEWBORNS		
VALUE	**YEOMANS*** (*n* = 146)	**RAMIN*** (*n* = 1,292)	**RILEY[†]** (*n* = 3,522)
Arterial blood			
pH	7.28 (0.05)	7.28 (0.07)	7.27 (0.069)
P_{CO_2} (mmHg)	49.2 (8.4)	49.9 (14.2)	50.3 (11.1)
HCO_3^- (mEq/L)	22.3 (2.5)	23.1 (2.8)	22.0 (3.6)
Base excess (mEq/L)	—[‡]	−3.6 (2.8)	−2.4 (2.0)
Venous blood			
pH	7.35 (0.05)	—	7.34 (0.063)
P_{CO_2} (mmHg)	38.2 (5.6)	—	40.7 (7.9)
HCO_3^- (mEq/L)	20.40 (4.1)	—	21.4 (2.5)
Base excess (mEq/L)	—[‡]	—	−2.4 (2.0)

Data are presented as mean values ±1 standard deviation.
*Data are from infants of selected patients with uncomplicated vaginal deliveries.
[†]Data are from infants of unselected patients with vaginal deliveries.
[‡]Data were not obtained.
Remin, S. M., Gilstrap III, L., Leveno, K. J., & Little, B. B. (1989). Umbilical artery acid–base status in the preterm infant. *Obstetrics and Gynecology, 74*, 256–258.
Riley, R. J., & Johnson, J. W. C. (1993). Collecting and analyzing cord blood gases. *Clinical Obstetrics and gynecology, 36*, 13–23.
Yeomans, E. R., Hauth, J. C., Gilstrap III, L. C., & Strickland, D. M. (1985). Umbilical cord pH, PCO₂, and bicarbonate following uncomplicated term vaginal deliveries. *American Journal of Obstetrics and Gynecology, 151*, 798–800.

▶ If the cord gas shows acidemia, what else is evaluated?[10]

The cord gases should be further evaluated for the type of acidemia that has occurred. Table 14.3 shows a range for normal cord blood gas values for premature infants.

- **Respiratory acidosis** is associated with insults to the fetus that are of short duration. The fetus is able to continue to compensate for these insults with normal physiologic responses. Examples are tight nuchal cords or other causes of cord compression that may occur just before delivery. With immediate and appropriate resuscitation, these infants generally make rapid adaptations to extrauterine life.
- Infants with **metabolic or mixed acidosis** generally have had a more profound or longer lasting insult that may include a poor prenatal environment. These infants require more intensive resuscitation and careful neonatal follow-up.

TABLE 14.3	NORMAL UMBILICAL ARTERY BLOOD pH AND BLOOD GAS VALUES IN PREMATURE INFANTS		
VALUE FOR ARTERIAL BLOOD	**YEOMANS*** (*n* = 77)	**RAMIN*** (*n* = 949)	**RILEY[†]** (*n* = 1,015)
pH	7.29 (0.07)	7.27 (0.07)	7.28 (0.089)
P_{CO_2} (mmHg)	49.2 (9.0)	51.6 (9.4)	50.2 (12.3)
HCO_3^- (mEq/L)	23.0 (3.5)	23.9 (2.1)	22.4 (3.5)
Base excess (mEq/L)	−3.3 (2.4)	−3.0 (2.5)	−2.5 (3.0)

Data are presented as mean values ±1 standard deviation.
*Data are from infants of selected patients with uncomplicated vaginal deliveries.
[†]Data are from infants of unselected patients with vaginal deliveries.
Dickinson, J. E., Eriksen, N. L., Meyer, B. A., & Parisi, V. M. (1992). The effect of preterm birth on umbilical cord blood gases. *Obstetrics and Gynecology, 79*, 575–578.
Ramin, S. M., Gilstrap III., L. C., Leveno, K. J., Burris, J., & Little, B. B. (1989). Umbilical artery acid–base status in the preterm infant. *Obstetrics and Gynecology, 74*, 256–258.
Riley, R. J., & Johnson, J. W. C. (1993). Collecting and analyzing cord blood gases. *Clinical Obstetrics and gynecology, 36*, 13–23.

Care of Infants Requiring Resuscitation at Delivery

▶ **What are the preparations to be made before delivery of an infant requiring assistance with adaptation?[6,7,9]**

Risk factors can identify many infants who may require resuscitation. For instance, the delivery of a preterm infant, an infant with meconium-stained amniotic fluid, or an infant with a nonreassuring fetal heart rate tracing may have a need for resuscitation at delivery. Maternal conditions that may indicate the need for resuscitation of the newborn include diabetes, chronic hypertension or preeclampsia, chorioamnionitis, or others that can affect placental perfusion. It is important to anticipate and be prepared for the possibility of neonatal resuscitation at birth.

> Although it is impossible to completely predict all infants who will need resuscitation, *a person trained to begin neonatal resuscitation should be present at every delivery.*

Individuals trained to continue resuscitations should be immediately available for all deliveries and present for high-risk situations.

Programs are available to train and certify personnel in neonatal resuscitation. Nurses who work in antepartal units, labor and delivery units, newborn nurseries, and postpartum or mother–baby units need training in neonatal resuscitation, much like the routinely required certification in adult cardiopulmonary resuscitation.

Each birth room needs to be stocked with the equipment, supplies, and medications for a complete resuscitation. The AAP neonatal resuscitation program is an excellent resource for guidelines for training personnel and supplying units.

▶ **What actions are required when an infant needs resuscitation?[5–7,9]**

Newborn infants who do not respond normally to the extrauterine environment are in need of further assessment:

- Take the infant to a radiant warmer, place the infant supine, and thoroughly dry the infant to stimulate respirations and reduce cold stress. Remove all wet towels or blankets from the infant.
- Suction the infant, if necessary. Remember to suction the mouth first, then the nose.
- Assess the infant according to the resuscitation triad: respiration, heart rate, and color. Assessment determines whether resuscitation is needed. Initiate those techniques in which you are skilled and obtain necessary help for other procedures.
- Remember to keep the mother and other family members informed of what is occurring, why it is occurring, and what is being done. Parents usually respond well to accurate information given in a timely manner.
- Documentation of newborn status and adaptation to the extrauterine environment is also a necessary component of the care of the newborn. Apgar scoring, blood gases, any need for resuscitation, and actions taken are to be documented.

SKILL UNIT 1 | PROCEDURE FOR OBTAINING UMBILICAL CORD BLOOD SAMPLES (ARTERIAL AND VENOUS)

This section details how to collect umbilical cord blood samples in a manner that achieves the most accurate results. Study this section and then attend a skill practice and demonstration session scheduled by your preceptor. You will need to demonstrate the procedure for collecting the specimen(s). The steps of the examination are listed at the end of this unit.

REMEMBER: *Check with the procedures at your institution for recommendations. At some institutions, cord segments are transported rapidly to the laboratory and the laboratory technician will draw the sample.*

ACTIONS	REMARKS

1. Collect supplies:
  • Heparin 1,000 U/mL
  • Two 3-mL syringes with 22- or 23-gauge needles and caps
  • Labels and lab slips as needed
  • Gloves
	Remember to use universal precautions when handling blood products.
	Prepare labels and requisition slips before delivery.
	Prepare one label marked *venous sample* and one label marked *arterial sample.*

2. Prepare syringes for sampling: Flush syringes with heparin solution and eject heparin and air from syringes. Recap (one-hand technique).	The goal is to coat the syringe with heparin to prevent clotting of the specimen.
3. Receive segment of cord for sampling.	The physician or midwife will double-clamp a 6- to 8-inch segment of cord immediately after delivery and hand it to you for sampling.
4. Obtain samples: With the bevel of the needle up, insert the needle into the smaller and darker artery and withdraw 1 to 2 mL (Fig. 14.1). Remove air and recap the needle using the one-handed recap procedure or a hemostat to hold the needle cap. Repeat the procedure to obtain a specimen from the larger vein.	The venous specimen will be pinker than the darker arterial specimen. It is important to recap the needle using techniques to prevent needlestick injuries.

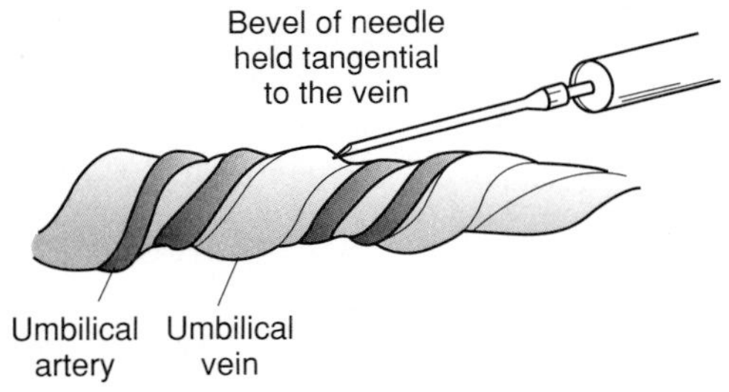

Bevel of needle
held tangential
to the vein

Umbilical   Umbilical
artery   vein

FIGURE 14.1

ACTIONS	REMARKS
5. Send the labeled specimens with the appropriate requisitions to the laboratory.	Cord segments and heparinized samples are stable for at least 30 to 60 minutes at room temperature. Sample and transport as soon as possible.

You will need to attend a skill session to practice this skill with the help of your preceptor. Mastery of this skill is achieved when you can do the following:
  • Assemble all necessary equipment for the procedure
  • Differentiate the arteries and vein in an umbilical cord
  • Demonstrate collection and labeling of 0.3 to 3.0 mL of venous and arterial blood sample using heparinized syringes

PRACTICE/REVIEW QUESTIONS

After reviewing Part 1, answer the following questions.

1. What is the 1-minute Apgar score for the baby described below? _____

   Heart rate: 126 bpm

   Respiratory effort: Crying

   Muscle tone: Active

   Reflex irritability: Grimace

   Color: Blue extremities

2. Do you anticipate that this baby will require resuscitation?

   a. Yes

   b. No

3. What is the 1-minute Apgar score for the baby described below? _____

   Heart rate: 96 bpm

   Respiratory effort: Slow, irregular

   Muscle tone: Flaccid

   Reflex irritability: No response

   Color: Blue

4. Do you anticipate that this baby will require resuscitation?

   a. Yes

   b. No

5. Which factor is most likely to cause a low Apgar score?

   a. A fall in maternal body temperature

   b. Visualization and suctioning of the infant's vocal cords

   c. Infant birth weight of more than 8 pounds

   d. An infant born at 41 weeks' gestation

6. List the steps of a recommended procedure for collection of umbilical cord blood gas samples.

   a. _____

   b. _____

   c. _____

   d. _____

   e. _____

7. An umbilical artery pH of 6.85 is considered abnormal.

   a. True

   b. False

8. Would you anticipate that an infant with a pH of 6.85 would need assistance with adaptation to extrauterine life?

   a. Yes

   b. No

PRACTICE/REVIEW ANSWER KEY

1. 8

2. b. No

3. 2

4. a. Yes

5. b

6. a. Collect supplies
   b. Prepare syringes
   c. Receive cord segment
   d. Obtain samples
   e. Send labeled samples

7. a. True

8. a. Yes

PART 2

Assessment of the Newly Delivered Mother

As you complete Part 2 of this module, you will learn:

1. Components and expected findings of the physical assessment of a newly delivered mother
2. Variations from normal findings during the early postpartum period and familiarity with common interventions
3. Nursing interventions that promote parent–infant attachment
4. Techniques to assist the mother with the initiation of breastfeeding in the immediate postpartum period
5. Necessary interventions for women with recovery complicated by surgery, anesthesia, infection, or pregnancy-related hypertension
6. Techniques to assist parents who have experienced a birth with neonatal complications
7. Ongoing needs of the newly delivered mother during postpartum hospitalization
8. General guidelines for discharge of mother and infant

When you have completed Part 2 of this module, you should be able to recall the meaning of the following terms. You should also be able to use the terms when consulting with other health professionals. The terms are defined in this module or in the glossary at the end of this book.

atony	lochia
dermatome	nipple confusion
eclampsia	rubra
en face	tubal ligation
hematoma	

Postpartum Assessment of the Mother

► **What are the components and expected findings of the physical assessment of a newly delivered mother?[4,5]**

The period after delivery of the placenta and continuing until maternal stabilization—the immediate postpartum period—is a time of rapid physiologic change that requires careful monitoring by the nurse. Although women can be cared for in a variety of settings (e.g., traditional recovery room; labor, delivery, recovery room [LDR]; labor, delivery, recovery, and postpartum room [LDRP]), components of care are unchanged.

To care for a newly delivered mother's postpartum needs, the nurse must know both the prenatal and intrapartum history. Although assessments and interventions begin immediately postpartum, an orderly, ongoing, and complete assessment is needed during the first postpartum hour.

Postpartum education is a component of care. Explanation of the findings of assessments and needed interventions by the nurse to the mother and support person continues the educational process begun antepartally.

General Assessment

Note the overall appearance of the mother, including skin color, motor activity, facial expression, speech, manner, mood, state of awareness, and interactions with others.

Vital Signs

- **Blood pressure**—Monitor at least every 15 minutes for the first hour. Findings should return to prelabor values.
- **Pulse**—Monitor every 15 minutes for the first hour. Postpartum pulse rates may be lower than labor values.
- **Respirations**—Monitor every 15 minutes for the first hour. Findings should return to prelabor values.
- **Temperature**—Monitor at least once during the initial postpartum hour. Temperature should be in normal range (below 100.4°F).

Uterus

Evaluation of the uterus includes assessment of fundal height and uterine tone. This evaluation is done with the vital sign evaluation, usually at least every 15 minutes, or more frequently as indicated by findings.

Procedure for Evaluation of Fundal Height

Starting well above the umbilicus, palpate firmly with the flat of the fingers and hand, midline in the abdomen, until the fundus of the uterus is felt. It might be helpful to cup the uterus with the hand to clearly outline its location and size. The fundal height is measured in relation to the umbilicus and is calculated in fingerbreadths above the umbilicus (e.g., 2 fingerbreadths above the umbilicus).

Normal Findings

In the immediate postpartum period, after delivery of the placenta, the fundus should be found midline in the abdomen, approximately 2 cm below the umbilicus. Within 12 hours, the fundus usually rises to approximately 1 cm above the umbilicus. By 24 hours postpartum, the fundus is usually palpable at the umbilicus. The fundus should descend 1 to 2 cm every 24 hours. This process is called "involution." Figure 14.2 indicates expected fundal height measurements during the postpartum period.

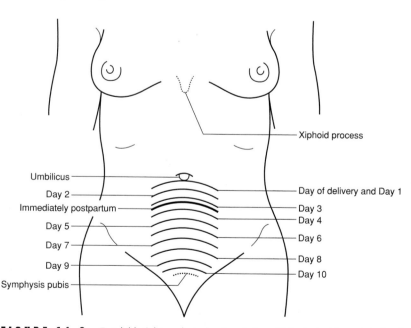

FIGURE 14.2 Fundal height and uterine involution. (Adapted with permission from Varney, H. [1997]. *Varney's midwifery* [3rd ed., p. 624]. Boston: Jones & Bartlett.)

Procedure for Evaluation of Uterine Tone

After assessing fundal height, palpate the tone of the uterus. A boggy uterus feels very soft and is often difficult to find.

Normal Findings

The uterus should be firm and midline.

Lochia

Observe *lochia* (vaginal bleeding) to identify the amount, color, and presence of any clots. Evaluate peripad for amount of saturation.

Normal Findings
Lochia should be red (***rubra***) and moderate in flow during the first hour. Flow should not exceed the saturation of two peripads in the first hour.

Bladder

Gently palpate the lower abdominal area just above the symphysis pubis to palpate for bladder fullness or tenderness.

Normal Findings
The bladder should not be palpable.

Perineum

With adequate lighting and exposure, evaluate for edema and signs of *hematoma* (a discolored or bruised and edematous area). If an episiotomy or laceration repair has been performed, observe for intact stitches.

Normal Findings
The perineum should be pink, without signs of bruising or findings of considerable edema. Inspection of an episiotomy or laceration repair should reveal approximated tissues with little edema.

Breasts

Inspect the nipples of mother planning to breastfeed.

Normal Findings
Nipples may be erect, flat, or inverted (Fig. 14.3).

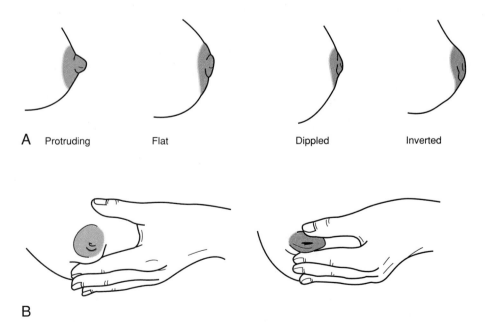

FIGURE 14.3 **A.** Nipple shapes. **B.** *Left:* The mother can help the baby to latch on to an inverted nipple if she places her thumb above the areola and her fingers below and pushes the breast against her chest wall. *Right:* The mother should avoid squeezing her thumb and fingers together. The nipple might invert further. (Adapted from Huggins, K. [1990]. *The nursing mother's companion* [Rev. ed., pp. 29, 65]. Boston: Harvard Common Press.)

Interventions in Case of Variations From Normal Findings

▶ **What are some variations from these normal findings in the postpartum period and how are they managed?**[4,5,12–18]

Findings of variations from normal on postpartum assessments require early interventions to prevent potentially serious consequences.

Vital Signs

Elevated Blood Pressure

Validate the reading by retaking the blood pressure. Notify the physician or midwife of readings of 140/90 mmHg or above or an elevation of 30 mmHg systolic or 15 mmHg diastolic above early pregnancy levels. Assess the patient for pain and provide pain relief as indicated.

Elevated blood pressure in the postpartum period can be a sign of pregnancy-related hypertension and preeclampsia. Patients diagnosed with pregnancy-related hypertension require vigilant monitoring in the early postpartum period.

Decreased Blood Pressure

Validate readings by retaking blood pressure. Assess for increased lochia flow. Notify the physician or midwife if blood pressure does not stabilize, is accompanied by excessive flow of lochia or signs of shock.

Elevated Temperature

Abnormal values must be evaluated to determine their cause. Dehydration after a lengthy labor with inadequate fluid intake is a common cause of early postpartum fever. Women who have had epidural anesthesia may have fever unrelated to infection. Notify the physician or midwife and infant care practitioner if maternal temperature is higher than 100.4°F.

Uterus

Increased Fundal Height

A fundus that is higher than 2 fingerbreadths above the umbilicus might indicate a distended bladder or a uterus that is filled with blood clots. After delivery of a large infant, the fundal height can be slightly elevated, and this may be a normal finding.

Assist the mother to empty her bladder. Catheterize only if the mother is unable to void. Reevaluate the fundal height. Massage the fundus in an attempt to expel any retained blood clots. Report increased fundal height that does not respond to these measures.

Decreased Uterine Tone

Some clinical situations that can predispose a newly delivered woman to uterine *atony* (decreased muscle tone of the uterus) are as follows:

- Prolonged labor
- Oxytocin induction/augmentation of labor
- Magnesium sulfate therapy or use of tocolytics for labor suppression
- Large infant or multiple gestation
- Cesarean section under general anesthesia (halogenated anesthetics)

> REMEMBER: In most cases, postpartum hemorrhage related to uterine atony cannot be predicted before delivery. Every newly delivered mother needs careful monitoring.

The finding of a boggy uterus requires the nurse to massage the uterus to prevent potentially profuse bleeding from the large maternal sinuses at the placental site. Explain the procedure to the woman and ask her to relax her abdominal muscles. Position the woman with her head supine and her knees flexed. Before massaging the uterus, attempt to locate its position in

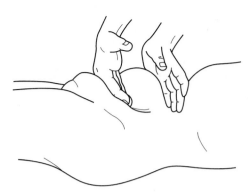

FIGURE 14.4 Placement of the hands for uterine massage.

relation to the umbilicus. To massage the uterus, cup one gloved hand midline on the abdomen near the umbilicus and begin massaging the area. The other gloved hand should be placed just above the symphysis pubis to stabilize the uterus, as shown in Figure 14.4. Moderate massage usually stimulates the relaxed uterus to contract. Massage the uterus only until firm. Downward pressure toward the vagina may be needed to expel clots. While massaging the uterus, continue to observe the perineum for the amount of bleeding and/ or size of expelled clots. If uterine massage does not result in a firm uterus, notify the primary care provider. Often, 10 to 20 U of oxytocin are ordered by the physician or midwife to be added to 1,000 mL of intravenous (IV) fluids (or given intramuscularly) to maintain a firmly contracted uterus. For many practitioners, this is a routine part of postpartum management. In addition, methylergonovine or 15-methyl-prostaglandin F_{2a} (a prostaglandin) may be ordered to ensure uterine contraction and prevent hemorrhage. For further discussion of postpartum hemorrhage, refer to Module 18.

Lochia

Increased Flow of Lochia

The most common cause of increased vaginal bleeding in the immediate postpartum period is uterine atony. Other causes that must be considered are retained placental fragments and bleeding from lacerations.

If excessive lochia flow is identified, massage the fundus until firm. Notify the physician or midwife if bleeding becomes heavy, if a pad is saturated within 15 minutes, or if large clots are expressed. Anticipate the need for an IV line, if not already available. Monitor vital signs, including blood pressure and pulse. Remember that in the postpartum period, significant blood loss can occur without a decrease in blood pressure. Medications, as discussed in the section on decreased uterine tone, may be ordered. If bleeding continues despite a firm uterus, notify the physician or midwife. Assessment of the perineum, vagina, and cervix for lacerations or evaluation of the patient for retained placental fragments may be necessary.

Bladder

Distended Bladder or Inability of Patient to Void

The sensation of needing to void might be decreased in the postpartum woman as a result of pressure on the bladder during labor and birth or because of the continued effects of regional (epidural or spinal) anesthesia. The bladder may become distended from IV fluids administered during labor or from the diuresis that normally occurs postpartum. A distended bladder can interfere with uterine contractility and lead to uterine atony and excessive vaginal bleeding. Many women are able to void when assisted to the bathroom, so this should be attempted before catheterization if there are no contraindications to ambulation. Avoid allowing the bladder to become overdistended, which can lead to loss of muscle tone and continued difficulty with voiding. Catheterization may become necessary. Remember that any catheterization increases the woman's risk for urinary tract infection.

Perineum

Perineal Edema or Hematoma Formation

For all newly delivered women, perineal care with warm water is comforting, promotes healing, and allows good visualization of the area. An ice pack to the perineum during the first 24 hours is recommended after episiotomies or repaired lacerations or if edema is present. After 24 hours, the use of warm, moist heat in the form of a sitz bath facilitates healing and reduces discomfort. Nonsteroidal anti-inflammatory drugs may be ordered by the physician or midwife to reduce the inflammatory response and promote healing. Analgesics may be required. After initial treatment with ice, sitz baths may be ordered.

Notify the physician or midwife of excessive perineal edema or symptoms of hematoma formation. Carefully document the size and location of affected area for comparison during resolution. Occasionally, hematomas must be surgically drained. Observe carefully for signs of distended bladder that may occur if edema is extensive and the patient is unable to void.

Breasts

Flat or Inverted Nipples in the Breastfeeding Mother

Flat nipples that cannot be made to protrude when gently squeezed just behind the nipple can cause difficulty with the infant latching onto the breast. A truly inverted nipple inverts further when this pinch test is attempted.

Breast shells should be worn by the mother to place pressure on the areola and encourage the nipple to protrude (Fig. 14.5). Shells are recommended during the last trimester of pregnancy, but can be used postpartum if the nipple problem is not identified until after delivery. A manual or electric breast pump can also be used immediately before nursing to attempt to make the nipples easier for the infant to grasp.

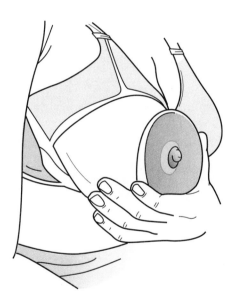

FIGURE 14.5   Breast shells may improve the nipple shape. (Adapted from Huggins, K. [1990]. *The nursing mother's companion* [Rev. ed., p. 30]. Boston: Harvard Common Press.)

Role of the Nurse in Postpartum Care

Promoting Bonding

▶ **What can the nurse do to promote infant attachment?**[4,5,17]

The bond between parents and their infant begins during pregnancy and continues to develop during infancy. Attachments to other family members also develop with the birth. All infants need this nurturing bond with others to thrive.

As parents get to know their newborn, certain behaviors typically emerge. A parent often first touches the newborn with fingertips only and slowly progresses to use of the entire hand to caress the infant. The mother or father will hold the baby so that the infant's face is directly in front of the parent's face, the ***en face*** position, at a distance of about 10 to 12 inches, the distance at which the newborn can most clearly see. The parent will also typically talk to the newborn in a higher pitch than normal conversation, a pitch that elicits a response from the newborn.

The nurse can promote this attachment to the infant in simple ways. Parents and family need access to their infant. Well newborns should remain in the mother's room. Many hospitals encourage this practice by assigning one nurse to both mother and infant and organizing care for both in the mother's room. If an infant must be cared for in the nursery, it is important that policy allows either parent to visit at any time and to call as needed.

Parents need opportunities to get to know their infant and to learn to feel confident in caring for the infant's needs. The nurse can arrange these opportunities and give positive reinforcement. For example, the father gains confidence and learns much more about his new infant if he is assisted in changing the baby's diaper than if the expert nurse does the job.

It is important for the nurse to observe the interactions between parents and infant during the postpartum stay and to notify pediatric and obstetric care providers of observed difficulties with attachment.

Breastfeeding

▶ **How can the nurse assist the mother in initiating breastfeeding in the immediate postpartum period?[15–18]**

Very few conditions exist that would contraindicate a mother's choice to breastfeed. Contraindications noted by AAP and ACOG in the Guidelines for Perinatal Care are as follows:
- Active tuberculosis in the mother before she has received adequate therapy
- Primary maternal infection with cytomegalovirus during the acute phase of the disease
- HBsAg-positive status (until the hepatitis B immune globulin and vaccine are given to the infant)
- HIV-positive status
- Active herpes infections in the breast area

The decision to breastfeed is often made early in the prenatal period. A discussion of the value of breastfeeding with the physician or midwife and an examination of the breasts to identify inverted nipples or other breast problems that might interfere with breastfeeding is an important part of prenatal education.

Initiation of breastfeeding during the first hour of the infant's life and frequent early nursing is associated with fewer problems with lactation.

A mother should be taught that the use of any medications while breastfeeding should be discussed with her physician, midwife, or primary care practitioner.

Artificial nipples (e.g., bottles, pacifiers) should be avoided during the early postpartum period to prevent the problem of nipple confusion. *Nipple confusion* describes the difficulty some infants display in learning to breastfeed after having been fed by bottle.

Routine supplementation with formula or water in the early postpartum period is unnecessary and can interfere with successful lactation.

Breastfeeding is a learned activity for both the mother and infant. This process takes time and assistance from knowledgeable care providers.

Assessments/Interventions for Breastfeeding

As soon as possible after birth and, if possible, during the first postpartum hour, determine the readiness of the mother and infant to breastfeed. During this first hour, the infant is typically in the quiet/alert state and is receptive to breastfeeding.

Assist the mother to a comfortable position. Sitting in an almost upright position is often a position that is good for early nursings. The mother can see her infant, and the nurse can easily observe the nursing couple. Use pillows to position the mother and infant comfortably. The infant should be positioned so that the infant's body faces the mother's body and the infant's head is in a straight line with his or her own body (Fig. 14.6). The cradle hold, the cross-cradle hold, and the football hold are all good positions for early nursings.

Have the mother gently stroke the infant's lower lip until the infant opens the mouth wide. While the infant's mouth is wide open, instruct the mother to quickly move the infant toward the breast. The mother can cup her breast with her hand to guide the breast, grasping the breast with four fingers below and the thumb above the areola (Fig. 14.6). Fingers need to be kept well back from the areola (the pigmented area of the breast that surrounds the nipple).

The infant should draw 0.5 to 1 inch of the areola into the mouth. At this first feeding, allow the infant to nurse on one breast for as long as the baby continues to actively nurse, then assist the mother to position the infant at the opposite breast. The infant may or may not vigorously nurse both breasts at this first feeding. Remind the mother to begin nursing with this second breast at the next feeding. Allow the infant to learn to nurse during this early

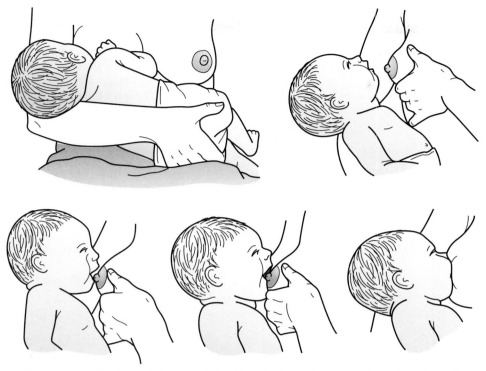

Assist the mother to position the infant's body to face the mother's body.

Show the mother how to grasp the breast with four fingers below and the thumb above.

Instruct the mother to touch the nipple to the infant's lower lip.

When the infant's mouth opens wide, instruct the mother to pull the baby in to latch on.

FIGURE 14.6 Positioning for breastfeeding. (Adapted from Huggins, K. [1990]. *The nursing mother's companion* [Rev. ed., p. 43]. Boston: Harvard Common Press.)

feeding. Duration of the feeding is not as important as is the stimulation of the breasts and the learning process.

Teach the mother to break the infant's suction by inserting the tip of her finger into the corner of the infant's mouth when feeding is complete.

Encourage the mother to nurse frequently during the hospital stay. Have her offer the breast every 2 to 3 hours and teach her the cues that the infant is waking and getting ready to feed. It is easier to learn to nurse a calm infant who is not crying with hunger.

Some infants do not readily nurse for several feedings. Explain to the mother that this is normal and that her baby is also tired from birth. Most infants nurse vigorously by 12 to 24 hours after birth. Continued difficulties should be referred to a lactation consultant or care provider experienced in lactation assistance. It is important that infants are feeding well before discharge from the hospital and that mothers know how to get assistance if needed.

Cesarean Birth

After a cesarean delivery, the woman should be cared for in a postanesthesia recovery room or an appropriately equipped LDRP room. Standards for care of this patient are no different from standards for any patient recovering from major surgery and anesthesia.

Routine separation of mother and infant is not necessary unless warranted by the condition of either the mother or the baby.

Assessments and interventions for the postpartum mother also apply after a cesarean delivery.

▶ **What special assessments or interventions are needed for the woman who has undergone cesarean birth?**[4,5,17,18]

For a discussion of intrapartum care for the woman experiencing a cesarean delivery, see Module 19.

Assessment of Recovery From Regional Anesthesia

As a component of the assessment of recovery from anesthesia, it is important for the nurse to know the type of anesthesia used and the specific medication. Length of action of the different anesthetics affects the recovery period.

For women who have received spinal or epidural anesthesia, the spinal level needs to be evaluated. A *dermatome* chart is helpful in this evaluation (Fig. 14.7). The chart is used to identify areas of the skin that correspond to the area of innervation in the spine. Assessment of the spinal level of the anesthesia may be performed by using an alcohol pad to touch the abdomen until sensation is identified by the woman. The level at which sensation is felt corresponds to the spinal level. As anesthesia wears off, the spinal level decreases. Ability to move the legs and sensation in the legs also indicates that the level of anesthesia is diminishing.

Interventions

While under the effect of a regional anesthetic, the newly delivered woman will not have the sensation of a full bladder, so the nurse must carefully evaluate the bladder for distention. Careful

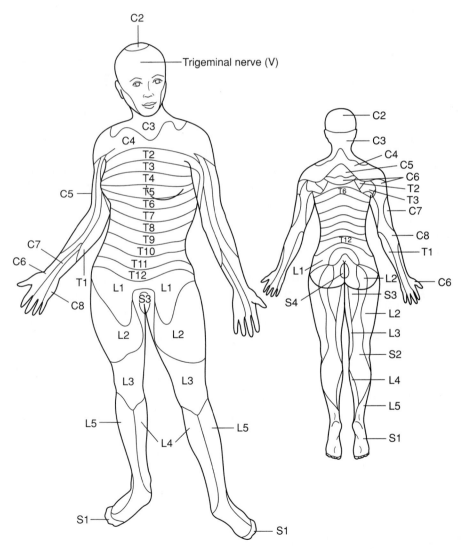

FIGURE 14.7 Segmental dermatome distribution of spinal nerves. *Abbreviations:* C, cervical segments; L, lumbar segments; S, sacral segments; T, thoracic segments. (Adapted with permission from Thibodeau, G. [1987]. *Anatomy and physiology* [p. 71]. St. Louis: Mosby.)

attention to positioning of the lower extremities to prevent injury is also important. Ambulation should not be attempted until full control of the legs returns. Even after motor control has returned, sensation in the lower body can be diminished. The temperature of bath water must be monitored to prevent burns.

Assessment of Recovery From General Anesthesia

Patients requiring general anesthesia for cesarean delivery are at a greater risk for aspiration. Therefore, recovery from general anesthesia occurs in a specially equipped recovery area so that the vital signs and respiratory status of the woman can be monitored closely. Nurses working in postanesthesia recovery rooms receive specialized training in the monitoring of these patients. In labor and delivery units, nurses receive this training or are assisted by anesthesia personnel.

Care of the Incision

Assess the status of the incision by evaluating the abdominal dressing.

Normal Findings

The dressing should be dry and intact, with no signs of bleeding or drainage. Note this finding in the chart.

Interventions

If any drainage is noted, chart the size and description of the drainage. (For example, "A 5-cm area of dark red drainage is noted on the left lower margin of the abdominal dressing.") Continue to inspect the dressing and notify the primary care provider of increased drainage.

Management of Pain

As anesthesia wears off during the early postpartum period, the patient might report pain or request pain medication. It is important for the nurse to know which medications the patient received during surgery and which medications the physician has ordered for the postpartum period. Some patients might have received spinal or epidural narcotics that will decrease pain during the postpartum period. Remember to adequately assess the report of pain, including perception of severity and location.

Normal Findings

Pain and/or discomfort are normal findings immediately after surgery; a goal of care is to reduce the severity of the pain.

Interventions

Medicate the postpartum cesarean-delivered mother as needed to achieve comfort. An adequately medicated person experiences fewer complications related to immobility than a person in pain and recovers more quickly from surgery. Comfort measures, such as positioning and massage techniques, should not be forgotten as means of decreasing discomfort.

Evaluation of Fluid Status

The cesarean-delivered mother will have an IV line and a Foley catheter. The rate of the IV infusion and the fluid infused will be ordered by the physician and should be monitored. During the early postpartum period, oxytocin is often added to the infusion.

The catheter drainage bag should be emptied on admission to the recovery area and again after 1 hour to determine the initial hourly output. Until the catheter is removed, the output should be monitored at least every shift, or more frequently as ordered by the physician.

Normal Findings

The IV site should be free of signs of inflammation or edema, and the fluids should infuse freely. The urine should be amber or straw colored and measure at least 30 mL per h.

Interventions

Maintain the IV infusion as ordered by the physician. Unless excessive blood loss has occurred, the rate of the infusion is typically 125 or 150 mL per hour. Notify the primary care provider if urine output is less than 30 mL per hour or if it is blood tinged after the first hour postpartum.

Sterilization

▶ What is the role of the nurse in postpartum sterilization?[19]

The decision for postpartum sterilization is most appropriately made during the antepartum period and includes the process of informed consent. Informed consent is obtained by the physician and includes information that the patient can understand about the risks and benefits of a procedure and any alternatives to the procedure. The woman is allowed the opportunity to ask questions and then make her decision. A permit for the procedure is the documentation of this process of education, decision, and consent.

Tubal ligation (the interruption of the course of the fallopian tube) may be performed in the immediate postpartum period if a regional anesthetic has been used for the delivery and if the condition of the mother and infant is satisfactory. If an anesthetic must be initiated for the surgery, the anesthesia care provider will consider the risks and benefits of the timing of this procedure. Some providers postpone tubal ligation for several hours and request that the patient be given nothing by mouth during this period.

Assessments

Preoperative assessments include a review of the permit and evaluation of the woman's status in the immediate postpartum period. Vital signs, fundal height, and lochia flow are evaluated. The woman's bladder should also be assessed for distention. The woman should be encouraged to empty her bladder immediately before being transferred to the operating room. Allow the woman the opportunity to ask questions about the procedure.

Postoperative Assessments

Refer to the assessments of a woman recovering from cesarean delivery. The incision is smaller, and pain is typically less severe. Often, women report pain localized to the right side of the abdomen after tubal surgery. A catheter in the bladder is not used for tubal sterilization. Therefore, the patient's bladder should be carefully assessed to prevent distention.

Interventions

The anesthesia care provider or obstetrician might order preoperative medications. It is important to notify the care provider of any variations from the normal postpartum assessments of the mother or any problems of the newborn before tubal ligation is performed. Postoperative interventions are also similar to care after a cesarean delivery. Pain can usually be managed with oral medications.

Obstetric, Medical, or Surgical Complications

▶ What are the components of the recovery care for a woman with puerperal infection or with preeclampsia?[5,17,18]

Women with obstetric, medical, or surgical complications need careful monitoring in the early postpartum period. *Puerperal infection* is a term used to describe any bacterial infection of the genital tract in the postpartum period. The pediatric care practitioner needs to be notified of infections in the mother, although mothers and infants are not routinely separated. The cure for preeclampsia is delivery. Usually, a woman rapidly improves after the birth; however, the risk for eclampsia (seizure activity in a preeclamptic woman) continues, especially in the first 24 hours.

Assessment of the Woman With a Genital Tract Infection

Infection during the birth process is most commonly chorioamnionitis, an infection of the fetal membranes that begins to resolve after delivery. Postpartum infections can include endometritis (an infection of the uterus) or a urinary tract infection. Prolonged rupture of the membranes, multiple vaginal examinations, and catheterization of the bladder are all risk factors for infection.

The vital signs of the newly delivered mother must be evaluated. An oral temperature of greater than 100.4°F is considered fever and should be reported to the physician or midwife. A single elevation of temperature may be related to dehydration, but needs to be followed closely with additional temperature readings. Other signs of infection can include a tender uterus or the typical signs of cystitis, burning or pain on urination, or suprapubic pain.

Interventions

The physician or midwife will consider the cause of the fever and, if infection is suspected, may order antibiotics. Fluids may also be ordered, either intravenously or by mouth. In addition, medication may be ordered to reduce fever. Monitoring of the course of the infection by evaluation of the temperature is important to determine the effectiveness of treatment.

Assessment of the Woman With Preeclampsia

Women with preeclampsia need careful assessment and monitoring of vital signs, especially blood pressure, and evaluation of reflexes in the early postpartum period. Reports of headache and visual changes by the mother are also important to consider in the overall assessment of recovery. Urinary output needs careful assessment. Less than 30 mL per hour (oliguria) is an abnormal finding.

Interventions

Blood pressure evaluation is important for these women. The physician or midwife will define parameters of blood pressure readings that are acceptable for this patient and those that require notification of the provider.

> Refer to Module 9 on hypertensive disorders of pregnancy for a more complete description of preeclampsia and the necessary assessments and interventions.

Perinatal Loss and Newborn Illness

▶ **How can the nurse assist parents who experience a perinatal loss or parents of an ill newborn?[5,17,19–23]**

The delivery of a stillborn infant or the birth of a newborn who requires the special care nursery is an event that produces enormous stresses for the new mother and her family. The perinatal nurse is often the person in the hospital setting who has contact with a family that has experienced a perinatal loss or the delivery of a sick newborn. In this role, the nurse must function as a patient care provider, a support person during the grief process, a patient advocate, and a facilitator information provider and coordinator of care.

> See Appendix C for key elements about effective pain management for the dying newborn.

▶ **What can help the parents who experience a stillbirth or the death of a newborn?[20–23]**

Many hospitals have developed programs to help care providers deal with the issues of perinatal loss and have instituted procedures to assist parents with the grief process through coordination of services and ongoing sensitive care.

Immediately after the delivery of a stillborn infant, both parents are in the shock phase of grief. The mother is concerned with her own personal health and safety, as after any delivery. Questions relating to the reason for the death arise and are often difficult or impossible to answer. The nurse's role during this initial phase is both to provide physical care for the mother and to assist with the process of grief.

To begin to grieve for the infant lost, it is necessary for the parents to create memories of the child. Parents should be offered adequate time to hold and touch the infant in a private setting. The family may wish to view the infant multiple times. The nurse can wrap the infant in a blanket and remain with the family, if needed or requested, to answer questions. It is common for parents to remark on the gender of the child, the perfection of hands or feet, and family resemblance—in effect, to claim the child as their own. Photographs can be taken, identification bracelets made, footprints made, handprints made, locks of hairs preserved, and certificates prepared, and all of these offered to the family. Sometimes parents initially refuse such mementos, but then ask for them weeks or months later. It is the responsibility of the unit to retain the memento packet if the parents initially decline. Naming the child is another activity that assists parents with this process of claiming the child who has died.

The nurse has ongoing responsibilities in coordinating care for this mother and her family. Decisions about location of the postpartum stay, notification of hospital staff who will be in contact with the mother, and notification of support services (e.g., social services, clergy, grief counselors) are tasks for the nurse. The mother may not wish to stay in the obstetric setting and prefer to recover during her postpartum stay in another area, away from the newborn nursery. It is important for all care providers to be aware of the family's loss. Each unit should devise a system for alerting other health care providers and staff that a loss has occurred. This will hopefully prevent awkward and painful encounters. The nurse must also facilitate and allow ample time for decisions to be made about disposition of the infant's remains.

Finally, perinatal nurses must consider their own feelings related to the loss. Just as parents search for the answers to why the loss occurred, so do the care providers. It is also common for nurses to avoid the family because of the uncertainty of how to help or feelings that medical care has failed this family. The belief that every pregnancy should have the outcome of a healthy infant is common, but not realistic. Nurses need to examine their role in good outcomes, while accepting the fact that poor outcomes cannot always be prevented. A hospital with a carefully considered plan for assisting families with perinatal loss also considers these needs of the care providers.

▸ How can the nurse help the parents of an ill newborn?[20,21]

Many of the suggestions for the care of parents who have experienced a perinatal loss are appropriate for parents of an ill newborn. These parents have lost their dream of a healthy infant. The nurse can expect the family to exhibit signs of the grief process.

As soon as possible, considering the condition of the mother and the infant, it is important for the parents to visit the newborn. Intensive care nurseries can be frightening for parents, and a nurse should be available to the parents to explain equipment, answer questions, and encourage interaction with the infant. Frequently, the intensive care nursery staff takes pictures of the newborn for the parents to have with them.

If the mother is discharged from the hospital before the infant, parents should be given the telephone number of the nursery and instructions to call or visit frequently. Some newborn intensive care units have programs to contact parents at frequent intervals to provide information on the infant's condition.

Care of the Mother During the Postpartum Hospitalization

▸ What are the mother's ongoing needs during postpartum hospitalization?[5,17]

The period of postpartum hospitalization can be as brief as a few hours, but is commonly at least a 24-hour stay. Women remain in the hospital during that time when intensive postpartum care is required and return to their home environments to recover completely. During the hospital stay, the newly delivered mother is often expected both to recover physically and also to demonstrate the capability to care for herself and her newborn. Rubin's identified periods of the postpartum, *taking in* and *taking on,* identify maternal readiness for self-care and infant care. During *taking in,* the mother is more passive and focuses primarily on her physical needs. In the *taking on* period, the mother begins to assume the care of herself and her infant. The mother is commonly discharged during the taking in period or the early taking on period and is not ready for assuming total care of herself or her infant. The family needs to understand the new mother's need for help with her care and the infant's care during this early phase of the postpartum period.

The educational needs of the new family have always been a concern and the responsibility of the postpartum and nursery nurse. As postpartum stays have become brief, opportunities for education have also decreased. New research supports the need for thorough prenatal education in postpartum and newborn care. In the early postpartum period, the newly delivered mother is only able to assimilate information that is reinforcement or review of that previously learned. Topics of education that are important for reinforcement of previous teaching include physical care of the mother, physical care of the infant, warning signs of problems of both infant and mother, infant nutrition, family adjustments, birth control, and needs for continued care. A simple technique that is effective for education of the new family is for the nurse to explain the care given as it is being provided. The woman has an immediate opportunity to ask questions.

The physical needs of mother and baby during the hospital stay include the needs of the mother for rest and nourishment. The nurse will be evaluating the continued recovery from delivery and monitoring the return to the prepregnant state. Variations from normal assessments should be discussed with the physician or midwife before discharge. Infant needs are similar and include the need for the establishment of nourishment. Whether the infant is breastfed or bottle fed, patterns of feeding need to be observed by the nurse and assistance provided to the parents.

▶ How can the postpartum nurse begin to prepare the mother for the transition to care at home?[5,17]

A well-organized and coordinated system of maternity care is needed to ensure that mothers and infants receive the follow-up care necessary to meet the needs of the early postpartum period. Health care systems are responding to these needs for follow-up care in a variety of ways. Home visits by specially trained home health nurses, sometimes called "perinatal community nurses," are available for some women. Follow-up phone interviews to identify problems is another method used by care systems.

Every mother, before discharge, needs to know how she can obtain further care for herself and her newborn. Schedules for needed follow-up visits for mother and infant are important. Written lists of emergency phone numbers are also helpful. This information needs to be discussed with the new family and should also be provided in writing.

PRACTICE/REVIEW QUESTIONS

After reviewing Part 2, answer the following questions.

1. It is not unusual to be unable to palpate the uterus immediately after delivery. During this time, the uterus is often boggy and difficult to locate.

   a. True

   b. False

2. A distended bladder is suspected if the fundal height is above the umbilicus and deviated to the right of the midline.

   a. True

   b. False

3. During the first postpartum hour, the vital signs should be evaluated at least every 15 minutes.

   a. True

   b. False

4. Excessive edema of the perineum should be reported to the physician or midwife.

   a. True

   b. False

5. It is not uncommon for the newly delivered woman to have brisk vaginal bleeding during the first postpartum hour.

   a. True

   b. False

6. A newly delivered mother must be separated from her ill infant. The nurse can facilitate attachment by:

   a. Arranging a visit to the nursery as soon as the mother is physically able

   b. Reassuring the woman that her infant is being well cared for by the nursery nurses

   c. Explaining to the woman that bonding with the infant can wait until the infant is well

7. A woman is concerned that her infant did not vigorously nurse at the first feeding and may be hungry. You tell the woman:

   a. She might have to supplement breastfeeding with formula until the infant begins to nurse more effectively

   b. Newborns are learning to nurse at the first feeding and will learn with time; colostrum will meet the newborn's nutritional needs

   c. You will let the pediatrician know about the problem

8. A mother who is breastfeeding should be taught to check with her physician, midwife, or primary care provider before taking any medications.

   a. True

   b. False

9. Breast shells should be worn if the woman who is breastfeeding has inverted nipples.

   a. True

   b. False

10. Fewer problems with breastfeeding occur if the infant nurses during the first hour of life.

    a. True

    b. False

11. Informed consent for sterilization includes:

    a. Information on the risks of the procedure

    b. Reasons to have the surgery done

    c. Alternatives to the surgery

    d. A decision by the woman to have the surgery done

    e. All of these

12. Immediately after a cesarean delivery, the newly delivered mother:

    a. Can return to her postpartum room

    b. Should be cared for in a recovery room or an appropriately equipped LDRP room

13. A family experiencing a perinatal loss will:

    a. Experience the grief process

    b. Have no special needs during the postpartum

    c. Request early discharge

14. Parents of an ill newborn require assistance with the grief process.

    a. True

    b. False

15. Postpartum education for the new family should include:

    a. Infant care

    b. Care of the new mother

    c. Infant feeding

    d. Contraception

    e. A, B, and C

    f. All of these

PRACTICE/REVIEW ANSWER KEY

1. b. False. Immediately after delivery, the uterus should be firm and easily palpable in the midline.

2. a. True

3. a. True

4. a. True

5. b. False

6. a

7. b

8. a. True

9. a. True

10. a. True

11. e

12. b

13. a

14. a. True

15. f

REFERENCES

1. Finster, M., & Wood, M. (2005). The Apgar score has survived the test of time. *The Journal of the American Society of Anesthesiologists, 102*(4), 855–857.
2. Blackburn, S. (2003). *Maternal, fetal, and neonatal physiology: A clinical perspective.* St. Louis: Saunders.
3. Apgar, V. (1953, July/August). A proposal of a new method of evaluation of the newborn infant. *Current Researches in Anesthesia and Analgesia, 32*(4), 260–267.
4. Leifer, G. (2005). *Maternity nursing: An introductory text* (9th ed). St. Louis: Elsevier Saunders.
5. Lowdermilk, D., & Perry, S. (2006). *Maternity nursing* (7th ed). St. Louis: Mosby.
6. Diehl-Svrjcek, B., & Price-Douglas, W. (2007 Winter). Neonatal resuscitation: The 2006 standards for evidenced based clinical practice. *Journal of Legal Nurse Consulting, 18*(1), 16–19.
7. American Heart Association and American Academy of Pediatrics (2006). *Neonatal resuscitation program textbook* (5th ed). Elk Grove, IL: Author.
8. American Academy of Pediatrics, American College of Obstetricians and Gynecologists. (2003). *Neonatal encephalopathy and cerebral palsy; defining the pathogenesis and pathophysiology.* Elk Grove Village, IL, and Washington, DC: Authors.
9. Cunningham, F. G., Leveno, K. J., Bloom, S. L., et. al. (2005). The newborn infant. In *William's obstetrics* (22nd ed). New York: McGraw-Hill.
10. ACOG Committee Opinion No. 348: (2006, November). Umbilical cord blood gas and acid base analysis. Washington, DC: Author.
11. Ross, M. G., & Gala, R. (2002). Use of umbilical artery base excess: Algorithm for the timing of hypoxic injury. *American Journal of Obstetrics and Gynecology, 187*(1), 1–9.
12. MacMullen, N. J., Dulski, L. A., & Meagher, B. (2005). Red alert; perinatal hemorrhage. *Maternal Child Nursing, 30*(1), 46–51.
13. ACOG Technical Bulletin No 76 . (2006). Postpartum hemorrhage. *Obstetrics and Gynecology, 108*(4), 1039–1044.
14. Borgeat, A., Ekatrdramis, G., & Schenker, C. A. (2003). Postoperative nausea and vomiting in regional anesthesia: A review. *Anesthesiology, 98*(2), 530–547.

15. Lawrence, R. A. (1998). *Breastfeeding—A guide for the medical profession* (5th ed.). St. Louis: Mosby.

16. Auerbach, K. (2000). Evidence-based care and the breastfeeding couple: Key concerns. *Journal of Midwifery and Women's Health, 45*(3), 205–211.

17. Simpson, K. R., & Creehan, P. (2001). *Perinatal nursing* (2nd ed.). Philadelphia: Lippincott.

18. American Academy of Pediatrics. American College of Obstetricians and Gynecologists. (2003). *Guidelines for perinatal care* (5th ed.). Elk Grove, IL, and Washington, DC: Authors.

19. Rothrock, J. (2004, September). Witnessing a surgical consent form. *Ask the Experts about Legal/Professional Issues for Advanced Practice Nurses.* From Medscape Nurses [On-line]. Available at: www.medscape.com/viewarticle/488418 .

20. Rybarik, F., & Bond, C. (2000). Conversations with a colleague: Documenting a neonate's death. *AWHONN Lifelines, 4*(2), 27–28.

21. Wolf-Gabor, S. (2000). Reflections of women's health: Individuality of grief. *AWHONN Lifelines, 4*(2), 72–73.

22. Gold, K. J., Dalton, V. K., Schwenk, T. L. (2007). Hospital care for patients after perinatal death. *Obstetrics and Gynecology, 109*(5), 1156–1166.

23. Silver, R. M. (2007). Fetal Death. *Obstetrics and Gynecology, 109*(1), 153–167.

SUGGESTED READINGS

ACOG Practice Bulletin No. 36. (2002, July). *Obstetric analgesia and anesthesia.* Washington, DC: American College of Obstetricians and Gynecologists.

American Academy of Pediatrics. (2005). Policy statement section on breastfeeding and the use of human milk. *Pediatrics, 115*(2), 496–506.

American College of Obstetricians and Gynecologists. (2007). Breastfeeding: Maternal and infant aspects. ACOG Committee Opinion No. 361. *Obstetrics and Gynecology, 109*(2), 479–480.

AWHONN Position Statement. (1999, June). *Issue: Breastfeeding.* Washington, DC: The Association of Women's Health, Obstetric and Neonatal Nurses.

AWHONN Position Statement. (1999, June). Issue: *The role of the nurse in the promotion of breastfeeding.* Washington, DC: The Association of Women's Health, Obstetric and Neonatal Nurses.

Askin, D. (2007 June/July). Physical assessment of the newborn part 1 of 2: Preparation through Auscultation. *Nursing for Women's Health, 11*(3), 292–313.

Askin, D. (2007 June/July). Physical assessment of the newborn part 2 of 2: Inspection through palpation. *Nursing for Women's Health, 11*(3), 304–313.

Biancuzzo, M. (2002). *Breastfeeding the newborn: clinical strategies for nurses* (2nd ed). St. Louis: Elsevier Health Sciences.

Dabrowski, G. (2007). Skin-to-skin contact: Giving birth back to mothers and babies. *Nursing for Women's Health, 11*(1), 64–71.

Donnelly, A., Snowden, H. M., Renfrew, M. J., & Woolridge, M. W. (2000). Commercial hospital discharge packs for breastfeeding women. *Cochrane Database System Review,* (2), CD002075.

Hale, T. W. (2004). Maternal medications during breastfeeding. *Clinical Obstetrics and Gynecology, 47*(3), 696–711.

Howard, C. R., & Howard, F. M. (2004). Management of breastfeeding when the mother is ill. *Clinical Obstetrics and Gynecology, 47*(3), 683–695.

Komara, C., Simpson, D., Teasdale, C., Whalen, G., Bell, S. & Giovanetto, L. (2007). Intervening to promote early initiation of breastfeeding in the LDR. *Maternal Child Nursing, 32*(2), 117–121.

Malkin, J. D., Garber, S., Broder, M. S., & Keeler, E. (2000). Infant mortality and early postpartum discharge. *Obstetrics and Gynecology, 96*(2), 183–188.

Martell, L. K. (2000). The hospital experience and the postpartum experience: A historical analysis. *Journal of Obstetric, Gynecologic, and Neonatal Nursing, 29*(1), 65–72.

Miller, L. C., Cook, J. T., Brooks, C. W., Heine, A. G., & Curtis, T. K. (2007). Breastfeeding education: Empowering future healthcare providers. *AWHONN's Nursing for Women's Health, 11*(4), 376–380.

Mohrbacher, N., & Stock, J. (2002). *La Leche League International: The breastfeeding answer book* (3rd ed). Schaumburg, IL: La Leche League International.

Renfrew, M. J., Lang, S., Martin, L., & Woolridge, M. W. (2000). Feeding schedules in hospitals for newborn infants. *Cochrane Database System Review,* (2), CD000090.

Ruchala, P. (2000). Teaching new mothers: Priorities of nurses and postpartum women. *Journal of Obstetric, Gynecologic, and Neonatal Nursing, 29*(3), 265–273.

Urbanski, P. (2000, June). Getting the *go ahead:* Helping patients understand informed consent. *AWHONN Lifelines, 4*(3), 45–49.

M O D U L E

15 *Liability Issues in Intrapartum Nursing*

BETSY B. KENNEDY ■ SUZANNE M. BAIRD ■ MARCELLA T. HICKEY

Objectives

As you complete this module, you will learn:

1. Why malpractice suits are a nursing concern
2. Common areas of litigation for intrapartum nurses
3. Components of informed consent
4. Circumstances that require consent
5. When informed consent is not necessary
6. Who may give consent for the treatment of an adult
7. When nurses are responsible for obtaining the patient's consent
8. Issues related to delegation of responsibility for obtaining informed consent
9. The functions of the chart
10. The relationship that exists between national standards of nursing practice and documentation of care
11. Information that must be documented in the chart by nurses during care of the woman in the intrapartum period
12. The general guidelines for documentation in a chart
13. Tips for countersigning notes, documenting verbal orders, and telephone triage
14. Strategies for avoiding malpractice claims
15. What to do if you are named in a lawsuit

Key Terms

When you have completed this module, you should be able to recall the meaning of the following terms. You should also be able to use the terms when consulting with other health professionals. The terms are defined in this module or in the glossary at the end of this book.

addendum	fraud
capacity	information
collusion	informed consent
confidentiality	malpractice
conservator	standard of practice
documentation	therapeutic privilege
emancipated	voluntariness

Introduction

The intrapartum nurse faces high risk for involvement in a malpractice suit.[1] The alarming number of cases alleging malpractice in obstetrics as a whole may be the result of a number of factors.[1,2]

- Childbirth is an intense, emotional experience and parents have high expectations for a "perfect" birth and newborn. Poor outcomes are not tolerated well.
- Parents may be well-informed consumers of health care.
- Obstetrics is a high-pressure, rapidly changing specialty. Accidents, errors in judgment, and negligence do occur.

The increasing number of nurses named in malpractice cases also reflects the increasing accountability and autonomy in nursing practice, as well as the overarching nursing shortage.[3,4]

This module is divided into four parts, reviewing the elements of malpractice and liability issues unique to intrapartum nurses; the elements of informed consent and possible exceptions; documentation; and professional strategies to avoid malpractice claims.

Components of Malpractice

▶ Why should nurses be concerned about malpractice?

The current **standards of practice** publicized by national professional nursing organizations hold the nurse accountable for nursing practice. These are the standards that the legal profession and courts use in malpractice cases. Therefore, a nurse can be sued for negligence and **malpractice**.

▶ What are malpractice and negligence?[5]

Malpractice is professional negligence, improper discharge of professional duties, or a failure to meet the standard of care of a professional that results in harm to another. **Negligence** is failure to act as a reasonable and prudent person, or conduct contrary to that of a reasonable person under the same or similar circumstances.

▶ Where are nursing standards found?

Nursing standards are found within state statutes (nurse practice acts), the American Nurses Association (ANA), national professional and specialty nursing organizations, the Joint Commission for Accreditation of Healthcare Organizations (JCAHO), documentary evidence, hospital policy and procedures, and testimony from expert witnesses.[6]

▶ What is standard of care?

"Standard of care" is a term used to determine what is "reasonable" under the circumstances and is defined as the degree of skill, care, and judgment used by an "ordinary, prudent" health care provider under similar circumstances.[6]

▶ What are the key elements of professional negligence suits?

In a lawsuit, the plaintiff must allege a negligence or malpractice claim including all of the following[7]:

- Was there a *duty* or a nurse–patient relationship established?
- Was there a *breach* in the standard of care?
- Are there *damages*?
- Are the damages due to or a direct result of the breach in the standard of care (*causation*)?

General Areas of Nursing Management Cited in Legal Cases[3,6,8]

- Inadequate documentation or lack of documentation
- Medication errors
- Violations of the standard of care

- Improper use of equipment
- Poor or inadequate communication
- Chain of command issues
- Failing to follow orders
- Inaccurate assessment and monitoring

Legal Issues Unique to Intrapartum Care

▶ **What are common allegations nurses in intrapartum care face?[1,9]**

Failure to Appreciate a Change in Maternal Status

Birth is an evolving process with changes in maternal physiologic status occurring throughout. Frequent, regular assessments are required during the intrapartum period. The purpose of these assessments is to determine if and when changes in maternal status occur and whether the assessment data fall outside the realm of normal. Nurses are often brought into a malpractice suit due to their failure to interpret and evaluate the patient's response to nursing and/or medical regimes. *Analyze the assessment data to determine nursing interventions, evaluate the effect of nursing and/or medical interventions and formulate a plan of care.*

Failure to Appropriately Administer Uterine Stimulants

When less-than-optimal pregnancy outcomes have occurred and uterine stimulants have been utilized during labor, a variety of issues may arise during litigation.

Common Allegations With Uterine Stimulants

- Fetal injury related to direct trauma associated with frequent, intense uterine contractions
- Failure to accurately assess maternal/fetal status
- Fetal injury related to hypoxia due to uterine hyperstimulation
- Fetal injury related to the use of uterine stimulants with evidence of a nonreassuring fetal status with electronic fetal monitoring
- Maternal and/or fetal injury related to the use of uterine stimulants when it was contraindicated
- Failure to fully inform patient regarding the risks and benefits of elective induction

Uterine hyperstimulation is a common theme in litigation when uterine stimulants have been used to induce or augment labor. In the literature, there are numerous definitions of uterine hyperstimulation that may be utilized by the plaintiff against care providers.

Common themes in the various definitions of uterine hyperstimulation include:

- Frequent uterine contractions
- Prolonged uterine contractions
- Increased resting tone
- Nonreassuring fetal status

Use caution when administering uterine stimulants to avoid uterine hyperstimulation. *The safest method for administration of any uterine stimulant is the use of the lowest possible dose that effects cervical change and labor progress. No matter how the uterine stimulant is ordered, titration of the dose should be based on uterine activity, fetal response, and cervical change.*

Failure to Initiate Appropriate Shoulder Dystocia Maneuvers

When shoulder dystocia is diagnosed by the physician and/or midwife, prompt interventions are required to decrease the risk of maternal–fetal injury and liability. Even though shoulder dystocia is unpredictable, the nurse may be named in a malpractice case due to the failure to identify risk factors, actions taken at delivery, and/or documentation of events. Refer to Module 18 for a complete discussion of shoulder dystocia.

Nursing actions that may decrease liability for the nurse when shoulder dystocia occurs include the following:

- Remain calm
- Call for nursing (RN)/physician (MD) assistance
- Call for the neonatal team and prepare for newborn resuscitation
- Avoid fundal pressure
- Provide firm suprapubic pressure
- Position patient for McRoberts maneuver

- Assist physician/midwife with patient positioning for additional maneuvers such as the all-fours Gaskin maneuver
- *State out loud the maneuvers you are assisting with. For example, "I am applying supra-pubic pressure."*
- Reassure the patient

Specific documentation to reduce liability risks include the following:
- Fetal assessment and/or attempts to obtain fetal assessment data during maneuvers
- Time when calls for help were sent out and when help arrived
- Timing and sequence of all maneuvers
- Timing of delivery—head to body time
- Health team members present during delivery
- Family members present during delivery
- Newborn resuscitation measures utilized
- Document as soon as possible after the delivery

> It may be helpful to discuss delivery events with health team members who were present to provide accurate documentation.

> Before the delivery, the nurse can decrease liability related to shoulder dystocia by documenting awareness of risk factors and by recognizing and reporting any delays in expected labor progress to the physician and/or midwife.

Failure to Provide Adequate Screening for Obstetric Maternal Triage (Telephone or Inpatient)

Common Allegations With Obstetrical Triage
- Failure to accurately assess maternal–fetal status (telephone and/or during triage)
- Failure to advise woman to seek medical treatment
- Failure to comply with Emergency Medical Treatment and Active Labor Act (EMTALA) requirements
- Failure to require a physician to assess maternal–fetal status
- Transfer and/or discharge of patient in active labor, with a high-risk complication or based on her inability to pay for medical expenses

EMTALA requires the following:
- Provision of an adequate medical screening examination for every patient
- Stabilization treatment within the capabilities of the institution to every patient with an emergency medical condition
- Transfer/discharge according to outlined guidelines[10,11]

Medical screening examinations may be done by a nurse if the following criteria are met[11,12]:
- Hospital and nursing policy specifically outline the scope of practice and requirements
- Nurses are educated and competent to complete the medical screening examination
- A discussion occurs between the nurse and physician regarding the assessment data
- Discharge orders from the physician are obtained and documented in the medical record

Telephone Triage

Telephone calls from patients are an everyday occurrence in today's health care world. These calls are a potential source of legal problems in two ways. First, an unqualified person might be providing health care information to the patient. Second, documentation of the interaction might be incomplete. Because diagnosing conditions by telephone cannot be done accurately or reliably, *it has been recommended that when calls come in to an intrapartum setting, the mother should be instructed to come in for evaluation or to contact their primary care provider.*[9] The primary care provider should make the assessment of the mother's condition and determine the plan. **IF telephone triage is done, there must be specific and consistent guidelines.** These guidelines may include the following[7]:
- What information should be obtained about the problem
- Who will handle the calls: nurse, nurse practitioner, midwife, or physician
- What problems require an immediate visit
- Where the patient will be seen
- The documentation required for each telephone contact

Bleeding in pregnancy, ruling out labor, abdominal pain, headache, fetal activity concerns, persistent nausea and vomiting, vaginal discharge, and breast complaints are clinical problems appropriate for development of telephone protocols.[6]

Appropriate documentation for telephone triage reflect the following:
- Date and time of contact
- The name of the caller (e.g., "patient Mary Smith" or "Joe Smith, husband of patient, Mary Smith")
- The care provider or practice name that manages the patient's care
- The reason for the call in the caller's words
- Pertinent information about the problem (e.g., signs/symptoms, onset, duration, frequency; actions that alleviate or increase them)
- Significant background information (e.g., prior history, chronic problems, allergies, current medications)
- Conclusions reached about the problem and its urgency
- Instructions given to the individual, including when to seek additional evaluation and care
- The person's response to instructions

It is critical to document the person's response to the instructions. A documented refusal to comply when there is an adverse outcome demonstrates the individual's contributory negligence to the situation. Also, a patient who requests a visit should be directed to the most expedient source of evaluation.

Failure to Initiate Chain of Command

Every perinatal unit should have a written chain of command policy/procedure. Nurses may become liable when a disagreement regarding clinical management occurs and they fail to initiate the chain of command. *Chain of command activation is recommended when there is potential for the maternal and/or fetal condition to rapidly deteriorate causing harm, and discussions with the appropriate physician or midwife have failed to provoke an agreeable action plan (Display 15.1).*

DISPLAY 15.1 EXAMPLE CHAIN OF COMMAND[13]

1. Conflict regarding nursing and medical management.
2. Conversation between primary nurse and physician/midwife.
3. Notification of charge RN.
4. Notification of nurse manager/supervisor.
5. Discussion by charge RN and/or nurse manager with physician/midwife.
6. Discussion by charge RN and/or nurse manager with Chief of Obstetrics.
7. Chief of Obstetrics discusses plan with physician/midwife.
8. Notification of Hospital Administrator by Nursing and/or Chief of Obstetrics.
9. Hospital Administrator assists with resolution of conflict.

Failure to Notify the Physician/Nurse-Midwife

There is a legal duty to communicate in a timely manner any significant, abnormal assessment data to the appropriate physician and/or midwife. Failure to communicate these findings may lead to poor outcomes and increase the chances for malpractice litigation.

Common breakdowns in RN to physician/midwife communication involve the following situations:
- Busy providing urgent care to patient
- Nurse is convinced physician/midwife will not act on assessment data
- Fear that physician/midwife will become angry regarding communication
- Nurse does not want to interrupt physician/midwife
- Nurse fails to see the relevance of assessment data
- Communication with physician who does not have surgical privileges
- Failing to persist in communication

Effective communication techniques that nurses, nurse midwives, and physicians can use include the following:

- Speak clearly
- Speak using a congenial tone
- Be courteous and professional
- Present facts in a methodical or chronological style—organization
- Ask for clarification if communication is unclear
- Communicate all relevant facts, abnormal findings, and specific concerns
- State your reasons if you disagree with a treatment plan
- If the mother or fetus (or both) are at risk, tell the physician to report to the hospital to assess the patient immediately, and document
- Inform the physician or provider if you plan to communicate up the chain of command

---

Example Documentation of Assertive Communication:

"Dr. _____, I'm really uncomfortable with the fetal heart rate, the variability has deteriorated, and there are decelerations. I have put on oxygen, repositioned the patient, and turned off the Pitocin, but the decelerations have continued. I think this patient needs your personal assessment regarding immediate delivery. I want you to come in now."

Failure to Appropriately Manage the Second Stage of Labor

Common allegations during the second stage of labor include the following:

- Failure to appreciate a nonreassuring fetal status
- Failure to notify the appropriate physician/midwife
- Failure to anticipate neonatal resuscitation needs

There are several options for management of the second stage of labor. When a patient has epidural anesthesia, coached closed glottis pushing when compete cervical dilation is assessed is very common. This method does not consider maternal desire to bear down with uterine contractions or the fetal station. Passive fetal descent or the "laboring down" method delays active pushing until the woman feels the urge to push. This delayed pushing option results in less fetal oxygen desaturation episodes, does not increase the risk of cesarean section or length of the second stage, and decreases the percentages of operative vaginal birth with forceps or vacuum.[14] Open glottis pushing has been found to be an effective alternative that does not involve the mother holding her breath and initiating the Valsalva maneuver, which can have negative effects on maternal hemodynamics and the fetal response.[14–16]

In planning for care of a patient in the second stage of labor, consider the following:

- Fetal response to uterine contractions and maternal pushing efforts
  - Baseline rate
  - Baseline variability
  - Presence of repetitive decelerations
  - Presence of accelerations appropriate for gestational age
- Maternal urge to push/bear down
- Fetal station and position of presenting part
- Maternal physiologic status (e.g., cardiac disease, fatigue)
- Ability to change maternal position

To decrease liability with second stage management:

- Consider AWHONN recommendations for second stage management.
- Accurately assess fetal status.
- Know where the delivering physician/midwife is located.
- Report any fetal and/or maternal concerns to the physician/midwife in a timely manner.
- Consider using delayed pushing method ("laboring down") with concerns regarding maternal and/or fetal status.
- Anticipate the need for neonatal resuscitation. Request neonatal resuscitation team to be present at delivery if indicated.
- Avoid the supine lithotomy position.
- Discourage the Valsalva maneuver with pushing.
- Support the woman's efforts.

If the physician/midwife orders "continuous fetal monitoring," the order should be carried out even if the patient is moved to another environment for birth (e.g., operative suite).

Failure to Recognize a Nonreassuring Fetal Status and Provide Appropriate Intrauterine Resuscitation

Failure by the nursing staff to recognize signs of fetal compromise may increase liability exposure, especially if an adverse perinatal outcome occurs.

Common allegations related to recognition and treatment of abnormal fetal heart rate (FHR) patterns include the following:

- Failure to accurately assess fetal status
- Failure to appreciate a deteriorating fetal status
- Failure to provide appropriate intrauterine resuscitation measures for the external fetal monitoring (EFM) pattern
- Failure to timely notify the physician/midwife regarding a nonreassuring fetal status
- Failure to require the physician/midwife to come in to assess fetal status

It is important to provide the appropriate intrauterine resuscitation indicated by the EFM pattern. These interventions may include, but are not limited to, the following:

- Repositioning the mother
- Administration of an intravenous fluid bolus
- Initiate oxygen at 10 L per minute via nonrebreather face mask
- Decrease in or discontinuation of oxytocin infusion
- Administration of terbutaline
- Assessment of cervical status for prolapsed cord, rapid change, and/or fetal descent
- Assessment of maternal blood pressure; comparison with baseline
- Notification of the physician/midwife

If the fetal heart rate pattern is nonreassuring, analysis to determine the cause can aid in development of a plan of care, guide interventions, and decrease liability. The following illustrates suggested progressive steps for EFM assessment[17]:

1. What is the baseline FHR?
2. Is the baseline rate within normal limits?
3. If not, what clinical factors (maternal or fetal) could be contributing to this baseline rate?
4. Is there evidence of baseline variability?
5. If not, does fetal scalp stimulation elicit an acceleration of the FHR appropriate for gestational age?
6. What clinical factors could be contributing to the baseline variability?
7. Are accelerations or decelerations present?
8. If decelerations are present, what type?
9. What are the appropriate interventions for this type of deceleration?
10. Does the FHR pattern suggest a chronic or acute maternal–fetal condition?
11. Is uterine activity normal in frequency, duration, intensity, and resting tone?
12. What is the FHR response to uterine activity?
13. If the FHR pattern is nonreassuring, what are the appropriate interventions to resolve the situation? Will they resolve the situation?
14. Is the FHR pattern such that notification of the physician/midwife or ancillary services (NICU, OR team) is warranted?

Ongoing fetal assessments should be made at the patient's bedside utilizing the printed strip instead of the surveillance computer screen.

If "continuous fetal monitoring" is ordered and there is difficulty in tracing the fetal heart rate continuously, documentation should reflect these difficulties and actions taken to attempt a continuous tracing. For example: *"Pt. repositioned on right side. Difficult to maintain continuous EFM tracing due to fetal movement. Plan to continue replacement of US to attempt continuous tracing. When tracing, EFM reassuring. Will place FSE with any nonreassuring EFM parameters."*

Components of Informed Consent

One of the many legal issues affecting medical and nursing practice is that of informed consent. Legally, professionals are required to obtain the patient's permission for procedures and treatments. It is crucial to understand the necessary content, applicability, and the professional nurse's role and responsibility in this area.

▶ What are the components of informed consent?[5]

There are three components of *informed consent*: capacity, information, and voluntariness. *Capacity* refers to the individual's age and competence. Eighteen is recognized as the legal age in most states. In some states, younger persons are considered *emancipated* if they (a) marry, (b) become a parent, (c) are economically independent, or (d) live in a separate setting from their parents. *Competence* refers to the individual's ability to make choices and understand the expected outcomes of a particular choice.

> States may vary in the requirements for informed consent. It is the responsibility of the care provider to know the laws regarding informed consent in their own state of practice!

Information refers to the content of the explanation given to the patient. Four standards may be applied by the courts to this portion of a consent.
1. The **professional standard** requires the practitioner to provide the information considered reasonable in the professional community. In other words, *information* is defined as what most professionals would tell most of their patients in similar circumstances.
2. The **reasonable patient standard** requires that risk factors and expected outcomes be presented as they relate to the individual.
3. The **subjective patient standard** is one held in some states. It requires that a patient be provided information about potential risks as they relate to the patient's lifestyle.
4. The **informed refusal standard** means the patient has received information about the risks of not consenting to treatments or diagnostic testing and yet refuses treatment or testing.

The information should include the following[5]:
- The nature of the individual's condition, the diagnosis, or suspected diagnosis
- The nature and purpose of the proposed treatment, including who will perform the treatment
- Expected outcomes and benefits
- Major risks, complications, and side effects of the proposed treatment
- Reasonable alternatives
- Possible consequences of refusing treatment

Voluntariness refers to the circumstances surrounding the individual giving consent. If force, fraud, duress, or collusion is present, the consent is invalid. Remember that an individual can withdraw consent for a particular procedure. Withdrawal can be given verbally, in writing, or by gesture (e.g., shaking head "no," withdrawing arm from nurse's hand). The procedure should be discontinued as soon as safely possible. Extenuating circumstances in a life-threatening situation can negate the patient's refusal of treatment.

> A lawsuit can be filed if it can be proved that the patient did not consent to a procedure or was poorly informed about it by the professional.

> **REMEMBER:** A positive outcome of a procedure does not protect you, the professional, from a lawsuit.

> **IMPORTANT CONCERNS:** Barriers of language, hearing impairment, and visual impairment must be addressed through interpreters and the use of available technology and services to assist the hearing and visually impaired.[6]

▶ Under what circumstances should consent be obtained?

Many professionals believe that consent must be obtained only for major interventions (e.g., surgery, chemotherapy). **This is incorrect.** A written format is not necessary for every contact, but the components of informed consent must be present. The patient can give consent verbally or by actions that imply consent (e.g., extending an arm for you to draw blood).

> Consent must be obtained whenever the patient is going to be touched by a care provider. Your failure to obtain consent constitutes battery.

▶ Are there exceptions to informed consent?

It is not absolutely necessary to obtain consent when delay will cause the patient's death or seriously jeopardize the patient's health.

▶ Under what circumstances may another individual give consent for treatment of an adult?

When an adult is mentally incompetent, comatose, or senile, a legal guardian, conservator, patient's attorney, or court may provide consent; these are the only sources for such consent. Family members do not automatically have the right to give consent. The court can overrule a competent adult's decision about a treatment. This is done when the state's interest of preservation of life is counter to the patient's wishes.[5]

NOTE: *The preservation of life concept is the basis for many court decisions involving the fetus and/or newborn after the age of viability has been achieved.*

EXAMPLE: *A patient who refuses a cesarean section when the fetus is at term and a placenta previa is evident.*

> *Therapeutic privilege* occurs when a health care provider does not fully inform a patient about a treatment or procedure because the health care provider decides complete disclosure would be harmful. This exception to informed consent is usually not recognized by the courts because of the potential for abuse.

▶ Who should obtain consent for treatment or a procedure?[5]

- Nurses are responsible for obtaining consent for nursing procedures.
- Nurses in an advanced practice role are responsible for obtaining consents for procedures they order or perform.
- Physicians are responsible for obtaining consent for medical procedures or treatments.

The advanced practice nurse and physician are responsible for obtaining consent because they are usually the only ones who can fulfill all the elements of informed consent. Nurses are frequently requested to witness informed consent. However, in some settings, the physician might delegate the task of obtaining consent for specific procedures to nursing personnel. **THE GUIDELINESS FOR OBTAINING CONSENT IN THESE CASES MUST BE SPECIFICALLY WRITTEN FOR THE PROCEDURE, AND APPROVED, AND SIGNED BY MEDICAL AND NURSING ADMINISTRATION. If the patient questions the information provided or refuses to sign the consent, you must not only refrain from trying to persuade the patient but are OBLIGATED, BOTH LEGALLY AND ETHICALLY, TO INFORM THE ATTENDING PHYSICIAN OF THE PATIENT'S INQUIRIES AND /OR REFUSAL TO SIGN. The physician is the ONLY person legally responsible for providing additional information or answering the patient's questions about the treatment.**

> Remember that a nurse simply obtaining a patient's signature for a consent form does not transfer the legal liability for informed consent from the physician to the nurse.

> *Confidentiality* refers to the legal and ethical duty of health care providers to protect patient information, whether in written form or not. Legal parameters for confidentiality privileges vary according to state.[5]

Guidelines for Documentation of Care

The following demonstrates how a professional nurse documents the provision of nursing care that meets the current national standards for nursing practice. One of the responsibilities of a professional group is to develop the standards that define and measure the practice of its members. In the area of intrapartum care, the Association of Women's Health, Obstetric and Neonatal Nurses (AWHONN) has developed the standards for nursing practice. One of the standards requires the documentation of the care provided for each patient. *Documentation* refers to accurate recording on the appropriate chart forms, observations, assessments, nursing actions, and outcomes. These documents serve as a legal record of the professional nursing care provided for each patient.

▶ What are the functions of the chart?[5]

The chart may be a written or computerized record and serves the following purposes:
- Provides an ongoing written record of the patient's status, the care provided, and the outcomes of the interventions
- Documents that appropriate standards of care were implemented by a qualified professional
- Provides a permanent legal record of the patient's course while in the health care system
- Serves as a means of communication from one care provider to another
- Can be used for reimbursement purposes
- Can be a source for research data
- Can be used for quality assurance monitoring

> DISCUSSION: Everyone has heard the saying "If it wasn't charted, it wasn't done." In practice, this may not always be the case, but omissions in documentation can be used to allege a breach of the standard of care. You may provide perfect care for the mother and baby, but if it was not charted, you cannot "prove" it in court. Care providers may testify that something was done, but the omission in documentation will be criticized in the courtroom. Remember that a legal proceeding may not take place until years after the care was provided and your memories of the care provided will have faded.

Components of the Nursing Portion of the Chart

▶ In the intrapartum setting, what should be documented in the nursing portion of the chart?[18]

From the time of admission until discharge from the unit, chart documentation should cite information on the woman and fetus, which includes the following:
- The nurse's assessment (observations)
- Interventions (actions)
- Outcomes of care (responses)
- Unusual incidents
    Specifically, you must take a history, do a review of systems, and perform a physical examination that meets the standards of practice as outlined by AWHONN and that incorporates hospital policies and unit guidelines.

Nursing Components of the Chart Include:

1. **Presenting complaint in the patient's words**
2. **History**
   - Family history: genetic and congenital abnormalities, mental retardation, metabolic problems, multiple births
   - Past medical history: allergies, diabetes, hypertension, herpes, HIV, exposure to tuberculosis, recent exposure to chickenpox
   - Previous obstetric history:
     Gravida _____
     Term _____
     Premature _____
     Abortion _____
     (Spontaneous) _____
     (Termination) _____
     Living _____
     Type of delivery, newborn weight, problems, gynecologic surgery or infections (group B streptococcus, herpes simplex)
   - Social history: smoking, alcohol intake, support person for labor, labor preparation classes
   - Course of this pregnancy: last menstrual period; expected date of confinement; weight gain; infections; gestational diabetes; hypertension; vaginal bleeding; results of ultrasound examinations, nonstress test, contraction stress test, amniocentesis, and laboratory studies; blood type; Rh status; antibody status; serology titer; rubella titer; hemoglobin/hematocrit; triple screen; HIV testing; and culture results for chlamydia, gonorrhea, and group B streptococcus
   - Current history: onset of uterine contractions, frequency, duration, quality; vaginal discharge; bleeding consistency and amount; status of membranes, intact, rupture time, color of fluid; fetal activity; oral intake of liquid, solids, time; current medications (including over-the-counter preparations, herbs, and illicit drugs) with dosage and time last taken; any concurrent symptoms of visual disturbance, headache, or dysuria; timing of last bowel movement and voiding
   - Care provider: name, title, date and time of notification and by whom
   - Infant care plans: feeding, breast/bottle; nursery care, rooming in; care provider; adoption plans
3. **Review of systems: notation of any loss of function; presence of prosthesis, dentures, glasses, contact lenses**
4. **Physical examination**
   - Height
   - Weight
   - Blood pressure
   - Pulse, respirations
   - Temperature
   - Uterine contraction, frequency, intensity, duration, and relaxation
   - Deep tendon reflexes
   - Urine dipstick results

In some settings, head, eyes, ears, nose, throat, breast, heart and lungs, abdomen (general), and extremities may be examined by other care providers according to unit policies. However, the nurse must be aware of the findings and their impact on the nursing assessment and care plan.

Fetal assessment includes fundal height, estimated weight, heart rate (includes baseline, accelerations, and periodic changes), position, and presentation.

Pelvic examination includes effacement, dilatation, station, presentation, condition of membranes, and if present, amniotic fluid amount, color, odor; results of Nitrazine or fern tests; and the collection of cultures when appropriate.

Your *continuous evaluation* of the patient must include evaluation of both maternal and fetal well-being. The record should reflect *why* nursing procedures and interventions were instituted and what the maternal and fetal responses were to them. When the care provider is notified of a deviation from normal, his or her response is to be noted in the record. Flowsheets, checklists, and charting by exception may be the norm for most units, but *it is essential to provide evidence of your critical thinking and clinical decision making in your doc-*

umentation. For example, if the nurse observes a change in the fetal status, a phone call may be made to the primary care provider. The nurse then attempts to deflect responsibility by documenting "Physician aware, no orders received"; "Midwife notified"; or "Dr. Smith called." There is no documentation of the conversation, the nurse's clinical reasoning, actions taken, or responses in the notation. Although no one advocates "overcharting" or "double charting," a narrative note is often the best way to provide evidence of your sound clinical judgment. Adequate space to accomplish this must be provided for in the documentation system.

You must develop the skills needed for clear documentation when you are in a stable situation. Then when an emergency situation occurs, you will be able to record the situation accurately. Summary notes are acceptable if contemporaneous charting is not possible, but the chronology must be correct.[19]

General Guidelines for Chart Documentation[8]

- Record only factual information.
- Make entries legible.
- Avoid gaps in documentation that can be filled in later or used for speculation about what happened.
- Use only standard abbreviations. Be aware of the official "Do not use" list.
- Include the date, time, and your (the recorder's) name and title.
- To correct an error, draw a line through the incorrect information, write "error" above it, write the date and time, and initial the entry. *The accurate information is entered as an* **addendum.**
- Enter an addendum at the next available space on the chart form. Use the current date and time for the new entry. The content can be referenced to the previous material.
- *When there is a delay in entering chart information, write the phrase "late entry" at the beginning of the note.* Enter the note at the next available space on the chart form. *Use the current date and time for the entry.* Explain the delay in recording the information and cross-reference it to the area of the record where it should have appeared in chronologic order.
- Never make entries for another person in the labor and delivery setting.
- Avoid biased language against the patient and other health care providers.
- Document discussions that affect the plan of care. Use quotation marks for patient statements if needed.
- An addendum made after the record is requested for legal action is suspect.
- Use documentation to demonstrate your sound clinical reasoning and critical thinking.
- *Remember, the record you create today is the one you may go into court with in the future.*

Electronic Charting

Although attitudes toward computerized clinical documentation vary, there is no doubt that it has become a norm.[20] It is important to remember that even when computerized charting is used, the nurse still has a responsibility to be complete and accurate, and to demonstrate evidence of sound clinical reasoning. There should always be a mechanism for entering narrative information.

Remember[21]:
- Never share your access code or password for the system.
- Access information ONLY as part of your job function.
- Do not ignore computer alerts about data entry or missing data.
- Use correct procedures for adding late entry information to a record.
- Take care to use your correct code and the patient's personal code.
- Maintain competencies in system use.

Countersigning Notes

When policies of an institution require the professional nurse to countersign or sign off for other personnel, consider the following[22]:
- Countersigning means that you reviewed the entry and consider it accurate.
- It also means that you approved the care provided by the other person.
- Make sure the note indicates who provided the care.

Communication Problems

JCAHO has identified miscommunication among caregivers as a primary cause of infant death and injury.[23] In the intrapartum setting, communication among all caregivers is essential. Communication occurs in the written record and verbally.

Verbal and Telephone Orders

Although technology has eliminated the need for telephone or verbal orders in many settings, this type of order may still be used. However, there are many opportunities for misinterpretation of orders. If a telephone or verbal order is unavoidable, most institutions have policies governing time frames for the practitioner cosigning the order (e.g., verbal orders for medications must be cosigned within 24 hours). When taking a verbal order, write down the order, restate the order verbatim, including the patient's name, and ask for confirmation. In charting the order, indicate "repeated and confirmed."[24]

Nurse-to-Nurse Communication, Nurse-to-Physician/Midwife Communication

Ultimately, all care providers have the same goal of a healthy mother and baby. It is important to remember this goal in communicating and collaborating with all members of the health care team. Using effective, standardized methods of communication such as SBAR (Situation, Background, Assessment, Recommendation) can enhance patient safety, improve outcomes, and reduce liability. The most common communication between nurses is report, hand-off, or hand-over, when care of the patient is transferred between shifts or units. The purpose of the hand-over is to pass along patient-specific information to ensure continuity of care and safety. *Shift reports should be standardized to minimize gaps in information that could contribute to inappropriate care of the patient.* The SBAR technique has been recommended as a framework for effective communication between nurses and between nurses and physicians or midwives (Display 15.2).[25,26]

DISPLAY 15.2	SBAR TECHNIQUE FOR EFFECTIVE COMMUNICATION BETWEEN NURSES AND OTHER NURSES, PHYSICIANS, OR MIDWIVES
S – Situation	*Who are you?* *What is your role in the care of the patient?* *Who is the patient?* *What is the reason for the call or transfer of care?* *(Examples: nonreassuring FHR pattern, bleeding, elevated blood pressure, transfer to another shift or unit)*
B – Background	*What is the clinical context?* *What is the patient's pertinent medical and obstetrical history?* *(Examples: gravida status, parity, gestational age, history of preeclampsia, previous cesarean delivery, plan of care)*
A – Assessment	*What is the current concern?* *What is your assessment of the situation?* *(Examples: Complete description of EFM parameters, vital signs, other symptoms, lab results, transferring care to the next shift)*
R – Recommendation	*What needs to be done to correct it?* *What are you requesting?* *(Examples: "I need you to come and assess the patient now"; "I need you to come and assess the EFM tracing now"; "I need this order changed"; "These labs need to be drawn in the next shift.")*

NOTE: *Be specific about your request and the time frame for response! Always clarify, confirm, and restate any orders given.*

Being well prepared to give a report during a hand-over or before making a call to the physician is important. If you are unsure of your assessment, discuss the situation with your charge nurse or preceptor.

Strategies for Avoiding Malpractice Claims

Ten Professional Strategies for Protecting Yourself From Malpractice Allegations[1,9,19,27]

1. **Review your institutional guidelines and policies.** Make sure they are current and reflect the best available evidence. Be certain they are in accord with current published standards and recommendations from national professional organizations and regulatory boards such as AWHONN, ACOG, ACNM, and JCAHO. Know them and use them.

2. **Perform only those skills you know to be within your scope of practice. Know the scope of practice for your role in providing care. Know your strengths and weaknesses. Work with your preceptors and charge nurse to gain experience and confidence in areas where you feel weak.**

3. **Stay current in obstetrics and with technological advances by attending continuing education conferences, seminars, and in-services.** This demonstrates a commitment to providing excellent, safe patient care, and to the practice of professional nursing.

4. **Be clear about who is managing the patient.** Everyone on the health care team should know at all times who is responsible for the patient. Communication is automatically improved if you know you are talking to the right person.

5. **Be a patient advocate and know how to use the chain of command.** To use the chain of command effectively, you must be confident in your assessments and clinical reasoning. Overcoming fear of conflict and being assertive is easier if you know the "HOW" and "WHY." Don't be afraid to advocate for the patient when you feel the outcome is dependent upon your actions.

6. **Learn and use good communication skills.** Technical expertise is expected, but communication skills can make the difference in whether or not you get sued. Whether communicating a plan of care to an oncoming shift during report, communicating with the patient and family, or communicating with a physician about a nonreassuring fetal monitor tracing, say what you mean.

7. **Document everything.** Your charting should be accurate and complete. Review your charting and imagine you were defending it in front of a jury.

8. **Get to know your patients.** Use your good communication skills with patients as well as other health care providers. Be mindful of both verbal and nonverbal communication. Patients who feel as if their needs are not being met, whether or not it is an accurate perception, become angry. Your interactions with the patient and family frame their perception of the quality of care they are receiving. Always treat patients with dignity and respect.

9. **Don't make excuses.** Certainly the nursing shortage has acquainted all of health care with the concept of "understaffing." Do not use this as an excuse for delivering poor quality care. The parents (and jury) will not care that you didn't have 30 minutes for lunch if there is a poor outcome for their newborn.

10. **THE GOLDEN RULE.** Of all strategies to avoid a malpractice claim, perhaps the most basic and most important is to use the golden rule we learn as children.

> *Treat others as you would like to be treated.*

What to Do if You Are Called to Testify

In-depth information about depositions or testifying in a malpractice suit is beyond the scope of this book. However, some broad guidelines are as follows[3,28,29]:

- Notify your professional insurance carrier.
- Notify your employer's risk manager.
- Engage your own counsel if necessary.
- Do not discuss the case with anyone except your insurance carrier, claims representative, attorney, or risk manager.
- Review the patient's chart and write down all aspects of the incident recalled.
- Know the patient's record inside and out.
- Review the institution's policy and procedure manual for the year in which the incident occurred.
- Have a current curriculum vitae documenting your continuing education.

PRACTICE/REVIEW QUESTIONS

After reviewing this module, answer the following questions.

1. List three components of informed consent.

    a. _____

    b. _____

    c. _____

2. List four circumstances that are considered in determining emancipation of a minor.

    a. _____

    b. _____

    c. _____

    d. _____

3. What four standards are applied to information provided to the patient? Describe the meaning of each standard.

    a. _____

    b. _____

    c. _____

    d. _____

4. List the type of information that should be included when obtaining informed consent.

    a. _____

    b. _____

    c. _____

    d. _____

    e. _____

    f. _____

5. When must the patient's consent be obtained?

    _____

    _____

    _____

6. Describe the exceptions to informed consent?

    _____

    _____

7. Who may give consent for treatment when an adult is mentally incompetent?

    _____

    _____

8. Under what circumstances are nurses clearly responsible for obtaining a patient's consent?

    a. _____

    b. _____

9. Who is responsible for obtaining consents for medical procedures or treatments?

    _____

10. State at least three important functions of the chart from a legal standpoint.

    a. _____

    b. _____

    c. _____

11. In general, what are the nurse's responsibilities for documentation in the chart?

    _____

    _____

12. When medications or procedures are withheld, what action should the nurse take?

    _____

    _____

13. How should an error in charting be corrected?

    _____

    _____

14. What three circumstances should be present when a professional nurse countersigns another person's notes?

    a. _____

    b. _____

    c. _____

15. State the precautions to be taken when accepting a verbal order.

    a. _____

    b. _____

    c. _____

16. In handling a telephone triage, what information is needed about the current problem?

    a. _____

    b. _____

17. List items to review in preparation for giving a deposition or testimony.

    a. _____

    b. _____

18. What criteria will be used to judge a nurse's practice?

    _____

19. List four of the areas of nursing management that are most often cited in legal actions.

   a. _____

   b. _____

   c. _____

   d. _____

20. List three reasons why intrapartum nurses face high risk for involvement in a malpractice suit.

   a. _____

   b. _____

   c. _____

21. Define *negligence*.

   _____

   _____

22. Define *malpractice*.

   _____

   _____

23. List seven sources of nursing standards.

   a. _____

   b. _____

   c. _____

   d. _____

   e. _____

   f. _____

   g. _____

24. List the four key elements in a malpractice suit.

   a. _____

   b. _____

   c. _____

   d. _____

25. List eight allegations faced by intrapartum nurses.

   a. _____

   b. _____

   c. _____

   d. _____

   e. _____

   f. _____

   g. _____

   h. _____

26. Describe the safest method for administration of uterine stimulants.

   _____

   _____

27. List five nursing actions to decrease liability in the event of a shoulder dystocia.

   a. _____

   b. _____

   c. _____

   d. _____

   e. _____

28. When is activation of chain of command recommended?

   _____

   _____

   _____

29. List six effective communication techniques.

   a. _____

   b. _____

   c. _____

   d. _____

   e. _____

   f. _____

30. The acronym SBAR stands for:

   S- _____

   B- _____

   A- _____

   R- _____

31. List 10 professional strategies for protection against malpractice.

   a. _____

   b. _____

   c. _____

   d. _____

   e. _____

   f. _____

   g. _____

   h. _____

i. _____

j. _____

PRACTICE/REVIEW ANSWER KEY

1. a. Capacity
   b. Information
   c. Voluntariness

2. a. Marriage
   b. Parenthood
   c. Economic independence
   d. Living in another setting

3. a. Professional standard—The practitioner provides the information considered reasonable in the professional community.
   b. Reasonable patient standard—The practitioner explains risk factors, expected outcomes, and alternatives as they relate to a reasonable person.
   c. Subjective patient standard—The practitioner provides information about risks as they relate to the patient's lifestyle.
   d. Informed refusal—The patient has received information about the risk of not consenting to treatment or diagnostic testing and yet refuses treatment or testing.

4. a. The nature of the individual's consideration
   b. The purpose of the treatment
   c. Expected outcomes
   d. Major risks
   e. Reasonable alternatives
   f. Possible outcomes of refusing treatment

5. Consent must be obtained whenever the patient is going to be touched by the care provider. This does not always mean written consent, but the components of informed consent must be present.

6. When delay will cause death or serious jeopardy to the patient's health.

7. Only a legal guardian, conservator, the patient's attorney, or a court

8. a. Before instituting a nursing procedure
   b. Before nurses in an expanded practice role order or perform procedures

9. The physician

10. Any three of the following:
    a. Provides an ongoing written record of the patient's status, care provided, and the outcomes of the interventions.
    b. Documents that appropriate standards of care were implemented by a qualified professional.
    c. Provides a permanent legal record of the patient's course while in the health care system.

d. Serves as a means of communication from one care provider to another.

11. Nurse's assessments, interventions, and the outcomes of care for the woman and the fetus

12. Document in the chart the reasons that the medication or procedure was not administered.

13. Draw a line through the incorrect information, write "error" above it, write the date and time, and initial the entry. The accurate information is entered as an addendum.

14. a. It is a requirement of the institution's policies and procedures.
    b. The nurse has reviewed the content of the note.
    c. The nurse approves the care provided to the patient.

15. a. Restate the order, including the patient's name.
    b. Ask for confirmation.
    c. Chart "repeated and confirmed."

16. a. Signs/symptoms, onset, duration, and frequency
    b. Actions that alleviate or increase the signs and symptoms

17. a. The patient's chart
    b. Policy and procedure manual enforced at the time of the incident

18. Current national standards as developed by national professional organizations such as AWHONN

19. Any four of the following:
    a. Incomplete documentation
    b. Medication errors
    c. Violation of national standards of practice
    d. Improper use of equipment
    e. Failure to notify the appropriate professionals when maternal or fetal status falls outside normal parameters
    f. Failure to follow physician orders, hospital policies, and hospital procedures
    g. Failure to recognize and respond to cases of fetal distress
    h. Failure to intervene appropriately in the presence of negligence on the part of the providers

20. Childbirth is an intense, emotional experience and parents have high expectations for a "perfect" birth and newborn.
    Poor outcomes are not tolerated well.
    Parents may be well informed consumers of health care.
    Obstetrics is a high-pressure, rapidly changing specialty; accidents, errors in judgment, and negligence do occur.

21. **Negligence** is the failure to act as a reasonable and prudent person; conduct contrary to that of a reasonable person under the same or similar circumstances

22. **Malpractice** is professional negligence, improper discharge of professional duties, or a failure to meet the standard of care of a professional that results in harm to another.

23. a. State statutes (nurse practice acts)
    b. American Nurses Association (ANA)
    c. National professional and specialty nursing organizations
    d. Joint Commission for Accreditation of Healthcare Organizations (JCAHO)
    e. Documentary evidence
    f. Hospital policy and procedures
    g. Testimony from expert witnesses

24. a. Duty
    b. Breach of duty (standard of care)
    c. Damages
    d. Causation

25. a. Failure to appreciate a change in maternal status
    b. Failure to appropriately administer uterine stimulants
    c. Failure to initiate appropriate shoulder dystocia maneuvers
    d. Failure to provide adequate screening for obstetric maternal triage (telephone or inpatient)
    e. Failure to initiate chain of command
    f. Failure to notify physician/midwife
    g. Failure to appropriately manage the second stage of labor
    h. Failure to recognize nonreassuring fetal status and provide appropriate intrauterine fetal resuscitation

26. Use the lowest possible dose that effects cervical change and labor progress.

27. Any five of the following:
    a. Remain calm
    b. Call for RN/physician assistance
    c. Call for neonatal team and prepare for newborn resuscitation
    d. Avoid fundal pressure
    e. Provide firm suprapubic pressure
    f. Position patient for McRoberts maneuver
    g. Assist physician/midwife with patient positioning for additional maneuvers such as the all-fours Gaskin maneuver
    h. State out loud the maneuvers you are assisting with. For example, "I am applying suprapubic pressure."
    i. Reassure patient

28. Chain of command activation is recommended when there is potential for the maternal and/or fetal condition to rapidly deteriorate causing harm, and discussions with the appropriate physician or midwife have failed to provoke an agreeable action plan.

29. Any six of the following:
    a. Speak clearly
    b. Speak using a congenial tone
    c. Be courteous and professional
    d. Present facts in a methodical or chronological style—organization
    e. Ask for clarification if communication is unclear
    f. Communicate all relevant facts, abnormal findings, and specific concerns
    g. State your reasons if you disagree with a treatment plan
    h. If the mother or fetus (or both) is at risk, tell physician to report to the hospital to assess the patient immediately—document
    i. Inform the physician or provider if you plan to communicate up the chain of command

30. Situation, Background, Assessment, Recommendation

31. a. Review institutional policies and guidelines
    b. Perform only those skills you know to be within your scope of practice
    c. Stay current in obstetrics and technologic advances through continuing education
    d. Be clear about who is managing the patient
    e. Be a patient advocate and know how to use chain of command
    f. Learn and use good communication skills
    g. Document everything
    h. Get to know your patients
    i. Don't make excuses for poor care
    j. Remember the "Golden Rule"

R E F E R E N C E S

1. Greenwald, L. M., & Mondor, M. (2003). Malpractice and the perinatal nurse. *Journal of Perinatal and Neonatal Nursing, 17*(2), 101–109.
2. Hamilton, E., & Wright, E. (2006). Labor pains: Unraveling the complexity of OB decision making. *Journal of Perinatal and Neonatal Nursing, 29*(4), 342–353.
3. Reising, D. L., & Allen, P. N. (2007). Protecting yourself from malpractice claims. *American Nurse Today, 2*(2), 39–43.
4. Croke, E. (2003). Nurses, negligence, and malpractice: An analysis based on more than 250 cases against nurses. *American Journal of Nursing, 103*(9), 54–63.
5. O'Keefe, M. E. (2001). *Nursing practice and the law.* Philadelphia: F. A. Davis.
6. Rostant, D. M., & Cady R. F. (Eds.). (1999). *Liability issues in perinatal nursing* (2nd ed., p. 328). Philadelphia: Lippincott.
7. Iyer, P. W.; American Association of Legal Nurse Consultants. (2003). *Legal nurse consulting principles and practice* (2nd ed., p. 261). Boca Raton, FL: CRC Press.
8. Austin, S. A. (2006). "Ladies and gentlemen of the jury, I present . . . the nursing documentation." *Nursing 2006, 36*(1), 56–62.
9. Simpson, K. R., & Knox, G. E. (2003). Common areas of litigation related to care during labor and birth: Recommendations to promote patient safety and decrease risk exposure. *Journal of Perinatal and Neonatal Nursing, 17*(2), 110–125.
10. Bitterman, R. A. (2001). *Providing emergency care under federal law: EMTALA.* Washington, DC: American College of Emergency Physicians.
11. Emergency Medical Treatment and Active Labor Act, 42 USC §1395dd. (1986).

12. Emergency Medical Treatment and Active Labor Act, Statutory Regulations, 42 CFR, pt 489. (1992).
13. Feinstein, N., & McCartney, P. (1997). *Association of Women's Health, Obstetric and Neonatal Nurses: Fetal heart monitoring principles and practices* (2nd ed.). Dubuque, IA: Kendall/Hunt.
14. Simpson, K. R., & James, D. C. (2005). Effects of immediate versus delayed pushing during second-stage labor on fetal well-being: a randomized clinical trial. *Nursing Research, 54*(3), 149–157.
15. Mayberry, L. G., Wood, S.H., Strange, L.B., et al. (2000). *Second stage labor management: promotion of evidence-based practice and a collaborative approach to patient care* (Practice Monograph). Washington, DC: Associate of Women's Health, Obstetric, and Neonatal Nurses.
16. Association of Women's Health, Obstetric and Neonatal Nurses. (2000). *Nursing management of the second stage of labor (Evidence-based clinical practice guidelines)*. Washington, DC: Author.
17. Association of Women's Health, Obstetric and Neonatal Nurses. (2003). *Standards and guidelines for professional nursing practice in the care of women and newborns* (6th ed., pp. 1–43). Washington, DC: Author.
18. Flores, J. A. Proper charting for nurses and other healthcare professionals. Male Nurse Magazine. Available from: www.malenursemagazine.com/charting.html. Retrieved August 18, 2007.
19. Rubeor, K. (2003). The role of risk management in maternal-child health. *Journal of Perinatal and Neonatal Nursing, 17*(2), 94–100.
20. Smith, K., Smith, V., Krugman, M., & Oman, K. (2005). Evaluating the impact of computerized clinical documentation. *CIN: Computers, Informatics, Nursing, 23*(2), 132–138.
21. Brent, N. J. (1997). *Nurses and the law: A guide to principles and applications* (pp. 65–84, 237–268). Philadelphia: WB Saunders.
22. Joint Commission on Accreditation of Healthcare Organizations. (2004). *Preventing Infant Death and Injury During Delivery, Sentinel Event Alert No. 30.* Oakbrook Terrace, IL: Author.
23. Trandel-Korenchuk, D. M., & Trandel-Korenchuk, K. M. (1997). *Nursing and the law.* (5th ed., pp. 166–173, 184). Philadelphia: Lippincott.
24. Joint Commission on Accreditation of Healthcare Organizations. (2006). Guidelines for accepting and transcribing verbal or telephone orders. *The Source, 4,* 6–10.
25. World Health Organization. (2007). Communication during patient handovers. *Patient Safety Solutions, 1*(3).
26. Joint Commission on Accreditation of Healthcare Organizations. (2005). The SBAR technique: Improves communication, enhances patient safety. *Joint Commission Perspectives on Patient Safety, 5*(2), 1–8.
27. Brous, E. A. (2004, June). 7 tips on avoiding malpractice claims. *Travel Nursing 2004.*
28. Brooke, P. S. (2006). So you've been named in a lawsuit: So what happens next? *Nursing, 36*(7), 44–48.
29. Shinn, L. J.; American Nurses Association, The Nursing Risk Management Series. (2001). *Yes, you can be sued.* Washington, DC: Author.

SUGGESTED READINGS

Angelini, D. J., & Mahlmeister, L. R. (2005). Liability in triage: Management of EMTALA regulations and common obstetric risks. *Journal of Midwifery and Women's Health, 50*(6), 472–478.

Hankins, G. D. V., MacLennan, A. H., Speer, M. E., Strunk, A., & Nelson, K. (2006). Obstetric litigation is asphyxiating our maternity services. *Obstetrics & Gynecology, 107*(6), 1382–1385.

Miller, L. A. (2005). Patient safety and teamwork in perinatal care. *Journal of Perinatal and Neonatal Nursing, 19*(1), 46–51.

Miller, L. A. (2006). Malpractice liability in perinatal care: That was then, this is now. *Journal of Perinatal and Neonatal Nursing, 20*(1), 76–78.

Murphy, E. K. (2003). Charting by exception. *AORN Journal, 78*(5), 821–823.

Simpson, K. R., James, D. C., & Knox, G. E. (2006). Nurse–physician communication during labor and delivery: Implications for patient safety. *Journal of Gynecologic, Obstetric, Neonatal Nursing, 35*(4), 547–556.

M O D U L E

16

Maternal Transport

E. JEAN MARTIN ■ SUSAN B. DRUMMOND

Objectives

As you complete this module, you will learn:

1. Advantages and disadvantages of maternal transport
2. Recommendations for the optimal time for maternal transport
3. What constitutes a high-risk maternal transport
4. Who should be involved in making the decision for maternal transport and a suggested process for implementing the referral
5. Composition of the transport team
6. Contraindications to maternal transport
7. Conditions warranting consultation and/or transport of the pregnant woman from a Level I or Level II community hospital to a high-risk Level III regional center
8. Responsibilities of referring and receiving centers
9. Appropriate documentation and records that should accompany a maternal transport patient
10. Nursing interventions designed to assist the mother and family through the transfer process at both the referring and receiving hospitals
11. Basic equipment needed for maternal transport
12. Specific liability issues related to transport
13. Information about a program to which hospitals involved in medical transport may voluntarily apply; the program provides evaluation of compliance with accreditation standards

Key Terms

When you have completed this module, you should be able to recall the meaning of the following terms. You should also be able to use the terms when consulting with other health professionals. The terms are defined in this module or in the glossary at the end of this book.

inborn neonate	mortality
morbidity	outborn neonate

Determining the Need for Maternal Transport

▶ **What is maternal transport?**

An essential component of any perinatal care system is the capability of providing interhospital transport of pregnant women and neonates.[1] *Maternal transport* refers to the process of transferring the pregnant woman under the supervision of skilled medical personnel from a Level I or Level II institution (referring hospitals) to a Level III institution (receiving hospital). Each situation is considered individually. The transfer can be accomplished by private vehicle, ambulance, rotary-wing aircraft (helicopter), or fixed-wing aircraft. The decision regarding the type of vehicle depends on the condition of the pregnant woman and fetus as well as distance. It is a decision that should be shared jointly by the referring care provider and flight nurse or receiving physician.

Advantages of Maternal Transport

During recent years, the transport of the premature or sick newborn to intensive care units of regional centers after birth has become widely accepted. These babies are often referred to as **outborn neonates,** in distinction to those born within the referral hospital (i.e., **inborn neonates**). The survival rates and quality of life for the high-risk neonate have improved significantly. However, documentation and research over the past 20 years have demonstrated a decreased mortality risk for very low birth weight infants transported to a hospital with a level III neonatal intensive care unit before delivery.[2] Morbidity and/or mortality are decreased by delivering an infant in a facility that has the equipment, staffing, and resources appropriate for optimal care.[3-5] Transport of the neonate involves not only the availability of a local neonatal intensive care unit, but also the complication risk during transport, the need for highly skilled personnel and specialized equipment, and the expense of the transport. In utero transport of selected risk pregnancies is strongly recommended. The outcome of an outborn neonate with major medical or surgical problems (which includes extreme prematurity) remains worse than that for an inborn infant. When possible, the primary emphasis should always be on prenatal diagnosis and subsequent maternal transfer. Even with advanced training and technologies, mothers usually make the best transport incubator.[6] Transport within regionalized perinatal care networks allows for benefits of high-technology maternity and fetal/neonatal care and services, while presumably reducing costs and decreasing duplication of services within a region.

Advantages include several considerations:

- If the baby is transferred in utero, the need for sophisticated equipment and the risk of neonatal problems during transport are reduced. Advanced testing and treatment at the center enables a more accurate assessment of when and how to deliver the baby.
- Advanced therapeutic techniques can be provided for the high-risk mother.
- If an ill or severely preterm baby is delivered, immediate steps can be taken to stabilize and treat the newborn without losing precious time during transport.
- The hospital stay of the mother and her newborn tends to be shorter, resulting in a reduction of hospital costs.
- Finally, maternal transport ensures that the mother and baby are together during the first few days after birth. This provides the opportunity for the mother and baby to become acquainted and attached to each other in the unique process of bonding.

Disadvantages of Maternal Transport

Probably the greatest concern in transferring the undelivered mother to the regional center is the physical separation from her family and friends. Because of this, it is important that a family member accompany the mother or follow in a car, if possible, at the time of transport. The woman and/or her neonate, after receiving specialized care at a referral center, may be returned to the original referring hospital for continuing care after the problems that required the transfer have been resolved. This may result in a decreased amount of time that the woman and neonate are separated from family and community.

> The referring nursing staff and transport personnel must help to reduce the disruption and stress for the pregnant woman and her family during transfer. Create a quiet private place to explain to the expectant woman and her family why the transfer is necessary and exactly how it is going to take place. Stress any positive aspect of the clinical situation (e.g., the baby is doing well presently).

The rate of admissions to neonatal intensive care units increases with a maternal transport system. A great percentage of these babies have extremely low birth weights. In the past, these babies did not survive. They require special care, which is met in tertiary care centers that have established maternal–fetal medicine programs. Administrative and fiscal considerations may necessitate a commitment of additional resources for such a program.[7]

Timing of Maternal Transport

▶ **When is the best time to transport the mother?**

Transport of the undelivered mother to a regional center should be considered in the following situations:

- It is anticipated that the infant might require intensive care not available at the referring hospital.
- The obstetric, medical, or surgical needs of the mother require diagnosis, treatment, and care using highly specialized equipment, skills, and staff not available at the referring hospital.

When possible, referral should be made while the mother and fetus are in a stable condition and delivery is not expected during the immediate 24-hour period. This presents a low risk for transferring the mother and fetus. It is optimum, of course, to refer early enough to allow beginning assessment and treatment at the receiving hospital, thus preventing a crisis situation for either mother or fetus when they reach the receiving hospital. Transport team members should be selected from appropriately trained, licensed health care providers.[8]

High-reliability perinatal units promote clinical practices based on nationally recognized guidelines and espouse a team philosophy of "safety first." One feature of such perinatal units is that "patients are transferred in a timely and reliable way" to facilities that can care for all potential problems rather then operating on the hope "that the disaster will not occur."[9] (Behavioral scientists define *high-reliability organizations* as those with "the ability to operate technologically complex systems essentially without error over long periods."[9])

Transfer of patients in early labor is recommended in the following circumstances:
- Time for transport will take less than 2 hours.
- The mother's condition is stable.
- Delivery is not anticipated for 4 to 6 hours.
- A professional attendant, such as a flight nurse, physician, or an experienced emergency medical technician, can accompany the mother.

High-risk transport situations include the following:
- The mother's condition is unstable.
- Time of delivery is unpredictable.

In high-risk transport situations, the decision as to whether the mother is stable enough for transport and who should accompany the mother should be made by the perinatal specialist and transport team experienced in such decision making.

In either of these high-risk situations, it is highly recommended that the mother be accompanied by the following:
- Referring physician or designate
- Nurse or neonatologist with the skill and experience to manage resuscitation and care of the newborn

---

NOTE: Maternal transport might be contraindicated in women who are too unstable at the time of the transport request. For example, a mother in premature labor who is dilated beyond 5 cm should be evaluated carefully. Decisions depend on the makeup of the transport team, distance, and time. Safety of the mother and the fetus are the primary considerations.

Other contraindications can include women with the following:
- Actively bleeding placenta previa
- Abruptio placentae
- Unstable fetal condition

Many times, the transport team will need to make critical decisions before leaving the referring hospital.

REMEMBER: *Critical factors in successful maternal transport are appropriate treatment of the mother before transport and attendance by skilled personnel.*

Conditions Requiring Transport to a Regional Center

▶ What conditions in the mother require referral to a regional center?

The majority of maternal transports will be carried out because of concern for a potentially compromised fetus. Prematurity remains the predominant cause of neonatal morbidity and mortality. In 2004, preterm births represented 12.5% of all births in the United States. This number is an 18% increase since 1990.[10] Preterm infants also constitute approximately 75% of neonatal mortalities. Statistics from selected regional centers indicate uniformly better outcomes for in utero fetal transport (i.e., the mortality risk for fetuses transported in utero is approximately half that of neonates transported after delivery).

The following conditions may require that the mother be transported to a regional center for high-risk care.[11,12]

Obstetric Complications

- **Preterm premature rupture of membranes occurring before 34 weeks' gestation or with a fetus estimated to weigh less than 2,000 g**

Maternal risks with preterm premature rupture of membranes:
- Infection
- Abruptio placentae (occurs in approximately 4% to 12% of these women).[13]

Fetal/neonatal risks with preterm premature rupture of membranes:
- Infection
- Complications of prematurity
- Respiratory distress
- Cord prolapse

Management varies with gestational age. A vaginal culture for group B streptococcus (GBS) should be obtained using a *sterile* cotton-tipped applicator on women when presenting with preterm premature rupture of membranes. Infection with GBS is responsible for serious neonatal morbidity and mortality.[14,15] See Appendix A for GBS discussion.

- Any condition in which the probability exists for the delivery of an infant less than 34 weeks' gestation or weighing less than 2,000 g, such as the following:
  - Severe preeclampsia or other hypertensive complications
  - Certain anticipated multiple births
  - Poorly controlled or severe diabetes mellitus
  - Severe intrauterine growth restriction
  - Some women with third trimester bleeding
  - Rh isoimmunization
  - Severe oligohydramnios

Medical Complications

- Infections that are likely to result in premature birth
- Severe organic heart disease
- Renal disease with deteriorating function or increasing hypertension
- Drug overdose
- Some women with carcinoma
- Morbid obesity
- Uncontrolled diabetes mellitus

Surgical Complications

- Trauma requiring intensive care or surgery beyond the capabilities of local facilities or where the procedure can result in the onset of premature labor

- Acute abdominal emergencies at less than 34 weeks' gestation or with a fetus estimated to weigh less than 2,000 g
- Thoracic emergencies requiring intensive care or surgical correction

Fetal Complications

- Fetal congenital anomalies diagnosed by ultrasound can dictate the need for maternal transport

NOTE: Transfer from a Level II institution should be considered for the following:
- *Any fetus anticipated to require long-term ventilation support after birth.*
- *Any fetus anticipated to require neonatal care at less than 28 to 34 weeks' gestation. (This will depend on the skilled personnel and advanced technology of the institution.[8])*
- *Suspected genetic disorder requiring further evaluation.[8]*

Other Considerations

After birth, many babies are cyanotic, often peripherally. Typically, cyanotic babies have the following characteristics[16]:
- Premature, have experienced a difficult delivery or ingested meconium, or had premature rupture of membranes
- Marked respiratory distress
- Radiographic evidence of lung disease
- Elevated P_{CO_2} levels
- P_{O_2} increases with 100% oxygen

On the other hand, a baby experiencing a cardiac abnormality usually has the following characteristics[16]:
- Term
- Normal delivery
- Little respiratory distress
- Cyanosis, which is central and disproportionate to distress; tongue and mucous membranes are blue
- No radiologic evidence of lung disease

When born with cyanotic congenital heart disease in a Level I or Level II hospital, a baby should be transported by a neonatal transport team immediately because he or she is only going to get worse. Most babies should be referred to a major pediatric cardiac unit. Most require surgical treatment.[11] **IT IS FAR BETTER TO ANTICIPATE THIS NEED WHEN POSSIBLE AND TRANSPORT THE MOTHER BEFORE DELIVERY.**

Glucocorticoid Therapy for Fetal Maturation

Preterm delivery continues to be a major cause of illness and death in infants. In March 1994, the National Institutes of Health (NIH) sponsored a consensus Development Conference on the Effect of Corticosteroids for Fetal Maturation on Perinatal Outcomes.[17] The consensus panel concluded that *giving a single course of corticosteroids* to pregnant women at risk for preterm delivery reduces the risk of death, respiratory distress syndrome (RDS), and intraventricular hemorrhage in their preterm infants. Such therapy brought about a significant and clear decrease in RDS in infants born between 29 and 34 weeks' gestation. For infants born between 24 and 28 weeks' gestation, only the severity of the disease was decreased, not the incidence.[18]

Antenatal glucocorticoid therapy promotes fetal lung maturation. Clinical studies reveal that glucocorticoids can accelerate lung maturation in immature fetuses. Administration of glucocorticoids (corticosteroids) such as betamethasone or dexamethasone to pregnant women 24 to 48 hours before delivery has been shown to stimulate surfactant production. Fetal lung alveoli remain expanded because of decreased surface tension within the alveoli.

Based on scientific studies, both prenatal glucocorticoids (betamethasone or dexamethasone) and postnatal surfactant therapy are effective in preventing RDS. Studies also demonstrate that combination therapy is often better than either treatment alone.

In 2000, the National Institute of Child Health and Human Development and the Office of Medical Applications of Research of the National Institutes of Health reconvened a consensus conference on antenatal steroids to address the issue of repeated courses of corticosteroids for fetal maturation. This consensus panel reaffirmed the 1994 consensus panel's recommendation.[18] Because of insufficient scientific evidence, the panel also recommended that repeat corticosteroid courses should not be routinely used.[18]

Clinical recommendations are as follows[18]:

- All pregnant women between 24 and 34 weeks' gestation who are at risk for preterm delivery within 7 days should be considered for antenatal treatment with a single course of corticosteroids. Optimal benefit from such therapy lasts 7 days.
- Treatment consists of two doses of 12 mg of **betamethasone** given intramuscularly 24 hours apart **OR** four doses of 6 mg of **dexamethasone** given intramuscularly 12 hours apart, as recommended by the consensus panel in 1994. There is no proof of efficacy for any other regimen.
- Because there are insufficient scientific data from randomized clinical trials regarding efficacy and safety, repeat courses of corticosteroids should not be used routinely. In general, this should be reserved for patients enrolled in randomized controlled trials. The use of corticosteroids after 34 weeks of gestation is not recommended unless there is evidence of fetal pulmonary immaturity.[19] For patients with preterm PROM before 32 weeks' gestation, a single course of antenatal corticosteroids should be administered to reduce the risks of RDS, perinatal mortality, and other morbidities.[13]

Fetal Echocardiography

The use of fetal echocardiography is currently evolving and requires extensive experience by the diagnostician to accurately diagnose some congenital cardiac abnormalities. A diagnosis by an inexperienced individual can be wrong or incomplete. When a cardiac abnormality is suspected in utero in a facility other than a tertiary care center, maternal transport is indicated.[16]

Responsibilities of the Referring and Receiving Centers

▶ **What steps should be taken by the referring physician and hospital in initiating the transport?**

The decision to transport the pregnant or laboring woman should be made jointly by her physician and the physician to whom the referral is being made. The situation should be discussed with the mother and/or her family.

In 1986, Congress enacted the Emergency Medical Treatment & Labor Act (EMTALA) to ensure public access to emergency services regardless of ability to pay. Section 1867 of the SSA imposes specific obligations on Medicare-participating hospitals that offer emergency services to provide a medical screening examination (MSE) when a request is made for examination or treatment for an emergency medical condition (EMC), *including active labor,* regardless of an individual's ability to pay. Hospitals are then required to provide stabilizing treatment for patients with EMCs. If a hospital is unable to stabilize a patient within its capability, or if the patient requests, an appropriate transfer should be implemented (www.cms.hhs.gov).

The following guidelines for the organization of the transport are divided into referring center responsibilities and receiving center responsibilities.[8]

Referring Center Responsibilities

- The referring care provider confers with the receiving physician by phone. This should assist the receiving physician in developing a treatment plan to maintain stabilization of the patient before and during transport. It is the referring center's responsibility to follow COBRA/EMTALA guidelines.[a]

---

[a]COBRA/EMTALA Statute: 42 USC 1395 federal regulation relating to the transfer and medical treatment of women in labor. Circumstances are delineated under which an individual may be transferred to another medical care facility, including the steps to be taken for stabilization and treatment before transfer.[12]

- An ambulance is the most appropriate vehicle for the majority of maternal transports. An alternative form of transportation should be agreed on by the referring and receiving physicians.
- The composition of the transport team should be a joint decision between the referring and receiving care providers based on the condition of the mother and/or fetus.
- If the transport is done by the referring hospital, the referring physician and hospital retain responsibility until the transport team arrives with the patient at the receiving hospital. If the transport team is sent by the receiving hospital, the receiving physician or designee assumes responsibility for patient care from the time the patient leaves the referring hospital.[1]
- *An up-to-date copy of the mother's prenatal record, hospital chart, laboratory data, and the mother's signed consent form for the transport are sent with her.*
- The mother is transported from the obstetric unit of the referring center or physician's office to the obstetric unit of the receiving hospital. This reduces the risk of unnecessary delays in the emergency room or admitting office.

NOTE: *A member of the mother's family should be encouraged to accompany her. If the mother requires care by the ambulance attendants, the family member may sit with the ambulance driver or follow in a car.*

▶ **What steps should be taken by the receiving physician and hospital in accepting the transport?**

Receiving Center Responsibilities

- The receiving center is responsible for providing referring physicians with access by telephone on a 24-hour basis to communicate with receiving obstetric and neonatal units.[1]
- The receiving physician is responsible for accepting the referring care provider's request for transport and for making preparations to receive the transport.
- Shared responsibility for the patient by the receiving physician and the referring provider begins on initial consultation and acceptance for the transfer. Full responsibility begins with admission to the receiving center.
- Every patient accepted by transport from a referring hospital should be seen by a physician within 30 minutes of arrival.
- Communication by telephone, letter, or fax with the referring care provider should occur after admission.
- If the patient is discharged undelivered, communication should occur before the discharge.
- A discharge summary including diagnosis, an outline of the hospital course, and recommendations for ongoing care of both mother and baby should be sent to the referring physician.
- The mother should return to the care of the referring care provider as soon as possible. Separation of mother and infant should be avoided when possible.
- If the mother needs to be referred to the receiving center or physician again, the referral process begins again with a physician-to-physician phone call.

REMEMBER: *Adequate documentation of the mother's health status is essential for developing a treatment plan at the receiving center. Send all available medical records and complete prenatal records, including any ultrasonography reports and laboratory test results.*

Nursing Care in Maternal Transport

▶ **How can the nurse assist the mother and her family through the transfer process?**

The process of being transferred from one hospital to another increases the mother's and family's awareness of the medical problems accompanying the pregnancy. At the same time, geographically distancing mothers and members of her family reduces the opportunity for mutual support. Coping abilities of both parties can suffer. It is important that communication between mother and father or other family members be facilitated throughout the stay at the high-risk center. Many transport teams have printed information for the mother and family that can be helpful.

Nursing Interventions Throughout the Stay at the Referring Hospital[20]

These interventions are aimed at preparing the family for the transport.

- Ensure that the woman and her family understand the reasons for the transfer. **Ask the woman to say why she is being transported.** *This is important.*
- Inform the family about the regional hospital to which the transfer is being made. Information should include the following:
  - The name of the physician and a primary nurse at the receiving hospital (sometimes this is unknown)
  - The type of care given at the receiving hospital (teaching facility or private hospital)
  - How the mother will be transported (e.g., ambulance, helicopter)
  - How long the trip will take
  - When the trip is to occur
  - Who will accompany her (check with the transport team to see if someone is allowed)
  - Hospital unit policies, including visiting hours and telephone numbers
  - How family members can travel to the receiving hospital by car or mass transportation
  - Cost of transport and whether covered by insurance
- Encourage the mother to discuss her fears and concerns with you. Be able to answer questions regarding her diagnosis and proposed plan of care.

Nursing Interventions at the Receiving Hospital[20]

> Patients/families under great stress have difficulty dealing with more than a few people. Ideally, one nurse should be assigned initially to assist the mother and her family.

- Welcome the woman and her family while orienting them to the unit.
- Review unit policies and encourage the mother's support person to visit as often as is appropriate.
- Facilitate telephone communication with family members as appropriate.
- Promote prebirth bonding of the mother and family to the fetus by discussing the fetus' unique characteristics, such as activity levels and times of quiet.

> Have the neonatal nurse practitioner or neonatologist speak to the mother and family members regarding their concerns for the premature infant.

> Parents need to be assisted to identify the fetus as a developing individual—a part of the family—even with a fetus who is greatly compromised during the pregnancy.

- After the infant's birth, promote parent–infant interaction at whatever level is appropriate. If the infant is in a neonatal intensive care unit (NICU), do the following:
  - Encourage parental visits.
  - Take a picture of the infant for family members to see.
  - Have the NICU nurse report to or write down information about the infant's progress.
  - Involve parents, when possible, with decisions about their baby's care.
  - Provide opportunities for parents to care for their baby at whatever level appropriate.
- Allow the mother and family to discuss their fears, concerns, and anxieties.
- Provide the family with some privacy during visits.
- Assist mother with the initiation of breastfeeding including the pumping and storage of breast milk if this is the mother's choice.
- Assist the family to contact the appropriate support services (e.g., social service, clergy, psychologists, parent groups).
- Facilitate continuity of care for infant and parents if the infant is transferred back to the referring hospital for final recovery closer to the parent's home.

Ensuring Safe Transport

Transport team members should have the collective expertise sufficient to provide the following, if necessary: (1) monitoring of blood pressure, uterine contractions, deep tendon reflexes, and fetal heart rate; (2) monitoring the administration of intravenous infusions and usage of tocolytic, antihypertensive, and anticonvulsant medications; and (3) care for a wide variety of emergency conditions, including delivery and neonatal resuscitation.[8]

▶ What basic equipment is needed for maternal transport?

Most ambulances have basic life support (BLS) equipment adequate for the majority of maternal transports. The referring physician should be familiar with the availability of BLS and advanced life support (ALS) ambulances in the area. Equipment should also be available for anticipated complications such as delivery, seizure, and hemorrhage. Organization and maintenance of additional transport equipment is the responsibility of the transport team. The Tennessee Perinatal Care System *Guidelines for Transportation*[8] lists additional equipment that may be necessary:

- Doppler
- Reflex hammer
- Infusion pump
- Medications
  - Oxytocin (Pitocin)
  - Methergine
  - Misoprostol
  - Magnesium sulfate
  - Calcium gluconate
  - Antibiotics
  - Tocolytic agents
  - Antihypertensive agents
- Oxygen masks (premature and newborn size)
- Infant positive-pressure bag and mask
- Suction catheter (#6, #8, and #10 F)
- Latex-free equipment and supplies must be available

An incubator must be capable of the following:

- Providing a stable, adjustable heat source
- Providing constant and adjustable oxygen
- Providing good visibility of the infant
- Being easily transported
- Providing easy access to the infant for care and treatment
- Operating on DC sources of electric power while in transport and AC sources for hospital use

> When preterm labor is a risk during transport, a birth kit from the referring hospital should be included—that is, suction catheters, suction bulbs, blankets, and a hat for the newborn.[21]
> In transporting a high-risk laboring mother who has the possibility of delivery before reaching the referral hospital, a *transport incubator* should be part of the equipment.

NOTE: *In all transport situations, the mother should be encouraged to avoid positions that compromise maternal blood flow. Keep the mother in a semi-Fowler's or left side-lying position. This displaces the gravid uterus off the vena cava, preventing compromised maternal circulation.*

An important step in the preparation for transfer is to carefully label any bag of intravenous fluid just before transport. In addition, the transport service must have a method of assuring that all medications and intravenous fluids are appropriately calculated.[22] Oxygen administration is advised in any clinical situation for which there is concern about potential fetal distress.

Specific Liability Issues Related to Transport[23]

Every nurse and provider involved in transport should be keenly aware of liability issues. Such sensitivity may serve to sharpen all facets of clinical practice to the benefit of both the patient and health care personnel.

Specific liability issues include the following:

- Use of treatment protocols or algorithms
- Lack of informed consent
- Failure to stabilize before transport

- Failure to diagnose or delay in diagnosing a problem more significant than what was relayed by the transferring hospital
- Equipment issues
- Delay in treatment or transfer
- Actual error (e.g., wrong drug or dose)
- Liability transfer from referring facility to receiving facility

The Commission of Accreditation of Medical Transport Systems (CAMTS) offers a program of voluntary evaluation of compliance with accreditation standards. This provides medical professionals involved with air and ground transport systems to improve services and can serve as a marker of excellence for federal, state, and local agencies, as well as to the public.[22] See "Resources of Note" for further information.

PRACTICE/REVIEW QUESTIONS

After reviewing this module, answer the following questions.

1. What is the primary advantage of transporting the high-risk mother to a regional center before the baby is born?

   _____

2. What is the primary disadvantage of transporting the high-risk mother to a regional center?

   _____

   _____

3. Describe a *low-risk* maternal transport situation.

   _____

   _____

   _____

4. Under what conditions should the *high-risk* woman in *early* labor be transported?

   a. _____

   b. _____

   c. _____

   d. _____

5. Describe a *high-risk* maternal transport situation.

   _____

   _____

   _____

6. The obstetric complications necessitating high-risk care involve conditions occurring before _____ weeks' gestation or an estimated birth weight below _____ g.

7. List several *obstetric complications* that require high-risk care and therefore maternal transport from community hospitals in some cases.

   a. _____

   b. _____

   c. _____

   d. _____

   e. _____

8. Briefly list *medical* and *surgical complications* necessitating high-risk care.

   Medical Complications

   a. _____

   b. _____

   c. _____

   d. _____

   e. _____

   Surgical Complications

   a. _____

   b. _____

   c. _____

9. What fetal situations necessitate the transfer of a mother from a Level II to a Level III institution?

   a. _____

   b. _____

10. Babies often experience cyanosis after birth, often peripherally. List three characteristics of cyanotic babies, who are generally not experiencing a cardiac abnormality.

    a. _____

    b. _____

    c. _____

11. A baby with a cyanotic congenital heart abnormality needs to be kept at the Level I or Level II hospital until he or she is stabilized. After stabilization, the baby may be transferred.

    a. True

    b. False

12. Cyanosis of mucous membranes and the tongue in a term baby who has no radiologic evidence of lung disease is suspicious for:

    a. Cardiac abnormality

    b. Peripheral cyanosis, common in many babies

13. Current recommendations from the NIH (2000) advise antenatal treatment for all pregnant women between _____ weeks' gestation and _____ weeks' gestation who are at risk for preterm delivery within _____ days and that they be considered for treatment with a single course of corticosteroids.

14. Corticosteroid therapy (e.g., betamethasone, dexamethasone) brings about a significant decrease in RDS in infants born between 29 and 34 weeks' gestation.

    a. True

    b. False

15. A *single course* of treatment with *betamethasone* consists of _____ doses of _____ mg given intramuscularly _____ hours apart.

16. A single course of treatment with *dexamethasone* consists of _____ doses of _____ mg given intramuscularly _____ hours apart.

17. The referring physician must initiate the transport by contacting the receiving physician.

    a. True

    b. False

18. A health professional should always accompany the mother during transport.

    a. True

    b. False

19. The mother's record and laboratory data should be sent to the high-risk center by mail.

    a. True

    b. False

20. The mother should be taken to the emergency room of the receiving hospital.

    a. True

    b. False

21. A discharge summary sheet should be sent to the referring care provider.

    a. True

    b. False

22. A woman who is a gravida 3, para 2, is at a Level I hospital in her 34th week of pregnancy. She is dilated 6 cm, and her preterm labor is complicated by severe preeclampsia. The receiving and referring physicians have agreed on maternal transport by helicopter to the high-risk regional center, which is 40 miles away. Who is the most appropriate member of the health team to accompany the patient? _____

    Why? _____

23. List eight nursing interventions that the nurse at the referring hospital can do to assist the mother and her family in the transfer to the high-risk regional center.

    a. _____

    b. _____

    c. _____

    d. _____

    e. _____

    f. _____

    g. _____

    h. _____

24. List eight nursing interventions designed to assist the mother in adjusting to the high-risk regional center after transfer.

    a. _____

    b. _____

    c. _____

    d. _____

    e. _____

    f. _____

    g. _____

    h. _____

25. List five specific liability issues related to transport.

    a. _____

    b. _____

    c. _____

    d. _____

    e. _____

PRACTICE/REVIEW ANSWER KEY

1. Survival rates and quality of life (long-term sequelae) for the high-risk neonate are improved.

2. The mother is separated from friends and family.

3. The low-risk transport situation is one in which the mother and fetus are in a stable condition and delivery is not expected during the immediate 24-hour period.

4. a. Transport will take less than 2 hours.
   b. The mother's condition is stable.
   c. Delivery is not anticipated for 4 to 6 hours.
   d. An experienced health professional can accompany the mother.

5. The high-risk transport situation is one in which the mother's or fetus' condition is unstable (e.g., actively bleeding with a placenta previa or in active labor and dilated 5 cm or beyond) and the time of delivery is unpredictable.

6. 34: 2,000

7. Answers should include:
   a. Premature rupture of membranes before 34 weeks' gestation or with a fetus thought to weigh less than 2,000 g
   b. Premature labor before 34 weeks' gestation
   c. Conditions in which the infant might deliver before 34 weeks' gestation or weigh less than 2,000 g (e.g., severe preeclampsia or hypertensive disorder, multiple gestation, poorly controlled or severe diabetes mellitus, intrauterine growth restriction with signs of fetal distress, bleeding in the third trimester, Rh isoimmunization, severe oligohydramnios)

8. **Medical complications**
   a. Infections that can result in premature birth
   b. Severe heart disease
   c. Renal disease with deteriorating function or increasing hypertension
   d. Drug overdose
   e. Some patients with carcinoma

   Surgical Complications
   a. Trauma that requires care or surgery beyond what the local hospital can provide
   b. Acute abdominal problems at less than 34 weeks' gestation or a baby weighing less than 2,000 g
   c. Thoracic emergencies

9. a. Any fetus anticipated to require long-term ventilatory support after birth
   b. Any fetus anticipated to require neonatal care at less than 30 to 34 week's gestation (this depends on the skilled personnel and advanced technology of the institution).

10. Any three of the following:
    a. Are premature, had a difficult delivery, experienced meconium passages in utero, had premature rupture of membranes
    b. Are in marked respiratory distress
    c. Have radiologic evidence of lung disease
    d. Have an elevated P_{CO_2} level
    e. Have P_{O_2} increases with 100% oxygen

11. b. False—The infant is going to get worse with time.

12. a

13. 24; 34; 7

14. a. True

15. 2; 12; 24

16. 4; 6; 12

17. a. True

18. b. False—This depends on the circumstances under which the mother is being transported. Occasionally, a private car may be used, in which case the health professional would not accompany the mother.

19. b. False

20. b. False

21. a. True

22. A physician
    This represents a high-risk maternal transport.

23. Any eight of the following:
    a. Ensure that the woman and her family understand the reasons for the transfer.
    b. Inform the family about the regional hospital to which the mother is being transferred.
    c. Give the names of the physician and a primary nurse at the regional center.
    d. Discuss the type of care given.
    e. Tell the mother how she will be transported and how long the trip will take.
    f. Tell her when the trip is to occur and who will be accompanying her.
    g. Familiarize her with the hospital unit policies, including visiting hours and telephone numbers.
    h. Discuss how family members can get to the regional center and where they might be able to stay.
    i. Allow the mother to discuss her fears and concerns with you.

24. Any eight of the following:
    a. Welcome the woman and her family while orienting them to the unit.

b. Review unit policies and promote visiting of the mother's support person as appropriate to her level of illness.

c. Facilitate telephone communication with family members as appropriate.

d. Promote prebirth bonding of the mother and family to the fetus by discussing the fetus' unique characteristics, such as activity levels and times of quiet.

e. Promote parent–infant interaction at whatever level is possible and appropriate.

f. Encourage the mother and family to discuss their fears, concerns, and anxieties.

g. Provide the family with some privacy during visits.

h. Assist the family to contact appropriate support services (e.g., social service, clergy, psychologists, parent groups).

i. Facilitate continuity of care for infant and parents if the infant is transferred back to the referring hospital for final recovery.

25. Any five of the following:
   a. Use of treatment protocols or algorithms
   b. Lack of informed consent
   c. Failure to stabilize
   d. Failure to diagnose or delay in diagnosing a problem more significant than what was relayed by the transferring hospital
   e. Equipment issues
   f. Delay in treatment or transfer
   g. Actual error (e.g., wrong drug or dose)
   h. When does liability transfer from the referring facility to the receiving facility

REFERENCES

1. American Academy of Pediatrics and the American College of Obstetricians and Gynecologists. (2003). Interhospital care of the perinatal patient. In *Guidelines for perinatal care* (5th ed., pp. 57–71). Washington, DC: Author.

2. American College of Obstetricians and Gynecologists. (2002). Perinatal care at the threshold of viability. *Practice Bulletin, 38,* 1–8.

3. Clement, M. S. (2005). Perinatal care in Arizona 1950–2002: A study of the positive impact of technology, regionalization and the Arizona Perinatal Trust. *Journal of Perinatology, 25,* 503–508.

4. Clement, M. S. (2002). Perinatal transport in Arizona. Office of Women's and Children's Health. Phoenix: Arizona Department of Health Services.

5. Hohoagschwandter, M., Husslein, P., Klebermass, K., Weniger, M., Nardi, A., & Langer, M. (2001). Perinatal mortality and morbidity: Comparison between maternal transport, neonatal transport and inpatient antenatal treatment. *Archives of Gynecology and Obstetrics, 265*(3), 113–118.

6. Ohning, B. L., & Driggers, K. P. (2001, May). Transport of the critically ill newborn. *EMedicine Journal, 2*(5). Available from: www.emedicine.com/ped/topic2730.htm.

7. Cowett, R. M., Coustan, D. R., & Oh, W. (1986). Effects of maternal transport on admission patterns at a tertiary care center. *American Journal of Obstetrics and Gynecology, 154*(5), 1098–1100.

8. Tennessee Perinatal Care System. (2006). *Guidelines for transportation* (5th ed.). Nashville: Tennessee Department of Health, Maternal and Child Health. Prepared by the Subcommittee on Perinatal Transportation of the Perinatal Advisory Committee.

9. Knox, G. E., Simpson, K. R., & Garite, T. J. (1999). Highly reliable perinatal units: An approach to the prevention of patient injury and medical malpractice claims. *Journal of Healthcare Risk Management, 19*(2), 24–27.

10. National Center for Health Statistics. (2004). Preliminary Births for 2004: Infant and Maternal Health. Available at: www.cdc.gov.

11. Rehm, N. E. (1987). Indications for maternal transport—The Utah experience. In Coulter, D. M. (Ed.), *Current concepts in transport: Neonatal, maternal, administrative* (3rd ed., pp. 297–298). Salt Lake City: Perinatal Transport Service, University of Utah Medical Center.

12. Strobino, D. M., Frank, R., Oberdorf, M. A., Shachtman, Kim, Y. J., Callan, N., & Nagey, D. (1993). Development of an index of maternal transport. *Medical Decisions Making, 13*(1), 64–73.

13. American College of Obstetricians and Gynecologists. (2007). Premature rupture of membranes. *Practice Bulletin, 80,* 1–13.

14. Centers for Disease Control and Prevention. (2002). Prevention of perinatal group B streptococcal disease: A public health perspective. *MMWR Morbidity and Mortality Weekly Report, 51*(RR-11), 1–22.

15. American College of Obstetricians and Gynecologists. (2002). Prevention of early-onset group B streptococcal disease in newborns. *Committee Opinion, 279,* 1–8.

16. Orsmond, G. S. (1995). Management of cyanotic heart disease. In Trautman, M. S. (Ed.), *Current concepts in transport. Neonatal syllabus* (7th ed., pp. 16–20). Salt Lake City: University of Utah.

17. National Institutes of Health. (1994, February 28–March 2). Effect of corticosteroids for fetal maturation on perinatal outcomes. *NIH Consensus Statement, 12*(2), 1–24.

18. National Institutes of Health. (2001, September 5). Antenatal corticosteroids revisited: Repeat courses. *NIH Consensus Statement Online 2000, 17*(2), 1–10.

19. American College of Obstetricians and Gynecologists (2002). Antenatal Corticosteroid Therapy for Fetal Maturation. *Committee Opinion, 273,* 1–3.

20. Davis, D. H., & Hawkins, J. W. (1985). High-risk maternal and neonatal transport: Psychosocial implications for practice. *Dimensions of Critical Care Nursing, 4*(6), 373–379.

21. Simpson, K. R., & Creehan, P. A. (Eds.). (2008). *Perinatal nursing* (3rd ed., p. 275). Philadelphia: Lippincott.

22. Commission on Accreditation of Medical Transport Systems. (2006). *Accreditation standards of the Commission on Accreditation of Medical Transport Systems* (7th ed.). Anderson, SC: Author.

23. Youngberg, B. (2001, February 28–March 3). Liability issues every transport nurse should consider. In *Current concepts in transport (syllabus)*. Annual Conference.

SUGGESTED READING

National Institutes of Health. (2001, September 5). Antenatal corticosteroids revisited: Repeat courses. *NIH Consensus Statement Online 2000, 17*(2), 1–10.

RESOURCES OF NOTE

Commission on Accreditation of Medical Transport Systems. (2006). *Accreditation standards of the Commission on Accreditation of Medical Transport Systems. Mission statement.* Anderson, SC: Author.

Conference. (Annual). *Current concepts in transport (neonatal, pediatric).* Sponsored by the Pediatric Education by the Pediatric Education Services at Primary Children's Medical Center, University of Utah, School of Medicine, Salt Lake City, Education Department. Phone: 801-588-4060.

Tennessee Perinatal Care System. (2006). *Guidelines for transportation* (5th ed.). Subcommittee on Perinatal Transportation of the Perinatal Advisory Committee. Tennessee Department of Health, Maternal and Child Health. Address: 425 5th Avenue North, 5th Floor, Cordell Hull Building, Nashville, TN 37247-4701.

M O D U L E

17

Intimate Partner Violence During Pregnancy

BETSY B. KENNEDY

BETSY B. KENNEDY

Objectives

As you complete this module, you will learn:

1. Direct and indirect effects of intimate partner violence against pregnant women
2. Risk factors for intimate partner violence
3. Victim and partner behaviors that may indicate a pattern of violence
4. Components of the cycle of violence
5. Health care provider's role in screening for pregnant victims of intimate partner violence
6. Defensive measures and safety plans for pregnant victims of intimate partner violence
7. Possible interventions and resources for pregnant victims of intimate partner violence

Key Terms

When you have completed this module, you should be able to recall the meaning of the following terms. You should also be able to use the terms when consulting with other health professionals. The terms are defined in this module or in the glossary at the end of this book.

acute violence stage
cycle of violence
domestic violence
honeymoon or reconciliation phase
intimate partner violence

intimate partner abuse
partner abuse
safety plan
tension-building phase
wife abuse/spousal abuse

Intimate Partner Violence

▶ **What is intimate partner violence (IPV)?**

Intimate partner violence (IPV), or abuse of a woman by a known perpetrator, has reached epidemic proportions. There are many myths and misconceptions about IPV, but the intrapartum nurse must be aware of truth surrounding this public health issue. Inevitably, an intrapartum nurse will care for women who are being abused at the hands of their partners. This type of violence may be known by other terms, listed in Display 17.1, but it is important to recognize that an intimate partner can be a current or former spouse, partner, boyfriend, or girlfriend.[1] The relationship between the woman and her abuser may be casual, cohabitating, engaged, or married. The violence that characterizes the relationship may be physical, sexual, emotional, or threatened.

| DISPLAY 17.1 | OTHER TERMS FOR INTIMATE PARTNER VIOLENCE |

Wife abuse/spousal abuse
Partner abuse
Domestic violence/abuse

Physical violence is an intentional use of force (actual or threatened) and may include:
- Pushing
- Slapping
- Punching
- Kicking
- Choking
- Beating
- Burning
- Biting
- Shaking
- Scratching
- Assault with a weapon (knife, gun, or other)
- Tying down or restraining
- Refusal to allow access to medical care when needed
- Leaving the woman in a dangerous place

Sexual violence includes acts such as:
- Degrading sexual comments
- Threatened force to compel the woman to engage in sexual acts against her will
- Intentionally hurting the woman during sex (including the use of objects intravaginally, orally, or anally)
- Pursuing sex with the woman when she is unable to avoid participation, unable to communicate unwillingness, or to understand the nature of the act
- Rape

Emotional or psychological *abuse* refers to acts of:
- Humiliation
- "Name calling"
- Intimidation
- Belittling
- Insulting
- Ridiculing
- Deliberately embarrassing (especially in public)
- Social isolation
- Withholding of finances or resources
- Controlling of activities

> *It is important to note that this is not a complete list. Abuse may include anything the victim perceives as threatening. The victim feels that she must comply with the abuser's wishes or things that are important to her, such as persons or objects, may be harmed.*

▶ How often does IPV occur?

IPV affects approximately 1.5 million women each year.[2] A common misconception is that IPV affects only a small percentage of pregnant women. Although the prevalence of abuse varies depending on the source and is probably underestimated (due to underreporting), it is thought that as many as 324,000 pregnant women are battered by their partners each year.[3] Therefore, IPV during pregnancy may be more common than routinely screened for complications of pregnancy such as gestational diabetes or neural tube defects, and even preeclampsia.[4]

> *Homicide is a horrifying but important contributor to the maternal mortality rate.*[5]

Although some practitioners and lay people may believe that pregnancy can offer some protection for a woman who has previously been abused, many women who experience IPV before pregnancy continue to be abused during pregnancy. From the research, it is unclear how the pattern of violence changes during pregnancy. Certainly pregnancy increases the amount of stress and arguing in a relationship, which may translate into increased risk for violence.[6] In addition, pregnancy may increase the frequency of sexual victimization of the woman.[6]

Risk Factors

▶ Who is at risk for violence during pregnancy?

It is a commonly held belief that women who experience violence come from poor and uneducated backgrounds; however, violence does not fit snugly into a single demographic group.

> *Victims of violence come from every age group, religion, ethnic and racial group, socioeconomic level, educational background, and sexual orientation.*[7]

Research has demonstrated a higher prevalence of violence during pregnancy in some groups of women. These factors associated with an increased incidence of violence are presented in Display 17.2

DISPLAY 17.2	DEMOGRAPHIC AND PSYCHOSOCIAL FACTORS ASSOCIATED WITH VIOLENCE IN PREGNANCY[7]

Adolescent pregnancy	Alcohol and drug use
Unintended pregnancy	Lack of social support
Delayed prenatal care	Sexually transmitted infections, including HIV/AIDS
Smoking	

Cycle of Violence

▶ What is the cycle of violence?

Walker described a cycle of violence that can be divided into three phases (Fig 17.1).[8] The nurse may see the pregnant victim in the tension-building phase or the reconciliation phase in the

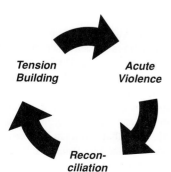

Tension Building **Acute Violence** **Reconciliation**

FIGURE 17.1 The cycle of violence.

intrapartum period. It is rare but not impossible that an acute episode of violence would take place in an intrapartum setting. The pattern can last for a long or short period of time, with the violence typically becoming more intense with each cycle.[8]

Tension-building phase—During this phase, the victim is compliant, but the abuser becomes angry with increasing frequency and intensity. There may be frequent threats of harm, humiliation, and intimidation.

Acute violence phase—This phase is marked by intentional use of force, including the behaviors listed previously, as well as sexual abuse. The abuse may increase in severity with each cycle.

Honeymoon or reconciliation phase—At this time, the victim is showered with apologies and affection by the abuser. The abuser gives assurances that the behavior will never happen again, makes excuses for the behavior, or even denies that violence occurred.

Effects of Violence in Pregnancy

Violence against anyone at any time can be devastating, but violence against a pregnant woman is of particular concern because harm may come to both mother and fetus.

The direct effects of violence in pregnancy can be severe. Maternal trauma and injury surely affects the well-being of the fetus. Maternal abdominal trauma can cause placental abruption, fetal fractures, rupture of the uterus, miscarriage (spontaneous abortion), hemorrhage, and even fetal death.

Studies have documented indirect effects of violence in pregnancy, including[5,7]:

- delayed or inadequate prenatal care
- exacerbation of chronic illnesses
- poor maternal weight gain
- chronic maternal anxiety and/or depression
- low birth weight

The fetal health is affected by the maternal stress response to abuse, both physical and emotional. The mother may increase patterns of smoking and alcohol or drug use to cope with the abuse, or be unable to keep scheduled prenatal appointments and carry out recommended prenatal health care advice.

It is important to remember that if the mother has other children at home, they may be at risk for adverse and even long-term effects of violence as well. IPV is associated with abuse of other members of the household, including children.[7]

Manifestations of Violence

▶ **What signs would one observe that might indicate a pattern of violence?**

Client and partner behaviors as well as physical indicators of violence are presented in Table 17.1.

Screening for Violence

Many professional organizations, including AWHONN, ACNM, and ACOG, endorse routine universal screening for intimate partner violence and provide guidelines for such screening; however, many providers still do not include screening as a part of their practice. During pregnancy, there is a unique opportunity for identification of violence against women.[7] Most women seek care when they are pregnant and have frequent visits with health care providers throughout the pregnancy. Pregnancy may also be a powerful motivator for women to change their situations and hope for a better future with a new baby. Even though women are in the peripartum setting for a relatively short period of time, there is an undeniable bond that can form between the mother and her nurse. There is a sense of advocacy, trust, and care that may foster the type of environment in which the woman feels comfortable enough to disclose abuse. Although screening should take place in an outpatient setting as well, the intrapartum period can be viewed as a screening "safety net."

TABLE 17.1	CLIENT AND PARTNER BEHAVIORS AND PHYSICAL INDICATORS OF VIOLENCE[7,9]
Client behaviors	• Frequent visits for care OR frequently missed appointments • Noncompliance with prescribed treatments • Reluctance to speak • Evasiveness in answering questions • Poor eye contact • Inconsistent descriptions of injuries • Flat affect • Anxiety • Poor self-care
Partner behaviors	• Always accompanies client • Answers questions for client • Criticizes client • May display irrational jealousy • May be hostile and demanding
Physical indicators	• Contusions, abrasions, lacerations, fractures, burns • Intraoral injuries, dental trauma • Headaches, fatigue • Sleep and appetite disturbances • Substance abuse • Repeated sexually transmitted infections • Choking injuries • Defensive injuries to forearms or binding injuries to wrists and ankles • Injuries to face, head, neck, chest, breast, abdomen, genitalia • Injury to central areas, easily covered by clothing • Depression, anxiety, panic attacks • Patches of hair loss • Eating disorders • Exacerbation in symptoms of chronic disease • Low maternal weight gain • Irritable bowel syndrome

Components of screening include[7]:

1. **A thorough review of the social, medical, and obstetric history**
2. Observation and documentation of behaviors of the mother and partner
3. Specific questioning of the mother about abuse with active listening and accurate documentation of responses

In a careful review of the mother's records, look for a history of abuse, depression, substance abuse, psychological symptoms, or a pattern of repeated visits for injuries, chronic pain, or other issues. Careful observation of the interaction of the mother with her partner may give warning signals for abuse. Review the manifestations of violence for both the mother and her partner in Table 17.1.

> *The mother can be experiencing abuse without ANY warning signs in her medical records or upon observation!*

Upon admission to the birth setting, ask the mother questions appropriate for screening during the initial assessment. Questions should be asked when the mother is apart from her partner, family, or friends. At an antepartum visit, this may be accomplished if the mother comes alone for an appointment or by placing pamphlets with information on abuse or a questionnaire in the women's restrooms. In the intrapartum setting, this is not always easy to do. Be creative in separating the mother from her partner for a brief interview if abuse is suspected. Research has shown that a face-to-face encounter is more effective at eliciting information than a questionnaire.[10]

> *Unfortunately, the women most at risk for adverse pregnancy effects from IPV are those who do not or cannot respond to questions about their circumstances.*[11]

▶ What kind of questions should the nurse ask the woman about IPV?

Proper and careful phrasing allows for comprehensive, specific questions. Examples of phrases used for screening are given in Display 17.3. Explain to the mother about confidentiality and the laws regarding reporting of abuse in the state. Ask questions and listen to the responses in a non-judgmental manner.

DISPLAY 17.3 EXAMPLES OF INTRODUCTORY STATEMENTS AND SCREENING QUESTIONS FOR IPV [7,9,10,12]

- "Because violence is so common in many women's lives and because there is help available for women being abused, I now ask every patient about domestic abuse."
- "I am so concerned about family violence that I now ask all of my patients about it, just like I ask about other health issues."
- "I would like to ask you a few questions about physical or emotional trauma because we know that these are common and affect women's health."
- HITS—Has your partner or any family member[13]:
  - Physically HURT you?
  - INSULTED or talked down to you?
  - THREATENED you with harm?
  - SCREAMED or cursed at you during the pregnancy?
- "Does your partner ever humiliate you, put you down, or shame you?"
- "Has someone made you worry about your safety or the safety of your child (children)?"
- "Since you've been pregnant, have you been kicked, hit, slapped, forced into sexual activities, or otherwise physically hurt by someone?"

> *It is important to remember that a woman may need to be asked about violence several times before she discloses abuse.*

There are numerous ways of screening for violence, including interview, computer self-interview, checklists, and the use of tools such as the Abuse Assessment Screen, the Women's Experiences with Battering Scale, the Conflict Tactics Scales 2, the Danger Assessment, and the Index of Spouse Abuse. The CDC provides a detailed list and samples of various screening tools on their website. (See Resources at the end of the module.)

Interventions

▶ What should the nurse do if the mother discloses abuse?

Follow specific steps if the mother discloses abuse.

Step One—Acknowledge the Abuse

If the mother discloses abuse, the most important thing to do is validate her concerns.

> *If the mother discloses abuse, DO NOT respond with questions such as "Why don't you leave?" or "Why do you stay with him/her?" This may make her feel that she is responsible for the violence.*[7]

The mother may feel alone and ashamed. It is important to respond to the disclosure appropriately. Use supportive statements such as:

- "You are not alone."
- "I'm glad you told me, we see lots of women in similar situations."
- "You don't deserve this; we can help."
- "It is not your fault."
- "There are resources available to help you."
- "I am concerned for your safety."
- "We can help you with information and resources."

AWHONN has outlined the helpful "ABCDE's" of responding to intimate partner violence (Display 17.4).

DISPLAY 17.4   ABCDES OF RESPONDING TO INTIMATE PARTNER VIOLENCE

- You are not **A**LONE.
- I **B**ELIEVE that violence is unacceptable.
- This is **C**ONFIDENTIAL.
- I will **D**OCUMENT.
- I will **E**DUCATE you.
- I will work to ensure your **S**AFETY.

See AWHONN website: www.awhonn.org

Step Two—Evaluate and Facilitate Treatment of Physical Complaints Related to Abuse

Notify the primary care provider and collaboratively complete a physical assessment and facilitate treatment of current and/or past injuries from abuse.

Step Three—Assess Immediate Threat to the Mother

It is important to determine if there is an immediate threat to the mother.

- Is the abuser present at the birth setting?
- Does the mother require hospitalization?
- If the mother is to be discharged, does she feel that the abuser will harm her that day?
- Are there weapons in the household?
- Are the mother's other children or loved ones in danger?
- Does the mother feel safe enough to go home?
- Does the mother need immediate counseling?
- Does the mother want immediate police assistance?

Step Four—Assist With the Development of a Safety Plan

If there is an immediate threat of harm to the mother, a safety plan should be developed. The plan gives the mother steps to follow if she is in a dangerous situation. It should include detailed information about defensive measures such as the following[7,12]:

- Finding easy access to an exit
- Practicing how to get away safely
- Having a bag packed and keys ready to leave
- Using code words for calling the police
- Having a planned destination if she needs to leave suddenly
- Having access to keys, money, and important documents

There are many resources and pamphlets available for assistance in development of a safety plan.

Step Five—Provide Information, Resources, and Referrals

Identify for the mother any available support systems at the birth setting. A staff social worker may be contacted to help with consultation. Resources in the community, support groups, shelters, legal aid, child protective services, hotline phone numbers, law enforcement, clergy, or other victim advocates should be described, including national resources. Try to recognize the specific and unique needs of the mother when making referrals.

> *Having brochures available and visible in the birth setting area lets the mother know that it is a safe place, even if she is not yet ready to disclose abuse.*[14]

Step Six—Document Assessments, Findings, and Actions

▶ What should the nurse document?

Accurate and appropriate documentation of findings in situations of intimate partner violence are of the utmost importance. The woman's medical records are frequently used in court and relied upon to be objective and legible.[7,9] The language used should be specific and not leave room for misinterpretation or undermine the woman's credibility. Use quotation marks in charting to document in the woman's own words.

> *Language used in charting should not be judgmental.*

Recommendations for information to be included in the documentation can be found in Table 17.2.

TABLE 17.2 DOCUMENTATION OF INTIMATE PARTNER VIOLENCE[7,9]	
PORTION OF ASSESSMENT	**RECOMMENDING INFORMATION TO RECORD**
Relevant history	• Chief complaint • Medical problems related to the abuse • Detailed account of abusive situation including name and relationship of abuser, date, time, location, weapon used, nature of threats and witnesses • Statements made by the woman about the abuse • Past history of abuse • Relationship of past or current abuse to chief complaint

Results of assessment and laboratory or diagnostic procedures	• Specific gynecologic, neurologic, psychologic findings related to IPV
	• Description of injuries in detailed manner (use a body map for location)
	• Relationship of diagnostic procedure to current or past abuse
	• Photograph injuries
	    Document consent for photographs
	    Label and date any photographs

Interventions	• Information provided • Resources identified • Options discussed • Safety assessment and planning • Referrals made • Mandatory reporting if applicable • Follow-up arrangements

▶ What does the nurse do if the woman denies abuse, but the nurse still suspects it?

If the woman denies abuse but it is strongly suspected, her "no" response should still be documented.[7] Respect her autonomy and review the available resources with her. Even though it may be frustrating, every time the woman is asked, she may come closer to disclosing her abuse. If the woman's account of an injury and the clinical findings are in conflict, note the difference in a narrative.

Mandatory Reporting

Studies have indicated that women, while feeling comfortable disclosing abuse to a health care professional, also feel threatened by possible retaliation if the health care provider reports the abuse.[15] It is for this reason that many groups oppose mandatory reporting of abuse, and currently only a few states have mandatory reporting laws.[16] Many states have laws regarding mandatory reporting of gunshot or knife wounds and these should be followed. In addition, if the mother states that her other children in the home are being abused or are at risk of abuse, the nurse should follow the state laws regarding reporting requirements.

> *Know your state's laws regarding mandatory reporting of IPV!*

Overcoming Barriers to Care

Many barriers exist for both nurses and victims in the identification and support of women experiencing violence during pregnancy.

▶ Why would the woman who is a victim of abuse not disclose it?

A woman who is being abused may have several reasons for not disclosing it, including the following:
- Fear of judgment and blame
- Fear that the health care provider will not believe her
- Shame
- Fear of escalation of abuse
- Threatened harm upon disclosure
- Lack of confidence in the system
- Lack of financial resources
- Uncertainty about how to bring the subject up
- Unawareness that what she is experiencing is IPV
- Lost hope for change
- Family, religious, or cultural pressure
- Belief that the baby will need its father

▶ What are the barriers to IPV screening for the nurse?

Nurses cite many reasons for their reluctance to ask women about IPV, including the following[17,18]:
- Lack of education and instruction in screening
- Lack of privacy with woman
- Lack of time for screening
- Language barriers; inability to find translator except for family member
- Personal history with abuse
- Lack of adequate referral services
- Fear of offending the woman
- Belief that the victim has responsibility for the abuse

The intrapartum period is a busy time and many nurses feel that they have too many other things to do for the mother and that IPV should have been addressed earlier. Some nurses may feel that it is the mother's own fault—that she has the responsibility to speak up if she is experiencing abuse—and that the problem will not be fixed, even if identified. Still others may have their own personal, painful experiences with violence that prohibit them from feeling comfortable asking the questions.

A commonly cited reason for not screening is the fear of offending the mother.[15] However, recent evidence has demonstrated that the majority of women feel that screening for abuse by a health care provider is acceptable.[15]

Certainly it can be difficult to ask mothers questions about abuse. But, efforts in educating nurses will likely increase their comfort in asking the mother difficult and uncomfortable question about abuse.

> *Asking women questions about violence should be as routine as asking about other behavioral risk factors such as smoking or alcohol use.*

RADAR

Sadly, even after disclosure of abuse, the woman may return to the abusive situation. This can be difficult for health care providers to understand and may discourage them from future screening. However, what is asked and said at the present encounter may have positive effects in the future.

Remember that nurses are an essential part of a collaborative team in identifying and assisting victims of IPV. The acronym "RADAR", developed by Alpert,[19] can help nurses to remember their responsibilities as it relates to IPV in any setting.

*R*EMEMBER to routinely ask mothers about IPV.

*A*SK the mother direct and specific questions in screening for IPV.

*D*OCUMENT the mother's injuries.

*A*SSESS the mother's safety.

*R*EVIEW with the mother all possible options.

PRACTICE/REVIEW QUESTIONS

After reviewing this module, answer the following questions.

1. Identify other terms commonly used for intimate partner violence (IPV).

    a. _____

    b. _____

    c. _____

2. List five examples of physical violence.

    a. _____

    b. _____

    c. _____

    d. _____

    e. _____

3. List five examples of psychological abuse.

    a. _____

    b. _____

    c. _____

    d. _____

    e. _____

4. List three examples of sexual violence.

    a. _____

    b. _____

    c. _____

5. Abuse frequently begins or increases during pregnancy.

    a. True

    b. False

6. Women who experience violence during pregnancy are poor and uneducated.

    a. True

    b. False

7. Describe the phases of the cycle of violence.

    a. Tension-building phase: _____

    _____

    _____

    b. Acute violence phase: _____

    _____

    _____

    c. Reconciliation phase: _____

    _____

    _____

8. List five direct or indirect effects of violence during pregnancy.

    a. _____

    b. _____

    c. _____

d. _____

e. _____

9. As the nurse caring for a woman in an intrapartum setting, what are some of the behaviors that might indicate a pattern of violence?

_____

_____

_____

_____

_____

10. As the nurse performing a physical assessment on a woman in the intrapartum setting, what are some of the physical indicators of violence?

_____

_____

_____

_____

_____

11. State two reasons why pregnancy is a unique opportunity IPV screening.

a. _____

b. _____

12. The three components of screening for IPV are:

a. _____

b. _____

c. _____

13. State two appropriate responses from the nurse in response to a woman's disclosure of abuse.

a. _____

_____

_____

b. _____

_____

_____

14. List two questions for the nurse to ask the woman in determining an immediate threat to safety.

a. _____

_____

_____

b. _____

_____

_____

15. What is the purpose of a safety plan?

_____

_____

_____

16. The nurse should document a detailed account of an abusive situation including:

a. _____

b. _____

c. _____

d. _____

e. _____

f. _____

g. _____

17. Consent should be obtained and documented for any photographs taken of the victim's injuries.

a. True

b. False

18. List six reasons why a woman experiencing abuse may not disclose it to a health care provider.

a. _____

b. _____

c. _____

d. _____

e. _____

f. _____

19. List four reasons why a nurse might feel uncomfortable asking questions to screen for IPV.

a. _____

b. _____

c. _____

d. _____

PRACTICE/REVIEW ANSWER KEY

1. Wife or spouse abuse; partner abuse; domestic violence

2. Any five of the following:
   a. Pushing
   b. Slapping
   c. Punching
   d. Kicking
   e. Choking
   f. Beating
   g. Burning
   h. Biting
   i. Shaking
   j. Scratching
   k. Assault with a weapon (knife, gun, or other)
   l. Tying down or restraining
   m. Refusal to allow access to medical care when needed
   n. Leaving the woman in a dangerous place

3. Any five of the following:
   a. Humiliation
   b. "Name calling"
   c. Intimidation
   d. Belittling
   e. Insulting
   f. Ridiculing
   g. Deliberately embarrassing (especially in public)
   h. Social isolation
   i. Withholding of finances or resources
   j. Controlling of activities

4. Any three of the following:
   a. Degrading sexual comments
   b. Threatened force to compel the woman to engage in sexual acts against her will
   c. Intentionally hurting the woman during sex (including the use of objects intravaginally, orally, or anally)
   d. Pursuing sex with the woman when she is unable to avoid participation, unable to communicate unwillingness, or to understand the nature of the act
   e. Rape

5. A. True

6. b. False

7. a. Tension-building phase—During this phase, the victim is compliant, but the abuser becomes angry with increasing frequency and intensity. There may be frequent threats of harm, humiliation and intimidation.
   b. Acute violence phase—This phase is marked by intentional use of force including the behaviors listed previously as well as sexual abuse. The abuse may increase in severity with each cycle.
   c. Honeymoon or reconciliation phase—At this time, the victim is showered with apologies and affection by the abuser. The abuser gives assurances that the behavior will never happen again, makes excuses for the behavior, or even denies that violence occurred.

8. Any five of the following:
   a. Maternal trauma
   b. Placental abruption
   c. Fetal fractures
   d. Uterine rupture
   e. Miscarriage
   f. Hemorrhage
   g. Fetal death
   h. Delayed prenatal care
   i. Exacerbation of chronic illnesses
   j. Poor maternal weight gain
   k. Chronic maternal anxiety and/or depression
   l. Low birth weight

9. Any of the following:
   a. Frequent visits for care or frequently missed appointments
   b. Noncompliance with prescribed treatments
   c. Reluctance to speak
   d. Evasiveness in answering questions
   e. Poor eye contact
   f. Inconsistent descriptions of injuries
   g. Flat affect
   h. Anxiety
   i. Poor self-care

10. Any of the following:
    a. Contusions, abrasions, lacerations, fractures, burns
    b. Intraoral injuries, dental trauma
    c. Headaches, fatigue
    d. Sleep and appetite disturbances
    e. Substance abuse
    f. Repeated STDs
    g. Choking injuries
    h. Defensive injuries to forearms or binding injuries to wrists and ankles
    i. Injuries to face, head, neck, chest, breast, abdomen, genitalia
    j. Injury to central areas, easily covered by clothing
    k. Depression, anxiety, panic attacks
    l. Patches of hair loss
    m. Eating disorders
    n. Exacerbation in symptoms of chronic disease
    o. Low maternal weight gain

11. a. Most women seek prenatal care when they are pregnant.
    b. Pregnancy is a powerful motivator for change.

12. a. A review of the medical and obstetric history
    b. Observation and documentation of behaviors of the mother and partner
    c. Direct questions to the mother about abuse with active listening and accurate documentation of her response

13. Any two of the following:
    a. "You are not alone."
    b. "I'm glad you told me; we see lots of women in similar situations."

    c. "You don't deserve this; we can help."
    d. "It is not your fault."
    e. "There are resources available to help you."
    f. "I am concerned for your safety."
    g. "We can help you with information and resources."

14. Any two of the following:
    a. Is the abuser present at the birth setting?
    b. Does she require hospitalization?
    c. If the mother is to be discharged, does she feel that the abuser will harm her that day?
    d. Are there weapons in the household?
    e. Are her other children or loved ones in danger?
    f. Does she feel safe enough to go home?
    g. Does she need immediate counseling?
    h. Does she want immediate police assistance?

15. The safety plan describes specific defensive measures for the victim to take when she is in a dangerous situation.

16. a. abuser's name and relationship to victim
    b. date
    c. time
    d. location
    e. weapon used
    f. nature of threat
    g. witnesses

17. a. True

18. Any six of the following:
    a. Fear of judgment and blame
    b. Fear that the health care provider will not believe her
    c. Shame
    d. Fear of escalation of abuse
    e. Threatened harm upon disclosure
    f. Lack of confidence in the system
    g. Lack of financial resources
    h. Unsure of how to bring it up
    i. Unaware what she is experiencing is IPV
    j. Lost hope for change
    k. Family, religious, or cultural pressure
    l. Belief that the baby will need its father

19. Any four of the following:
    a. Lack of education and instruction in screening
    b. Lack of privacy with woman
    c. Lack of time for screening
    d. Language barriers, unable to find translator except for family member
    e. Personal history with abuse
    f. Lack of adequate referral services
    g. Fear of offending the woman
    h. Belief that the victim has responsibility for the abuse

REFERENCES

1. Saltzman, L. E., Fanslow, J. L., McMahon, P. M., & Shelley, G. A. (1999). *Intimate partner violence surveillance: Uniform definitions and recommended data elements, version 1.0.* Atlanta: National Center for Injury Prevention and Control, Centers for Disease Control and Prevention.

2. Tjaden, P., & Thoennes, N. (1998, November). *Prevalence, incidence, and consequences of violence against women: Findings from the National Violence Against Women Survey* [research in brief]. Washington, DC: U.S. Department of Justice, Office of Justice Programs.

3. Gazmararian, J. A., Peterson, R., Spitz, A. M., Goodwin, M. M., Saltzman, L. E., & Marks, J. S. (2000). Violence and reproductive health: Current knowledge and future research directions. *Journal of Maternal Child Health, 4*(2), 79–84.

4. Gazmararian, J. A., Lazorick, S., Spitz, A. M., Ballard, T. J., Saltzman, L. E., & Marks, J. S. (2006). Violence and reproductive health: Current knowledge and future research directions. *Journal of the American Medical Association, 275*, 1915–1920.

5. McFarlane, J., Campbell, J. C., Sharps, P., & Watson, K. (2002). Abuse during pregnancy and femicide: Urgent implications for women's health. *Obstetrics and Gynecology, 100*(1), 27–36.

6. Martin, S. L., Harris-Britt, A., Li, Y., Moracco, K. E., Kupper, L. L., & Campbell, J. C. (2004). Changes in intimate partner violence during pregnancy. *Journal of Family Violence, 19*(4), 201–210.

7. Centers for Disease Control, Division of Reproductive Health, National Center for Chronic Disease Prevention and Health Promotion. (N.D.). *Intimate partner violence, a guide for clinicians.* Atlanta. Available at: www.cdc.gov/reproductivehealth/violence/IntimatePartnerViolence/index.htm Accessed September 27, 2007.

8. Walker, L. E. (1984). *The battered woman syndrome.* New York: Springer.

9. Brigham and Women's Hospital. (2004). *Domestic violence: A guide to screening and intervention.* Boston: Author.

10. McFarlane, J., Christoffel, K, Bateman, L., Miller, V., & Bullock, L. (1991). Assessing for abuse: Self-report versus nurse interview. *Public Health Nursing, 8*, 245–250.

11. Yost, N. P., Bloom, S. L., McIntire, D. D., & Leveno, K. J. (2005). A prospective observational study of domestic violence during pregnancy. *Obstetrics and Gynecology, 106*(1), 61–65.

12. American College of Obstetrics and Gynecology. (1995). *Domestic violence* [ACOG technical bulletin no. 209]. Washington, DC: Author.

13. Bardwell, J., Sherin, K., Sinacore, J. M., Zitter, R., & Shakil, A. (1999). Screening for domestic violence in family medicine: development of the verbal HITS scale. *Journal of Advocate Health Care, 1*, 5–7.

14. Griffin, M. P., & Koss, M. P. (2002, January 31). Clinical screening and intervention in cases of partner violence. *Online Journal of Issues in Nursing, 7*(1), manuscript 2. Available at www.nursingworld.org/ojin/topic17/tpc17_2.htm

15. Renker, P. R., & Tonkin, P. (2006). Women's views of prenatal violence: Acceptability and confidentiality issues. *Obstetrics and Gynecology, 107*(2, part 1), 348–354.

16. Association of Women's Health, Obstetrical and Neonatal Nursing (AWHONN). (2001). Opposition to mandatory reporting of intimate partner violence. Available at www.awhonn.org/awhonn/content.do?name=05_HealthPolicyLegislation/5H_PositionStatements.htm.

17. Yonaka, L., Yoder, M. K., Darrow, J. B., & Sherck, J. P. (2007). Barriers to screening for domestic violence in the emergency department. *The Journal of Continuing Education in Nursing, 38*(1), 37–45.

18. Janssen, P. A., Holt, V. L., Sugg, N. K., Emanuel, I., Critchlow, C. M., & Henderson, A. D. (2003). Intimate partner violence

and adverse pregnancy outcomes: A population based study. *American Journal of Obstetrics and Gynecology, 188*(5), 1341–1347.

19. Alpert, E. J., Freud, K. M., Park, C. C., Patel, J. C., & Sovak, M. A. (1992). *Partner violence: How to recognize and treat victims of abuse*. Waltham: Massachusetts Medical Society.

SUGGESTED READINGS

Association of Women's Health, Obstetrical and Neonatal Nursing: www.awhonn.org

Centers for Disease Control: www.cdc.gov/
Family Violence Prevention Fund: http://endabuse.org/
JCAHO: www.jcaho.org/
National Domestic Violence Hotline: (800) 799-SAFE (7233)
National Domestic Violence Hotline for hearing impaired: (800) 787-3224
National Domestic Violence Hotline Website: www.ndvh.org/
National Institutes of Health: www.nih.gov/
National Coalition Against Domestic Violence: www.ncadv.org/
Nursing Network on Violence Against Women, International: www.nnvawi.org

M O D U L E

18

Intrapartum Emergencies

S U Z A N N E   M .   B A I R D   ■   B E T S Y   B .   K E N N E D Y

Objectives

As you complete this module, you will learn:

1. The importance of rapid nursing responses and collaborative care during intrapartum emergencies
2. Risk factors for umbilical cord prolapse
3. Steps to take when a prolapse of the umbilical cord is suspected or has occurred
4. Risks of shoulder dystocia to both the mother and the baby
5. Factors that indicate a possible shoulder dystocia
6. Primary collaborative measures to relieve a shoulder dystocia
7. Techniques for McRoberts maneuver and suprapubic pressure
8. Guidelines for documenting an occurrence of shoulder dystocia
9. Current theoretical knowledge and pathophysiologic alterations that occur with an amniotic fluid embolism
10. Symptoms of amniotic fluid embolism
11. Supportive therapies for the women experiencing a possible amniotic fluid embolism
12. Priorities for treatment of an obstetric hemorrhage
13. The "classic" symptoms of placental abruption
14. Etiologies of placental abruption
15. Criteria for classification of placental abruption
16. Treatment issues for placental abruption based on severity of symptoms
17. Incidence and risk factors for uterine rupture
18. Possible signs that a uterine rupture has occurred
19. Diagnostic criteria for postpartum hemorrhage
20. Predisposing factors for postpartum hemorrhage
21. Manipulative and pharmacologic measures to treat postpartum hemorrhage
22. The importance of maintaining family-centered care even during unexpected and emergency situations
23. The usefulness of team drills to improve outcomes in intrapartum emergencies

Key Terms

When you have completed this module, you should be able to recall the meaning of the following terms. You should be able to use the terms when consulting with other health professionals. Terms are defined in this module or in the glossary at the end of this book.

abruptio placentae (placental
  abruption)
amniotic fluid embolism (AFE)
anaphylactoid syndrome
McRoberts maneuver

obstetric hemorrhage
prolapsed cord
shoulder dystocia
suprapubic pressure
uterine rupture

Intrapartum emergencies are rare, but can be associated with significant maternal and fetal morbidity and mortality. It is important to know how to respond rapidly and appropriately. This module reviews selected issues and nursing care associated with emergencies in the intrapartum period, including cord prolapse, shoulder dystocia, amniotic fluid embolism, and hemorrhagic complications such as placental abruption, uterine rupture, and immediate postpartum hemorrhage. Other intrapartum emergencies such as fetal nonreassurance (Module 6), uterine hyperstimulation (Module 7), and eclamptic seizure (Module 9) are discussed in other modules.

Prolapsed Cord

Umbilical cord prolapse (UCP) may occur any time the maternal pelvis is not completely filled by the presenting fetal part. It occurs most often in fetal malpresentation, breech or transverse lie, or when the presenting part is not engaged. The umbilical cord can prolapse as a result of obstetrical manipulation such as artificial rupture of membranes, amnioinfusion, external version, or placement of internal monitors. Other described risk factors for UCP include a low-lying placenta, a preterm fetus, multiple gestation, polyhydramnios, grand multiparity, and maternal pelvic abnormality.

> A *prolapsed cord* means that the umbilical cord lies beside or below the presenting part of the fetus. This occurs in 0.1% to 0.6% of all pregnancies.[1]

A prolapsed cord can:
- Extend through the vaginal opening (overt; Fig 18.1)

> If the cord extends through the vagina, cover it with a sterile gauze pad moistened with saline solution to keep it from drying out.

- Be palpable at the cervix (funic presentation; Fig 18.2)

> In breech presentations, if membranes rupture spontaneously, a vaginal examination should be performed immediately to feel for the presence of a prolapsed cord.

- Be hidden and not palpable (occult; Fig 18.3)

> Prompt recognition of UCP can minimize the effects of fetal hypoxia due to cord compression.

The fetal heart rate monitor may demonstrate bradycardia or persistent variable decelerations.

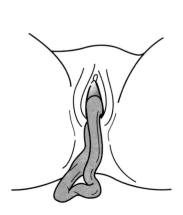

FIGURE 18.1 Prolapse of cord through the vaginal opening.

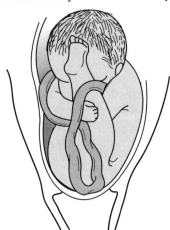

FIGURE 18.2 Prolapsed cord can be felt at the cervical opening.

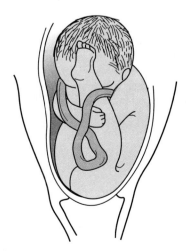

FIGURE 18.3 Hidden prolapsed cord.

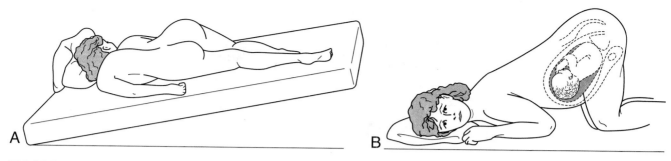

FIGURE 18.4 **A.** Sims position in Trendelenburg. **B.** Knee–chest position.

▶ **What should the nurse do after detecting or suspecting a prolapsed cord?**

---

1. **Notify the primary care provider at the slightest suspicion of a prolapsed cord.**
2. Place the mother in a position that uses gravity to reduce compression of the cord by the presenting part (Fig. 18.4).
3. Perform a sterile-gloved vaginal examination. Place two fingers on either side of the cord or both fingers on one side of the cord to avoid compressing the cord and exert upward pressure against the presenting part to relieve pressure on the cord.
4. DO NOT HANDLE THE CORD because it can cause the cord to spasm, shutting off the fetal blood supply.
5. Continue to monitor the fetus with external fetal monitoring (EFM); apply a fetal scalp electrode if necessary.
6. Begin measures for intrauterine fetal resuscitation including oxygen, delivered at 10 L by face mask, and increased (or initiation of) intravenous fluid administration.
7. If the cord extends through the vagina, cover it with a sterile gauze pad moistened with saline solution to keep it from drying out.
8. Educate and support the mother and family about the emergency and interventions.
9. Document events, interventions, and responses as soon as possible.

A prolapsed cord in a viable fetus requires prompt delivery, which usually means a cesarean section. Preparation for this should begin immediately. If the mother is completely dilated and the fetus is in a cephalic presentation, a forceps or vacuum-assisted birth may be attempted.

> Perinatal mortality rates with UCP have decreased to less than 10% due to more liberal use of cesarean delivery and improved neonatal resuscitation techniques.[1,2]

Shoulder Dystocia

Management of shoulder dystocia in the absence of a primary care provider is discussed in Module 13. This discussion focuses on the responsibilities of the nurse when the birth attendant is present.

> *Shoulder dystocia* occurs when the fetal head is delivered, but the anterior shoulder is impacted or "stuck" on the pubic arch. Shoulder dystocia complicates up to 3% of vaginal deliveries.[3]

Shoulder dystocia cannot be reliably predicted or prevented. However, antepartum and intrapartum risk factors for shoulder dystocia include[3]:
- Instrumented delivery (use of vacuum or forceps)
- Excessive maternal weight gain/weight

- Short maternal stature
- Postterm pregnancy
- Abnormal pelvic structure
- Previous delivery complicated by shoulder dystocia
- Previous macrosomic infant
- Maternal diabetes mellitus
- Prolonged labor

If one of these risk factors is present, be prepared to act rapidly. Shoulder dystocia is associated with significant maternal and fetal morbidity.

Risks to the Mother
- Postpartum hemorrhage
- Third- or fourth-degree episiotomy/laceration
- Uterine rupture

Risks to the Baby
- Brachial plexus injury
- Clavicular fracture
- Hypoxia
- Death

> **NOTE:** *The fetal pH drops by an estimated 0.14 per minute during delivery of the trunk; therefore, timing between delivery of the head to body is important to the fetal acid–base balance.*[4,5]

A team approach to managing shoulder dystocia is essential. All staff should be prepared to respond emergently should a shoulder dystocia occur. If a shoulder dystocia is anticipated based on risk factors, then preparation is important. Alert the anesthesia staff to be present for delivery for the mother's pain management needs and neonatal staff for possible help with resuscitation of the newborn at delivery. The mother's bladder should be emptied by catheterization to prevent obstruction of delivery and potential trauma.

▶ What should the nurse do if shoulder dystocia occurs?

In the event of a shoulder dystocia, the mnemonic "HELPERR" may be helpful for those in attendance.[4]
- Call for <u>HELP</u>—nurse
- <u>EVALUATE</u> for episiotomy—birth attendant
- <u>LEGS</u>—McRoberts maneuver—nurse
- Suprapubic <u>PRESSURE</u>—nurse
- <u>ENTER</u> maneuvers—birth attendant
- <u>REMOVE</u> the posterior arm—birth attendant
- <u>ROLL</u> the patient—all fours—nurse (Gaskins Maneuver)

Primary measures to relieve shoulder dystocia include the McRoberts maneuver and suprapubic pressure. They are considered to have the lowest risk with the highest rate of effectiveness. The *McRoberts maneuver* is accomplished by positioning the mother's thighs on her abdomen. This straightens the sacrum and decreases the angle of incline of the symphysis pubis, making it easier to deliver the anterior shoulder (see Figs. 13.8A, B, and C). Lowering the bed and side rails makes it easier to accomplish these measures, but precautions should be taken to protect the mother. Apply suprapubic pressure with a hand over the anterior fetal shoulder with downward and lateral motion (see Fig. 13.9). Direct downward and lateral motion can be better achieved by standing on a step stool.

> A combination of the McRoberts maneuver and suprapubic pressure may relieve more than 50% of shoulder dystocia cases.[4]

Secondary and tertiary measures are employed by the birth attendant if the shoulder dystocia is not relieved. Alternative positions, including "all fours," may be used and has a high success rate, but may be difficult to accomplish if the mother has received regional anesthesia.[6] Desperate measures, only used in "last resort" situations, include cephalic replacement, symphysiotomy, and deliberate fracture of the clavicle.

> The ACOG recommends antepartum screening for risk factors for shoulder dystocia and consideration of elective cesarean delivery if the estimated fetal weight is above 5,000 g (4,500 g for diabetic mothers).[7]

▶ What should be documented about the occurrence of a shoulder dystocia?

Accurate documentation of the event is essential because shoulder dystocia is one of the most frequently litigated occurrences in obstetrics.[8]

Nursing documentation of the event should include the following:

- Specifics about maneuvers performed, the order in which they were performed, who directed the maneuvers, and attempts to assess fetal status during the event
- Duration of the event (specifically the time from delivery of the fetal head to the delivery of the body)
- Team members involved
- Which arm was impacted
- Umbilical cord pH
- Resuscitation measures for the newborn

IMPORTANT: NEVER USE FUNDAL PRESSURE DURING SHOULDER DYSTOCIA BECAUSE OF SIGNFICANT RISK OF INJURY TO BOTH MOTHER AND BABY.

Be prepared to thoroughly assess the newborn at delivery for signs of brachial plexus injury. (See Module 14 for newborn assessment.) The members of the team involved in the event should also take time to speak with the mother and family after the event to educate, explain, and support.

Amniotic Fluid Embolism

▶ What is an amniotic fluid embolism?

Amniotic fluid embolism (AFE) is the entrance of amniotic fluid, fetal cells, hair, or other debris into the maternal circulation, signaling a series of rapid, complex pathophysiologic events that lead to life-threatening maternal symptoms.

> *The diagnosis of "anaphylactoid syndrome of pregnancy" has been proposed to take the place of AFE, because the exposure to fetal tissue is common, but only a small percentage of women respond with a massive release in endogenous mediators leading to maternal and fetal decompensation.[9]*

Even though AFE is a rare event in obstetrics, it is a leading cause of maternal mortality in developed countries.[9]

NOTE: *The incidence of AFE is estimated to be 1 in 8,000 to 30,000 pregnancies.[10,11]*

NOTE: *The maternal mortality rate with a diagnosis of AFE is between 60% and 80%, with only 15% of patients surviving neurologically intact. This is due to the severe cerebral hypoxia associated with symptoms.[9]*

AFE is usually described as having two phases.[12,13]

Phase I
- Amniotic fluid enters the maternal circulation
- Triggered release of endogenous chemical mediators
- Pulmonary vasospasm and intense vasoconstriction
- Pulmonary hypertension

- Hypoxia
- Capillary damage to myocardial and pulmonary vasculature
- Heart failure with acute respiratory distress

Phase II
- Initiation of the clotting cascade
- Hemorrhage
- Disseminated intravascular coagulation (DIC)

▶ **What are the most common symptoms of an AFE?[9]**

Signs and symptoms of AFE are listed in Table 18.1.

TABLE 18.1 SYMPTOMS OF AFE AND RATE OF OCCURRENCE[9]		
SYMPTOMS OCCURRING FREQUENTLY (in 80% to 100% of cases)	**SYMPTOMS OCCURRING WITH MODERATE FREQUENCY (in 20% to 80% of cases)**	**SYMPTOMS OCCURRING INFREQUENTLY (in less than 20% of cases)**
Hypotension	Dyspnea	Bronchospasm
Fetal distress	Seizure, tonic–clonic	Transient hypertension
Pulmonary edema or acute respiratory distress syndrome	Atony	Cough
Cardiopulmonary arrest		Headache
Cyanosis		Chest pain
Coagulopathy		

▶ **Can an AFE be predicted or prevented?[9]**

AFE is considered an unpredictable and unpreventable event and the cause is unknown. A 10-year national registry that tracked cases to identify risk factors and outcomes may offer a better understanding of the event. Forty-one percent of patients with AFE in the registry had a known allergic reaction to substances and AFE was more likely to occur in women carrying a male fetus. There was no identifiable relationship to age, race, or ethnicity.

▶ **When does amniotic fluid embolism usually occur?[9]**

In the national registry data, 70% of the women diagnosed with AFE were in labor, 19% of cases occurred during cesarean delivery, and 11% of cases occurred during the early postpartum period. AFE has also been reported to occur during amnioinfusion, termination of pregnancy, and abdominal trauma.

▶ **What should the nurse do if the mother exhibits signs of amniotic fluid embolism?[12]**

Nursing care for the woman experiencing a possible AFE is focused on supportive therapy.
- **Immediately notify the birth attendant, physician, and anesthesia and neonatal resuscitation staff (if patient is undelivered) and obtain a crash cart.**
- Continuously monitor the fetus if the mother is undelivered and anticipate an emergency cesarean delivery and neonatal resuscitation.
- Administer high-concentration oxygen by face mask to maintain normal saturation. **Anticipate** and prepare for intubation and ventilation.
- Call a code and initiate cardiopulmonary resuscitation (CPR) if the patient experiences cardiac arrest. If the mother does not respond to CPR, **anticipate** a perimortem cesarean section. Neonatal outcome is linked to the time interval between maternal cardiopulmonary collapse and delivery.
- Initiate intravenous access with large-bore cannula. **Anticipate** central line placement and/or multiple peripheral lines.

- Treat hypotension with positioning and crystalloid boluses. **Anticipate** the need for blood product replacement, vasopressor agents, and inotropic agents.
- **Anticipate** pulmonary artery catheterization in patients who are hemodynamically unstable.
- **Anticipate** arterial line placement for continuous blood pressure analysis and access for blood gases and laboratory examination.
- Prepare the mother and family for transfer to an intensive care environment or tertiary care center after initial stabilization.

Obstetric Hemorrhage

The following intrapartum emergencies are grouped together because they are all associated with complications from blood loss. Obstetric hemorrhage is the single most significant cause of maternal mortality worldwide, with one death occurring every 4 minutes.[14] It is associated with serious maternal morbidity, including acute respiratory distress syndrome (ARDS), acute renal failure, and disseminated intravascular coagulation (DIC). Although the maternal physiologic adaptations to pregnancy (Display 18.1) should allow for compensation of blood loss at delivery, if bleeding continues, previously effective compensatory mechanisms to maintain cardiac output (systemic vasoconstriction, tachycardia, and increased myocardial contractility) begin to fail and symptoms of shock and impaired organ perfusion appear.

| **DISPLAY 18.1** | HEMATOLOGIC ADAPTATIONS DURING PREGNANCY[15,16] |

- Increased blood volume to 6 to 7 L
  - Increased plasma volume 40%
  - Increased red blood cell volume
- Increased efficiency of clotting
- Impaired fibrinolysis

Estimated blood loss (EBL) can be extremely difficult to determine for every health care provider, especially when blood may be mixed with amniotic fluid. Rely on visual inspection and follow laboratory values as ordered (Table 18.2).

TABLE 18.2	CLASSIFICATION OF HEMORRHAGE[17]	
CLASS	**BLOOD LOSS**	**PATIENT SYMPTOMS**
I	900 mL (15%)	Pregnant patient is usually not symptomatic unless accompanied by hypovolemia (e.g., preeclamptic patient)
II	1,200–1,500 mL (20%–25%)	Tachycardia
		Tachypnea
		Narrowing pulse pressure—if pressure drops to ≤30 mmHg, evaluate for other signs of bleeding
		Delayed capillary refill >1–2 seconds after blanching palm at base of fingers at ulnar margin
III	1,800–2,100 mL (30%–35%)	Hypotension
		Marked tachycardia
		Tachypnea
		Skin—cold, clammy
IV	≥2,400 mL blood loss (40%)	Symptoms of profound shock
		• BP may be absent
		• Peripheral pulses may be difficult to palpate
		• Oliguria or anuria

> *Remember that by the time the pregnant woman exhibits signs of compromise such as dizziness, hypotension, and oliguria, the amount of blood loss is significant!*

General nursing considerations for obstetric hemorrhage are as follows[18]:
- Monitor intake and output every hour until stable
- Obtain intravenous access—two large-bore intravenous catheters (may require multiple intravenous lines for moderate to severe hemorrhage)
- Infuse crystalloid solutions to support circulatory status
- Use positioning to optimize cardiac output
- Place Foley catheter—urine output should not fall below 30 mL/h
- Obtain order for typing and cross-matching of blood
- Prepare for blood component therapy
- Monitor laboratory coagulation study findings
- Monitor maternal vital signs frequently until stable
- Monitor fetal status and employ intrauterine resuscitation techniques as needed
- Monitor arterial oxygenation saturation of hemoglobin (SaO_2) until stable
- Monitor and manage maternal pain status—notify anesthesia team as needed
- Prepare for emergency delivery or surgical intervention
- Prepare for possible invasive monitoring
- Prepare for possible maternal resuscitation
- Notify neonatal team of potential delivery if applicable

Blood component therapy may be required for women with significant hemorrhage. Commonly used blood products are described in Table 18.3.

TABLE 18.3 COMMONLY USED BLOOD PRODUCTS[19]		
BLOOD PRODUCT	**VOLUME PER UNIT (mL)**	**EFFECT**
Packed red blood cells	240	Increases hematocrit 3% per unit
Platelets	50	Increases platelets 5,000–10,000 per unit
FFP (factor V, VIII, fibrinogen)	250	Increases fibrinogen 10 mg/dL per unit
Cryoprecipitate (factor VIII)	40	Increases fibrinogen 10 mg/dL per unit

> *It is important to know and monitor for the desired effects of blood product administration.*

Because the management of obstetrical hemorrhage may involve the administration of blood products, the issue of the woman's refusal due to cultural or religious beliefs is a possibility. It is important to ensure the woman's wish is not confused with a lack of desire for all other interventions. Options to maintain cardiac output and oxygen transport such as autotransfusion and/or cell saving may be viewed as acceptable.

Placental Abruption

▶ **What is abruptio placentae?[20]**

Placental abruption is a premature separation of the normally implanted placenta from the uterus (Fig. 18.5). The fetus is deprived of essential blood and oxygen as the separation occurs.
It may be:
> **Revealed**—blood collects between the decidua and the membranes and passes out the cervix and vagina.
> **OR**
> **Concealed**—blood collects behind the placenta and there is no vaginal bleeding noted.
It is a rare but serious complication, with risks for both mother and fetus.

NOTE: The incidence of placental abruption varies but is approximately 1 in 100 pregnancies and may even be higher because not all placentas are pathologically examined.[20]

Suspicion of abruption may be based on symptoms before delivery, but a definitive diagnosis comes with inspection of the placenta after delivery.

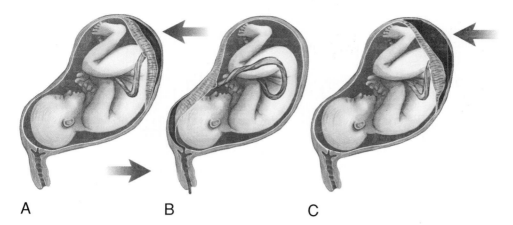

A   B   C

FIGURE 18.5   Placental abruption. **A.** Partial with concealed hemorrhage. **B.** Partial with apparent hemorrhage. **C.** Complete with concealed hemorrhage. (From Orshan, S. A. [2008]. *Maternity, Newborn, & Women's Health Nursing.* Philadelphia: Lippincott Williams & Wilkins.)

▶ What are the classic symptoms of abruption?[16]

Presentation of placental abruption varies widely and depends on the location and degree of separation. Hallmark signs and symptoms of placental abruption include the following:
- Uterine tenderness/backache
- History of sharp, abdominal pain
- Vaginal bleeding
- Dark, "port-wine"–stained amniotic fluid
- Increased uterine tone—described as "board-like"
- Uterine irritability, uterine hypertonus, and/or frequent uterine contractions
- Maternal tachycardia
- Nonreassuring fetal status leading to fetal death

Placental abruption can be classified according to clinical assessments and laboratory findings and is defined in Table 18.4.

The fetal heart rate monitor may reveal a nonreassuring pattern with late decelerations in the fetal heart rate (FHR), fetal bradycardia, or fetal tachycardia (Fig. 18.6).

TABLE 18.4	GRADING OF PLACENTAL ABRUPTION[21]	
GRADE	**MATERNAL EFFECTS**	**FETAL EFFECTS**
1	Slight vaginal bleeding Uterine irritability Blood pressure unaffected Fibrinogen level normal	Heart rate pattern normal
2	Vaginal bleeding mild to moderate Uterine irritability, tetanic or frequent uterine contractions Elevated heart rate Blood pressure maintained Fibrinogen level may be decreased	Heart rate pattern with signs of fetal compromise
3	Vaginal bleeding moderate to severe; may be concealed Uterus tetanic and painful Maternal hypotension Fibrinogen levels often <150 mg/dL Other coagulation deficits present such as thrombocytopenia, clotting factor depletion	Heart rate pattern nonreassuring and/or fetal death has occurred

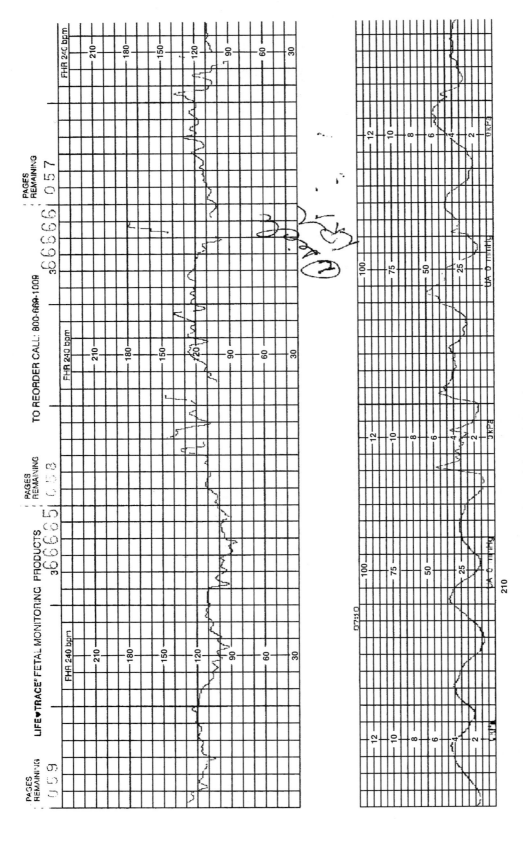

FIGURE 18.6 Electronic fetal monitoring tracing with evidence of placental abruption.

When there is more than a 50% separation of the placenta (Grade 3), the risk for fetal death is very high.

▶ Why does placental abruption occur?[20]

The primary etiology of placental abruption is unknown. Common factors that have been linked with abruption are as follows:

Strongly Linked
• Previous placental abruption—15- to 20-fold in subsequent pregnancies
• Cocaine and drug use
• Chronic hypertension with preeclampsia

Linked
• Cigarette smoking
• Multiple gestations
• Chronic hypertension OR preeclampsia
• Premature rupture of membranes (PROM)
• Chorioamnionitis

Other Possible Links
• Maternal thrombophilias
• Maternal age and parity
• Trauma, sudden uterine decompression—rupture of amniotic membranes, falls, motor vehicle crash, violence

▶ What should the nurse do if a placental abruption is suspected?[20]

Obstetric management of placental abruption is individualized based on the gestational age and the severity of the maternal and fetal symptoms. For example, severe placental abruption with maternal and fetal compromise at any viable gestational age is aggressively managed to achieve delivery as soon as possible. If symptoms are mild and gestational age is preterm (20 to 34 weeks), a stable mother and fetus are managed conservatively to optimize neonatal outcome. If mother is at term or near term and stable, and fetal status is reassuring, vaginal delivery may be achieved.

Mild Symptoms
• Prepare to administer corticosteroids to promote fetal lung maturity if pregnancy is at less than 32 weeks' estimated gestational age (EGA)
• Closely monitor both maternal and fetal status
• Be prepared for a high-risk newborn

Moderate/severe Symptoms
• Anticipate central line placement
• Administer oxygen via nonrebreather face mask at 10 L/min
• Initiate continuous pulse oximetry
• Continuously monitor fetal status
• Prepare for blood product replacement
• Anticipate cesarean delivery

In cases of severe placental abruption that result in fetal death, the mother is allowed to delivery vaginally as long as she remains stable.

Remember that there is a significant risk for coagulopathy such as DIC if the fetus is dead. Be vigilant in monitoring the mother's vital signs and blood loss.

Uterine Rupture

▶ What is a uterine rupture?[21]

Uterine rupture (Fig. 18.7) is defined as the symptomatic disruption of the layers of the uterus that is characterized by one or more of the following symptoms:

- Hemorrhage
- Bladder injury
- Uterine damage (resulting in hysterectomy)
- Any portion of the fetal–placental unit outside of the uterus
- Nonreassuring fetal tracing.

> *True uterine rupture, which requires emergency intervention, should not be confused with uterine scar dehiscence, which may be asymptomatic.*

▶ How often does uterine rupture occur?[22,23]

The overall incidence of uterine rupture is approximately 1%. It is most commonly associated with vaginal birth after prior cesarean delivery. Conditions associated with uterine rupture include the following:

- **Uterine scars—prior cesarean delivery,** prior rupture, trauma, abortion, instrumentation injury, myomectomy, uterine perforation
- **Induction of labor, excessive uterine stimulation**
- Uterine or fetal anomalies
- Prior invasive molar pregnancy
- History of placenta percreta or increta
- Malpresentation
- Obstructed labor

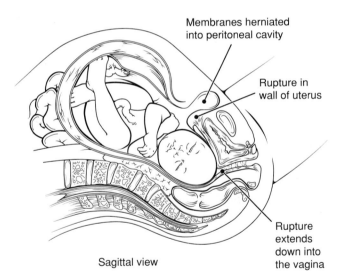

Membranes herniated into peritoneal cavity

Rupture in wall of uterus

Rupture extends down into the vagina

Sagittal view

> *The incidence of uterine rupture may likely increase due to the rising rate of cesarean deliveries.[24]*

> **Induction of labor is associated with higher rates of uterine rupture. Use agents for cervical ripening and/or induction of labor with EXTREME CAUTION and avoid uterine hyperstimulation.**

FIGURE 18.7 Uterine rupture.

For a discussion of vaginal birth after cesarean delivery (VBAC) and trial of labor (TOL), refer to Module 19.

▶ What is first sign/symptom of uterine rupture?[22]

A nonreassuring or abnormal fetal heart rate tracing may be the first manifestation of uterine rupture in a laboring patient. It may be described as an abrupt decrease in FHR, late and/or severe variable decelerations, absent fetal heart rate baseline variability, fetal tachycardia or bradycardia, or an erratic fetal heart rate pattern. Any time an electronic fetal monitor strip exhibits these signs, uterine rupture may be suspected and the physician should be notified to assess the mother immediately (Fig. 18.8).

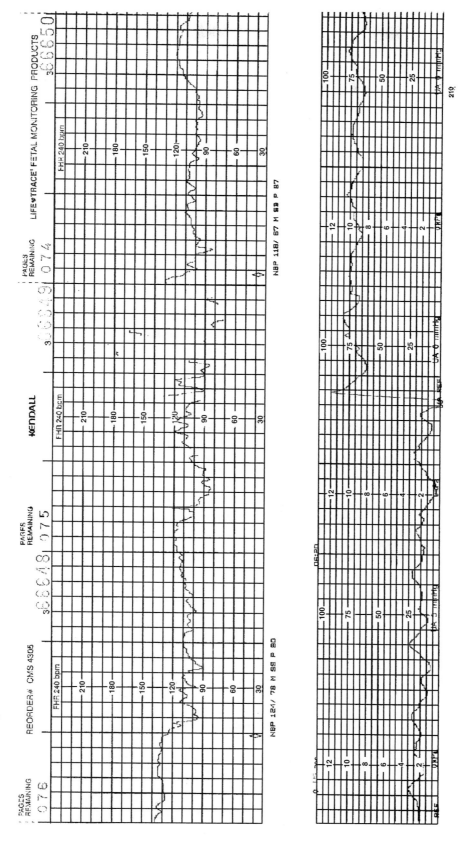

FIGURE 18.8 External electronic fetal monitor tracing prior to diagnosis of uterine rupture.

▶ **What other signs and symptoms might indicate a uterine rupture has occurred?**[22,23]

Other signs of uterine rupture may include:
- *Abrupt change in uterine activity*—an increase or cessation of uterine contractions
- *Loss of fetal station or no fetal descent*
- *Palpable fetal parts*
- *Vaginal bleeding*—bright red
- *Symptoms of maternal shock*—hypotension, tachycardia
- *Maternal pain*—described as ripping or tearing sensation that is independent of uterine contractions, sudden sharp abdominal pain

> *NOTE: If the mother has regional anesthesia for labor, she may not be able to report a sensation of pain, but may have other intense feelings such as anxiety and restlessness.*

▶ **What should the nurse do if a uterine rupture is suspected?**

- Notify the attending physician immediately
- Notify the anesthesia team, the operating room team, and the neonatal team to prepare for immediate delivery
- Discontinue oxytocin
- Prepare patient for emergency cesarean delivery if vaginal delivery is not imminent
- Administer oxygen by nonrebreather face mask at 10 L per minute
- Position patient in left or right lateral recumbent position
- Administer crystalloid IV fluid bolus
- Anticipate blood product replacement
- Continuously monitor fetal status
- Prepare for a high-risk newborn

Postpartum Hemorrhage

▶ **What is a postpartum hemorrhage (PPH)?**

Postpartum hemorrhage (PPH) is defined as blood loss of more than 500 mL after birth, a 10% change in maternal hematocrit between admission and postpartum, and/or the need for transfusion. Average blood loss during delivery is presented in Display 18.2.

DISPLAY 18.2 AVERAGE BLOOD LOSS DURING DELIVERY[15]

Vaginal delivery: 300 to 500 mL
Cesarean delivery: 900 to 1,100 mL

PPH occurs in 4% to 6% of pregnancies and is primarily caused by uterine atony.[25] Uterine atony has many different etiologies, including:
- grand multiparity
- overdistention of the uterus (large fetus, multiple gestation, polyhydramnios)
- precipitous labor or delivery
- prolonged labor
- oxytocin induction or augmentation
- previous history of uterine atony
- full bladder after delivery

> PPH can occur *early* in the first 24 hours after delivery, or *late,* between 24 hours and 6 weeks postpartum.

▶ **How does uterine atony lead to postpartum hemorrhage?**

After delivery of the placenta, uterine contraction causes the myometrial fibers to constrict the spiral arterioles and control blood loss. If the uterus is unable to contract, increased blood loss will occur.

Other causes of early and late PPH may include the following[25]:

Early Causes
- Lacerations
  - Lower genital tract (perineal, vaginal, cervical, periclitoral, labial, periurethral, rectal)
  - Upper genital tract (broad ligament)
  - Upper urinary tract (bladder, urethra)
- Retained placental fragments
- Invasive placentation (placenta accrete, placenta increta, placenta percreta)
- Uterine rupture
- Uterine inversion
- Coagulation disorders (hereditary, acquired)

Late Causes
- Infection
- Retained placental fragments
- Placental site subinvolution
- Coagulation disorders

> *BE AWARE of any predisposing factors for PPH in the intrapartum period and BE PREPARED for a rapid response.*

▶ What should the nurse do in the event of a PPH?[18]

After delivery, if the mother is having continued, excessive vaginal bleeding, first empty the bladder and perform uterine massage. If the uterus is "boggy"—soft and not contracted—compression can help to lessen the bleeding and express clots. Thorough assessments at appropriate intervals in the postpartum period are essential in identifying postpartum hemorrhage. Review postpartum care in Module 14. The birth attendant may perform a bimanual pelvic examination of the uterine cavity for retained placental fragments and an inspection of the perineum, vagina, and cervix for laceration.

> *NOTE: Blood flow from the placenta to the uterus is 600 mL/min, so there is great potential for significant blood loss in a short period of time.*[26]

Oxytocin may be given prophylactically after delivery of the placenta to contract the uterus. Dosing for oxytocin and other uterotonic medications, along with nursing considerations, are presented in Table 18.5.

TABLE 18.5 UTEROTONIC MEDICATIONS [18,25]

MEDICATION	DOSE	ROUTES	FREQUENCY	SIDE EFFECTS	CONTRAINDICATIONS
Oxytocin (Pitocin)	10–40 U in 1 L normal saline or lactated Ringer's solution, delivered at around 200 mU/min	IV, IM, IMM	Continuous IV solution, NO bolus, monitor fluids	Nausea and vomiting, water toxicity	
Methylergonovine (Methergine)	0.2 mg	IM, IMM, no IV	q2–4 hours for up to 5 doses	Nausea and vomiting, hypertension, myocardial ischemia	Hypertension, coronary insufficiency
15-methyl PGF2alpha (Carboprost, Hemabate)	0.25 mg	IM, IMM	15–90 min (maximum of 8 doses)	Nausea, vomiting, diarrhea, flushing, fever, vasospasm, bronchospasm	Asthma patients; cardiac, pulmonary, renal, or hepatic disease
Misoprostol (Cytotec)	Varies	Oral (600 μg), vaginal, rectal (400–100 μg)	Varies	Hyperpyrexia in high oral doses	

If manipulative and medication measures fail to control the bleeding, more invasive techniques may be used. Vaginal packing, angiographic arterial embolization, and surgical options can be successful in treating refractory bleeding. Be prepared for rapid transfer to the surgical suite if necessary.

The Importance of Maintaining Family-Centered Care

Although any number of complications can place the mother in a dangerous emergency situation, remember that this is still a birth experience. Every effort must be made to keep the mother and her family and support person informed and educated. This requires skills that keep the mother and support person always in focus. Although usually there is no warning, if a complication is anticipated based on risk factors, the mother can be adequately educated ahead of time. If this is not possible, then a collaborative debriefing should be done to inform the mother and family what has happened, what was done, and why. When possible, the mother should be allowed contact with her newborn to facilitate attachment.

Strategies for Success in Intrapartum Emergencies

An intrapartum emergency not only causes fear and anxiety for the mother, it can also be stressful for the health care team. The potential for errors is great. A rapid, multifaceted response from the team is essential to success during intrapartum emergencies.[27] The potential importance and effectiveness of periodic team drills to improve health care provider responses in emergencies has been established.[27,28] JCAHO has recommended the use of drills since 2004 for common obstetric emergencies such as those presented in this module.[29]

Mock drills may also be used effectively for emergency cesarean births.

▶ **How can mock drills help the response to intrapartum emergencies?[27–29]**

Drills for obstetric emergencies can potentially
- increase the preparedness of the team
- increase the confidence of the team
- increase the effectiveness of the team
- increase patient safety
- reduce health care provider anxiety
- promote collaborative care
AND
- improve outcomes for mothers and babies

Although there is little information available on how to prepare for emergency drills in obstetrical situations, it is reasonable for the team to do the following[28]:
- Choose the most commonly experienced intrapartum emergencies
- Develop a list of roles and responsibilities of members
- Develop algorithms or protocols for the order and assignment of interventions
- Ensure a way to record the drill (scribe or video) for feedback
- Set reasonable goals for implementation
- Document and share successful programs for all to reap the benefits

Ultimately, hospital and birth setting systems will be improved and a safety net will be in place for emergencies.

PRACTICE/REVIEW QUESTIONS

After reviewing this module, answer the following questions.

1. Explain the first step that you would take when a prolapsed cord is detected.

   _____

2. If you suspect a prolapsed cord and the membranes rupture spontaneously, what should you do? _____

   _____

3. If the cord extends through the vagina, what should you do? _____

   _____

4. Why is it not advisable to handle a prolapsed cord?

   _____

   _____

5. State five situations in which the danger of a prolapsed cord exists, necessitating a vaginal examination.

   a. _____

   b. _____

   c. _____

   d. _____

   e. _____

6. Shoulder dystocia occurs when _____

   _____

   _____

7. Shoulder dystocia can be predicted and prevented.

   a. True

   b. False

8. Antepartum and intrapartum risk factors for shoulder dystocia include:

   a. _____

   b. _____

   c. _____

   d. _____

   e. _____

   f. _____

9. List the risks of shoulder dystocia to both the mother and the baby.

   Mother   Baby

   _____   _____

   _____   _____

   _____   _____

   _____   _____

10. List actions to take if you anticipate a shoulder dystocia may occur.

    a. _____

    b. _____

    c. _____

11. Match the interventions for shoulder dystocia (Column A) with the provider (Column B)

    Column A   **Column B**

    _____ 1. Call for help.   a. nurse

    _____ 2. Evaluate for episiotomy   b. birth attendant
                                            (midwife
    _____ 3. McRoberts maneuver   or physician)

    _____ 4. Suprapubic pressure

    _____ 5. Manipulative maneuvers

    _____ 6. Remove posterior arm

    _____ 7. Roll mother to "all fours"

12. McRoberts maneuver is accomplished by positioning the mother's _____ on her _____. This makes it easier to deliver the anterior shoulder by _____ and _____ _____.

13. Documentation of the occurrence of a shoulder dystocia should include all of the following:

    a. _____

    b. _____

    c. _____

    d. _____

    e. _____

    f. _____

14. Fundal pressure should never be used due to significant risks to the mother and the baby.

    a. True

    b. False

15. Amniotic fluid embolism is the entrance of _____ _____ into the maternal circulation followed by a series of pathophysiologic events.

16. Maternal mortality with a diagnosis of AFE is _____.

17. Most AFEs occur during the immediate postpartum period?

    a. True

    b. False

18. The most common symptoms of AFE are:

_____

_____

_____

19. If the intrapartum mother is not responding to CPR after a cardiac arrest caused by an AFE, a _____

_____may be performed to improve neonatal outcome.

20. List the maternal signs and symptoms of a Class II hemorrhage (1200 to 1500 mL blood loss):

a. _____

b. _____

c. _____

d. _____

21. Maternal hypovolemic shock symptoms do not appear until approximately 40% of the circulating blood volume is lost.

a. True

b. False

22. The classic signs of a placental abruption are:

a. _____

b. _____

c. _____

d. _____

e. _____

f. _____

23. If the mother is experiencing mild to moderate vaginal bleeding, frequent uterine contractions, and an elevated heart rate and the fetus demonstrates a change in heart rate baseline (tachycardia or bradycardia) and late decelerations, the placental abruption would likely be classified as:

a. Grade 1

b. Grade 2

c. Grade 3

24. List five factors associated with placental abruption.

a. _____

b. _____

c. _____

d. _____

e. _____

25. For the mother at 31 weeks' gestation with mild symptoms of placental abruption the nurse would anticipate administration of _____ to enhance fetal lung maturity.

26. A 28-year-old woman at 30 weeks' gestation has severe abdominal pain and palpable fetal parts outside the uterus. By definition, a disruption of the layers of the uterus allowing any portion of the fetal–placental unit outside is known as _____

_____.

27. Rank the following according to the highest incidence of uterine rupture with a history of a previous cesarean delivery.

a. no labor

b. induction with prostaglandin

c. induction without prostaglandin

d. spontaneous labor

28. Changes in the electronic fetal monitor tracing which may indicate a uterine rupture include

_____

_____

29. Postpartum hemorrhage (PPH) is defined as blood loss greater than _____mL after birth, or a _____% change in admission and postpartum maternal hematocrit.

30. Explain how uterine atony may cause postpartum hemorrhage.

_____

_____

_____

31. A 20-year-old gravida 3 is having continued, excessive bleeding 45 minutes after a spontaneous vaginal delivery of a baby girl. The first two nursing actions should be

a. _____

b. _____

32. Oxytocin may be given after delivery at a dose of _____ U mixed in _____ _____ infused per IV line at around _____ U/min to prevent postpartum hemorrhage.

33. Methergine should not be used in patients with _____ _____or _____.

34. Administration routes for Cytotec include

_____

_____

PRACTICE/REVIEW QUESTION ANSWER KEY

1. Place the mother in a position that reduces compression of the cord by the presenting part. Use the extreme Trendelenburg or modified Sims position.

2. Perform a vaginal examination. If you encounter a prolapsed cord, leave your hand in the vagina, holding up the presenting part to alleviate compression on the cord.

3. Do not touch it. Cover the cord with a sterile gauze pad moistened with saline solution. Place the mother in the knee-chest or Sims position and call the primary care provider.

4. Handling the cord can cause it to go into spasms, shutting off the fetal blood supply.

5. a. When there is unexplained fetal distress (especially when the presenting part is high)
    b. When membranes rupture with a high presenting part
    c. When membranes rupture in a woman with a malpresentation
    d. When the baby is very premature
    e. In a twin gestation

6. The fetal head is delivered, but the anterior shoulder is impacted on the pubic arch.

7. b. False

8. Any six of the following:
    a. Excessive maternal weight gain/weight
    b. Short maternal stature
    c. Postterm pregnancy
    d. Abnormal pelvic structure
    e. Previous delivery complicated by shoulder dystocia
    f. Previous macrosomic infant
    g. Maternal diabetes mellitus
    h. Prolonged labor
    i. Need for instrumented delivery

9. Mother—postpartum hemorrhage, third- or fourth-degree episiotomy, uterine rupture
   Baby—brachial plexus injury, clavicular fracture, hypoxia, death

10. a. Alert anesthesia staff to be present for the mother's pain management needs.
    b. Alert neonatal staff to be present to help with resuscitation of the newborn as needed.
    c. Empty the mother's bladder by catheterization to prevent possible obstruction or trauma.

11. 1. a
    2. b
    3. a
    4. a
    5. b
    6. b
    7. a

12. Thighs, abdomen, straightening the sacrum, decreasing the angle of incline of the symphysis pubis.

13. a. Specific maneuvers employed, order and number of attempts
    b. Duration of the event, time from delivery of the fetal head to the delivery of the body
    c. Team members involved
    d. Fetal arm impacted, left or right
    e. Umbilical cord pH
    f. Resuscitation measures for the newborn

14. a. True

15. Amniotic fluid, fetal cells, or other debris

16. 60% to 80%

17. b. False

18. Hypertension, fetal distress, pulmonary edema or ARDS, cardiopulmonary arrest, cyanosis and coagulopathy.

19. Perimortem cesarean section

20. a. Tachycardia
    b. Tachypnea
    c. Narrowing pulse pressure
    d. Delayed capillary refill

21. a. True

22. a. Uterine tenderness or abdominal pain
    b. Vaginal bleeding
    c. Increased uterine contractions
    d. Rigid, board-like abdomen
    e. Nonreassuring fetal status
    f. Maternal tachycardia

23. b. Grade 2

24. Any five of the following:
    a. Trauma
    b. Uterine or umbilical cord anomaly
    c. Maternal hypertension
    d. Cigarette smoking
    e. Maternal age and parity
    f. Cocaine use
    g. Premature rupture of membranes
    h. Placement of an intrauterine pressure catheter

i. Previous cesarean delivery

j. Maternal thrombophilia

25. Corticosteroids

26. Uterine rupture

27. b, c, d, a

28. Abrupt decrease in FHR, late or severe variable decelerations, or an erratic FHR

29. 500 mL, 10%

30. Uterine atony can cause postpartum hemorrhage since the uterine vessels are not compressed when the uterine muscle is in a relaxed state.

31. Empty her bladder and perform uterine massage

32. 10 to 40 U in 1 L normal saline or lactated Ringer's at about 200 mL per hour

33. Hypertension or coronary insufficiency

34. Oral, vaginal, or rectal

REFERENCES

1. Lin, M. G. (2006). Umbilical cord prolapse. *Obstetrical and Gynecologic Survey, 61*(4), 269–277.

2. Boyle, J. J., & Katz, V. L. (2005). Umbilical cord prolapse in current obstetric practice. *Journal of Reproductive Medicine, 50,* 303–306.

3. Kwek, K., & Yeo, G. S. H. (2006). Shoulder dystocia and injuries: prevention and management. *Current Opinion in Obstetrics and Gynecology, 18,* 123–128.

4. Baxley, E. G., & Gobbo, R. W. (2004). Shoulder dystocia. *American Family Physician, 69*(7), 1707–1714.

5. Beer, E., & Folgera, M. G. (1998). Time for resolving shoulder dystocia. *American Journal of Obstetrics and Gynecology, 179,* 1376–1377.

6. Bruner, J. P., Drummond, S. B., Meenan, A. L., & Gaskin, I. M. (1998). All-fours maneuver for reducing shoulder dystocia during labor. *Journal of Reproductive Medicine, 43,* 439–443.

7. American College of Obstetricians and Gynecologists. (2002). *Shoulder dystocia* [Practice bulletin No. 40]. Washington, DC; Author.

8. Simpson, K. R., & Knox, G. E. (2003). Common areas of litigation related to care during labor and birth: Recommendations to promote patient safety and decrease risk exposure. *Journal of Perinatal and Neonatal Nursing, 17*(2), 110–125.

9. Clark, S. L Hankins, G. D., Dudley, D. A., Dildy, G. A., & Porter, T. F. (1995). Amniotic fluid embolism: Analysis of the national registry. *American Journal of Obstetrics and Gynecology, 172,* 1158–1189.

10. Steiner, P. E., & Luschbaugh, C. C. (1941). Maternal pulmonary embolism by amniotic fluid. *Journal of the American Medical Association, 117,* 1245–1254.

11. Morgan, M. (1979). Amniotic fluid embolism: A review. *Anesthesia, 34,* 20–32.

12. Schoening, A. M. (2006). Amniotic fluid embolism: Historical perspectives and new possibilities. *Maternal Child Nursing, 31*(2), 78–83.

13. Moore, J., & Baldisseri, M. R. (2005). Amniotic fluid embolism. *Critical Care Medicine, 33*(10 Suppl.), S279–S285.

14. American College of Obstetrics and Gynecologists. (2006). *ACOG technical bulletin #76.* Washington, DC: Author

15. Jansen, A. J. G., van Rhenen, D. J., Steegers, A. A. P., & Duvekot, J. J. (2005). Postpartum hemorrhage and transfusion of blood and blood components. *Obstetrical and Gynecological Survey, 60*(10), 663–671.

16. Lockwood, C. J. (2006). Pregnancy-associated changes in the hemostatic system. *Clinical Obstetrics and Gynecology, 49*(4), 836–843.

17. Baker, R. (1977). Hemorrhage in obstetrics. *Obstetrics and Gynecology Annual, 6,* 295.

18. MacMullen, N. J., Dulski, L. A., & Meagher, B. (2005). Red alert: Perinatal hemorrhage. *Maternal Child Nursing, 30*(1), 46–51.

19. Martin, S. R., Strong, T. H. (2004). Transfusion of blood components and derivatives in the obstetric care patient. In *Obstetric Intensive Care Manual* (2nd ed.). Foley, M. R., Strong, T. H., & Garite, T. J. (Eds.). New York: McGraw-Hill.

20. Oyelese, Y., and Ananth, C. V. (2006). Placental abruption. *Obstetrics and Gynecology, 108*(4), 1005–1016.

21. Francois, K. E., & Foley, M. R. (2007). Antepartum and postpartum hemorrage. In *Obstetrics: Normal and Problem Pregnancies* (5th ed.). Gabbe, S. G., Simpson, J. L., & Niebyl, J. R. (Eds.). New York: Churchill Livingstone.

22. Ayers, A. W., Johnson, T. R. B., & Hayashi, R. (2001). Characteristics of fetal heart rate tracings prior to uterine rupture. *International Journal of Obstetrics and Gynecology, 4,* 235–240.

23. Toppenberg, K. S., & Block, W. A. (2002). Uterine rupture: What family physicians need to know. *American Family Physician, 66*(5), 823–828.

24. Murphy, D. J. (2006). Uterine rupture. *Current Opinion in Obstetrics and Gynecology, 18,* 135–140.

25. American College of Obstetricians and Gynecologists. (2006). Postpartum Hemorrhage, ACOG Practice Bulletin No. 76. *Obstetrics and Gynecology, 108*(4), 1039–1047.

26. You, W. B., & Zahn, C. M. (2006). Postpartum hemorrhage: Abnormally adherent placenta, uterine inversion, and puerperal hematomas. *Clinical Obstetrics and Gynecology, 49*(1), 184–197.

27. Skupski, D. W., Lowenwirt, I. P., Wienbaum, F. I., Bridsky, D., Danek, M., & Eglinton, G. S. (2006). Improving hospital systems for the care of women with major hemorrhage. *Obstetrics and Gynecology, 107*(5), 977–983.

28. Simpson, K. R. (2005). Emergency drills in obstetrics. *Maternal Child Nursing, 30*(3), 220.

29. Joint Commission on Accreditation of Healthcare Organizations. (2004). JCAHO *Sentinel Event Alert #30.* Sentinel Event Alert. Oakbrook Terrace, IL: Author.

SUGGESTED READING

Sorensen, S. S. (2007). Emergency drills in obstetrics: Reducing risk of perinatal death or permanent injury. *JONA's Healthcare Law, Ethics and Regulation, 9*(1), 9–16.

Young, W. (2005). Shoulder dystocia drill [videotape]. Atlanta: American College of Obstetricians and Gynecologists.

M O D U L E

19

Caring for the Woman Undergoing an Instrumented or Operative Delivery

BETSY B. KENNEDY ■ SARAH BRANAN

Objectives

As you complete this module, you will learn:
1. Indications for operative vaginal deliveries and cesarean sections
2. Indications and contraindications for operative vaginal deliveries, that is, vacuum-assisted deliveries and forceps-assisted deliveries
3. Risks and benefits of vacuum-assisted deliveries and forceps-assisted deliveries
4. Nursing considerations for operative vaginal deliveries and cesarean sections
5. The most common types of forceps and their uses
6. Types of cesarean births
7. Guidelines for identifying appropriate VBAC candidates
8. Indications for and risks of cesarean birth
9. Roles of the nurse during the preoperative, intraoperative, and postoperative period
10. Ways to promote family centered care for the woman experiencing operative birth

Key Terms

When you have completed this module, you should be able to recall the meaning of the following terms. You should be able to use the terms when consulting with other health professionals. Terms are defined in this module or in the glossary at the end of this book.

cephalopelvic disproportion (CPD)
cesarean birth
cesarean delivery upon maternal request
cesarean hysterectomy
classic incision
dystocia
emergency cesarean delivery
forceps-assisted birth
low segment transverse incision
low segment vertical incision
primary cesarean delivery
repeat elective cesarean delivery
shoulder dystocia
trial of labor (TOL)
vacuum-assisted birth (vacuum extraction)
vaginal birth after cesarean (VBAC)

Although most women desire and set a goal for a spontaneous vaginal birth, occasionally complications arise in the second stage of labor necessitating a choice between an instrumented or operative vaginal delivery and cesarean birth. Operative deliveries, that is, cesarean section and vaginal birth assisted by vacuum or forceps, are modifications in the mode of delivery implemented by the primary care provider in certain circumstances to reduce maternal or fetal risk.

Vacuum-Assisted Birth (Vacuum Extraction)

Vacuum-assisted birth is achieved by the use of a vacuum cup attached to the fetal head (occiput anterior). Suction is used to create negative pressure and an artificial caput (chignon), ensuring a snug fit of the cap onto the head (Fig. 19.1). The birth attendant uses *gentle traction* while the mother is actively pushing with contractions to help the fetal head descend and shorten the second stage of labor.

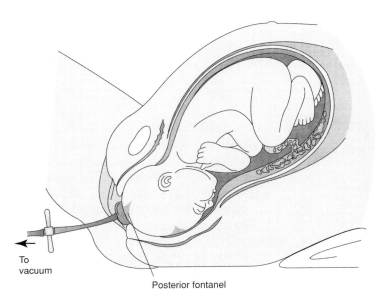

To vacuum

Posterior fontanel

FIGURE 19.1 Vacuum extraction (From Pillitteri, A. [2007]. *Maternal & child health nursing: Care of the childbearing & childrearing family* [5th ed.]. Philadelphia: Lippincott Williams & Wilkins.)

▶ **Why is the vacuum used to assist birth?**[1]

The vacuum may be used in a variety of situations. Some of the most common scenarios are summarized in Display 19.1.

DISPLAY 19.1 INDICATIONS FOR VACUUM EXTRACTION[1]

Prolonged second stage of labor
Fetal compromise (non-reassuring status)
Maternal benefit
- Poor pushing effort (secondary to exhaustion or analgesia/anesthesia)
- Cardiac, pulmonary, cerebrovascular or neurologic disease

NOTE: *Operative vaginal deliveries (vacuum and forceps assisted) occur in approximately 10% to 15% of all deliveries. The rate of use of the vacuum has increased over the last two decades, and has now surpassed that of forceps; however, the overall percentage of instrumented deliveries has remained constant.*[1,2]

For vacuum-assisted birth to be successful[1,2]:
- The fetus must be in a vertex (cephalic) presentation and engaged, with the head position known
- The membranes must be ruptured to ensure proper placement
- The mother's cervix should be completely dilated to avoid potential lacerations

Contraindications to vacuum use include[1,2]:
- face or breech presentation
- severe maternal or fetal compromise requiring rapid delivery
- evidence of cephalopelvic disproportion (CPD)
- congenital anomalies of the fetal head
- gestational age less than 34 weeks or estimated fetal weight less than 2,000 g
- live fetus with a known bleeding disorder

▶ What are the risks of vacuum-assisted birth?

The fetus/newborn commonly experiences cup marks, bruising, and minor lacerations (Fig. 19.2). *These effects are lessened with the use of a soft cup as opposed to a rigid one.*

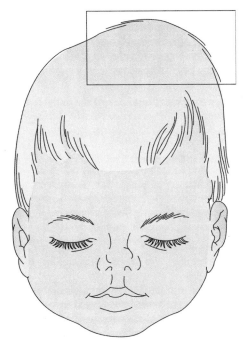

FIGURE 19.2 Caput succedaneum. (From Pillitteri, A. [2007]. *Maternal & child health nursing: Care of the childbearing & childrearing family* [5th ed.]. Philadelphia: Lippincott Williams & Wilkins.)

More serious risks include[3]:
- cephalohematoma
- subgaleal hematoma
- retinal hemorrhage
- intracranial hemorrhage
- skull fractures

Scalp avulsions, abrasions, blistering, bruising, and other trauma are more likely to occur when the vacuum is applied for a prolonged period of time (longer than 20 minutes) or with excessive suction (maximum pressure force should not be longer than 10 minutes).[4]

BE PREPARED: Shoulder dystocia may be more frequently encountered with vacuum extraction, but it is also associated with a prolonged second stage, one of the indications for use of the vacuum. Adverse long-term effects of vacuum-assisted birth, as opposed to other modes of delivery, have not been demonstrated in the literature. The use of the vacuum on the preterm fetus has not been sufficiently studied, but it *is usually contraindicated in gestational ages less than 34 weeks.*[1]

Maternal complications are rare, but may include pain, extension of episiotomy, bladder trauma, perineal lacerations, and soft tissue injuries to the vulva, vagina, cervix, and anal sphincter.[2,4]

▶ What is the nurse's responsibility in a vacuum-assisted birth?

The nurse's role in a vacuum-assisted birth is twofold: educating the mother and family about the procedure and supporting the birth attendant. Nursing actions are summarized in Display 19.2.

DISPLAY 19.2   NURSING ACTIONS: VACUUM-ASSISTED BIRTH[4-7]

---

1. **Educate the mother and her support person about the procedure and prepare her for vaginal birth.**
   - Verify consent for delivery
   - Place the mother in lithotomy position to provide for optimal traction
   - Empty the mother's bladder to decrease the risk of trauma
   - Remind the mother that she must still push with uterine contractions
   - Ensure adequate pain relief for the mother (generally no additional medication other than that which is normally needed is required)
   - Tell the mother that the baby will probably have a finding of caput succedaneum (Fig. 19.2). This is considered to be a normal finding (it gradually resolves, usually within 24 hours of delivery).
2. **Prepare the room for the procedure, assemble necessary equipment, and support the birth attendant as needed.**
   - Connect sterile tubing to the suction machine
   - Set suction at 0.6–0.8 kg/cm^2 (550–600 mmHg)
3. **Assess the fetal heart rate (FHR) throughout the procedure and document findings.**
   - Continuous electronic fetal monitoring (EFM) may be used
   - If EFM is not used, the FHR should be auscultated and documented every 5 minutes
4. **Be prepared for emergent delivery if necessary.**
   - Alert the charge nurse that vacuum-assisted delivery will be attempted
   - Ensure the capability to perform an emergent cesarean section if necessary
5. **Note and document the time of the first application of the vacuum.**
   - Cup detachment is common, most expert practitioners advocate a limit of 2–3 detachments before the procedure is abandoned
   - The maximum total time of vacuum application should not exceed 20 minutes, the time of maximum pressure force should not be longer than 10 minutes, but manufacturer's recommendations should be observed
   - Steady traction should only be applied during contractions while the mother is actively pushing, without rocking or torque movements.
6. **Assess the neonate after birth for signs of trauma at the site of the vacuum application.**
   - Continue to observe the infant during the immediate postpartum period for signs of cerebral trauma
   - Report (and document) to neonatal care staff that a vacuum was used at delivery
7. **Assess the immediate postpartum mother for signs of perineal trauma, lacerations, or increased bleeding.**
8. **Document the events of delivery accurately.**

▶ What are the advantages of vacuum-assisted delivery?

The vacuum is generally preferred over forceps for operative vaginal delivery because it is easier to apply and there is less associated maternal trauma.[6]

Forceps-Assisted Birth

Obstetrical forceps are metal blades (tongs) designed to curve around the fetal head and help to facilitate delivery. Forceps are shaped to fit the fetal head and maternal pelvis using blades that are curved to provide the best traction in a variety of situations. The blades are joined with a locking pin, screw, or groove to limit compression of the fetal skull.[2]

Incidence of forceps-assisted delivery varies according to birthing facility and the skill and experience of the birth attendant. The incidence has decreased in the last few decades as practitioners opt for the use of the vacuum or cesarean section.[3]

► Why are forceps used?

Forceps are used for a variety of situations, similar to the indications for use of the vacuum (see Display 19.1). Forceps may also be used in cases of malpresentation for rotation of the fetal head. Other indications for use of forceps instead of the vacuum are listed in Display 19.3. Under these conditions, forceps delivery is considered safer than vacuum-assisted delivery.[6]

DISPLAY 19.3	SPECIFIC INDICATIONS FOR FORCEPS-ASSISTED DELIVERY[1]

Assisted delivery of the head in a breech delivery (singleton or twin gestation)
Preterm fetus
Face presentation
Suspected coagulopathy or thrombocytopenia of the fetus
Maternal conditions that prohibit pushing (cardiac, respiratory, cerebrovascular or neurologic disease)
Instrumented delivery with mother under general anesthetic
Cord prolapse in the second stage of labor
Controlled delivery of the head during a cesarean section

► What are the advantages of forceps-assisted birth?[6]

Although vacuum-assisted birth is now more common, forceps have some advantages. Advantages of a forceps-assisted delivery include[6]:
* Less failure than vacuum-assisted delivery
* Quicker than vacuum-assisted delivery

► Are there different kinds of forceps?

There are different forceps applications for use in several situations.
* *Outlet forceps* are used when the fetal head is visible at the vaginal introitus without separating the labia to guide and control delivery.
* *Low forceps* are used when the leading part of the fetal head is at least +2 station.
* In *midforceps* application, the fetal head is engaged but above +2 station. Figure 19.3 illustrates the application of outlet forceps on the fetal head.

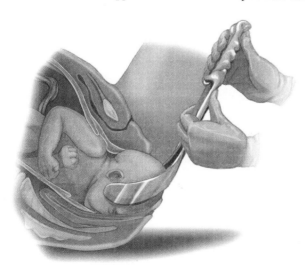

FIGURE 19.3 Forceps-assisted delivery: application of the forceps to the fetal head. (From Orshan, S. A. [2008]. *Maternity, newborn, & women's health nursing.* Philadelphia: Lippincott Williams & Wilkins.)

NOTE: High forceps applications are no longer a part of current obstetric practice due to the high incidence of maternal and fetal injury.[1]

There are a variety of forceps in use today. The more common types and their uses are found in Display 19.4

DISPLAY 19.4 COMMON TYPES OF FORCEPS[2]

Simpson or Elliot forceps are used for outlet vaginal deliveries and are designed for application to the molded fetal head.

Kielland or Tucker-McClane forceps are used for rotational deliveries and are appropriate for application to the fetal head with little or no molding.

Pieper forceps which have a reverse pelvic curve are used for breech deliveries.

As with vacuum-assisted birth, for forceps-assisted delivery to be safely attempted,

- the membranes must be ruptured
- the cervix must be completely dilated
- the mother's bladder should be empty
- adequate anesthesia should be provided for the mother
- the fetal head must be engaged and the fetal head position must be known

    Knowledge of the presenting part is essential and may be confirmed by vaginal examination and ultrasound. CPD should not be present. The operator should be experienced with the type of forceps used. In addition, the facility should be capable of performing a cesarean section.[1,2]

    Nursing considerations in care of the mother undergoing a forceps-assisted birth are similar to those of vacuum assisted birth. They are summarized in Display 19.5.

DISPLAY 19.5 NURSING ACTIONS: FORCEPS-ASSISTED BIRTH[4,5,7]

---

1. **Educate the mother and her support person about the procedure and prepare her for vaginal birth.**
   - Verify consent for delivery
   - Place the mother in lithotomy position to provide for optimal traction
   - Empty the mother's bladder to decrease the risk of trauma
2. **Ensure adequate pain relief for the mother.**
   - Forceps application is more invasive than vacuum application and the mother may require increased analgesia or anesthesia
3. **Prepare the room for the procedure, assemble necessary equipment, and support the birth attendant as needed.**
   - Locate the type of forceps requested by the birth attendant
   - Frequent checks for proper placement will be done by the birth attendant
4. **Assess the fetal heart rate (FHR) throughout the procedure and document findings.**
   - Fetal bradycardia may be observed due to head compression and should be transient
   - Continuous electronic fetal monitoring (EFM) may be used
   - If EFM is not used, the FHR should be auscultated and documented every 5 minutes
5. **Be prepared for emergent delivery.**
   - Alert the charge nurse that a forceps-assisted delivery will be attempted
   - Alert the neonatal resuscitation staff if necessary
   - Ensure the capability to perform an emergent cesarean section if necessary
6. **Assess the neonate after birth for:**
   - Bruising or abrasions at the site of application
   - Cerebral/ocular trauma or skull fracture
   - Nerve damage (facial palsy) related to pressure on the cranial nerve (VII) from the forceps
7. **Assess the immediate postpartum mother for:**
   - Vaginal and cervical lacerations, bruising, hematoma (third and fourth degree episiotomies and lacerations are more commonly associated with forceps-assisted delivery)
   - Increased bleeding
   - Urinary retention from bladder trauma
8. **Report (and document) to neonatal care staff that forceps were used at delivery**

Maternal morbidity after forceps-assisted birth includes an increased risk for postpartum infection because of the invasive nature of the procedure. Other significant maternal risks include lacerations to the vagina and cervix, extension of episiotomy, uterine rupture, bladder trauma, fracture of coccyx, hemorrhage, increased vaginal bleeding, uterine atony, and anemia.[4] *Notify the primary care provider immediately if the woman has symptoms of hematoma formation or increased bleeding.* The mother may require more analgesia in the postpartum period and a longer hospital stay than with a spontaneous or vacuum-assisted birth.

Review postpartum assessment in Module 14.

> If forceps delivery is attempted but not achieved, then a cesarean birth is indicated.

Nursing Management Concerns

1. The birth attendant makes the decision about the use of vacuum or forceps to assist in delivery; *however, you have the independent responsibility to evaluate the decision.* You may be held responsible for not initiating the chain of command if an inappropriate attempt at operative vaginal delivery is made.
2. Although you are not directly responsible for obtaining informed consent for nonemergent operative vaginal delivery, you must be certain to document that the mother understands the procedure, the risks, and the benefits.
3. Document in the medical record the condition of the mother and newborn at birth.

Cesarean Birth

Cesarean birth is achieved through a surgical incision in the mother's abdomen. The purpose of the procedure is to preserve the health and well-being of the mother or the fetus. The rate of cesarean birth has risen over the last decade and it is one of the most commonly performed surgical procedures.

> *In 2004, 1.2 million births, or 29.1% of all live births in the United States were by cesarean delivery.[8] Preliminary data for subsequent years also show a further increase in the cesarean birth rate.[9]*

▶ Why has the cesarean birth rate increased?

Reasons for the increase in cesarean delivery rates are varied but are known to be associated with the following[8]:

1. Increased fear of litigation on the part of health care providers.
2. Increased use of electronic fetal monitoring (EFM) with decreased tolerance of suspected fetal compromise in labor.
3. Decreased tolerance of the fetal risks associated with a potentially hazardous vaginal delivery (e.g., vaginal breech delivery, vaginal twin delivery, forceps-assisted delivery, large estimated fetal weight).
4. Increased safety of anesthesia and operative care (use of antibiotics and a safe blood supply).
5. Increased numbers of high-risk pregnancies.
6. Potential pelvic floor damage related to labor and delivery resulting in future urinary and fecal incontinence.
7. Increased respect for the mother's autonomy in decision making about the mode of birth.
8. Increased numbers of labor inductions.
9. Increased use of regional anesthesia.
10. Increased number of repeat cesarean deliveries.

Many of the factors contributing to the increase in the cesarean delivery rate are interrelated and all likely play some part in the phenomenon. There have been many initiatives to decrease the cesarean birth rate and all involve education of mothers *and* healthcare providers. Selected interventions that may have an impact are summarized in Display 19.6.

DISPLAY 19.6 | EFFORTS TO REDUCE THE CESAREAN BIRTH RATE [10,11]

Education of women regarding:
- Home environment for latent or early labor
- Reasons for admission
- Techniques to manage pain during labor
- Techniques to enhance labor
- Facts about VBAC
- Advantages of vaginal birth
- The importance of choosing a care provider
- Development of a personal birth plan and discussion of plan with provider

Education of birth attendants regarding:
- Development of admission criteria
- The importance of assessments in determining labor status
- Individualized rationale for labor interventions
- Avoidance of automatic interventions
- Support of "one-on-one" care during labor
- Support and encouragement of positioning and nonpharmacologic pain relief measures
- Establishment of criteria for elective cesarean delivery and trial of labor

Lowering the incidence of cesarean birth is a complex issue. There may not be an "ideal" rate that encompasses the multiple factors involved in making the decision for a cesarean delivery. [12]

▶ **What are the different types of cesarean birth?**

There are two types of cesarean surgical techniques.

1. The **classic incision** is made on the upper part of the uterus in the vertical midline (Fig. 19.4A). The classic incision is rarely used, except in an emergency situation requiring extremely quick access to the fetus or if alternate access to the fetus is needed.

2. **Low-segment cesarean incisions** may be done with either a **low transverse incision or a low vertical incision** (Figs. 19.4B, C).

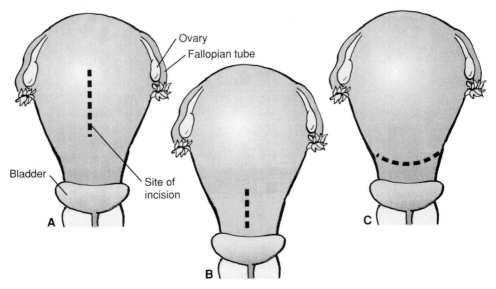

FIGURE 19.4 Cesarean birth uterine incisions. **A.** Classic. **B.** Low vertical. **C.** Low transverse. (From Orshan, S. A. [2008]. *Maternity, newborn, & women's health nursing.* Philadelphia: Lippincott Williams & Wilkins.)

*NOTE: The incision that is visually apparent on the mother's skin **may not be the incision on the uterus!***

The low transverse incision is the most popular incision for mothers and physicians for the following reasons[13]:

1. The scar may be hidden in the pubic hair.
2. The incision is easier to perform and repair.
3. Less risk of uterine rupture in future pregnancies. (Lower uterine segment is less contractile)
4. Less associated blood loss and postoperative infection.

A *cesarean hysterectomy*, removal of the uterus after delivery of the fetus, may be performed in an obstetric emergency such as uterine hemorrhage, uterine rupture, or placenta accreta. Such conditions are rare.

NOTE: Placenta accreta is an abnormal adherence of the placenta to the myometrium that may result in risks of prematurity for the fetus and severe hemorrhage for the mother.

Important Terms

Primary cesarean—a woman's first cesarean birth.

Repeat elective cesarean—a subsequent cesarean birth in the absence of any obstetric or maternal medical indications.

Vaginal Birth After Cesarean (VBAC)

▶ What is a VBAC?

Vaginal birth after cesarean (VBAC) has been a topic of much discussion since the 1980s. It was once thought that "once a cesarean, always a cesarean" due to the risk of uterine rupture. However, with the rise in the cesarean delivery rate, there were concerns over the complications of repeated surgeries and subsequent pregnancies. Studies have since demonstrated a VBAC success rate of 60% to 80%.[14] Currently, VBAC is considered an accepted part of obstetric practice, with careful maternal selection and management.[15] Appropriate selection for a trial of labor (TOL) after a previous cesarean birth is paramount. The mother should have no other contraindications to labor and birth.

General Considerations for Maternal Selection[15,16]

Knowledge of Prior Uterine Incisions
- A low-segment transverse uterine incision has the lowest risk of uterine rupture.
- No more than two prior low transverse cesarean births.
- Previous classic fundal uterine incision is a contraindication for trial of labor
- The maternal pelvis should be clinically adequate, with no history of prior uterine rupture.

Setting for Delivery
- There must be an ability to perform an emergency cesarean delivery if needed.
- Appropriate surgical staff, anesthesia staff, and support staff must be available.
- Due to potential uterine rupture and subsequent blood loss, blood products should be readily available.
- Due to potential neonatal compromise, neonatal resuscitation staff must be readily available.

Anticipated Family Size
- With multiple cesarean deliveries, the risk for placental abnormalities including placenta previa and placenta accreta increases dramatically.
- Future family planning should be discussed with the mother when the risks and benefits of VBAC are discussed.

Factors associated with VBAC success include:[15]
- history of a previous vaginal birth with spontaneous, augmented, or induced labor
  OR
- current pregnancy presentation in spontaneous labor.

Frequently Asked Questions About TOL and VBAC

▶ Can a mother attempting trial of labor and vaginal birth after cesarean have labor induced?

In appropriately selected and counseled mothers, with one prior cesarean delivery, labor induction or augmentation is a reasonable option.[15,17]

> **EXTREME CAUTION SHOULD BE USED IN MANAGING THE MOTHER WHO IS ATTEMPTING A VBAC WITH INDUCTION OR AUGMENTATION OF LABOR. EXCESSIVE USE OF OXYTOCIN AND HYPERSTIMULATION SHOULD BE AVOIDED. The nurse is the primary and consistent observer at the mother's bedside and must be knowledgeable of and comfortable with the guidelines for oxytocin management. Additionally, assertiveness and patient advocacy may be needed. Charge nurses should make assignments and adjust staffing as necessary.**

▶ Is a mother who has had two or more prior cesareans a candidate for a TOL and VBAC?

The American College of Obstetricians and Gynecologists (ACOG)[14] advocates VBAC as an option for mothers with a history of two or more cesarean deliveries ONLY if they have had a prior vaginal delivery.[14] More recent data suggest similar risks of uterine rupture and success rates among women with a history of multiple cesarean deliveries and only one prior cesarean delivery. Therefore some consider that trial of labor and vaginal birth after cesarean are viable options.[14]

▶ Is a mother with twins a candidate for TOL and VBAC?

Recent studies have indicated that there is no increased maternal risk for morbidity and similar success rates for mothers with single gestation as compared to those with twin gestations. This indicates that it may be an appropriate delivery option, but further research is needed.[15]

Nursing Management Concerns

- Current opinion, based on the available literature and evidence, is that mothers with a history of a previous cesarean delivery should be monitored continuously (with external fetal monitoring [EFM]). If they are undergoing cervical ripening, this should be done in an inpatient setting as opposed to an outpatient setting.
- There is no need for an intrauterine pressure catheter (IUPC) to be placed simply because the mother is attempting a VBAC. *Intrauterine pressure catheters should be used for obstetric indications.*
- VBAC attempt is not a contraindication for using epidural anesthesia, but *recognize that pain associated with a uterine rupture may be masked or atypical in presentation.* Signs of uterine rupture are discussed in Module 18.

Cesarean Birth Upon Maternal Request

There is a growing rate of cesarean births for which there are clear medical or obstetric indications.[18] These procedures, commonly referred to as "maternal choice" cesareans, are done primarily for convenience and pose ethical concerns for some care providers. Reasons offered for maternal choice cesarean births may include the ability to schedule the timing of the birth, decreased risk of future maternal pelvic floor problems, fear of labor (pain, complications), and desire for control. Current evidence does not show a significant difference in maternal or neonatal outcomes in women experiencing primary cesarean birth upon maternal request and those with a planned vaginal birth.[19] However, it is imperative that mothers and practitioners talk about the risks of a surgical procedure versus the natural process of birth and implications for future pregnancies. The procedure should be highly individualized, performed after 39 weeks' gestation or fetal lung maturity confirmation, and consistent with ethical principles.[8]

Indications/Risks for Cesarean Birth

Cesarean birth is done to benefit the fetus as well as the mother. Labor and birth complications are the most common reasons for cesarean birth. Relative contraindications include a nonviable fetus or a dead fetus. In these cases the maternal risks of surgery cannot be justified.

▶ What are the indications for a cesarean birth?[13]

Cephalopelvic disproportion (CPD)—CPD is an inadequate maternal pelvis in relation to the fetal head. A history of maternal pelvic trauma, fetal macrosomia (estimated birth weight greater than 4,000 to 4,500 g) can suggest a finding of CPD.

Fetal malpresentation—(see Module 2) Transverse and shoulder presentations make vaginal delivery difficult and potentially dangerous. Breech presentations may also be considered too dangerous to attempt vaginal delivery. Vaginal breech deliveries are dependant on the skill and experience of the birth attendant.

Labor dystocia—Labor dystocia may be associated with CPD or fetal malpresentation, but can also include inadequate, ineffective uterine contractions and incomplete cervical dilitation without fetal descent (failure to progress, or failed induction). Soft tissue dystocia or obstructed labor due to excessive maternal adipose tissue or tumors may also necessitate a cesarean delivery.

Nonreassuring fetal status—A nonreassuring FHR pattern may indicate that the fetus is not well oxygenated and thus requires careful evaluation and possible surgical intervention.

Congenital fetal anomalies—Some fetal anomalies such as conjoined twins and gastrosch require controlled delivery and immediate intervention by neonatal staff.

Obstetric indications—Umbilical cord prolapse, placenta previa, abruptio placentae, multiple gestation, uterine rupture, hemorrhage are conditions which contraindicate vaginal birth or may require a rapid birth.

Maternal medical indications—Hypertensive disorders, active herpes lesions, diabetes mellitus, uterine or vaginal abnormalities, cardiac disease may require a surgical birth.

▶ What are the maternal and fetal risks of a cesarean birth?

Although cesarean birth seems to have been "normalized" as a viable birth option, it is a major surgical procedure and not without risks and complications (Display 19.7). Cesarean birth is of great benefit to babies and mothers in certain circumstances and some studies have demonstrated that operative delivery has improved neonatal outcomes.[20]

DISPLAY 19.7 MATERNAL RISKS IN CESAREAN DELIVERY [10,13,20,21]

Anesthetic complications (aspiration, airway mishaps, and respiratory failure)
Laceration and injury to bowel, bladder
Hemorrhage
Wound complications (dehiscence)
Infection (uterine, bladder)
Thromboembolic complications
Increased risk for placenta previa and uterine rupture in subsequent pregnancies
Increased length of stay in the hospital
Increased costs
Increased chance of rehospitalization
Impaired maternal newborn interaction (related to pain, fatigue, medication effects, difficulty breastfeeding)
Disruption of support network
Increased recuperation time
Negative emotional consequences of failure to achieve vaginal birth (anger, depression, grief, lowered self-esteem, altered body image, psychosomatic symptoms)

Neonatal risks include respiratory problems such as delays in neonatal transition, transient tachypnea, mild respiratory distress syndrome (RDS), iatrogenic prematurity (if gestational age is not certain), and lacerations occurring during surgery.[20]

Anesthesia for Cesarean Birth

▶ **What type of anesthesia is used for a cesarean birth?**

Anesthesia selection for cesarean birth depend on the mother's current status and medical history, fetal status, and urgency of the procedure. The majority of women who undergo operative birth are administered regional anesthesia (spinal or epidural block).

Regional Anesthesia
- Has a lower risk of airway problems and allows the mother to be awake and aware during the birth experience.
- Allows the mother to communicate with her support person and interact with her newborn after delivery.

General endotracheal anesthesia is usually reserved for emergency problems requiring immediate delivery or in cases of maternal conditions that contraindicate regional anesthesia.

NOTE: *Fetal cord blood gases collected at a cesarean birth can demonstrate a lower pH in women administered regional anesthesia, but infants born to mothers under general endotracheal anesthesia have lower Apgar scores.*[22]

Nursing Considerations for Care of the Mother Undergoing Cesarean Birth

The nurse involved in the care of the mother experiencing a cesarean birth may take on varied roles. Most often, the labor nurse is the one who prepares the mother, is in the operating room with the mother, and cares for her in the immediate postoperative period. In the operating room, this nurse is referred to as the *circulating nurse*. A nurse may take on the role of the *surgical nurse*. The surgical nurse is "scrubbed in," prepares the instrument kit, and assists the surgeon during the procedure with sterile instruments, sutures, and supplies.

More recently, some obstetric nurses are expanding their practice to include first assisting at or with cesarean deliveries.[23] The first assistant:
- is knowledgeable about the procedure and the sequence of events
- is skilled at instrument handling
- is a clear and effective communicator with the surgical team
- provides adequate exposure and visualization of the surgical site while safely handling tissues
- assists with delivery of the fetus and placenta
- assists with the repair of the surgical incision

Education and certification for first assistants varies according to institutional requirements and certifying agency.

Elective, Unanticipated, and Emergency Cesarean Births

Nursing care may need to be modified depending on whether the cesarean is planned or unanticipated, or even an emergency. If the procedure is planned (elective), then the mother and family can be prepared with teaching. If the procedure is unanticipated, the mother must still be prepared, and opportunity given for a decision to be made. Answer questions and allow the mother to express any concerns.

NOTE: *Informed consent for the cesarean surgical procedure must be obtained by the birth attendant, midwife, or physician.*

If the procedure is deemed an emergency, try to support the patient and family under extreme circumstances. With an emergency cesarean birth, the time from decision to incision is rapid, from 10 to 30 minutes.[24] During this time, many essential nursing tasks must be accomplished, but communication with the mother and her family (or support person) is of the utmost importance. The mother may have overwhelming stress and anxiety about the emergency procedure and for the safety of her baby. Expect to spend time after the procedure talking with the mother and her family about the events that led to the emergency situation.

Phases of Nursing Care

▶ What are nursing responsibilities during a cesarean birth?

To provide care to the mother undergoing a cesarean birth, obstetric and surgical principles must be combined.

> *The standards of care for the surgical and recovery areas in the birth setting are the same as those of the operating suites in a hospital![24-26]*

Nursing care responsibilities during cesarean birth can be divided into three parts.[4]

DISPLAY 19.8 NURSING CONSIDERATIONS DURING CESAREAN BIRTH

Preoperative care

- Complete initial assessment per unit guidelines.
- Initiate 20- to 30-minute baseline fetal heart rate tracing per electronic EFM. If in active labor or tracing is not reassuring then continue monitoring until mother is scrubbed and prepped.
- Apply appropriate identification bracelets to mother and prepare newborn identification bracelets.
- Initiate preoperative teaching for the mother, support person, and family about expected care, procedures, sensations, and noises before, during, and after the operative birth.
- Draw and send ordered preoperative labs, view results (type and screen, CBC, coagulation panel).
- Ensure NPO status.
- Witness consent for cesarean birth.
- Insert an intravenous line, at least 18 gauge, or ensure patency of existing line and initiate fluids.
- Shave the abdomen.
- Insert an indwelling Foley catheter, delay until after placement and dosing of epidural if possible.
- Administer preoperative medications if ordered.
- Safely transport the mother to the surgical suite.
- Document according to unit guidelines.

Intraoperative care

- Assist with transfer to operating table.
- Assist anesthesia personnel with initiation of anesthetic as needed.
- Ensure lateral positioning of the mother with a hip wedge.
- Continue EFM until abdomen is prepped, if needed. Fetal scalp electrode is removed after abdominal prep.
- Ensure appropriate placement and securing of the mother's arms on arm boards.
- Align the mother's legs and secure with appropriate restraint.
- Apply appropriate grounding device according to manufacturer's recommendations.
- Scrub and prepare abdomen according to unit guidelines.
- Verify that suction and electrocautery units are working properly.
- Ensure neonatal resuscitation equipment is in working order and all supplies are available.
- Notify other health care and surgical team members, intensive care nursery, or pediatric staff as necessary to be present for delivery.
- Position support person at the mother's head, behind the sterile screening drape.
- Assist with gowning and gloving of surgical staff as needed.
- Perform initial and subsequent sponge, needle and instrument counts according to unit guidelines.
- Participate in OR "time out" or other procedure to correctly identify patient, purpose, procedure, and participants.
- Document the events of surgery including incision, time of delivery and the completion of the procedure.
- Support mother and support person as needed.
- Support and assist surgical and anesthesia staff as needed.
- Support and assist neonatal staff as needed.
- Obtain umbilical cord blood samples and other pathologic samples such as the placenta, as required.
- Assist with placement of abdominal dressing.
- Note maternal and newborn status before transport to postanesthesia recovery unit (PACU).
- Safely transport the mother to the PACU.
- Document according to unit guidelines.

display continues on page 512

Postoperative care

- Ensure proper PACU equipment is available and functional.
- Perform and document postoperative assessments according to unit guidelines.
- Initial and ongoing assessments to include:
  Respiratory status: patency, oxygen needs, rate, quality and depth of respirations, oxygen saturations, and auscultation of lungs.
  Circulatory status: blood pressure, pulse, ECG, and skin color.
  Level of consciousness: Orientation to person, place and time, response to stimulation.
  Obstetric status: position and character of fundus, abdominal dressing, amount and color of lochia, maternal–newborn attachment, breastfeeding desires.
  Motor status: Level of sensation, movement
  Intake and output: intravenous fluids, urine output and estimated blood loss
  Pain scale: mother's reports of pain and medications given
- Facilitate interaction and closeness for the new family after delivery.
- Discharge from PACU care after recovery period is complete, after collaboration with anesthesia provider and birth attendant, if mother is stable according to unit guidelines.
- Document according to unit guidelines.

Family-Centered Care

▶ How can the mother's family be involved in a cesarean birth?

Despite the cesarean birth, the mother and her family should be offered the same opportunities for participation and bonding.[24] If possible, the mother's support person should be allowed to attend the birth, but may not be allowed to accompany the mother if she is undergoing general anesthesia. The support person, with consent of the anesthesia team, should be allowed to sit at the mother's head in the surgical suite to talk to her, support her, hold her hand, and hold the newborn. The support person is behind the sterile screening drape, but can still communicate with the circulating nurse. In the PACU, when the mother is fully awake and stable, she should be allowed to see her newborn.

Opportunities for support person participation during an operative birth include:
- Being present for education about operative birth
- Being in attendance at administration of regional anesthetic
- Being in attendance at operative delivery when appropriate
- Staying as near as possible if not allowed into surgical suite
- Holding newborn in surgical suite
- Accompanying newborn to the nursery
- Being present at all possible times with the mother for emotional support

Even though a cesarean birth experience may not be what the mother expected or desired, it can still be positive and meaningful with the appropriate nursing support, education, and reassurance.

PRACTICE/REVIEW QUESTIONS

After reviewing this module, answer the following questions.

1. What constitutes an operative delivery?

   _____

   _____

   _____

2. For a mother undergoing an operative delivery, the intrapartum nurse should educate the mother and her support person about the procedure and prepare them for delivery.

   a. True

   b. False

3. The nurse cannot be held responsible if an inappropriate attempt at an operative delivery is made by the birth attendant.

   a. True

   b. False

For questions 4 through 13, match the following terms with the correct answer.

a. forceps

b. vacuum

c. outlet forceps

d. low forceps

e. midforceps

f. Simpson of Elliott forceps

g. Kielland or Tucker McClane forceps

h. Pieper forceps

i. 20 minutes

j. 10 minutes

4. Used when the leading part of the fetal head is at +2 station _____

5. Metal blades designed to curve around the fetal head and help facilitate delivery _____

6. Used for outlet vaginal deliveries _____

7. A cup with a suction device attached that when placed on the fetal head and suction is increased a seal is formed allowing gentle traction to be applied to facilitate delivery of the fetal head _____

8. Used for breech deliveries _____

9. Used when fetal head is visible at the vaginal introitus without separating the labia to guide and control delivery _____

10. Used when the fetal head is engaged but above +2 station _____

11. Used for rotational deliveries _____

12. The maximum total time of vacuum application should not exceed _____.

13. The time of maximum pressure force from vacuum application should not exceed _____.

14. List the indications for the use of vacuum extraction or forceps.

    a. _____

    b. _____

    c. _____

    d. _____

15. List the conditions that a vacuum or forceps can be used.

    a. _____

    b. _____

    c. _____

    d. _____

16. List five contraindications for vacuum use.

    a. _____

    b. _____

    c. _____

    d. _____

    e. _____

17. List the more common risks to the fetus from a vacuum-assisted birth.

    a. _____

    b. _____

    c. _____

18. List five of the more serious risks to the fetus using a vacuum to assist with delivery.

    a. _____

    b. _____

    c. _____

    d. _____

    e. _____

19. During a vacuum assisted delivery if EFM is NOT being used the nurse should auscultate and document the FHR every 10 minutes.

    a. True

    b. False

20. Shoulder dystocia may be more frequently encountered with vacuum extraction.

    a. True

    b. False

21. The advantages of using a vacuum as opposed to forceps include _____ and _____.

22. List three things that the nurse should include in the documentation during an operative delivery.

    a. _____

    b. _____

    c. _____

23. List the nursing actions during a vacuum-assisted delivery.

    a. _____

    b. _____

    c. _____

    d. _____

    e. _____

24. List the possible maternal complications from a vacuum-assisted delivery.

    a. _____

    b. _____

    c. _____

    d. _____

    e. _____

25. List three indications for when a forceps delivery is considered safer than vacuum-assisted delivery.

    a. _____

    b. _____

    c. _____

26. After a delivery using forceps, the neonate should be assessed for:

    a. _____

    b. _____

    c. _____

27. After a delivery using forceps the mother should be assessed for:

    a. _____

    b. _____

    c. _____

    d. _____

    e. _____

28. State the purpose of a cesarean birth.

    _____

29. List five possible reasons for the increase in cesarean birth rate.

    a. _____

    b. _____

    c. _____

    d. _____

    e. _____

30. List three indications for a cesarean birth.

    a. _____

    b. _____

    c. _____

31. List five maternal risks of cesarean birth.

    a. _____

    b. _____

    c. _____

    d. _____

    e. _____

32. List three neonatal risks of cesarean birth.

    a. _____

    b. _____

    c. _____

33. List four of the advantages of using regional anesthesia for a cesarean birth.

    a. _____

    b. _____

    c. _____

    d. _____

34. A low-segment transverse uterine incision has the highest risk of uterine rupture.

    a. True

    b. False

35. Factors associated with VBAC success include _____ and _____.

PRACTICE/REVIEW ANSWER KEY

1. Operative delivery includes cesarean birth and vaginal birth assisted by vacuum or forceps.

2. a. True

3. b. False

4. d. Low forceps

5. a. Forceps

6. f. Simpson or Elliott forceps

7. b. Vacuum

8. h. Pieper forceps

9. c. Outlet forceps

10. e. Midforceps

11. g. Kielland or Tucker McClane forceps

12. i. 20 minutes

13. j. 10 minutes

14. a. prolonged second stage of labor
    b. Fetal compromise (nonreassuring status)
    c. poor pushing effort (secondary to exhaustion or analgesia/anesthesia)
    d. cardiac, pulmonary, cerebrovascular, or neurologic disease

15. a. vertex presentation
    b. engaged with the fetal head position known
    c. membranes must be ruptures
    d. mother's cervix should be completely dilated

16. a. face or breech presentation
    b. several maternal or fetal compromise requiring rapid delivery
    c. evidence of CPD
    d. congenital anomalies of the fetal head
    e. gestational age less than 34 weeks

17. a. cup marks
    b. bruising
    c. minor lacerations

18. a. cephalohematoma
    b. subgaleal hematoma
    c. retinal hemorrhage
    d. intracranial hemorrhage
    e. skull fractures

19. b. False

20. a. True

21. a. easier to apply
    b. less associated maternal trauma

22. a. FHR throughout the procedure
    b. the time of the first application of the vacuum or forceps
    c. a report to neonatal care staff that a vacuum or forceps was used during delivery

23. a. Educating the mother and support person about the procedure and prepare her for vaginal birth
    b. Prepare the room for the procedure, assemble the necessary equipment, and support the birth attendant as needed
    c. Assess the fetal heart rate throughout the procedure
    d. Be prepared for emergent delivery if necessary
    e. Note and document the time of the first application of the vacuum.

24. a. pain
    b. extension of episiotomy
    c. bladder trauma
    d. perineal lacerations
    e. soft tissue injuries to the vulva, vagina, cervix, and anal sphincter

25. Any three of the following
    a. Assisted delivery of the head in breech delivery
    b. Preterm fetus
    c. Face presentation
    d. Suspected coagulopathy or thrombocytopenia of the fetus

e. Maternal conditions that prohibit pushing
    f. Instrumented delivery with mother under general anesthesia
    g. Cord prolapse in the second stage of labor
    h. Controlled delivery of the head during s cesarean section

26. a. bruising or abrasions at the site of application
    b. cerebral or ocular trauma or skull fracture
    c. nerve damage (facial palsy)

27. a. vaginal and cervical lacerations
    b. bruising
    c. hematoma
    d. increased bleeding
    e. urinary retention from bladder trauma

28. To preserve the health and well-being of the mother or the fetus

29. Any five of the following
    a. Increased use of EFM with decreased tolerance of fetal compromise in labor
    b. Decreased tolerance of fetal risks associated with potentially hazardous delivery
    c. Increased safety of anesthesia and operative care
    d. Increased numbers of high risk pregnancies
    e. Potential pelvic floor damage related to labor and delivery
    f. Urinary and fecal incontinence
    g. Increased respect for the mother's autonomy in decision making about mode of birth
    h. Increased numbers of labor inductions
    i. Increased use of regional anesthesia
    j. Increased number of repeat cesarean deliveries
    k. Increased fear of litigation

30. Any three of the following:
    a. Cephalopelvic disproportion
    b. Fetal malpresentation
    c. Labor dystocia
    d. Nonreassuring fetal status
    e. Congenital fetal anomalies
    f. Obstetric indications
    g. Maternal medical indications

31. Any five of the following:
    1. Anesthetic complications
    2. Laceration and injury to bowel or bladder
    3. Hemorrhage
    4. Wound complications
    5. Infection
    6. Thromboembolic complications
    7. Increased risk for placenta previa and uterine rupture in subsequent pregnancies
    8. Increased length of hospital stay
    9. Increased costs
    10. Increased chance of rehospitalization

11. Impaired maternal newborn interaction
12. Disruption of support network
13. Increased recuperation time
14. Negative emotional consequences of failure to achieve vaginal birth

32. a. respiratory problems
    b. iatrogenic prematurity
    c. lacerations occurring during surgery

33. a. lower risk of airway problems
    b. allows the mother to be awake and aware of the birth experience
    c. mother is able to communicate with her support person
    d. mother is able to interact with her newborn after delivery

34. b. False

35. history of previous vaginal delivery with spontaneous, augmented, or induced labor; current pregnancy presenting in spontaneous labor

REFERENCES

1. American College of Obstetricians and Gynecologists. (2000). *Operative vaginal delivery* [Practice bulletin No. 17]. Washington, DC: Author.
2. Incerpi, M. H. (2007). Operative delivery. In DeCherney, A. H., Nathum, L., Goodwin, T. M., & Laufner, N. (Eds.), *Current diagnosis and treatment in obstetrics and gynecology* (10th ed., pp. 462–476). New York: McGraw-Hill.
3. Miskovsky, P., & Watson, W. J. (2001). Obstetric vacuum extraction: State of the art in the new millennium. *Obstetrical and Gynecological Survey, 56*(11), 736–751.
4. Kendrick, J. M., & Simpson, K. R. (2001). Labor and birth. In Simpson, K. A., & Creehan, P. A., (Eds.), *Perinatal nursing* (2nd ed., pp. 346–359). Philadelphia: Lippincott.
5. Simpson, K. R., & Knox, G. E. (2003). Common areas of litigation related to care during labor and birth: Recommendations to promote patient safety and decrease risk exposure. *Journal of Perinatal and Neonatal Nursing, 17*(2), 110–125.
6. Patel, R. R., & Murphy, D. J. (2004). Forceps delivery in modern clinical practice. *British Medical Journal, 328,* 1302–1305.
7. Nichols, C. M., Pendlebury, L. C., & Jennell, J. (2006). Chart documentation of informed consent for operative vaginal delivery: Is it adequate? *Southern Medical Journal, 99*(12), 1337–1339.
8. National Institutes of Health. (2006). NIH state-of-the-science conference statement on cesarean delivery on maternal request. NIH Consensus Science Statements. Available at: http://consensus.nih.gov.
9. Hamilton, B. E., Martin, J. A., & Ventura, S. J. (2006). *Births: Preliminary data for 2005* [National vital statistics reports; vol. 55, no. 11]. Hyattsville, MD: National Center for Health Statistics.
10. Loudermilk, D. L. (2006). Labor and birth at risk. In Loudermilk, D. L. & Perry, S. E. (Eds.) *Maternity nursing* (pp. 769–818). St. Louis: Mosby.
11. Williams, D. R. (2006). Preserving vaginal birth. *Journal of Midwifery & Women's Health, 51*(4), 239–241.
12. Walker, S. P., McCarthy, E. A., Ugoni, A., Lee, A., Lim, S., & Permezel, M. (2007). Cesarean delivery or vaginal birth: A survey of patient and clinician thresholds. *Obstetrics and Gynecology, 109*(1), 67–72.
13. Cunningham, G., Leveno, K. J., Bloom, S. L., et al. (Eds.). (2005). Cesarean delivery and peripartum hysterectomy. In *Williams's Obstetrics* (22nd ed.). (pp. 587–607). New York: McGraw-Hill.
14. American College of Obstetricians and Gynecologists. (2004). *Vaginal birth after previous cesarean delivery* [ACOG Practice Bulletin]. Washington, DC: Author.
15. Cahill, A. G., & Macones, G. A. (2007). Vaginal birth after cesarean delivery: Evidence-based practice. *Clinical Obstetrics and Gynecology, 50*(2), 518–525.
16. Fang, Y. M. V., & Zelop, C. M. (2006). Vaginal birth after cesarean: Assessing maternal and perinatal risks: Contemporary management. *Clinical Obstetrics and Gynecology, 49*(1), 147–153.
17. American College of Obstetricians and Gynecologists. (2002). *Induction of labor for vaginal birth after cesarean delivery* [ACOG committee opinion #271]. Washington, DC: Author.
18. Miekle, S. F., Steiner, C. A., Zhang, J., & Lawrence, W. L. (2005). A national estimate of the elective primary cesarean delivery rate. *American Journal of Obstetrics and Gynecology, 105*(4), 751–756.
19. Visco, A. G., Viswanathan, M., Lohr, K. N., et al. (2006). Cesarean delivery on maternal request: Maternal and neonatal outcomes. *Obstetrics and Gynecology, 108*(6), 1517–1529.
20. Buhimschi, C. S., & Buhimschi, I. A. (2006). Advantages of vaginal delivery. *Clinical Obstetrics and Gynecology, 49*(1), 167–183.
21. Simpson, K. R., & Thorman, K. E. (2005). Obstetric "conveniences": Elective induction of labor, cesarean birth on demand, and other potentially unnecessary interventions. *Journal of Perinatal and Neonatal Nursing, 19*(2), 134–144.
22. Bloom, S. L., Spong, C. Y., & Weiner, S. J. (2005). Complications of anesthesia for cesarean delivery. *Obstetrics and Gynecology, 106,* 281–287.
23. Tharpe, N. (2007). First assisting in obstetrics: A primer for women's healthcare professionals. *Journal of Perinatal and Neonatal Nursing, 21*(1), 30–38.
24. American Academy of Pediatrics and American College of Obstetricians and Gynecologists. (2002). *Guidelines for perinatal care* (5th ed.). Elk Grove Village, IL: Author.
25. Association of Women's, Obstetric, and Neonatal Nurses. (2003). *Standards and guidelines for professional nursing practice in the care of women and newborns* (6th ed.). Washington, DC: Author.
26. Joint Commission on Accreditation of Healthcare Organizations. (2000). *Comprehensive accreditation manual for hospitals.* Oak Park, IL: Author.

ABO incompatibility a lack of compatibility between two groups of blood cells having different antigens because of the presence of one of the type antigens (A, B, or both) and its absence in the other

abruptio placentae premature separation of a normally implanted placenta; the separation can be partial or complete

abuse physical, sexual, emotional, or threatened violence against another

accelerations, fetal an increase in the fetal heart rate (FHR; onset to peak in less than 30 seconds) from the most recently calculated baseline. The duration of the acceleration is defined as the time from the initial change in FHR from the baseline to the return of the FHR to the baseline

> **At 32 weeks gestation and beyond**, an acceleration has an acme of 15 bpm above the baseline with a duration of 15 seconds or more, but less than 2 minutes
>
> **Before 32 weeks gestation**, an acceleration has an acme of 10 bpm above the baseline and with a duration of 10 seconds or more, but less than 2 minutes
>
> **Prolonged accelerations** last 2 minutes or more but less than 10 minutes
>
> If an acceleration lasts 10 minutes or longer, it is a baseline change

acidemia buildup of acid in the blood

acidosis condition in which there is a disturbance in the acid–base balance of the body, resulting in an accumulation of acids or an excessive loss of bicarbonate

active immunity protection from a disease resulting from the development within the body of substances that keep a person immune; this could result from having the disease or by the injection of an organism or products of an organism

active management of labor protocol for the augmentation of labor that includes strict criteria for inclusion, early amniotomy, high dose oxytocin infusion for ineffective contraction patterns

addendum statements added to the chart after the original documentation of an event; may contain additional facts about the situation or correct misinformation in the first entry

AIDS acquired immunodeficiency syndrome

alanine aminotransferase (ALT) an enzyme that contributes to protein metabolism; specifically, it catalyzes the reversible transfer of an amino group from glutamic acid to pyruvic acid to form alanine; the old term for this enzyme was *serum glutamic-pyruvic transaminase* (SGPT); this enzyme is present in the liver; during viral hepatitis and in cases of hepatocellular necrosis, marked elevations are seen

algorithm a logical progression that, for example, outlines sequential steps to be taken in the diagnosis and management of a disease

alpha-fetoprotein (AFP) test determination of fetal antigen levels during pregnancy; elevated levels in amniotic fluid are associated with neural tube defects, and low levels may be associated with Down syndrome

17-Alpha hydroxyprogesterone caproate (17P) a naturally occurring metabolite of progesterone and is sometimes used to treat women with a history of preterm birth

amniocentesis puncturing the amniotic sac using a needle so that amniotic fluid can be obtained for testing

amniotic fluid embolus (AFE) entrance of amniotic fluid, fetal cells, hair, or other debris into the maternal circulation initiating a series of rapid, complex events that lead to life-threatening maternal symptoms

amniotic fluid index (AFI) a method of reporting amniotic fluid volume

amniotic phosphatidylglycerol (PG) a class of compounds found in amniotic fluid that can be analyzed to determine fetal pulmonary maturity

amniotomy puncturing the amniotic sac, allowing amniotic fluid to escape; this is sometimes done during active labor

anaphylactoid syndrome proposed term for **amniotic fluid embolus**

anoxia deficiency of oxygen; *see also* **hypoxia**

antibody protein substances developed in response to the presence of an antigen; antibodies, which the body produces to inhibit or destroy the antigen, are part of the body's defense against foreign substances such as bacteria and viruses

antigen a substance that, when introduced into a host, is capable of producing antibodies; an antigen can be introduced into the host body, or it can be formed within the body; bacteria and viruses are examples of antigens

antiphospholipid antibodies antibodies directed against phosphorated polysaccharides of fatty acids; associated with immune mediated illnesses such as lupus and rheumatoid arthritis

antiretroviral therapy treatment with drugs designed to prevent the HIV virus from replicating in HIV-infected persons

Apgar score assessment tool used to determine a newborn's adaptation to the extrauterine environment

arborization fernlike appearance

ARC AIDS-related complex, which is a milder form of the immune deficiency causing a disease process

arterial embolization procedure to obstruct a blood vessel. May be used to control hemorrhage.

aspartate aminotransferase (AST) an enzyme that contributes to protein metabolism; specifically, it is important in the biosynthesis of amino acids because it catalyzes the reversible transfer of an amino group between glutamic and aspartic acid; the old term for this enzyme was *serum glutamic-oxaloacetic transaminase* (SGOT); when cell damage occurs (e.g., in the liver), AST is released into the tissues and bloodstream

asphyxia decrease in the body's oxygen along with an increase in the carbon dioxide content caused by interference with respiration

assisted delivery manual extraction of the fetus with a vacuum device or forceps

augmentation increasing contractions by chemical stimulation to help labor progress

auscultation method of assessment of the fetal heart rate, accomplished by listening and counting the rate

avulsion a forced tearing of tissues.

AZT azidothymide (chemical name), ZVD (zidovudine, generic name), and Retrovir (brand name); a nucleoside analog reverse transcriptase inhibitor drug commonly used to treat HIV infection; special precautions are recommended for dentistry

bacterial vaginosis a bacterial infection of the vagina, characterized by a foul-smelling, grayish vaginal discharge that exhibits a characteristic fishy odor when 10% potassium hydroxide is added

ballottement a sign that can be determined during abdominal examination of the pregnant woman; when the fingers tap lightly over a fetal part, it "bounces" back under the fingers; this sign can also be felt during a vaginal examination

baroreceptors specialized tissue located in the carotid arch and aortic sinus; cells in these areas are sensitive to stretching of surrounding tissues caused by increased blood pressure; when pressure is increased, these areas communicate this change to the brain, which responds by reducing the heart rate and cardiac output in an attempt to reduce blood pressure

base deficit (BD) the amount of bases used by the body in an attempt to normalize a reduced pH (neutralize the acid); illustrates the degree of change in the bicarbonate concentration of the body

baseline fetal heart rate the mean fetal heart rate rounded to increments of 5 bpm during a 10-minute segment, excluding periodic and episodic changes, periods of marked variability and segments of the baseline that differ more than 25 bpm; baseline must be for a minimum of two minutes in any 10 minute segment; normal range is between 110 and 160 bpm

baseline variability fluctuations of the fetal heart rate of two cycles per minute or more; visually quantified as the amplitude from peak to trough in beats per minute; the categories of variability are as follows:

absent amplitude range is undetectable (appears as straight line)

minimal amplitude range is detectable, but 5 bpm or fewer

moderate (normal) amplitude range is 6 to 25 bpm

marked amplitude range is more than 25 bpm

baseline uterine tone amount of tone remaining in the uterus between contractions, usually between 5 and 15 mm Hg; can be measured only by an intrauterine pressure catheter

β-adrenergic agonist substance that attaches to specific receptor sites in the smooth muscle and this inhibits the chemical reaction necessary for smooth muscle to contract

β-adrenergic receptors specific sites on smooth muscle cells (e.g., the cells of the myometrium) where chemicals (agonists) can couple to produce a chemical reaction

β-mimetic drugs unique chemical substances that are able to bind to β-receptor sites on smooth muscle cells, causing a depressant or relaxing effect on the contracting ability of that cell; such cells are found in the myometrium of the uterus; β-mimetic drugs belong to a group of chemicals called "agonists"

biparietal diameter (BPD) the largest transverse diameter of the fetal head; measures the distance between the parietal bones

bradycardia, fetal baseline FHR less than 110 bpm

Braxton-Hicks contractions intermittent painless contractions of the uterus; occur more frequently toward the end of the pregnancy and can sometimes be mistaken for true labor

capacity the age and competence of an individual required for giving informed consent

caput succedaneum swelling produced on the presenting part of the fetal head during labor; can be mistaken for the bag of waters

carrier individual who is capable of transmitting a disease to another person; many times, carriers are not sick and have no idea that they are capable of spreading a disease

catecholamines group of chemicals that mediate physiologic and metabolic responses associated with sympathetic nervous system functioning

CD4⁺ T cell critical subpopulation of regulatory T lymphocytes involved in the induction of most immunologic functions; depletion of this subset of T lymphocytes is the key element in profound immunosuppression seen in HIV infection

cephalic replacement May be used in the management of shoulder dystocia. Includes rotation of the baby's head back to occiput anterior, flexing of the baby's head, and firm pressure to push the baby's head back into the vagina. A cesarean section is then performed to deliver the baby. Also called the Zavanelli maneuver.

cephalopelvic disproportion (CPD) a condition that develops when the infant's head is of size, shape, or position that it cannot pass through the mother's pelvis

cervix the "neck," or lowest part, of the uterus that extends into the vagina; during labor, the cervix dilates, allowing the fetus to pass through it

cervical ripening softening of the cervix, occurs normally as physiologic process before labor or can be accomplished artificially by use of dilators and medications.

cesarean birth manual removal of the fetus, placenta, and membranes through an abdominal incision

primary cesarean delivery a woman's first cesarean birth

emergency cesarean delivery emergency operative birth in the setting of life-threatening complications for either mother or fetus

cesarean delivery on maternal request cesarean birth in the absence of any obstetric or maternal medical indications, *also* **elective cesarean delivery**

repeat cesarean delivery subsequent cesarean births

repeat elective cesarean birth a subsequent cesarean birth in the absence of any obstetric or maternal medical indications

cesarean hysterectomy removal of the uterus during a cesarean birth; the cervix, fallopian tubes, and ovaries may also be removed

cesarean incision the abdominal incision created to remove the fetus, placenta, and membranes

classic incision incision on upper part of the uterus in the vertical midline

low-segment transverse incision transverse incision made on the lower part of the uterus, just above the symphysis pubis

low-segment vertical incision vertical incision made on the lower part of the uterus

chancroid lesions that appear as red and ulcerated papules; may be associated with syphilis

chemoreceptors specialized tissue, located in the aortic and carotid bodies and in the medulla, that are sensitive to decreases in oxygen, carbon dioxide content, and pH in the blood; they recognize these changes, initiating responses that assist the body in compensating for these problems

chorioamnionitis infection of one of the membranes forming the amniotic sac, which holds the fetus during the pregnancy

cleft palate congenital defect in which an opening is left in the roof of the mouth (the palate); during fetal development, this area fails to close and a communicating passageway between the mouth and nasal cavities is left

clonus spasmodic alteration of contraction and relaxation of a foot or hand

collusion secret agreement or cooperation between or among individuals for illegal or deceitful actions

conduction anesthesia (regional anesthesia) form of anesthesia that is given centrally (i.e., in the spinal canal) or peripherally (i.e., in the skin) to block pain impulses without causing a loss of consciousness

confidentiality protection of patient information in all forms

confirmatory test a highly specific test designed to confirm the results of an earlier screening test

conservator person appointed by a court to manage the personal and legal affairs of an incompetent adult

contraction(s) shortening or tightening of a muscle; often used to describe the activity of the uterus that brings about dilatation of the cervix and descent of the fetus during labor

corticosteroids synthetic hormones, such as betamethasone or dexamethasone, given to women in preterm labor to enhance fetal lung maturity

corticotropin-releasing factor (CRF) neuropeptide released by the hypothalamus to stimulate the release of corticotrophin by the anterior pituitary

corticotrophin-releasing hormone chemical released by the cortex response to stress; may play a role in determining the length of gestation

cultural competence conscious motivation to develop cultural awareness, knowledge, skill in encounters with those from other cultures.

cycle of violence describes three phases of violence, including

tension-building phase the victim is compliant, but the abuser becomes angry with increasing frequency and intensity, with increased frequency of threats of harm, humiliation and intimidation

acute violence phase intentional use of force which may increase in severity with each cycle

honeymoon or reconciliation phase victim is showered with apologies and affection by the abuser, abuser gives assurances that the behavior will never happen again, makes excuses for the behavior, or even denies that violence occurred

cytokines substances produced by the immune system in response to infection; also, recent findings indicate that cytokines (e.g., interlukin-1β seem to play a role in labor initiation

decelerations, fetal heart rate

early decelerations in association with a uterine contraction, a visually apparent, gradual (onset to nadir 30 seconds or greater) decrease in the FHR with return to baseline; the nadir or low point of the deceleration occurs at the same time as the peak of the contraction

late decelerations in association with a uterine contraction, a visually apparent, gradual (onset to nadir 30 seconds or greater) decrease in the FHR with return to baseline; the onset, nadir, and recovery of the deceleration occur after the beginning, peak, and end of the contraction, respectively

variable decelerations abrupt (onset to nadir less than 30 seconds), visually apparent decrease in the FHR below the baseline; the decrease in FHR is 15 bpm or more, with a duration of 15 seconds or more, but less than 3 minutes

prolonged decelerations visually apparent decrease in the FHR below baseline; deceleration is 15 bpm or more, lasing 2 minutes or more but less than 10 minutes from onset to return to baseline; if the deceleration lasts longer than 10 minutes, it is a baseline change

decidua the lining of the uterus that envelopes the impregnated ovum to form part of the placenta

dehiscence Separation of a surgical wound.

dermatome the area of skin supplied with afferent nerve fibers by a single posterior spinal root

diabetic ketoacidosis (DKA) severe metabolic disturbance that occurs in the absence of insulin; life-threatening emergency that, left untreated, may result in coma and death

diabetogenic producing diabetes symptoms

dipping when the presenting part has descended into the false pelvis but is not through the pelvic inlet

direct fetal monitoring *see* internal fetal monitoring

disseminated intravascular coagulation (DIC) a grave disorder in blood clotting resulting from the overstimulation of the body's clotting processes; initially, generalized intravascular clotting occurs, succeeded by a deficiency in clotting factors and subsequent hemorrhaging; signs of hemorrhage may appear beneath the skin or mucous membranes, as evidenced by ecchymosis or petechiae

dizygotic pertaining to or derived from two separate zygotes (fertilized ova), as in a twin gestation resulting from two different fertilized ova

documentation recording, in written or electronic format, actions and decisions regarding patient care

domestic violence actual or threatened abuse of an intimate partner; *also* intimate partner violence, partner abuse, spousal abuse, wife abuse

doula supportive companion who accompanies a laboring woman to provide emotional, physical, and informational support and acts as an advocate for the woman and her family

Down syndrome congenital condition accompanied by moderate to severe mental retardation

dysmature condition in which the fetus or newborn is abnormally small or large for its gestational age; implies failure to achieve maturity in structure or function

dysrhythmia irregularity in the heart rate that can be a result of an electrical abnormality, congenital anomaly, or injury; can be a transient and benign problem or a continuous and serious condition; most fetal dysrhythmias are benign

dystocia abnormal labor as seen in very slow cervical dilatation or fetal descent or a complete halt in progress, which can be due to maternal or fetal conditions

early decelerations *see* decelerations, fetal heart rate

eclampsia pregnancy-related hypertensive disease accompanied by hypertension, proteinuria, edema, tonic and clonic convulsions, and coma; can occur during pregnancy or shortly after delivery

EIA an enzyme immunoassay test for HIV infection; has 99% sensitivity when performed under optimal laboratory conditions on serum specimens from persons infected for 12 weeks or more (formerly called *ELISA*)

emancipated released from parental care and responsibility; freed from the power of another individual

embolism obstruction of a blood vessel by foreign substances or a blood clot (as in erythroblastosis fetalis)

endemic a disease that is indigenous to a geographic area or population

endogenous originating within the body

endogenous insulin insulin that is secreted from the pancreas (within the body)

endothelin-derived releasing factor (EDRF) substance that acts as a vasorelaxor in the vascular smooth muscle

endothelium layer of epithelial cells that lines the cavities of the heart and of the blood and lymph vessels

en face face to face

Engerix-B currently licensed hepatitis B vaccine that is the result of genetic engineering; the usual schedule of doses is at birth, and then at 1 and 6 months of age; may be given in an alternate four-dose schedule at birth, 1, 2, and 12 months; a recent CDC advisory also recommends administration before 2 months of age, at 2 to 4 months, and at 6 to 18 months

enteric precautions procedures followed in the care of certain patients that are intended to reduce the risk of contamination of personnel or other patients from potentially infected intestinal waste

epigastric pain pain occurring in the right upper quadrant of the abdomen and that is the result of hepatic edema and hemorrhages in the liver capsule

epinephrine a substance produced by the adrenal medulla gland predominantly; it is produced synthetically and is used therapeutically as a vasoconstrictor, cardiac stimulant, and bronchiole relaxant

episodic fetal heart rate changes those that do not occur in relation to a contraction

erythroblastosis condition of hemolytic disease of the newborn characterized by anemia, jaundice, and enlargement of the liver and spleen

esophageal atresia closure or absence of the esophagus

euglycemia normal level of glucose in the blood

exogenous insulin insulin that comes from a source outside the body

external fetal monitoring *also* "indirect or noninvasive fetal monitoring"; this method involves the use of an ultrasonic transducer and tocodynamometer to monitor fetal heart tones and contractions, respectively; these are held in place by belts

fetal anencephaly condition in the fetus in which there is an absence of the brain and spinal cord

fetal attitude relation of fetal parts to each other; the basic attitudes are flexion and extension; for example, when the baby's head is bent toward its chest, the head is in an attitude of flexion

fetal bradycardia See bradycardia, fetal

fetal fibronectin (fFN) glycoprotein produced by the chorion, found at the junction of the membrane and the uterus

fetal hydrocephaly condition in the fetus in which there is an increased accumulation of cerebrospinal fluid within the ventricles of the fetus' brain; this leads to rapid head growth; it is a result of interference with normal circulation and absorption of the fluid

fetal karyotype chromosomal contents found in the cell nucleus of the fetus

fetal lie relationship of the body of the fetus to the body of the mother; fetal lies are longitudinal or transverse

longitudinal lie fetal body from head to toe is parallel to the length of the mother

transverse lie fetal body lies at right angles to the mother's body

fetal monitoring type of electronic monitoring in which information about the fetal heart rate and the contraction pattern are continually assessed; *see also* external fetal monitoring

fetal position position of the fetus within the uterus in relation to the maternal pelvis

fetal presentation within the uterus, the lowest part of the fetus that comes first, either the head, buttocks, or, rarely, the shoulders

fetal reserve amount of oxygen provided to the fetus above that which is needed; oxygen supplied minus the oxygen needed

fetal scalp electrode spiral electrode attached directly to the presenting part of the fetus; determines the fetal heart rate by counting R waves in the fetal ECG; this results in a tracing that allows variability to be assessed; part of the internal monitoring system

fetal tachycardia increase in the baseline fetal heart rate to greater than 160 bpm

floating when the presenting part is entirely out of the pelvis and can be moved by the examiner

fontanelle spaces where the sutures of the skull bones meet; "soft spots" on the baby's head

forceps assisted birth *see* assisted delivery

fraud intentional deception of an individual to gain that person's cooperation in surrendering their property or legal rights

fulminant occurring with great rapidity

Gaskin maneuver Positioning of a laboring woman on her hands and knees or "all fours" to reduce a shoulder dystocia. Named after Ina May Gaskin, MA, CPM, founder and director of the Farm Midwifery Center.

gap junctions intracellular channels that allow movement of small molecules or ions for communication between cells

gestational hypertension blood pressure elevation detected for the first time after midpregnancy (20 weeks); elevated pressures are transient, there is no progression to preeclampsia and the woman is normotensive by 12 weeks postpartum

gluconeogenesis synthesis of glucose from noncarbohydrate sources, such as amino acids and glycerol; occurs primarily with the liver and kidneys when carbohydrate supply is low

glycogenolysis the splitting up of glycogen in the liver, which yields glucose

grand multipara woman who has had five or more live births

group B streptococcus gram-positive bacteria that can be a cause of both meningitis and sepsis in the neonate

HAART highly active antiretroviral therapy; a combination of antiretroviral medications that work well against HIV

Havrix vaccine used against hepatitis A

HBV hepatitis B virus

hemoglobin A_{1c} (HbA_{1c}) measurement of the percent of glycosylation (linkage of hemoglobin to glucose) that occurs in red blood cells

hemorrhage rapid loss of large amounts of blood, may be internal or external

hematoma Localized collection of clotted or partially clotted blood.

hepatitis B immune globulin (HBIG) substance that supplies antibodies needed to provide immediate protection against hepatitis B

hepatocellular carcinoma (HPC) cancer of the liver

Heptavax B plasma-derived hepatitis B vaccine that is no longer produced in the United States

herpes simplex virus (HSV) type 1 serologic subtype of the herpes virus strain that primarily infects nongenital areas of the body, mainly mucocutaneous tissue of the mouth; however, HSV-1 can cause genital herpes infections as well

herpes simplex virus (HSV) type 2 virus that causes infections in the genital organs; it is the second most common venereal disease; when it occurs in the pregnant woman, it has been associated with spontaneous abortion, stillbirths, congenital malformations, and serious infections in the neonate

HIV the human immunodeficiency virus that causes AIDS

HIV-1 one of five known retroviruses; discovered in 1984 and once called human T-cell lymphotrophic virus type III

HIV-2 one of five known retroviruses; discovered in 1986 and once called human T-cell lymphotrophic virus type IV

HIV DNA PCR preferred virologic method for diagnosing HIV infection in infants

HIV infection acquiring of HIV in the blood and other body fluids and tissues; the individual may have no symptoms whatsoever

HIV RNA test *also* viral load or just RNA; a blood test that measures the amount of HIV virus in a person's blood plasma

home uterine activity monitoring monitoring of uterine activity using a portable external fetal monitoring system and telephone module to transfer data to a monitoring center

horizontal transmission transmission of microscopic organisms (e.g., viruses) from one sexual partner to another

HTLV-III a retrovirus known as human T-cell lymphotropic virus type III; a more specific name for HIV-1

hydatidiform mole result of a degeneration of the early developing placenta; multiple grape-like cysts develop, along with rapid growth of the uterus and bleeding

hydralazine (Apresoline) an arterial vasodilator used as an antihypertensive agent in the treatment of severe preeclampsia

hydramnios presence of excessive amounts of amniotic fluid (2,000 mL or more) in the uterus

hydrops edema in the fetus

hyperbilirubinemia excessive amounts of bilirubin in the blood; prenatal conditions in the mother such as diabetes, infections, drug ingestion, and blood incompatibility between mother and fetus can predispose the newborn to hyperbilirubinemia; certain neonatal conditions such as obstruction of the biliary duct or the lower bowel can also predispose the newborn to this condition; treatment to lower and stabilize bilirubin levels is necessary because excessive levels can lead to brain damage

hyperglycemic hyperosmolar nonketotic syndrome (HHNS) occurs in type 2 diabetes and is characterized by extreme hyperglycemia, absence of ketones, severe dehydration, and decreased consciousness

hyperpnea breathing that is deeper and more rapid than expected

hypertonic uterus labor contractions that last longer than 90 seconds; caused by overstimulation of the uterus

hyperventilation increased inspiration and expiration of air as a result of rapid or deep breathing, which leads to the reduction of carbon dioxide in the blood; symptoms include dizziness, light headedness, and tingling in the fingers and around the mouth

hypocalcemia abnormally low levels of calcium in the blood

hypoglycemia abnormally low levels of glucose in the blood

hypopharynx laryngopharynx, the bottom part of the pharynx that connects the throat to the esophagus

hypothermia having a body temperature below normal

hypoxemia decreased oxygen content in the blood

hypoxia insufficient availability of oxygen to meet the body's metabolic needs

iatrogenic caused by treatment or diagnostic procedures

idiosyncratic abnormal susceptibility to an agent, such as a drug, which is peculiar or unique to the individual

IgM immunoglobulin M; special proteins produced by the lymphatic system against foreign substances shortly after their invasion; they are larger in size than IgG molecules and incapable of crossing the placenta to any great extent; blood levels rise within days of an infection and fall to a nondetectable level within a few months

ileus intestinal obstruction

immune serum globulin (ISG) substance that contains proteins capable of acting as antibodies and thus potentially confers some passive immunity to the individual receiving it

immunization becoming immune or the process of rendering a patient immune

immunogenicity ability to stimulate the formation of antibodies

inborn neonate infant whose birth occurred within the birth center or hospital

indirect fetal monitoring *see* external fetal monitoring

induction artificially starting labor and ensuring ongoing labor, usually through oxytocin administration

information as a legal term, refers to the content of the explanation given to the patient

informed consent legal term describing a process by which patients are given specific information regarding procedures, may be written or verbal

inoculate introduce a substance (the inoculum) into the body that can produce a disease or an immunity to the disease, depending on the circumstances and the substance; inoculate is sometimes a cultured substance

internal fetal monitoring *also* called direct and invasive fetal monitoring; type of electronic monitoring in which the fetal heart rate is monitored by the use of a helix electrode and the laboring woman's contraction pattern is monitored by the use of an intrauterine pressure catheter

intrauterine pressure catheter catheter inserted into the uterine cavity alongside the presenting part of the fetus, allowing baseline uterine tonus and contraction intensity to be assessed; is part of the internal monitoring system

ketosis excess of ketone bodies in the blood; in uncontrolled diabetes mellitus, there is a great increase in fatty acid metabolism and impaired or absent carbohydrate metabolism, resulting in the increased production of ketone bodies

late deceleration *see* deceleration, fetal

late preterm birth infants delivered between 34 and 36 weeks' gestation

lecithin:sphingomyelin ratio (L/S ratio) complex and fairly lengthy test used to assess lung maturity in the fetus; a ratio of 2.0 or higher usually indicates mature lungs

leptin protein found in the plasma that reduces food intake and increases energy expenditure

lithotomy position in which the woman lies on her back with her thighs drawn up toward her chest, her knees flexed, and her legs extended out to the side

lochia discharge of blood, mucus, and tissue from the uterus during the postdelivery period

L/S ratio *see* lecithin:sphingomyelin ratio

macrophages type of white blood cell involved in the immune response by destroying/ingesting foreign material, debris, or dead cells

macrosomia large body size, including enlargement of organs such as the liver and spleen

malpractice failure of a professional person to act in accordance with current accepted professional standards or failure to foresee possibilities and consequences that a professional person, having the necessary skills and training to act professionally, should foresee no matter what the motivation

maturity-onset diabetes of youth (MODY) relatively mild, non–insulin-requiring form of diabetes mellitus beginning at a younger age than usual

McRobert's maneuver positioning of the mother's thighs on her abdomen to straighten the sacrum and decrease angle of incline of the symphysis pubis making it easier to deliver the anterior shoulder in the case of shoulder dystocia

meconium dark green or black material present in the large intestine of the near-term or term fetus; also the first stool passed by the newborn

meconium aspiration syndrome (MAS) syndrome caused by the inhalation of meconium or meconium-stained amniotic fluid into the lungs

mentum chin

microangiopathy disease of small blood vessels in which the basement membrane of the capillaries thickens or thrombi form in the arterioles and capillaries

microcephaly congenital deformity in the fetus in which the head is abnormally small in relation to the body; mental retardation is often associated with this condition

midpelvis most important plane of the pelvis because it has the least room

molding normal overlapping of skull bones of the baby so that the head will fit through the pelvis during labor

monozygotic pertaining to or derived from a single zygote (fertilized ovum), as in a twin gestation occurring from a single fertilization ovum

Montevideo units measurement of uterine activity made when an intrauterine pressure catheter is in place

morbidity state of disease; cases of disease in relation to a specific group or population

mortality death rate; ratio of number of deaths to a specific group or population

multipara woman who is in other than her first labor

multiple gestation pregnancy with more than one fetus; an example is twins

nasopharynx part of the pharynx situated above the soft palate (postnasal space)

necrotizing enterocolitis a serious illness involving necrotic lesions of the intestines; occurs primarily in preterm or low birth weight neonates

neonatal resuscitation actions to restore or enhance breathing and circulation in the newborn

nephropathy disease of the kidney caused by microvascular changes

neuropathy disease of the nervous system involving peripheral nerve dysfunction

newly born refers to an infant during the brief period of the first few minutes to hours of life

noninvasive fetal monitoring *see* external fetal monitoring

nosocomial infections that are hospital acquired, in contrast with community-acquired infections

nuchal cord umbilical cord with one or more loops around the neck of the infant; commonly present and ordinarily does no harm

nullipara woman in labor for the first time

nulliparous having never given birth to a child

obstetric hemorrhage significant loss of blood during the antepartum, intrapartum, or antepartum periods

occiput back of the fetal skull, below and behind the posterior fontanelle

oligohydramnios abnormally small amount of amniotic fluid; an AFI of 5 cm or less

oliguria severely decreased urinary output (less than 400 mL in 24 hours)

opportunistic infection infection developing in the host organism because of a lowered immune capability

organogenesis time of organ development, which occurs 17 to 56 days after conception

oropharynx central portion of the pharynx lying between the soft palate and upper portion of the epiglottis

outborn neonate infant whose birth occurred outside the birth center or hospital and who is then admitted

oxytocin hormone that stimulates the uterus to contract or a drug (Syntocinon or Pitocin) that imitates the natural hormone

palliative care *also called* comfort care; care aimed at prevention and relief of suffering, support for best possible quality of life for patients and their families

paracrine type of hormone function in which the hormone synthesized and released from endocrine cells binds to receptors in nearby cells, affecting their function

parous having had at least one child, either alive or dead at birth

partner abuse *see* domestic violence

parturition the act or process of giving birth

passive immunity immunity to a disease produced by injection of material containing the antibodies against a specific disease

pathogen microorganism or substance capable of producing disease

pelvic planes imaginary flat surfaces passing across parts of the true pelvis at different levels; used to describe dimensions of various parts of the pelvis

perinatal time between 20 weeks' gestational age and 28 days after birth

perinatal morbidity frequency or rate of disease among fetuses or infants between 20 weeks' gestational age and 28 days after birth

perinatal mortality death of a fetus or infant between 20 weeks' gestational age and 28 days after birth

perinatal transmission transmission of diseased blood elements that occurs during the perinatal period or during birth

periodic fetal heart rate changes transient fetal heart rate changes associated with contractions

placenta the spongy structure attached to the wall of the uterus throughout pregnancy through which nutrients and oxygen pass from the mother's blood to the fetus and through which waste products from the fetus pass into the mother's blood

placenta accreta placenta abnormally adhered to the myometrium of the uterus

placenta battledore placenta with the umbilical cord inserted at the edge

placenta circumvallate placenta encircled with a dense, raised, white nodular ring

placenta previa abnormal implantation of the placenta in the lower uterine segment; classification of the type of previa is based on how close the placenta lies to the cervical opening (os)

    total placenta previa completely covers the os

    partial placenta previa covers a portion of the os

    marginal placenta previa close to the os

plasma fluid part of the blood

plasma-derived vaccines vaccines that are produced from the pooled serum of infected individuals

Pco$_2$ partial pressure of carbon dioxide (quantity of CO_2 in the blood)

Po$_2$ partial pressure of oxygen (quantity of O_2 in the blood)

polydipsia excessive thirst, caused by dehydration

polyphagia excessive hunger, caused by tissue loss and the state of starvation that occurs with the inability of the cells to utilize glucose

polyuria frequent urination seen in diabetes because water is not reabsorbed by the renal tubules owing to the osmotic activity of glucose

postprandial after meals

postterm infant an infant with a gestational age of more than 42 weeks; *also* postmature

preeclampsia disease occurring during pregnancy (after 20 weeks or during the first week after delivery) with the development of high blood pressure in addition to protein in the urine, edema, or both

preexisting diabetes diabetic state present before pregnancy

pregestational diabetes diabetic state present before pregnancy

premature rupture of membranes (PROM) spontaneous rupture of membranes before the onset of labor, regardless of gestational age

preterm infant with a gestational age of less than 37 weeks; the term *premature* is sometimes used (*see also* late preterm birth and very preterm birth)

preterm birth delivery of an infant at less than 37 week gestation

preterm premature rupture of membranes (PPROM) rupture of membranes before term (37 completed weeks gestation) with or without the onset of labor

prevalence proportion of individuals in a population having a disease

primigravida woman who is pregnant for the first time

primipara woman who has given birth to her first child, whether or not the child is living or was alive at birth

prodromal time in which a symptom indicates the onset of a state (e.g., labor or a disease)

progesterone hormone produced by the ovaries when a woman is not pregnant and by the placenta during pregnancy; it has many important functions, including preventing the uterus from contracting during pregnancy

proinsulin precursor of insulin

prolapsed cord condition in which the umbilical cord slips down along the side of the fetal presenting part or comes ahead of the presenting part

proliferative retinopathy new blood vessel formation near the optic disk that can extend to growth in the vitreous chamber, rupture, and vitreous hemorrhage; in addition, fibrous tissue is generated and adheres to the posterior vitreous membrane and can lead to retinal detachment

prolonged acceleration *see* acceleration, fetal

prolonged deceleration *see* deceleration, fetal

prophylaxis observing procedures or steps to prevent a disease or harmful effect

prostacyclin hormone synthesized in the endothelial lining of the blood vessels; a potent vasodilator and inhibitor of platelet aggregation

prostaglandins group of chemical substances (derivatives of fatty acids) present in many tissues; stimulate the uterus to contract

proteinuria presence in the urine of abnormally large quantities of protein, usually albumin; by definition, occurs with a reading of 2+ on a random urine specimen or when there is 500 mg of protein in a 24-hour specimen (less than 250 mg of protein per day is excreted in the healthy adult)

pyelonephritis inflammation of the kidney caused by an infective process

pyloric stenosis condition found in the infant in which the opening from the stomach to the small intestines is narrowed so much that partially digested food cannot pass in a normal manner; a characteristic sign of this is highly forceful vomiting

Recombivax B synthetic, genetically engineered vaccine for hepatitis B

relaxin hormone secreted by the corpus luteum; acts on smooth muscle of the uterus to produce relaxation of muscle fibers

replication process of duplicating or reproducing (e.g., replication of an exact copy of a polynucleotide strand of DNA or RNA)

restitute movement of the newborn head once it is born wherein the neck untwists and the head turns approximately 45 degrees to resume its normal relationship with the shoulders, which are in an anteroposterior position at the pelvic outlet

retinopathy damage to the retina of the eye caused by the microvascular deterioration from elevated blood glucose levels

retrovirus unique virus form that contains an enzyme, reverse transcriptase, enabling it to synthesize DNA in the cells of a host; this DNA then enters the nucleus of that cell and becomes part of it; the viral DNA (genes) therefore becomes duplicated along with the host's cell genes, and new generations of cells are produced; these new generations contain the virus's genetic material

Rh incompatibility lack of compatibility between two groups of blood cells having different antigens; caused by the presence of the Rh factor in one group and its absence in the other

safety plan action plan giving a victim of abuse steps to follow in a dangerous situation, including detailed information about defensive measures

scotomata presence of specks or spots in the vision disturbing vision temporarily; suggestive of lesions in the retina or visual pathway

semi-Fowler's position semisitting position in which the patient is positioned at approximately 45 degrees

sensitivity probability that a test will be positive when infection or a specific condition is present

seroconversion process of blood serum developing an antibody response to a specific antigen (e.g., a virus or bacteria)

seronegative the absence of a primary infection with a specific agent, or the disappearance of antibodies after treatment or absence of antibodies usually found in a given disease/syndrome

seropositive producing a positive reaction to serologic tests

seroprotective level of antibody response that indicates protection (immunity) after exposure or vaccination

serous exudate accumulation of a fluid, having the nature of serum, in a cavity or on a surface

serum that part of blood that remains after clotting has occurred

shoulder dystocia difficult delivery of the shoulders of the fetus

sinciput brow or forehead of the fetus

sinusoidal pattern baseline pattern that demonstrates a regular undulating pattern above and below the fetal heart baseline; can be a sign of severe fetal anemia or fetal asphyxia or may be the effect of certain medications

spaces used in conduction anesthesia the spinal cord is covered by three layers; the outermost layer is the dura, the middle layer is the arachnoid, and the inner layer is the pia

  arachnoid space between the middle and inner layer covering the spinal cord and contains the spinal fluid

  extradural space (epidural, peridural) space found outside the outermost covering of the spinal cord into which chemicals may be injected for the purpose of inducing anesthesia

  subdural space space found between the outermost and the middle layer of the spinal cord

specificity probability that a test will be negative when the infection or specific condition is not present

spina bifida congenital defect in the walls of the spinal canal caused by lack of union between parts of the vertebrae; as a result, the membranes of the spinal cord are pushed through the opening, forming a tumor

spiral electrode *see* fetal scalp electrode

standards of practice accepted published professional levels of care for which the individual professional is held accountable; the legal profession and courts use these in malpractice cases

steroids chemical compounds that make up, among other things, hormones found in humans; many drugs are composed of steroids

STI sexually transmitted infection

strip graph tracing produced on graph paper by the electronic fetal monitor; allows fetal heart rate and contraction patterns to be continually assessed

Sugaleal Potential space between the periosteum (skull) and the epicranial aponeurosis (scalp). A subgaleal hemorrhage is a potential complication of vacuum assisted birth. It can be associated with intracranial hemorrhage or skull fracture and must be distinguished from caput succadaneum and cephalohematoma.

SUDS single-use diagnostic system; the only HIV-1 rapid test that is licensed by the Food and Drug Administration for use in the United States

suprapubic pressure pressure applied above the maternal symphysis pubis with a hand over anterior fetal shoulder with downward and lateral motion to relieve shoulder dystocia

surfactant mixture of phospholipids (primarily lecithin and sphingomyelin) secreted by alveolar cells into the alveoli and respiratory air passages, which reduces the surface tension of pulmonary fluids and contributes to the elastic properties of pulmonary tissue

sutures spaces between the bones of the fetal skull, which are covered by membranes

Symphysiotomy Transection of the firm ligaments between the left and right symphyseal bones, may be used in the event of a shoulder dystocia to gain pelvic circumference and facilitate of the baby's anterior shoulder. The procedure can be done rapidly, under local anesthesia.

tachycardia, fetal baseline fetal heart rate greater than 160 bpm

term infant infant with a gestational age of 38 to 42 weeks

therapeutic privilege withholding information about a treatment or medication when the individual's health would be significantly jeopardized by full disclosure of the information

thermoregulation regulation of temperature, especially body temperature

thrombocytopenia abnormal decrease in the number of blood platelets, usually caused by the destruction of erythroid tissue in bone marrow, which can be brought about by certain neoplastic diseases or an immune response to a drug; bleeding disorders are a consequence

thrombophlebitis inflammation of a vein; associated with the formation of a blood clot

thromboxane produced primarily by the platelets; potent vasoconstrictor; stimulates platelet aggregation

tocodynamometer part of an external monitoring system that provides information about the laboring woman's contraction pattern by detecting changes in the shape of her abdominal wall directly above the uterine fundus

tocolytic effect of quieting or inhibiting smooth muscle activity; the myometrium of the uterus is composed of smooth muscle

tocolytic therapy process of administering medications for the purpose of inhibiting uterine contractions

trial of labor labor with uterine contractions after a previous cesarean birth

trophoblastic disease disease resulting from degeneration in the early development of the placenta; a hydatidiform mole results

tubal sterilization operative procedure using ligation, surgical closure, and/or cauterization to render the fallopian tubes incapable of sperm or ova transport

tumor necrosis factor-α protein that has a wide range of proinflammatory actions; usually considered a cytokine

ultrasonic transducer part of the external monitoring system that monitors fetal heart rate by detecting movement within the fetal heart as the heart valves open and close; similar to sonar

uterine atony loss of normal tone of the muscles of the uterus; results in relaxation of the muscles that normally control postpartum uterine bleeding

uterine dystocia abnormal labor or difficult labor

uterine tonus degree of muscle tone within the uterus; *see also* baseline uterine tonus

uterine rupture symptomatic disruption of the layers of the uterus

vacuum-assisted birth (vacuum extraction) birth of infant assisted by the placement of vacuum device to provide gentle traction and guidance of the fetal head

vacuum-assisted delivery *see* assisted delivery

vagal stimulation stimulation of the vagus nerve; can be caused by intubation of neonate

vaginal birth after cesarean (VBAC) vaginal birth after a previous cesarean birth

Vaqta vaccine against hepatitis A

variability *see* baseline fetal heart rate variability

variable deceleration *see* deceleration, fetal

vasopressor substance or medication that causes vasoconstriction

velamentous cord insertion major vessels found in the cord separate in the membranes at a distance from the edge of the placenta where they are surrounded only by a fold of amnion

vertex top of the skull between the anterior and posterior fontanelles

vertical transmission transmission of microscopic organisms (e.g., viruses) to the fetus and newborn either through breaks in the placental barrier during pregnancy or at the time of birth

very preterm birth infants delivered before 32 weeks' gestation

vibroacoustic stimulation process of fetal stimulation using sound; objective is to elicit a fetal startle or movement that is then used to evaluate fetal status

viral replication process of a virus reproducing itself

viremia (viremic) state of having viruses in the blood

virulent very poisonous; infectious

voluntariness circumstances surrounding an individual's giving consent

Western blot test supplemental laboratory test that detects specific antibodies to components of a virus; mainly used to validate repeatedly reactive enzyme immunoassays (EIA) or enzyme-linked immunoassays (ELISA) for HIV infection; is highly specific when strict criteria are used to interpret the results; when a repeatedly reactive EIA or ELISA and a positive Western blot test occur, it is highly predictive of HIV infection, even in a population with a low prevalence of infection

wife abuse *see* domestic violence

Sexually Transmitted Infections

Anne Moore

Introduction

Sexually transmitted diseases (STDs) or sexually transmitted infections (STIs) pose multiple threats in pregnancy. Maternal infection with an STD is often associated with spontaneous abortion, fetal anomalies, stillbirth, preterm labor, and low birth weight, as well as increased neonatal morbidity and mortality and long-term adverse health consequences in childhood.

Most of the diseases outlined in this appendix are defined as STDs. Although not currently categorized as such, bacterial vaginosis (BV), and candidiasis (monilia) are included in this appendix because of the potential adverse perinatal events associated with them. Group B streptococcus (GBS) infection is addressed in Appendix E. Infections with human immunodeficiency virus (HIV), hepatitis B virus (HBV), hepatitis C virus (HCV), herpes simplex virus 1 and 2 (HSV-1 and HSV-2, respectively), and human papilloma virus (HPV) have no associated cures or vaccines. A vaccine for the prevention of the four most common types of HPV has recently become available under the trade name Gardisil, but it is currently not recommended for use in pregnancy.

During admission of the laboring woman, careful attention to her prenatal history, physical examination, and laboratory workup can identify the presence of an unresolved, untreated, or undertreated STD or the potential for such. When such risk is diagnosed, therapies and preventive strategies for the birthing process and postpartum can be integrated into the mother's nursing and medical management. Newborn evaluation and appropriate therapy can be instituted immediately. The challenge is to identify the risk! Subsequent education during the postpartum period will affect the mother's understanding of the infection, self-care, and prevention. It is especially important that the mother appreciates any need for special newborn care, including early symptoms and the need for prompt medical attention.

Bacterial Vaginosis

Bacterial vaginosis (BV) is a condition in which normal hydrogen peroxide–producing (H_2O_2) lactobacillus, predominant in the healthy vagina, are replaced with anaerobic bacteria, mostly *Gardnerella vaginalis*, *Mobiluncus* species, and *Mycoplasma hominis*.

Although not considered a definitive STD, BV has epidemiologic elements consistent with those of an STD.

Epidemiology

- The prevalence of BV in pregnant women is similar to that in the general population, about 12% to 21%.[1]

- In the United States, BV is found in approximately 51% of African-American women, 32% of Hispanic women, and 23% of Caucasian women.[1]
- BV infection during pregnancy is associated with spontaneous preterm birth, preterm rupture of membranes, chorioamnionitis, and postpartum endometritis.[2]
- Research in pregnant and nonpregnant women suggests that BV in the lower genital tract is associated with an increased risk of infection in the upper genital tract; upper genital tract involvement may be one mechanism by which infection leads to inflammation, uterine contractions, and subsequent preterm labor.[3]
- It is uncertain whether BV should be classified as an STI or whether it is simply a situation of abnormal microbial colonization.[4]

Clinical Features

- The vagina harbors both Gram-positive and Gram-negative bacteria. However, only relatively few different types of bacteria are found in large numbers in the healthy vaginal environment. Lactobacilli are a dominant bacteria and contribute to the maintenance of a healthy vaginal environment with a pH of 3.8 to less than 4.5.
- The absence of normally occurring (endogenous) vaginal lactobacilli is important in the acquisition of BV. The absence of these lactobacilli correlates with a loss of vaginal acidity (pH greater than 4.5) seen in BV.[4]
- Hormonal changes, specifically estrogen loss, (e.g., during menstruation and pregnancy) appear to play a significant role in decreasing colonization of lactobacilli.[4]
- Risk factors consistently associated with BV (and other STIs) include smoking (this may simply be a marker for sexual behavior, however), racial origin, contraceptive practice (oral contraceptive use), and sexual activity.[4]
- BV is seen somewhat more frequently in conjunction with other STIs and occurs more often in women who are sexually active than in women who are not.[1]
- Many women and their infants who harbor anaerobic bacteria such as *G. vaginalis*, *Mobiluncus* species, and *Mycoplasmas* never manifest any signs of infection or adverse outcomes.[1] Additionally, some women do not normally colonize H_2O_2-producing lactobacilli.
- BV is more strongly associated with age greater than 25 years. This is contrary to most STIs, whose highest rates are almost always in women younger than 25.[1,4]
- The pathogenesis associated with BV (and other vaginal infections) is believed to result, in part, from enzymes and endotoxins that weaken the amniotic membrane, leading to bacterial

penetration of the intrauterine environment and subsequent infection and labor stimulation.[3,4]

- Causal relationships between BV and infertility, pelvic inflammatory disease, miscarriage, postpartum endometritis, and other gynecologic conditions are unknown and under investigation.[1,4]

Perinatal Consequences

- Forty percent of preterm births are associated with an etiology related to infection, but just how much of the infection incidence is related to BV is unknown.[4]
- Findings indicate that as many as 80% of early preterm births (24 to 28 weeks' gestation) are associated with intrauterine infection.[3]
- African-American women experience a disproportionate incidence of preterm birth. BV and other vaginal infections and low birth weight account for 40% of those births.[3,4]
- Preterm birth and low birth weight are major contributors to infant mortality, as well as infant and early childhood morbidity.
- The presence of BV increases a woman's susceptibility to HIV infection.[4]

Screening/Diagnosis

- A detailed gynecologic and obstetric history should accompany a workup for BV.
- Diagnosis is not difficult and is usually made according to Amsel criteria; that is, three of the following four elements must be present to make the diagnosis. The four criteria are (1) the presence of a thin homogeneous discharge (usually profuse and grayish-white in color), (2) a vaginal pH of greater than 4.5, (3) a positive "whiff" test (fishy odor), and (4) the presence of "clue" cells under microscopic examination (called a "wet prep").
- Vaginal cultures are unreliable and generally not used.
- Half of all women who meet the current criteria for the diagnosis of BV are asymptomatic.
- Evidence does not support routine screening for BV in all pregnant women.
- Currently, *universal* testing is not recommended for *nonpregnant* women because there is a high rate of recurrence, concern regarding microbial resistance development, and a lack of documentation of the effectiveness of prepregnancy detection/ treatment for preterm birth prevention.[5]
- Some experts recommend screening for BV in high-risk pregnancies (women who have previously delivered a premature infant) at the time of the first prenatal visit.[2,6] Adverse outcomes with BV appear to be much more significant when infection is present before 20 weeks' gestation.
- The American College of Nurse-Midwives advocates BV testing for all women during the first prenatal visit. Testing should be a standard part of care for women who have a history of previous preterm birth, a diagnosed STI, or bleeding in the current pregnancy—regardless of whether symptoms are present or not.[5]
- The Centers for Disease Control and Prevention (CDC) recommends evaluation and treatment for all symptomatic pregnant women.[2]

Treatment

NOTE: All pregnant women who have symptomatic BV require treatment.[2]

- There is no consensus regarding the approach to the treatment of BV. The recommendations that follow are according to 2006 CDC guidelines.[2]
- Treatment regimens are as follows:
  - Metronidazole 250 mg orally, three doses daily for 7 days
  - Metronidazole 500 mg orally, twice daily for 7 days
  - Clindamycin 300 mg orally, twice daily for 7 days

NOTE: *Oral doses are preferred. Vaginal administration of drugs has less systemic efficacy for the treatment of upper genital infection.*

- Follow-up evaluation is as follows:
  - Retesting in nonpregnant women is currently not considered necessary.[2]
  - In pregnant women, especially high-risk pregnant women who are asymptomatic, follow-up testing is recommended 1 month after treatment is completed to ensure that therapy was successful. This may prevent adverse pregnancy outcomes.[2]

Candidiasis vaginalis (Monilia)

Candidal vulvovaginal infection is a common fungal infection usually caused by one of three *Candida* species: *C. albicans, C. glabrata,* or *C. tropicalis. C. albicans* is the causative agent in 80% to 90% of infections, but the other two species are increasingly being associated with infection.[7]

Epidemiology

- Candidiasis is the second most common vaginal infection in women (BV being the most common).[7]
- Approximately 75% of women have at least one infection in their lifetime, and approximately 45% experience two or more episodes.[2]
- Epidemiologic data on the disease are incomplete. It is not reportable, and often self-treated or self-diagnosed without the benefit of microscopy or culture.

Clinical Features

- Symptoms include pruritus, vaginal discharge, vaginal soreness, vulvar burning, painful intercourse (dyspareunia), and painful urination (dysuria).
- Erythema in the vulvovaginal area; thick, white patches adhering to the vaginal walls; or a thin, watery discharge may be observed on inspection.
- It is generally not considered a sexually transmitted disease; however, it appears to be sexually associated because there is increased frequency of the infection at the time women become sexually active.
- Risk for acquiring vulvovaginal candidal infection is associated with uncontrolled diabetes and use of certain antibiotics.
- Candidal organisms are ubiquitous in nature and part of the microbial flora in humans. Pregnancy may predispose some women to candidiasis due to significant increases in estrogen, which alter glycogen content in the vagina. Although various species of *Candida* normally inhabit the vagina, any change in vaginal homeostasis may permit an overgrowth of fungi, resulting in infection.

Perinatal Consequences

- Vulvovaginal candidiasis commonly occurs during pregnancy. The organism can be cultured from the vagina in approximately 25% of women nearing term.[8]
- Maternal vaginal infection does not appear to have any association with preterm birth.[8]
- *Candida* species may be transmitted to the newborn from the vagina during birth.
- The clinical manifestations in the newborn vary depending on the location and extent of the infection. Thrush is an infection of the buccal mucosa, gingiva, and tongue. *Candida* also can appear as diaper dermatitis.[9]
- Newborns and especially infants with very low birth weight (VLBW) have qualitative and quantitative deficiencies in humoral and cellular immunity. This can allow *Candida* to penetrate lymphatics, blood vessels, and other tissues, resulting in disseminated infection.[9]

Screening/Diagnosis

- Maternal diagnosis is most frequently done by microscopic examination of vaginal discharge to visualize the yeast and mycelia or pseudohyphae. A Gram stain and culture can also be done. *Note that a positive culture in the absence of symptoms should not lead to treatment.* As has been stated, *Candida* species are a part of many women's vaginal flora.[2]
- Newborn evaluation *of local infection* can be done by microscopic examination (wet prep) of the local site. Newborn disseminated *candidiasis* is diagnosed by blood culture.

Treatment

Maternal Treatment

A number of over-the-counter (OTC) treatments are available to women and provide greater than 80% cure rates in women with uncomplicated infection. The CDC recommends 7 day therapies.[2]

Examples of OTC vaginal creams include the following:

Clotrimazole (Gyne-Lotrimin, Mycelex) 1% cream, 5 g per vagina at bedtime for 7 days

Miconazole (Monostat), 2% cream, 5 g per vagina for 7 days

Terconazole (Terazol) 0.4% cream, 5 g per vagina for 7 days

NOTE: *Oral fluconazole (Diflucan) is contraindicated in pregnancy.*

Newborn Treatment[5]

- Treatment varies with the location and extent of infection and the infant's age.
- *Thrush* is usually treated with nystatin (Mycostatin) suspension, 1 to 2 mL given orally four times a day for 5 to 10 days.
- Candida *diaper dermatitis* is treated with nystatin ointment three times a day for 7 to 10 days. Nystatin with a corticosteroid (mycology ointment) is used in severe cases.
- Systemic or disseminated candidal infection is treated with amphotericin B. This is the mainstay of therapy for the newborn infant and is well tolerated by the VLBW infant.

Chlamydia

Chlamydia is a bacterium whose most common strains infect the mucosal epithelium (preferentially infects the squamocolumnar junction of the cervix) of the genital tract, causing infection of the cervix, destruction of the host cell, and, when untreated, infection of the upper genital tract.

Epidemiology

- Chlamydia is the most common bacterial STI in the United States and is common in pregnant women. Infection in pregnancy can have serious maternal and newborn consequences.[10]
- Between 3 and 4 million new cases are estimated to occur in the United States each year. The World Health Organization (WHO) reports that 90 million infections are detected annually worldwide. Infection is significantly underreported because of its asymptomatic nature. Simple, cost-effective screening tests are not available.[11]
- The highest rates are seen in persons under age 25.
- Prevalence rates are higher among women of childbearing age in STI clinics; urban, inner-city poor women; and non-Caucasian women.
- Undiagnosed, untreated infection may lead to pelvic inflammatory disease (PID), which is a major cause of infertility among women. Estimates are that one third of infections result in PID. Ectopic pregnancy is another adverse outcome.
- Many infected men and women are asymptomatic.
- Newborns can acquire the infection through vertical transmission during delivery.
- Despite effective therapy, approximately 155,000 infants are born to infected mothers annually.[8] Consequences are more damaging to the reproductive health of women than of men.[10] Untreated partners, noncompliance in treatment, reinfection, and lack of prenatal care all play a role.

Clinical Features[8]

- Risk factors are age younger than 25, the presence or history of other STIs, multiple sexual partners, and a new partner within 3 months.
- Epithelial tissues of the urethra, rectum, conjunctiva, and the nasopharynx are susceptible to infection.
- Infection of cervical epithelial tissue may extend to the endometrium, salpinx, and peritoneum (PID).
- Perinatal transmission may be transplacental (intrauterine) or through exposure to maternal secretions such as breastmilk; however, transmission most commonly occurs through exposure to maternal blood and vaginal secretions at the time of delivery.
- This infection is clinically similar to gonorrhea.
- Recent research indicates a threefold to fivefold increased risk of acquiring HIV when chlamydia infection is present. As many as 70% of women may have no symptoms.
- Signs of local (cervical) infection are mucopurulent discharge and a friable cervix. Bleeding occurs when the cervix is touched (e.g., in obtaining a Pap smear or simply swabbing with a cotton-tipped applicator).

Perinatal Consequences

- Approximately 50% of infants delivered vaginally of an infected mother become infected.[4,8]

- As many as one third of infected infants develop conjunctivitis. [4,8]
- Afebrile pneumonia in infants up to 3 months of age is often caused by maternally transmitted chlamydial infection. The infection often occurs weeks after hospital discharge.
- Effective prenatal screening and maternal treatment would prevent neonatal infection. However, reinfection during pregnancy is not uncommon, especially among adolescents and inner-city minority young women.
- Clinical studies implicate recent chlamydial infections in pregnant women with adverse pregnancy outcomes such as premature and preterm labor and rupture of membranes. [10]
- Genitourinary infection at 24 weeks' gestation has been found to be associated with a two- to threefold increased risk of subsequent preterm birth. [12]

Screening/Diagnosis

- Diagnosis is made by swab specimens from the endocervix or vagina or through urine testing. Culture, enzyme immunoassay (EIA) nucleic acid hybridization or nucleic acid amplification testing (NAAT) may be used depending on the source of the sample.
- The CDC recommends the following[2]:
  - Screening all sexually active women younger than 25 years of age at least annually
  - Performing annual screening of women ages 25 and older who have one or more risk factors (new or multiple sex partner and lack of barrier contraception)
  - Testing all women with cervical infection and all pregnant women
- When screening/testing for chlamydia, one should also test for gonorrhea in susceptible adults and neonates.

Treatment

Maternal Treatment[2,8,13,14]

- Appropriate completed treatment prevents transmission to sex partners and to infants during birth.

NOTE: *Treatment of the infected individual and partner should be done at the same time. Both partners should abstain from intercourse until treatment is completed.*

- Recommended treatment regimens are as follows[2]:
  Azithromycin, 1 g orally in a single dose
  OR
  Amoxicillin, 500 mg orally three times a day for 7 days

NOTE: *Doxycycline and ofloxacin are contraindicated in pregnancy.*

- Reculture in 3 weeks, preferably with NAAT (Nucleic Acid Amplification Test) to ensure therapeutic cure.

Neonatal Treatment[14]

- The recommended regimen for ophthalmia neonatorum caused by *C. trachomatis* is as follows:
  - Erythromycin base, 50 mg/kg per day, orally, divided into four doses daily, for 10 to 14 days. Topical treatment is ineffective and not recommended. Data for the use of a course of azithromycin remain unclear.[2]

Gonorrhea

Gonorrhea is a bacterial infection of the mucous membranes of the genitourinary tract; it is caused by the gram-negative bacterium *Neisseria gonorrheae*.

Epidemiology

- It is estimated that there are 600,000 new cases of gonorrhea annually in the United States.[15]
- The disease is transmitted almost exclusively by sexual contact.
- The presence of gonorrhea is a marker for the possibility of concomitant chlamydial infection owing to the clinical similarities.
- The prevalence during pregnancy may be as high as 7%.[8]
- Risk factors include adolescence, drug abuse, prostitution, and poverty, as well as being single or having other STDs.
- Adolescents experience some of the highest rates.
- Newborns may acquire the infection during delivery through an infected birth canal.

Clinical Features[8]

- The risk of a woman being infected by an infected male partner is approximately 50% per episode of vaginal intercourse. The risk of a male being infected by an infected female is 20% per episode of vaginal intercourse.
- Although rectal intercourse is an effective mode of transmission, oral–genital transmission is rare.
- Immunity is not conferred by infection.
- Most cases either resolve spontaneously or are treated and resolve within a few weeks.
- Most infections are symptomatic, but asymptomatic infections do occur.
- Signs and symptoms are painful urination (dysuria), usually without frequency or urgency; purulent cervical discharge; bleeding upon swabbing the cervix; and cervical, uterine, or adnexal tenderness.
- Disseminated gonococcal infection results from gonococcal bacteremia and has been cited as occurring in 0.5% to 3.0% of infected individuals. In pregnant women, stillbirth and spontaneous abortion are risks.

Perinatal Consequences[8,16]

- Gonococcal infection may result in adverse pregnancy outcomes in any of the trimesters. Preterm delivery, premature rupture of membranes, chorioamnionitis, and postpartum infection are associated with infection at the time of delivery.
- Ophthalmia neonatorum is the most common form of gonorrhea in infants and occurs through vertical transmission from an infected mother during delivery. Without prompt treatment, blindness can occur as a result of corneal ulceration and perforation.
- Isolation of an infected infant is recommended until treatment has been in effect for 24 hours.

Screening/Diagnosis

- Laboratory diagnosis depends on identification of *N. gonorrheae* at an infected site.
- A screening test for gonorrhea is recommended at the first prenatal visit, and a repeat test should be done after 28 weeks' gestation in high-risk populations.[8]

- Repeat testing in the third trimester is recommended in any pregnant woman who tested positive at an earlier workup because reinfection is common.[8]
- Diagnosis can be determined through culture, nucleic acid hybridization tests, and NAAT of the endocervix, vagina, or urine (source determined by assay).
- **Syphilis and chlamydia screening is strongly recommended in any individual who has tested positive for gonorrhea because these infections are commonly found concomitantly with gonorrheal infection.**
- **All pregnant women at risk or living in an area with a high incidence of gonorrhea should be screened at the first prenatal visit. Consider rescreening in the third trimester for those at continued risk.[17]**

Treatment

- For uncomplicated gonococcal infections during pregnancy, treatment consists of ceftriaxone, 125 mg intramuscularly (IM; single dose); **or** cefixime, 400 mg orally (single dose): **or** spectinomycin, 2 g IM (single dose).[2,8]
- Intrapartum prophylaxis for the newborn is instituted by the instillation of a 1% aqueous solution of silver nitrate onto the conjunctiva soon after delivery. Topical application of erythromycin or tetracycline ointment can also be used.
- Both parents of an infected infant should be screened and treated for chlamydia.

Herpes Simplex Virus Infection

The herpes simplex virus (HSV) invades sensory or autonomic nervous system ganglia and is expressed as an infection of mucosal surfaces such as the oropharynx, cervix, and vulva. Acute infection (often asymptomatic) is followed by a remission period. It is essentially a chronic infection with frequent or rare exacerbations. Two types of the virus, HSV-1 and HSV-2, differ to some degree in biologic, biochemical, and antigenic properties. HSV-1 is generally associated with infection "above the waist," whereas HSV-2 is associated with genital and neonatal infections.[18,19] Up to 50% of first cases of genital herpes are caused by HSV-1. Recurrence is less frequent with genital HSV-1 infection than it is with HSV-2.

Epidemiology

- Genital herpes is the second most prevalent sexually transmitted viral infection in the world. Unfortunately, it is incurable, and at present, no effective vaccine exists.[20]
- Approximately 50 million people have been infected with genital herpes.[2] **However, most infected individuals are asymptomatic and have never been diagnosed.** The true prevalence rate is much higher than that reported.[2,18]
- The virus can be transmitted through intimate contact and sexual activity, as well as during vaginal birth.
- An individual with herpes oral infection can transmit HSV-1 by means of oral sex to male or female genitalia.
- The majority of genital and neonatal infections are caused by HSV-2.
- Women are more easily infected with HSV-2 than men.[18]
- Higher incidences occur in adolescents and young women (early 20s).[18]

- Risk factors are age, duration of sexual activity, race, previous genital infections, and number of sexual partners.
- It is estimated that each year, 800,000 pregnant women are infected with genital herpes.[21]

Clinical Features[18,22]

- Transmission of genital herpes occurs most often by individuals who are not aware they are carrying the virus.
- Neonatal infection and an increased risk of contracting HIV are serious consequences of infection. Genital ulcerative lesions are vulnerable to infection with other STDs (e.g., syphilis, HIV).[22]
- Lesions of HSV are often multiple, quite painful, and have the appearance of wet blisters or crusted vesicles.
- Fever, malaise, inguinal lymphadenopathy, and dysuria are common, although they by no means always accompany an initial HSV-2 genital infection. Symptoms usually peak in 4 to 5 days and can last as long as 2 to 3 weeks.
- After an initial infection, recurrences can be frequent and triggered by menstruation, stress, trauma, and ultraviolet light rays (sun exposure).
- Over time, symptoms are usually less acute and frequency of outbreaks is reduced.
- Many individuals experience *prodromal symptoms* of tingling, burning, itching, tenderness, or a swelling sensation followed by the herpes outbreak of lesions in about 24 hours.[22]
- **Primary genital infection** may by symptomatic or asymptomatic (subclinical). Clinical confirmation depends on the absence of **HSV-1** and **HSV-2** antibodies at the time the individual acquires the genital infection due to **HSV-1** or **HSV-2**.
  - When systemic symptoms (malaise, fever, and myalgia) occur with herpetic infections, it is generally thought to be a primary infection reflecting a high viremic load.
  - Without therapy, these lesions resolve completely in about 3 weeks.
  - Shedding of the virus from the cervix occurs intermittently in infected women, regardless of whether symptoms are present.
- **Nonprimary first-episode genital HSV** may be symptomatic or asymptomatic. This diagnostic designation is assigned when the development of genital herpes infection/lesion(s) occurs in an individual who has preexisting antibodies, indicating previous exposure at some point in time.
  - Prior HSV-1 infection provides *some* protection from an HSV-2 infection.
  - Nonprimary first-episode infections usually do not have quite as severe clinical symptoms that characterize a symptomatic primary infection
- **Recurrent infection** may be symptomatic or asymptomatic.
  - Individual patient response varies widely in terms of frequency, severity, duration of symptoms, and amount of viral shedding.
  - Usually, herpetic blisters or ulcers are confined to the genital region.
  - Symptoms tend to be local, not systemic.
  - **Shedding of the virus from the genital tract is intermittent, occurring in both symptomatic and asymptomatic individuals.**

- Viral quantity tends to be lower when no lesion is present, but a susceptible partner can be infected. This is what makes this STI so difficult to prevent.

Perinatal Consequences[18,19,22,23]

- Maternal–fetal (vertical) transmission appears to be related to gestational age.
- The rate of vertical transmission is reduced in the presence of preexisting maternal HSV-2 antibodies. However, having HSV-1 antibodies does not appear to reduce vertical transmission.
- There is a 30% to 50% transmission rate of genital herpes to the neonate from an infected mother when the infection is acquired near the time of delivery.[2]
- The rate of transmission is low (less than 1%) among women with recurrent infections or if the infection is acquired during the first half of pregnancy.[2]
- Transmission is higher among women with recurrences because this is more common than an initial outbreak during this time and recurrences are often asymptomatic with few visible lesions.[2]
- Vaginal delivery should be avoided in any woman with sign/symptoms of an outbreak; the potential for transmission to the neonate is high.

NOTE: When maternal infection is primary but asymptomatic, cervical shedding of the virus also incurs a risk of preterm delivery and possible HSV transmission to the newborn.

- Neonatal infections can develop as three different entities.[23,24]
  1. Localized to the skin, eye, or mouth (SEM disease)
  2. Systemic, causing encephalitis with or without skin lesions
  3. Disseminated in organs such as the lungs, liver, adrenal glands, skin, or central nervous system (CNS)
- Neonatal mortality occurs rarely if ever, when infection is localized to the skin, eyes, or mouth. Mortality is about 50% to 85% with CNS involvement and disseminated disease.[24]
- Breastfeeding is contraindicated only if an obvious herpetic lesion is on the breast.

NOTE: The herpes virus is acquired by direct contact. Family members with oral lesions can infect the newborn by hand/mouth contact.

- Mothers with active lesions should be careful when handling their babies.

Screening/Diagnosis

- Weekly late third trimester screening is **not** recommended for women with a history of herpes. Many, if not most, newborns develop HSV infection in the absence of a maternal history of the disease.
- The Pap and Tzank tests are not recommended as screening tests.
- PCR assays for HSV DNA are more sensitive than viral cell cultures of the lesion(s).[25] When cultures are performed, a Dacron swab is generally used for collection. The vesicles should be scraped (unroofed) to sample the fluid within; moist ulcers and crusts are scraped well. Specimens are placed in viral transport media.[18]
- The availability of reliable, type specific serologic test for HSV-1 or HSV-2 antibodies has increased detection of asymptomatic individuals.[26] Results reflect the presence/absence of IGG antibodies, indicating past infection/exposure. IGM testing is NOT recommended as the information regarding CURRENT infection status should be determined by culture/polymerase chain reaction.

Many practices are recommending routine serologic tests in conjunction with routine prenatal laboratory testing to provide insurance that transmission to the neonate by an asymptomatic mother is reduced. If results are HSV-2 IGG positive, suppressive antiviral therapy can be introduced in late gestation, further minimizing the risk of exposure. Serologic testing should be offered to pregnant women whose partner(s) have a history of genital HSV infection (as should) counseling to discordant couples to reduce the risk of transmission during pregnancy.[2]

Treatment[2,18,19,22]

- The goal of management is to reduce or prevent neonatal risk of exposure to HSV during the later half of pregnancy and during delivery.
- Studies demonstrate that antiviral therapy (oral or parenteral) shortens the course of infection and the duration of viral shedding.
- The ACOG treatment recommendations are summarized as follows.[18] Based on limited or inconsistent scientific evidence (Level B):
  - Symptomatic women with primary HSV during pregnancy should be treated with antiviral therapy.
  - *Cesarean delivery should be performed on women with first-episode HSV who have active genital lesions at delivery.*
  - For women at or beyond 26 weeks' gestation with a first episode of HSV occurring during the current pregnancy, antiviral therapy should be considered.
- Based on consensus and expert opinion primarily[2]:
  - Cesarean delivery should be performed on women with recurrent HSV infection who have active genital lesions or prodromal symptoms at delivery.
  - Expectant management of patients with preterm labor or preterm premature rupture of membranes and active HSV may be warranted.
  - For women at or beyond 36 weeks' gestation who are at risk for recurrent HSV, antiviral therapy also may be considered.
  - *In women with no active lesions or prodromal symptoms during labor, cesarean delivery should not be performed on the basis of a history or recurrent disease.* In addition, nongenital herpetic lesions (e.g., on the thigh or buttocks) should be covered with an occlusive dressing. The woman can then deliver vaginally.
- Avoiding the use of fetal scalp electrodes (FSE) in fetal monitoring, forceps- or vacuum-assisted deliveries, and artificial rupture of membranes during labor may minimize the risk of transmission.[2,27]
- The CDC recommends using oral acyclovir (class C) during pregnancy if a first episode of HSV infection occurs. Acyclovir given in late pregnancy reduces the incidence of ceasarean section in women with recurrent outbreaks by reducing the frequency of recurrences at term.[2,23]
- Two class B antiherpetic drugs, famciclovir (Famvir) and valacyclovir (Valtrex), with their increased bioavailability, involve less frequent dosing to achieve the same therapeutic results as acyclovir. However, currently only acyclovir is FDA approved

for use during pregnancy. The CDC has maintained a drug registry for women treated with acyclovir during pregnancy. To date, no increase in fetal abnormalities has been shown.[28]

- Vaccines are under research.

Human Papillomavirus Infection

Human papillomavirus (HPV) infection is an infection of the skin and mucous membranes of the anogenital tract. There are more than 150 types of HPV. Some viral strains result in visible external genital warts, or *condylomata acuminata,* and occur in both men and women.

Epidemiology

- Genital HPV is the most prevalent STD in the United States. Approximately 80% of the sexually active population is infected with HPV. This can be manifested in active (visible warts, cervical abnormalities) or latent/subclinical infection.[22]
- Studies repeatedly show high levels of infection in women, with the highest levels among young women (under age 24).[29]
- Fewer data are available on HPV among men; however, levels of current infection in men appear to be similar to those in women.[29] For both men and women, the infection is more common than current reporting reveals.
- Data on actual prevalence are difficult to gather because reporting of HPV is based on visible lesions and some testing measures (e.g., Pap smears and subsequent workup) but many patients have no symptoms and remain undiagnosed.
- Thirty-three types of HPV have been identified that infect the genital tract. Certain types are strongly associated with cervical, penile, and anal cancer.[2,30]

Clinical Features

- HPV infections are transmitted primarily by sexual contact with an infected partner. Lesions are highly contagious.
- Considerable evidence exists that HPV is the main infectious etiologic agent in the sexual transmission of a carcinogen, which can lead to cervical cancer.[5]
- Many of the risk factors that place a woman at risk for HPV infection also characterize risk factors for cervical cancer.[2]
- *Strong risk factors for cervical cancer and its precursors* include age at first intercourse (16 years or younger), a history of multiple sexual partners, a history of genital HPV infection or another STI, the presence of other genital tract neoplasia, and prior cervical tissue changes such as a squamous intraepithelial lesion. Additional risk factors include active or passive smoking, immunodeficiency (as in HIV infection), poor nutrition, and a current or past sexual partner with risk factors for STIs.[31]
- Nonsexual transmission *may* occur, but is uncommon; the virus has been detected on underwear, sex toys, tanning salon benches, and wet towels and has been cultured from gloves, instruments, and specula. The inability to culture HPV eliminates the possibility of documenting infectability.[32]
- The incubation period ranges from 3 weeks to 8 months, with an average of 3 months.
- Infection can by symptomatic or asymptomatic. In symptomatic cases, irritation, bleeding, pruritus, and often, fleshy, pink, warty raised lesions are present singularly or in clusters on affected areas, such as the surface of the perineum, introitus, vagina, cervix, and anus.
- The diagnostic spectrum of HPV infection ranges from clinically visible lesions to subclinical infection as seen by colposcopy to latent infection in which HPV DNA is diagnosed with tissue evaluation.
- Viral types 16, 18, 31, 33, 35, and 45 have a strong correlations with cervical dysplasia, high-grade squamous intraepithelial lesions, and invasive cancer,[22] as well as with types 51, 52, 56, 58, 59, and 68. High-risk versus low-risk typing is typically performed by "reflex testing" in the presence of an abnormal pap test. It is now known that more than 95% of all cervical cancers are caused by high-risk HPV.
- On Pap smear screening, the spectrum of abnormality may begin with atypia, progress to mild dysplasia to severe dysplasia or carcinoma in situ, and conclude with invasive cancer of the cervix.
- Cervical cancer typically presents in women over age 30 and is attributed to the persistence of high risk HPV.
- Studies comparing HPV prevalence and annual incidence rates for cervical cancer suggest that only up to 3% of HPV-positive women will go on to develop cervical cancer within 20 to 50 years; most women who are HPV positive at any one point in time are not at great risk.[33]
- Most HPV infections appear to be temporary and are probably cleared by an active cell-mediated immune response. However, reactivation to reinfection is possible.[34]
- Evidence suggests the following[32]:
  - Barrier methods of contraception lower the incidence of cervical neoplasia, probably because of lessened exposure to HPV.
  - Exposure to cigarette smoking is associated with increased risk.
  - Increased intake of micronutrients and other dietary factors such as carotenoids and folic acid are associated with decreased risk.
  - Education about risk factors for cervical cancer may lead to behavioral modification, resulting in diminished exposure.

Perinatal Consequences

- Genital warts tend to grow more rapidly during pregnancy.
- Perinatal viral transmission of types 6 or 11 through aspiration of infected material during delivery can cause laryngeal papillomatosis (juvenile onset of recurrent respiratory papillomatosis [JORRP]) in infants and children. The rate of infection is unclear. Studies indicate higher incidence for children delivered vaginally compared with those delivered by means of cesarean section.[22] One estimated overall incidence of JORRP is 600 to 700 cases annually.[35]
- Although the transmission rate to the newborn's oropharynx may be high (Cunningham cites one study at 30%), it is significant to note that most of the infants cleared the virus in 5 weeks.[8] Thomas cites infection rates at 2% to 5% within the first 5 years of life. The lesions can develop in 2 to 3 months. Clinical signs are stridor, hoarseness, abnormal cry, cough, and respiratory distress.[22]
- Occasionally, clusters of condylomata acuminata on the perineum are so profuse that they interfere with vaginal delivery when performing an episiotomy is deemed necessary (the lesions tend to bleed profusely).[22]

Screening/Diagnosis[22,31,36-38]

- Screening and diagnostic methods have become more efficient and include the following:
  - Direct visualization of condylomata and biopsy

NOTE: Although condylomata acuminata are easily seen on external surfaces with the naked eye, HPV disease on the cervix usually requires magnification (colposcopy) and the application of acetic acid for identification.

  - Pap smear with directed biopsy
  - Adjuvant HPV DNA testing

Treatment

Maternal Treatment

- Genital HPV lesions may regress without treatment. It is not currently possible to predict who will have a spontaneous remission or when that could occur. Regression rates for cervical intraepithelial neoplasia (CIN) are cited from composite data as analyzed by Östör.[36] He states that the approximate likelihood of regression of CIN1 is 60%, persistence is 30%, progression to CIN3 is 10%, and progression to invasive cancer is 1%. Corresponding approximations for CIN2 are 40%, 40%, 20%, and 5%, respectively. The likelihood of CIN3 regressing is 33%, and the likelihood of progressing to invasion is greater than 12%.[36] There may be no single "best" treatment, and for some patients a combination of treatments may be appropriate, depending on the site and extent of infection, response to treatment, and patient choice.[31] Resources and the expertise of the health care provider play a pivotal role.
- No evidence exists that treatments eradicate or affect the natural course of HPV infection. The goal of treatment for visible genital warts is simply removal.[22]
- Examination and treatment of partners is unnecessary as part of the woman's treatment plan. Partner treatment should be based on that individual's choice and may often be related to psychosocial and emotional health.[22] If the patient is lesbian or bisexual, female partners should be treated.
- Treatment options include the following[2,22]:
  - Topical medication such as Podofilox 0.5% (Condylox) solution or gel and Imiquimod (Aldara) cream, which can be applied by the patient at home (although Podophillin is contraindicated in pregnancy due to its anti-mitotic properties). Imiquimod, an immune response modifier, while not currently approved, is pregnancy category C.
  - Trichloroacetic acid (TCA) or bichloracetic acid (BCA)—commonly used but must be applied by a care provider
  - Cryotherapy—freezing that destroys targeted tissue
  - Laser vaporization—surgery using a high-intensity light
  - LLETZ—large loop excision of the transformation zone: removal of affected tissue using a hot wire loop (also called LEEP)
- Trichloroacetic acid (TCA) and bichloroacetic acid (BCA) have been approved by the FDA for use during pregnancy.
- The HPV vaccine is approved for use in females aged 9 to 24. The "Gardisil" vaccine (Merck) is a quadrivalent vaccine which provides immunity to HPV types 6 and 11—most commonly associated with external genital warts; and types 16 and 18—most commonly associated with cervical dysplasia.

Although the vaccine is currently listed as pregnancy category B, it is not recommended for use during pregnancy due to the limited amount of data.[39]

Newborn Treatment

- Both medical and surgical approaches may be used in treating laryngeal papillomatosis in the newborn.

Syphilis

Syphilis is a complex STD caused by the spirochete *Treponema pallidum*. Infectivity is high, with 60% of individuals acquiring the disease during the first exposure to a partner with a primary lesion. Maternal infection may be transmitted to the fetus (congenital syphilis).

Epidemiology

- Syphilis in the United States currently is characterized by geographic concentration, with southern states experiencing the highest rates.[40] It disproportionately affects populations living near or below the poverty level, as well as those involved in high-risk activities such as prostitution, illicit drug use, and multiple sexual partners.
- The number of cases of primary and secondary syphilis increased in the United States from 2000 to 2005, with a total of almost 9,000 reported cases.[40]
- Rates of primary and secondary syphilis were higher among women aged 20 to 24 and men aged 35 to 39.[40]
- Maternal infection is primarily found in the young and unmarried and among those who receive inadequate or no prenatal care.[41]
- Untreated maternal infection results in perinatal death in up to 40% of cases; If syphilis is acquired before pregnancy, up to 70% of fetuses may be infected.[40]
- Racial/ethnic minority populations have the highest rates of congenital syphilis.
- Failure of health care provider adherence to congenital syphilis screening recommendations may also result in congenital syphilis.

Clinical Features[8,41-43]

- The disease is divided into primary, secondary, and latent phases.
- The incubation period for primary syphilis ranges from 10 to 90 days. A chancre usually develops 3 to 4 weeks after exposure.
- The chancre of *primary syphilis* occurs at the site of inoculation and appears as a red, painless ulcer with raised edges and a granulation base (button appearance). Cervical chancres are common in exposed pregnant women, probably because of the friable cervix, which is easily infected. The chancre persists for 2 to 6 weeks and heals spontaneously. Often, nontender, enlarged inguinal lymph nodes can be palpated.
- *Secondary syphilis* occurs about 4 to 10 weeks after the primary chancre has healed. In approximately 15% of women, a chancre may still be present. This secondary stage involves more widespread dissemination of the *T. pallidum* and is therefore characterized by symptoms of systemic involvement: low-grade fever, sore throat, headache, malaise, adenopathy, and rashes on

mucosal and skin surfaces. Alopecia, mild hepatitis, and kidney involvement may develop.

- The lesions of secondary syphilis may be mild and even go unnoticed. Some women develop characteristic genital lesions of secondary syphilis called *condylomata lata*. They appear as white, raised, and moist lesions and are highly infectious. These lesions resolve in 3 to 12 weeks, and the disease enters the latent phase.
- *Latent syphilis* refers to infection in individuals who have reactive serologic tests but no clinical manifestations. *Latency* is divided into *early* (1 year or less from the beginning of infection) and *late* (more than 1 year from the beginning of infection). Infectiousness continues throughout these periods.
- *Tertiary syphilis* develops after years of untreated disease. The skeletal, nervous, and cardiovascular systems may be seriously affected.
- The clinical course of syphilis is not affected by pregnancy.
- Pregnancy outcomes are drastically affected by syphilis. Transmission of the disease largely depends on the duration of maternal disease.
- The most affected infants are those *conceived* in mothers with primary or secondary syphilis. The less affected are those infants *conceived* in mothers with early-late or late-stage disease.[43]

Perinatal Consequences[8,41–44]

- Syphilis causes infection in both the unborn and newborns.
- A two- to fivefold increase in the risk of HIV transmission occurs in the presence of syphilis.[44] Direct contact with a syphilitic lesion (chancre) found on external genitalia, vagina, anus, rectum, and lips and in the mouth has a very high infection occurrence.
- The risk of prematurity, perinatal death, and congenital infection is directly related to the stage of maternal syphilis during pregnancy. Untreated early syphilis of 4 years' duration or less results in higher rates of dead or diseased infants and a significantly increased possibility of neonatal death. Adverse consequences of late latent syphilis of more than 4 years' duration are lessened, but stillbirth rates are high.[40]
- The infection can be transmitted to the fetus in utero, presumably by a transplacental route or during delivery by newborn contact with a genital lesion.
- It was formerly believed that fetal infection did not occur before the fourth month of pregnancy. This has been disproved through electron microscopy, silver staining, and immunofluorescent techniques. Infection can cause fetal morbidity during early gestation (e.g., spontaneous abortion at 9 and 10 weeks' gestation).
- Pregnancy outcomes in the presence of untreated syphilis are commonly spontaneous abortion during the second or third trimester, stillbirth, nonimmune hydrops, premature delivery, and perinatal death.
- *Most infants delivered to mothers with untreated syphilis, irrespective of disease stage or duration, do not have clinical or laboratory evidence of infection at birth. If left untreated, these infants may develop clinical signs and symptoms months or years later.*[41]
- The infection *is not* transmitted via breastfeeding *unless* an infectious lesion is present on the breast.[40]

Screening/Diagnosis[2,8,41–43,45]

Diagnostic workup and treatment of syphilis infection in the pregnant woman require a thorough understanding of the natural history of the disease and how it relates to stages (primary, secondary, and latency), clinical progressions and relapse, and the proper evaluation of therapeutic results.[43] Laboratory techniques, their degrees of accuracy, and available applicability at given stages of the disease are essential. Recently, rapid tests for syphilis have become available that may be useful in worldwide disease detection and control.[46] The following statements highlight some key points.

- Establishing the diagnosis in a pregnant woman is essentially the same as that for a nonpregnant woman.
- Dark-field microscopic examination to identify spirochetes is the most accurate method of diagnosing syphilis. However, serology is the most common method of confirming infection.
- Two basic types of serology are used: the nonspecific antibody test and the specific antitreponemal antibodies test.
- Diagnosis of syphilis in the pregnant woman is most often made by serologic screening at the first visit and repeated at 28 to 32 weeks' gestation. Approximately 90% of states have statutes that require antepartum testing for syphilis; there is variation in the number of tests required and in the timing of the tests.[47]
- In high-risk populations, for which there may be limited prenatal care, a rapid plasma reagin (RPR) card test screening should be performed at confirmation of pregnancy.[48]
- Women in high-risk areas, those with a positive serology, and those previously untested should have a third trimester serology screen for syphilis.
- Nonspecific antibody tests include the rapid plasma reagin (RPR) and the Venereal Disease Research Laboratory (VDRL). The tests are reported as reactive or nonreactive. A positive test is reported as reactive with a titer. These tests are positive in the majority of women with primary syphilitic lesions and in all women with secondary syphilis. *However, it should be noted that most will be positive only after 4 to 6 weeks of initial infection.* These tests are not highly specific; therefore, a second confirmatory test is performed on anyone with an initial positive test.
- The confirmatory test is based on identification of treponemal antibodies: fluorescent treponemal antibody absorption test (FTA-ABS) or the microhemagglutination assay for antibodies to *T. pallidum* (MHA-TP). The MHA-TP has replaced the FTS-ABS in most clinical laboratories.[45] The WHO's recommendations suggest that treponemal antigen-based enzyme immunoassays (EIAs) are an appropriate alternative to the combined VDRL/RPR and MHA-TP screen. It is a single screening test and is being used in many laboratories.[45]

NOTE: Approximately 15% of individuals with primary syphilis will be seronegative at initial testing.[9] This is due to the prozone phenomenon, which is the result of an excess amount of anticardiolipin antibody present in a patient's serum, which interferes with the test chemically. Therefore, repeat testing should be performed on anyone at risk of recent infection.

- False-positive nontreponemal tests are relatively common and can be caused by recent febrile illness; intravenous drug use; autoimmune disease such as systemic lupus erythematosus; and viral (Epstein-Barr and hepatitis), protozoal, or mycoplasmal infection. A false-positive reaction may also be seen in elderly patients, those with malignancy or other chronic diseases, and even in pregnant women.[41]

- Treponemal antibody tests FTA-ABS and MHA-TP rarely give false-positive results. Once positive, these tests remain positive for life in most individuals.

- *When there is not a documented history of adequate treatment, a negative VDRL/RPR or EIA result does not mean that treatment is not needed. Inadequate treatment may lead to nonresolution of infection and relapses that can result in congenital infection.*[45]

Diagnosis of Fetal Syphilis

- Evidence of the disease in the fetus is usually not seen until about 18 weeks' gestation.[42]

- Prenatal diagnosis is possible using ultrasonography, which can identify fetal hydrops when maternal syphilis is documented. There may be ultrasound evidence of other fetal complications from syphilis including encephalitis, bone deformities, hepatomegaly, endocarditis, and chorioretinitis. The syphilitic placenta can be very large, but is without edema.[49]

- Most often, the diagnosis depends on testing after birth, at which time serology testing, physical examination, and laboratory testing are used.

- Detection of spirochetes in amniotic fluid and in fetal blood through cordocentesis can also be done.

Diagnosis of Congenital Syphilis

- Syphilis is confirmed by the demonstration of spirochetes in lesions, body fluids, or tissue using dark-field microscopy, immunofluorescence, or histologic examination.[41]

- PCR technique is highly specific for detecting *T. pallidum* in amniotic fluid and neonatal serum and spinal fluid.[8]

- The two most common clinical findings are hepatosplenomegaly and jaundice.[42]

- Serologic testing of maternal serum is preferable to testing the neonate's serum because a low maternal titer owing to late infection may result in a negative test on the neonate when, in fact, the infection exists in an early stage.[2]

- Infants born to mothers who have reactive treponemal and nontreponemal tests must be evaluated through a serum. No reliable IgM tests exist.[2]

Treatment

Maternal Therapy[2,8]

- Benzathine penicillin is the drug of choice for both acquired and congenital syphilis.

- There are no proven alternatives to penicillin treatment during pregnancy. Erythromycin may affect a maternal cure but not prevent congenital syphilis. Currently, it is not recommended for infected pregnant women.

- Penicillin desensitization is recommended for pregnant women with penicillin allergy. This requires hospitalization and careful monitoring, but is usually successful. Desensitization produces a temporary tolerance of penicillin, but does not prevent future allergic reactions.

- Recommended treatment according to CDC guidelines is as follows[2]:

Primary: Secondary: Early latent (1 year or less):	Benzathine penicillin G 2.4 million units IM
Late latent (more than 1 year): unknown duration	Benzathine penicillin G 7.2 million units IM. TOTAL: 3 doses of 2.4 million units at 1 week intervals.

- A treatment reaction occurring in up to 60% of patients treated for early syphilis in pregnancy is called the Jarisch-Herxheimer reaction. Manifestations include fever, chills, hypotension, tachycardia, and myalgia, which occur within a few hours of treatment and resolve by 24 to 36 hours. Pregnant women may experience frequent uterine contractions and even premature labor. Nonreassuring fetal heart rate patterns and decreased fetal activity can occur. The reaction usually occurs when spirochetes are abundant and it is self-limited.[6,8]

Treatment of Congenital Syphilis

- The CDC recommends that every infant with suspected or proven congenital syphilis have a cerebrospinal examination before treatment.[2]

Symptomatic infants: Infants with abnormal spinal fluid examination:	Aqueous penicillin G Administered as 50,000 U/kg IV every 12 hours for the first 7 days of life. This is followed by 50,000 U/kg for 10 days **OR** aqueous procaine penicillin G, 50,000 U/kg IM each day *so that a total of 10 days of treatment is completed.*
Asymptomatic positive:	Benzathine penicillin G, 50,000 U/kg IM for a single dose

Infants born to mothers treated with erythromycin for syphilis during pregnancy should be treated as though they have congenital syphilis.[8]

Trichomonas (Trichomoniasis)

Trichomonas vaginalis is a vaginal infection caused by a flagellated protozoan and is spread through sexual activity.

Epidemiology

- The Vaginal Infections and Prematurity Study Group identified a 13% infection rate in 14,000 women who had cultures done at midpregnancy. The highest incidence was found in African-American women, with a lower rate for Hispanic and Caucasian women.[50]

- Approximately 5 million new cases occur each year in men and women; it is especially prevalent in the 16- to 35-year-old age group.[2]

Clinical Features[8]

- Women may be asymptomatic. Common symptoms include foul-smelling or frothy green (yellow/green) vaginal discharge, pruritus, and redness. Occasionally, abdominal pain, dysuria, and dyspareunia are experienced.
- In men, the infection tends to be asymptomatic, but occasionally, urethritis epididymitis and prostatitis can occur.
- BV is a common coinfection in pregnant women diagnosed with trichomonas.

Perinatal Consequences[3,8]

- Numerous clinical studies have shown associations between vaginal infections and preterm premature rupture of membranes, preterm delivery, and low birth weight. However, there is currently not evidence that treatment of the infection lowers the risk. Common infections such as *Trichomonas,* chlamydia, and BV continue to be evaluated and future treatments may include adjunctive anti-inflammatory therapies.

Screening/Diagnosis[8]

- FDA approved tests include:
  - The OSOM Trichomonas Rapid Test—an immunochromatographic capillary flow dipstick technology
  - The Affirm VP III—nucleic acid probe test
    Both are performed on vaginal discharge samples and have a sensitivity of more than 83% and a specificity of more than 97%. Both tests provide information in less than 1 hour.
- Wet mount preparation for microscope examination is the most common technique. This can be done immediately in an office setting, and sensitivity is considered approximately 60% to 70%.

Treatment[2,6,8]

- Metronidazole 2 g PO single dose (category B in pregnancy)
- Tinidazole 2 g PO single dose (category C in pregnancy)
- Although a *vaginal* preparation of metronidazole exists, the CDC does not recommend its use in treating *Trichomonas* as the protozoans may reside in the urethra as well as Bartholin's and Skene's glands*; oral* administration is the effective treatment method.
- The CDC cites that metronidazole may be used during pregnancy. Extensive experience with metronidazole in pregnant women demonstrates that the drug does not appear to be associated with an increased teratogenic risk.
- Alcohol consumption should be avoided while taking metronidazole and for a few days after the last dose because it may induce nausea/vomiting.
- Sexual partners should be treated, and sexual intercourse should be avoided until both partners have completed treatment.
- A test of cure is not recommended.

REFERENCES

1. Allsworth, J. E., & Peipert, J. F. (2007). Prevalence of bacterial vaginosis: 2001-2004 National health and nutrition examination survey data. *Obstetrics and Gynecology, 109*(1), 114–120.
2. Centers for Disease Control and Prevention. (2006). 2006 guidelines for treatment of sexually transmitted diseases. *MMWR Morbidity and Mortality Weekly Report, 47*(RR-1), 1–100.
3. Riggs, M. A., & Klebanoff, M. A. (2004). Vaginal infections and preterm birth. *Clinical Obstetrics and Gynecology, 47*(4), 796–807.
4. Morris, M., Nicoll, A., Simms, I., Wilson, J., & Catchpole, M. (2001). Bacterial vaginosis: A public health view. *British Journal of Obstetrics and Gynecology, 108*, 439–450.
5. ACNM Clinical Bulletins. (1999). Clinical Bulletin No. 4—December 1998. Bacterial vaginosis in pregnancy. *Journal of Nurse-Midwifery, 44*(2), 129–134.
6. Donders, G. G. (2006). Management of genital infections in pregnant women. *Current Opinions in Infectious Disease, 19,* 55–61.
7. Andrist, L. C. (2001). Vaginal health and infections. *Journal of Obstetric, Gynecologic and Neonatal Nursing, 30*(3), 306–315.
8. Cunningham, F. G., Leveno, K. J., Bloom, S. L., Hauth, J. C., Gilstrap, L. C., & Wenstrom, K. D. (Eds.). (2006). *Williams obstetrics* (22nd ed.). New York: McGraw-Hill.
9. Edwards, M. S. (2002). The immune system: Part three. Fungal and protozoal infections. In Fanaroff, A. A. & Martin, R. J. (Eds.), *Neonatal-perinatal medicine: Diseases of the fetus and infant* (Vol. 2., 7th ed., pp. 745–748). St. Louis: Mosby.
10. Rahangdale, L., Guerry, S., Bauer, H. M., Packel, L., Rhew, M., Baxter, R., et al. (2006). An observational cohort study of chlamydia trachomatis treatment in pregnancy. *Sexually Transmitted Diseases, 33*(2), 106–110.
11. Weinstock, H., Berman, S., & Cates, Jr., W. (2004). Sexually transmitted diseases among American youth: Incidence and prevalence estimates, 2000. *Perspectives in Sexual Reproductive Health, 36,* 6–10.
12. Andrews, W. W., Goldenberg, R. L., Mercer, B., Iams, J., Meis, P., Moawad, A., et al. (2000). The Preterm Prediction Study: Association of second-trimester genitourinary chlamydia infection with subsequent spontaneous preterm birth. *American Journal of Obstetrics and Gynecology, 183*(3), 662–668.
13. Miller, J. M., & Martin, D. H. (2000). Treatment of *Chlamydia trachomatis* infections in pregnant women. *Drugs, 60*(3), 597–605.
14. Edwards, M. S. (2002). Part two: Postnatal bacterial infections. In Fanaroff, A. A. & Martin, R. J. (Eds.), *Neonatal-perinatal medicine: Diseases of the fetus and infant* (Vol. 2., 7th ed., pp. 724–726). St. Louis: Mosby.
15. Centers for Disease Control and Prevention. (2004). *Sexually transmitted disease surveillance 2004.* Atlanta: US DHHS, National Center.
16. Centers for Disease Control and Prevention. (2000). Gonorrhea—United States, 1998. *MMWR Morbidity and Mortality Weekly Report, 49*(24), 538–542.
17. Miller, J. M., Maupin, R. T., Mestad, R. E., & Nsuami, M. (2003). Initial and repeated screening for gonorrhea during pregnancy. *Sexually Transmitted Diseases, 30*(9), 728–730.
18. American College of Obstetricians and Gynecologists. (1999). *Management of herpes in pregnancy* [ACOG Practice Bulletin Number 8]. Washington, DC: Author.
19. Sandhous, S. (2001). Genital herpes in pregnant and nonpregnant women. *The Nurse Practitioner, 26*(4), 15–35.
20. Patrick, D. M., Dawar, M., Cook, D. A., Krajden, M., Ng, H. C., & Rekart, M. L. (2001). Antenatal seroprevalence of herpes simplex virus type 2 (HSV-2) in Canadian women. *Sexually Transmitted Diseases, 28*(7), 424–428.
21. Centers for Disease Control and Prevention. (2004) STI fact sheet. Available at: www.cdc.gov/std/STDFact-STDs&Pregnancy.htm
22. Thomas, D. J. (2001). Sexually transmitted viral infections: Epidemiology and treatment. *Journal of Obstetric, Gynecologic, and Neonatal Nursing, 30*(3), 316–323.
23. Baker, D. (2007). HSV in pregnancy. *Current Opinion in Infectious Disease, 20,* 73–76.

24. Handsfield, H. H., Waldo, A. B., Brown, Z. A., Corey, L., Drucker, J. L., Ebel, C. W., et al. (2005). Neonatal herpes should be a reportable disease. *Sexually Transmitted Disease, 32*(9), 521–525.

25. Wald, A., Huang, M. L., Carrell, D., Selke, S., & Corey, L. (2003). Polymerase chain reaction for detection of herpes simplex virus DNA on mucosal surfaces: Comparison with HSV isolation in cell culture. *Journal of Infectious Disease, 188,* 1345–1351.

26. Whittington, W. L., Celum, C. L., Cent, A., & Ashley, R. L. (2001). Use of a glyco-protein G-based type-specific assay to detect antibodies to herpes simplex virus type 2 among persons attending sexually transmitted disease clinics. *Sexually Transmitted Diseases 28,* 99–104.

27. Brown, Z. A., Wald, A., Morrow, A. M., Selke, S., Zeh, J., & Corey, L. (2003). Effect of serologic status and cesarean delivery on transmission rates of herpes simplex virus from mother to infant. *Journal of the American Medical Association, 289,* 203–209.

28. Stone, K. M., Reiff-Eldridge, R., White, A. D., Cordero, J. F., Borwn, S., Alexander, E. R., et al. (2004). Pregnancy outcomes following systemic acyclovir exposure: Conclusions from the International Acyclovir Registry, 1984–1999. *Birth Defects Research (Part A) 70,* 201–207.

29. Centers for Disease Control and Prevention. (2001). *Tracking the hidden epidemics: Trends in STDs in the United States, 2000* (pp. 10–19). Atlanta: Author. Available at: www.cdc.gov/nchstp/dstd/disease-info.htm.

30. Centers for Disease Control and Prevention, Division of STD Prevention. (1999). *Prevention of genital HPV infection and sequelae: Report of an External Consultants' Meeting* (pp. 1–35). Atlanta: Department of Health and Human Services.

31. National Cancer Institute. (2002). *Cervical cancer (PDQ®): Prevention summary of evidence: significance and evidence of benefits.* Available at: www.cancer.gov/cancer_infor...409fa2-ff12-41e7-9f5d-2911d566d242.

32. The Association of Reproductive Health Professionals. (2001, March). *Human papillomavirus (HPV) and cervical cancer.* AHRP Clinical Proceedings (pp. 1–32). Washington, DC: Author.

33. Bristow, R. E., & Montz, F. J. (1998). Human papillomavirus: Molecular biology and screening applications in cervical neoplasia—A primer for primary care physicians. *Primary Care Update OB/GYNs, 5*(5), 238–246.

34. Czelusta, A. J., Yen-Moore, A., Evans, T. Y., & Tyring, S. K. (1999). Periodic synopsis: Sexually transmitted diseases. *Journal of the American Academy of Dermatology, 41*(4), 614–623.

35. American Social Health Association (ASHA). (1999, Spring). HPV and JORRP. *HPV News, 9*(1), 1–12.

36. Östör, A. G. (1993). Natural history of cervical intraepithelial neoplasia: A critical review. *International Journal of Gynecological Pathology, 12*(2), 186–192.

37. American Social Health Association (ASHA). (2000, Winter). The vaccine marathon. *HPV News, 10*(4), 1–12.

38. National Cancer Institute. (2001). *Human papillomaviruses and cancer.* Fact Sheet 3.20. Available at: http://cis.nci.nih.gov/fact/3-20.htm.

39. Zimmerman, R. K. (2007). HPV vaccine and its recommendations, 2007. *The Journal of Family Practice, 56*(2), S1–S5.

40. Centers for Disease Control and Prevention. (1998). Primary and secondary syphilis—United States, 1999. *MMWR Morbidity and Mortality Weekly Report, 50*(7), 113–117.

41. Sanchez, P. J., & Wendel, G. D. (1997). Syphilis in pregnancy. *Clinics in Perinatology, 22*(1), 71–90.

42. Gilstrap, L. C., & Faro, S. (1997). Syphilis in pregnancy. *Infections in pregnancy* (2nd ed., pp. 135–149) New York: John Wiley & Sons.

43. Wicher, V., & Wicher, K. (2001). Pathogenesis of maternal-fetal syphilis revisited. *Clinical Infectious Diseases, 33*(3), 354–363.

44. Centers for Disease Control and Prevention, Division of Sexually Transmitted Diseases. (2001, May). *Syphilis elimination: History in the making.* Available at: www.cdc.gov/nchstp/dstd/FactSheets/SyphilisFacts.htm.

45. Young, H. (2000). Guidelines for serological testing for syphilis. *Sexually Transmitted Infections, 76*(5), 403–405.

46. Peeling, R. W. (2006). Testing for sexually transmitted infections: A brave new world? *Sexually Transmitted Infections, 82,* 425–430.

47. Hollier, L. M., Hill, J. Sheffield, J. S., & Wendel, Jr. G. D. (2003). State laws regarding prenatal syphilis screening in the United States. *American Journal of Obstetrics and Gynecology, 189,* 1178–1183.

48. Centers for Disease Control. (2006). STD Treatment Guidelines, Special Populations. Available at: www.cdc.gov/std/treatment/2006/specialpops.htm.

49. Bailão, L. A., Osborne, N. G., Rizzi, M. C. S., Bonilla-Musoles, F., Duarte, G., & Bailão, T. C. R. S. (2006). Ultrasound markers of fetal infection, Part 2: Bacterial, parasitic, and fungal infections. *Ultrasound Quarterly, 22,* 137–151.

50. Cotch, M. F., Pastorek, J. G., II, Nugent, R. P., Yerg, D. E., Martin D. H., & Eschenbach, E. A. (1991). (Vaginal infections and prematurity study group). Demographic and behavioral predictors of *Trichomonas vaginalis* infection among pregnant women. *Obstetrics & Gynecology, 78,* 1087.

APPENDIX B

Treatment of Diabetes During Pregnancy and Review of Diabetic Ketoacidosis

Mary Copeland Myers ■ *Donna Jean Ruth*

The three hallmarks in the treatment of diabetes during pregnancy are as follows:
1. Medical nutritional therapy
2. Exercise
3. Pharmacologic therapy—insulin or glyburide

Careful attention to each component is essential to optimizing glucose control.

Medical Nutritional Therapy

Medical nutritional therapy (MNT) is an essential component of successful diabetic management. Adherence to the plan is often challenging for pregnant women but is essential for successful management. To facilitate adherence, the MNT needs to be sensitive to culture, ethnicity, and financial considerations. Each patient needs an *individualized plan* appropriate to her lifestyle and diabetic management goals. Monitoring of blood glucose, HbA$_{1c}$, lipids, blood pressure, and renal status is included in the MNT plan.

Goals may differ depending on whether the patient has type 1, type 2, or gestational diabetes. The overall goals are:
1. Achieve and maintain euglycemia, a lipid and lipoprotein profile that reduces the risk for vascular disease, and promotes normal blood pressure levels.
2. Prevent or slow the rate of development of chronic complications of diabetes.
3. Address individual nutritional needs by including personal and cultural preferences and the individual's willingness to change.
4. Maintain normalcy and pleasure in eating by only limiting food choices when supported by evidenced base research.[1]

The recommended amount of calories must be individualized. During pregnancy with a singleton fetus, caloric requirements increase by approximately 300 kcal/d. The most appropriate recommended calorie intake depends on pregravid weight (Table B.1).[2]

TABLE B.1 RECOMMENDATIONS FOR CALORIC INTAKE DURING PREGNANCY

BODY WEIGHT	CALORIE REQUIREMENTS (kcal/kg)
<90% of ideal body weight	30–40
Ideal body weight	30–35
>120% above ideal body weight	24

The recommended distribution of calories is 40% to 50% complex high-fiber carbohydrates, 20% protein, and 30% to 40% primarily unsaturated fat. For obese women, carbohydrate restriction to 35% to 40% of calories has been shown to decrease maternal glucose values and improve maternal and fetal outcomes.[2] Most plans consist of three meals and two to four snacks each day. Consistency in times and amounts of food assist in preventing hypoglycemia. An evening snack assists in preventing overnight accelerated ketosis. Calorie distribution should be 10% to 20% at breakfast, 20% to 30% at lunch, 30% to 40% at dinner, and the remaining 30% for snacks.[2]

Carbohydrate monitoring, either by carbohydrate counting, exchanges, or experienced-based estimates is a key strategy. Currently, carbohydrate counting is the most popular and allows great flexibility.[3] Adequate energy intake must be provided for appropriate weight gain during pregnancy. A minimum of 175 g of carbohydrates should be provided. Ketonemia from ketoacidosis or starvation ketosis must be avoided.[1] Many methods for teaching meal planning exist. The choice of method must be individualized for each woman. **The exchange list method and carbohydrate counting method are commonly used.**

The Exchange List Method

- This method was developed and published by the American Dietetic Association and the American Diabetes Association.
- Foods are listed based on calorie and macronutrient composition.
- Foods in each list can be exchanged for other foods in the same list.
- The meal plan specifies when and how many exchanges for each group can be eaten at each meal or snack.

The Carbohydrate Counting Method

- This method is endorsed by the American Diabetes Association.
- It offers greater flexibility in food and choices.
- More self-monitoring of blood glucose and decision making by the patient is required.
- Emphasis is on the total amount of carbohydrate in each food, not the type of carbohydrate.
- The patient must count the total amount of carbohydrate in each food item.

To calculate the required carbohydrates per day:
1. Calculate the amount of calories the patient requires each day.
2. Calculate the percentage of carbohydrates the patient needs based on the required calories per day.
3. Divide the number of calories by 4 because there are 4 calories per gram of carbohydrate.

Example:
1. Patient's weight is 66 kg × 30 kcal/kg per day = 1,980 kcal/d
2. If 50% of diet is carbohydrates, divide 1,980 by 2 = 990 kcal in carbohydrates
3. Divide 990 kcal by 4 (4 kcal per carbohydrate) = 247 g of carbohydrates per day

The many variations in carbohydrate counting include counting carbohydrate servings, counting carbohydrate exchanges, counting carbohydrate grams, counting carbohydrates plus proteins, and counting total available glucose (TAG), which includes carbohydrates, protein, and fat. Three levels of carbohydrate counting have been identified and are based on the increasing level of complexity and skills required for each level (Table B.2).[4] Evidence-based research does indicate that there is not sufficient evidence to recommend the use of glycemic index or glycemic load but foods high in fiber are encouraged. *Although many hospitals diets continue to be ordered based on calorie levels based on the "ADA diet," since 1994, the ADA has not endorsed any single meal plan. Hospitals should consider implementing a diabetes meal planning system that provides consistency in carbohydrate content of specific meals.*[1]

TABLE B.2	THREE LEVELS OF CARBOHYDRATE COUNTING
LEVEL OF CARBOHYDRATE COUNTING	**REQUIREMENTS**
Level 1 (basic)	Counting consistent amounts of carbohydrates at each meal and snack
Level 2 (intermediate)	Level 1 + learning the relationship between food, medication, activity, and blood glucose
Level 3 (advanced)	Level 1 + level 2 + learning to match insulin to carbohydrate intake using a carbohydrate:insulin ratio

Exercise

Because metabolism is affected by exercise, the pregnant woman with diabetes must be aware of the impact of exercise on her diabetes. Maternal fitness and sense of well-being may be enhanced by exercise.

Because of the physiologic changes that occur with pregnancy, diabetic women should be aware of the following:
- The impact of pregnancy on exercise
- The impact of exercise on diabetes

For women without obstetric or medical complications, cardiorespiratory and muscular fitness can be maintained during pregnancy with moderate levels of physical activity. Pregnancy causes physiologic changes in the cardiovascular, respiratory, mechanical, thermoregulatory, and metabolic systems. Women should be encouraged to exercise for 30 minutes or more each day.[2] Walking, stationary bicycling, low-impact aerobics, and swimming are recommended.[5] Heart rates during exercise should not exceed 140 bpm. During exercise in individuals *without diabetes, the plasma insulin normally decreases, along with an increase in plasma counterregulatory hormones* (Table B.3). This allows hepatic glucose production and lipolysis to match glucose utilization during exercise. However, in individuals *with type 1 diabetes, these hormonal adaptations are absent and the insulin is exogenous* (by injection). Therefore, too little insulin with an excess release of counterregulatory hormones during exercise may cause a rise in already elevated glucose levels. It can even precipitate diabetic ketoacidosis (DKA). On the other hand, excess exogenous insulin can prevent the increased mobilization of glucose and produce hypoglycemia (see Table B.3). With type 2 diabetic and gestational diabetic patients, exercise benefits include an improvement in carbohydrate metabolism and insulin sensitivity.

TABLE B.3	EFFECTS OF EXERCISE		
TYPE OF PATIENT	**INSULIN**	**COUNTER-REGULATORY HORMONES**	**BLOOD GLUCOSE LEVEL**
Type 1 diabetic (exogenous insulin)	Too little	Excess release	Hyperglycemia (DKA is possible)
	or Too much Decreased	Absent adaptation Increased	Hypoglycemia Normal blood glucose
Nondiabetic (endogenous insulin)			

General guidelines that should be followed during exercise include the following:[5,6]
- Before initiating an exercise program, all patients should have a medical evaluation, be educated on benefits and risks of exercise, and understand the potential effects of exercise on glucose levels.
- Ensure metabolic control before exercising. Exercise is safe when glucose levels are between 90 and 140 mg/dL. If blood glucose is above 250 mg/dL, the urine should be checked for ketones. If positive for ketones, exercise should be delayed

until glycemic control is obtained and ketones are resolved. If ketones are negative but blood glucose is above 300 mg/dL, be cautious with exercise.

- Exercise programs should last no more than 45 minutes.
- Meals should be consumed 1 to 3 hours before the exercise program.
- Insulin should be given in the abdomen and not injected into active muscles. Decrease the bolus insulin if its peak coincides with the exercise period.
- Monitor blood glucose before and after exercise. Identify when changes in the insulin regimen or diet are necessary. Learn the way the body responds to different types of exercise.
- Monitor necessary food intake. Eat extra carbohydrates as needed to prevent hypoglycemia and always have carbohydrates available during and after exercise.
- Include a warm-up an cool-down period with each exercise session.
- Avoid exercising in the supine position after the first trimester to prevent aortocaval compression and hypotension.

Additional new recommendations include[7]:

- To improve glycemic control, assist with weight control, and reduce the risk of cardiovascular disease, aerobic physical exercise should be performed for at least 150 min/week. The activity should be distributed over at least 3 days per week with no more than 2 consecutive days without physical activity.
- If without contraindications, women with type 2 diabetes should be encouraged to perform resistance exercise three times a week, targeting all major muscle groups, progressing to 8 to 10 repetitions at a maximum weight.

Insulin and Treatment Regimens

Insulin is formed from a substance called "proinsulin." It is a hormone produced by the β cells of the islets of Langerhans in the pancreas. When the pancreas is stimulated by elevated blood glucose, the proinsulin molecule is broken apart into insulin and the connecting peptide referred to as "C-peptide." These two molecules are then secreted into the bloodstream in equal amounts. *Because insulin has a short half-life, the C-peptide level can be measured to monitor endogenous insulin production and to determine the type of diabetes an individual has. Normal daily insulin secretion in a healthy, non-pregnant woman is 0.5 to 0.7 U/kg each day.*

The goal of insulin therapy is to mimic the physiologic profile of insulin secretion. In a person without diabetes, insulin is released gradually throughout the day to counteract ongoing hormonal influences. This is called the **basal rate.** When food is ingested, a quick release of insulin occurs. This is called the **bolus.** Insulin management involves developing a regimen to provide exogenous insulin when it is necessary.

Proper use of exogenous insulin must be formulated based on the type of insulin selected and the amount of insulin prescribed. Currently, there are more than 20 types of insulin products. Insulin can be delivered by the common syringes, insulin pens, jet injectors, or insulin pumps. Research is currently focusing on the insulin patch and inhaled insulin. As of January 2006, pork insulin was no longer manufactured or marketed in the United, and in 1998, beef insulin was discontinued. Recombinant human insulin and insulin analogs have replaced animal-derived insulin.[8] Insulin is usually classified based on the peak effect and on duration of action.

The most common types of insulin used during pregnancy are as follows:

Examples	Type of Insulin
• Humalog (lispro) NovoLog (aspart)	Rapid-acting
• Humulin R Novolin R	Short-acting = Regular
• Humulin N Humulin L Novolin N Novolin L	Intermediate-acting = NPH
• Lantus (glargine)	Long-acting

The major complication of insulin therapy is hypoglycemia.

The choice of insulin for each patient is individualized. For patients with a regular schedule and set mealtimes, usually regular and NPH insulin are used. This choice involves only two injections each day. For patients with a hectic schedule and irregular mealtimes, usually Humalog and Glargine are used or Humalog and NPH. The combination of Humalog and Glargine allows for flexibility because Humalog is given immediately before each meal; however, it involves four injections each day. See Table B.4 for characteristics of Lispro, Aspart, regular, NPH, and Glargin insulin.[9]

TABLE B.4 ACTION OF INSULIN[9]

INSULIN	ONSET OF ACTION (hr)	PEAK ACTION (hr)	THERAPEUTIC DURATION (hr)	APPEARANCE
Lispro	15 min	30–90 min	3–5	Clear
Novolog	15 min	40–50 min	3–5	
Regular	30–60 min	50–120 min	5–8	Clear
NPH				Cloudy
Humulin N & Novolin N	1–3	8	20	
Humulin L & Novolin L	1–2.5	7–15	18–24	
Lantus	1	none	24	Cloudy

The currently available concentrations of insulin in the United States are **U-100** and **U-500**. **U-100** is the most commonly used. The choice of insulin should be made based on the patient's individual needs. Fixed mixtures of NPH and regular insulin, such as 70/30 or 50/50, are available, but their use is not encouraged during pregnancy because the fixed combinations do not allow flexibility in adjustments for tight control.

The total dose of insulin is calculated based on the patient's weight, blood glucose values, and caloric intake. When insulin therapy is started in the first trimester, the initial total dose is usually calculated at approximately 0.8 U/kg per day. The insulin requirement increases throughout pregnancy as a result of increasing hormones (Table B.5).[10]

TABLE B.5	INSULIN REQUIREMENTS DURING PREGNANCY[9,10]
GESTATIONAL PERIOD	**INSULIN REQUIREMENT (U/kg)**
Preconception	0.6
First trimester	0.8
Second trimester	1.0
Third trimester	1.2
Obese woman and type 2 diabetic patients may require up to 2.0 U/kg because of the high degree of insulin resistance.	

Many insulin regimens can be used to obtain glycemic control. These include a single-dose injection, a two-injection regimen, a three-injection regimen, a four-injection regimen, or a continuous subcutaneous insulin infusion by an insulin pump.

> The common insulin regimens are as follows:
> 1. Regular and NPH insulin
> 2. NPH and Humalog
> 3. Humalog and Glargine
> 4. Insulin pump with Humalog

The two-injection regimen with regular and NPH insulin consists of two thirds of the dose in the morning, with one third of the dose in the evening (Table B.6). Of the morning dose, one third is regular insulin and two thirds is NPH. Of the afternoon dose, half is regular insulin and half is NPH.

TABLE B.6	CALCULATION OF INSULIN FOR TWO-INJECTION REGIMEN OF REGULAR AND NPH INSULIN		
TIME OF DAY	**TOTAL DAILY DOSE**	**REGULAR INSULIN**	**NPH INSULIN**
Morning dose	⅔	⅓	⅔
Evening dose	⅓	½	½

With the **four-injection regimen involving Glargine and Humalog,** half of the dose is Glargine and half of the dose is Humalog. The Humalog dose is divided into three doses and given immediately before meals. One third is given as the breakfast dose, one third is given as the lunch dose, and one third is given as the supper dose. The Glargine dose can be given at any time of the day but always the same time of day. *It cannot be mixed with other insulins* (Table B.7).

TABLE B.7	CALCULATION OF INSULIN FOR FOUR-INJECTION REGIMEN	
TIME OF DAY	**HUMALOG (½ Total Daily Dose)**	**GLARGINE (½ Total Daily Dose)**
Breakfast	⅓	All at any time of day
Lunch	⅓	BUT always the same
Dinner	⅓	time

Last, with the **continuous subcutaneous infusion using the insulin pump,** a basal rate is programmed into the pump to deliver a set rate of insulin throughout the day; the rate may be altered depending on the time of day and the patient's activity. *Most patients have three basal rates.* The first is a low rate from midnight to approximately 4 AM to prevent nocturnal hypoglycemia. The second is an increased rate from 4 AM until approximately 10 AM to counteract the increased release of the cortisol and growth hormone that causes the dawn phenomenon. The third is an intermediate rate from 10 AM until midnight. The patient activates the pump to deliver a bolus of insulin with each meal to cover the glycemic response to food.[5]

Oral antidiabetic agents are not the drugs of choice to use during pregnancy for preexisting diabetes. Although research has been done to compare the use of glyburide (an oral diabetogenic medication) with insulin use among women with gestational diabetes, its use during pregnancy has *not* been approved by the U.S. Food and Drug Administration. In addition, metformin has been studied in the first trimester for women with polycystic ovary syndrome; however, at this time, it is not approved for use in gestational diabetes. *The ADA and ACOG both recommend insulin over other agents for glycemic control in pregnant women with preexisting diabetes.*

Diabetic Ketoacidosis

Diabetic ketoacidosis is a medical emergency that represents a state of acute diabetic decompensation. Prompt recognition and immediate and effective treatments are necessary to optimize both maternal and fetal health. DKA in pregnancy occurs most commonly in women who are insulin dependent but it is important to note that DKA has also occurred in pregnant women who have not been previously diagnosed with diabetes and they develop DKA.

Physiologic Changes That Predispose Women to DKA

Some of the normal physiologic changes that occur in the maternal system due to pregnancy will predispose diabetics to developing DKA. This is often referred to as the *diabetogenic effect of pregnancy*. These include:

- **Decreased ability to buffer acids**—the normal state of acid–base balance in pregnancy is a compensated respiratory alkalosis. This means the kidneys are secreting increased amounts of bicarbonate to maintain a normal pH in the blood and tissues. When there are increased acids produced during DKA, there is less buffer available to maintain the normal balance and increased vulnerability to metabolic acidosis occurs.
- **Increased insulin resistance**—during pregnancy insulin resistance is increased. This is the result of maternal hormones that impair/decrease the effectiveness of maternal insulin. These hormones include human placental lactogen, progesterone, estrogen, cortisol, and placental insulinase.
- **Increased insulin requirements**—as pregnancy progresses, insulin requirements also increase because of the increased insulin resistance. Adjustments in insulin doses may not keep up with the insulin requirements and the result is hyperglycemia and potentially DKA. These women need to maintain close contact with providers so that the insulin doses are adjusted to meet the increasing demand. This fact may also account for the fact that there is a higher incidence of DKA in the second and third trimesters.[11]

Factors That May Precipitate DKA

There are a variety of causes that can precipitate the development of DKA during pregnancy and these include:

- **Infections**—this can be a very common cause so it is important to identify and treat any infections during pregnancy. When women present with DKA a source of infection should be assessed and tested for.
- **Acute illness and stress** that can affect normal homeostasis. This may include women who have hyperemesis.
- **Medications**—especially β-adrenergic drugs given to inhibit labor and steroids given to enhance fetal lung maturity. Magnesium sulfate may be a better choice for tocolysis. If steroids are given for fetal lung immaturity, close monitoring of maternal blood glucose and adjustments to insulin dosages should be done.
- **Insulin pump failure**—this has been reported as a precipitating factor; however, it is difficult to assess how commonly this occurs.
- **Noncompliance with treatment**—this can be for many reasons including late access to prenatal or diabetic care and inadequate understanding of the physiologic changes of pregnancy that make the development of DKA much more common in pregnancy.

Pathophysiologic Effects of DKA (Maternal)

DKA is the result of inadequate insulin action, overproduction of glucose by the liver, and increased production of ketones (which are acids). These changes lead to derangements in the maternal system that are life-threatening for both mother and fetus.

- **Hyperglycemia**—decreased action of insulin and insulin resistance results in decreased glucose uptake by the cells. The result is increased maternal serum glucose levels.

- **Dehydration**—the hyperglycemia increases serum osmolarity and because of the increase in osmolarity into fluid moves from the tissue into the bloodstream. When the amount of glucose exceeds the renal threshold, glucose will be spilled into the urine. Glucose in the urine acts as a diuretic pulling water and electrolytes with it. The result is significant dehydration—both at the cellular level and in intravascular volume.
- **Hypovolemia**—the result of the dehydration is hypovolemia, decreased tissue perfusion, possible renal failure, hypovolemic shock, and death if the dehydration is not quickly corrected.
- **Electrolyte imbalances**—buffers are depleted as the acidosis develops. Electrolytes are also lost with the vomiting (which often occurs in women who are acidotic). Decreases in potassium, sodium, chloride, magnesium, and bicarbonate are to be expected.
- **Ketosis**—the lack of insulin results in cells that are glucose deprived. Fats are broken down as an alternative energy source for the cells. The result of this fat metabolism is ketones, which are acids. This breakdown of fats occurs rapidly during DKA. The amount of ketones produced is more than can be used by the cells, so the ketones accumulate and contribute to the development of the acidosis.

Effects of DKA on the Fetus

Maternal DKA can have potentially life threatening effects on the fetus, the most significant being fetal death. There are several processes that contribute to the fetal condition. Maternal hypovolemia leads to decreased perfusion of the placenta and fetus. Maternal acidemia also decreases uterine blood flow, reduces tissue perfusion, and decreases the amount of oxygen available to the fetus. With the increase in ketone production, ketoacids breakdown and these breakdown products (which are acids) readily cross the placenta leading to fetal metabolic acidosis.[12] All efforts should be directed at correcting the maternal condition.

IMPORTANT NOTE: Delivery should not be considered until the maternal condition is stabilized and corrected. The correction of the maternal condition usually results in correction of the fetal condition.

DKA = Dehydration, Ketosis, and Acidosis

These women usually present with malaise, nausea and vomiting, poor skin turgor, dry mucous membranes, increased heart rate, increased respiratory rate, and fruity odor on their breath. Altered mental status, from drowsiness up to coma, is possible. Assessment of the fetal monitor strip reflects the maternal status. It is common to see fetal tachycardia, minimal to absent variability, and late decelerations. Stabilization and treatment of the mother are the priority on admission.

NOTE: DKA can occur in pregnancy with only mild elevations in maternal glucose levels.

Treatment

The hallmark treatments for DKA are hydration and insulin therapy.
- **Rehydration**—fluid replacement is the most important component in the treatment of DKA. Often the fluid deficits may be as high as 8 to 10 L. Multiple formulas exist for estimating the fluid deficit and use of these formulas can serve as a useful

guide in the initial volume resuscitation. Large-bore IV access or placement of a central line allows for rapid volume replacement and should be done as soon as possible when the diagnosis of DKA is present. Initially volume replacement is 1 L of normal saline over the first hour followed by 250 to 500 mL/h until at least 75% of the deficit is corrected. Correction of the deficit can be assessed by looking for a return to normal hemodynamic parameters including heart rate, blood pressure, and respiratory rate. Once maternal glucose levels reach 250 mg/dL the replacement fluid should be continued with an IV solution that contains 5% glucose. Some recommend that solutions with lactate, such as D5LR be avoided as the lactate may contribute to the acidosis.

- **Insulin Therapy**—should begin once IV hydration has begun. Remember that these women are very insulin resistant so they may require larger amounts of insulin to treat the hyperglycemia. The recommended insulin therapy for DKA is regular insulin given as an IV infusion. Multiple formulas exist for determining the initial dose required. Adjustments to the dose will be based on maternal glucose levels. If glucose levels do not decrease by 20% to 25% after the first hour of IV insulin infusion the dose should be doubled.[11,12] When the glucose levels fall to 250 mg/dL, the mainline IV should be changed to a glucose-containing solution to avoid the hypoglycemia. While insulin is infusing, maternal glucose levels should be monitored every 1 to 2 hours with adjustments in insulin dosage as necessary. There are some computer programs available that will do this based on set criteria and formulas. These programs may be very useful in standardizing treatment.

- **Electrolyte Replacement**—close monitoring of electrolyte levels is essential. Replacement of potassium should begin if adequate renal function can be established. Potassium replacement should begin once fluid replacement and insulin therapy have been initiated. Hypokalemia can cause life threatening cardiac arrhythmias so ECG monitoring should be done on all women in DKA. The goal is to achieve a K^+ level of 4 to 5

mEq/L. Replacement of other electrolytes such as chloride and magnesium should be guided by the maternal serum values. Replacement with sodium bicarbonate is controversial and it's use should be avoided.[11,12]

REFERENCES

1. American Diabetes Association. (2007). Nutrition recommendations and interventions for diabetes. *Diabetes Care, 30*(Suppl 1), S48–S65.
2. Gabbe, S. G., & Graves, C. R. (2007). Management of diabetes mellitus complicating pregnancy. In J. Queenan (Ed.), *High-risk pregnancy* (pp. 98–109). Washington, DC: American College of Obstetricians and Gynecologists.
3. Roberts, S. S. (2007). Carb counting: A flexible way to plan meals. *Diabetes Forecast,* 25–26.
4. American Diabetes Association. (2005). Carbohydrate counting: The basics. *Clinical Diabetes, 23,* 123–124.
5. Harris, G. D., & White, R. D. (2005). Diabetes management and exercise in pregnant patients with diabetes. *Clinical Diabetes, 23,* 165–168.
6. Sigal, R. J., Kenny, G. P., Wasserman, D. H., & Castaneda-Sceppa, C. (2004). Physical activity/exercise and type 2 diabetes. *Diabetes Care, 27,* 2518–2539.
7. American Diabetes Association. (2007). Standards of medical care in diabetes-2007. *Diabetes Care, 30,* S4–S41.
8. U.S. Food and Drug Administration. (2005). *Frequently asked questions about importing beef or pork insulin for personal use.* Available at: www.fda.gov/cder/drug/beefandporkinsulin/default.htm. Retrieved May 19, 2007.
9. U.S. Food and Drug Administration. (2002). *Insulin preparation.* Available at: www.fda.gov/fdac/features/2002/chrt_insulin.html. Retrieved May 19, 2007.
10. Langer, O., Anyaebunam, A., & Brustman, L. (1988). Pregestational diabetes: Insulin requirements throughout pregnancy. *American Journal of Obstetrics and Gynecology, 159,* 616–662.
11. Ramin, K. (1999). Diabetic ketoacidosis in pregnancy. *Obstetrics and Gynecology Clinics, 26*(3), 481–488.
12. Carroll, M. A., & Yeomans, E. R. (2005). Diabetic ketoacidosis in pregnancy. *Critical Care Medicine, 33*(10), 1–11.

APPENDIX C

To Comfort Always: Caring for the Dying Newborn*

Mary Jo Gilmer ■ *Angel Carter*

> **To Cure Sometimes**
> **To Relieve Often**
> **To Comfort Always**
>   **—Hippocrates**

Self-Assessment Quiz

	True	False
1. Chronically ill newborns become tolerant of painful procedures.	☐	☐
2. A fetus can feel pain as early as 20 weeks gestation.	☐	☐
3. Newborns experience less pain than adults because of immature neurologic systems.	☐	☐
4. Morphine is never the drug of choice to treat pain because of the side effect of respiratory depression.	☐	☐
5. Newborns in ICUs are subjected to up to 130 procedures every 24 hours, many of which are painful.	☐	☐
6. Dying newborns need 130 cal/kg per day for maintenance nutrition.	☐	☐
7. All families should be at the bedside of a dying newborn.	☐	☐

Answers may be found at the end of this appendix, just before the references. If you answered all statements correctly, you are well on your way to providing excellent comfort care for the dying newborn.

Cure Sometimes

Infants with lethal conditions may be stillborn, die within a few minutes of birth, or may live several hours to days or even months. In many circumstances, the exact timetable cannot be accurately predicted. It is important, therefore, to attend to preparing the family *as soon as possible* for the experience to come, while preserving the moments that they may have with their baby. Advanced preparation is essential to ensure the minutes, hours, or days of their baby's life are experienced as meaningful and memorable.[1] Providing families with information regarding the likely course of their infant's brief life facilitates discussions regarding what the family can do for the infant, allowing them to perform basic parenting tasks, even as their baby dies.

Case Report

Baby Abigail was born at 38 weeks to a 28-year-old mother via a spontaneous vaginal delivery. She weighed 6 pounds. Mom is married and has one other child, reported to be a "healthy 2-year-old." Abigail was diagnosed at 18 weeks' gestation with anencephaly. Mom and dad were "devastated" with the diagnosis, although reportedly "did research" and had a modified birth plan available. Her delivery was unremarkable and she had adequate heart rate and respiratory effort at birth. No resuscitative efforts were performed, and she was wrapped and placed in mom's arms shortly after delivery. Mom and Dad had requested that a hat be placed on the baby's head after confirmation of the prenatal diagnosis, before their viewing of their baby. Based on prior conversations with their care providers, the parents requested that Abigail forego admission to the NICU and that they be allowed to take her with them to mother's postpartum room. Should Abigail continue to survive, they desired to bathe her, dress her, feed her, and, if possible, take her home. They also wanted Abigail's brother to make a brief visit. Abigail was transferred with mom to the postpartum floor. Mom reported that Abigail was "hungry" and attempted breastfeeding, which appeared to satisfy the baby. Dad stated that Abigail became restless and cried when her diaper was wet or dirty, and that changing her diaper "made her happy." Big brother held Abigail while other family members took photos. The family minister performed a blessing. At 9 hours of age, Abigail's skin began to "look purple-ish," she lost interest in feedings, and became lethargic. Within a few hours, mom reported that Abigail looked "uncomfortable." An assessment noted that Abigail's respirations had become difficult and she appeared agitated. A call to the NICU staff brought about an order for ativan and she subsequently appeared more comfortable. At 13 hours of age, her respirations were markedly slowed, became shallow and intermittent, and soon ceased. She remained in Mom's arms during confirmation of her absent heart rate. Mom and Dad requested private time to be with Abigail, during which time they bathed and dressed her. After a few hours, they wished for other family members, including Abigail's brother, to hold and spend time with Abigail. They requested "extra blankets" be wrapped around her so that she not "feel cold." During this time, staff members gathered items for the memory box including her hand and foot prints, another hat, and other keepsake items. Abigail's parents were added to the Bereavement Follow-Up program and they attended the Remembering Ceremony sponsored by the hospital in the year after her death.

* This text is based on the appendix originally written by Francine R. Margolius for the 3rd edition of this book. Her contribution is gratefully acknowledged.

Occasionally, some families choose not to have their baby with them as their baby is dying, for many reasons, including cultural, religious, and/or psychosocial. Care should be taken in exploring the wishes of the family while providing enough information for the family to make a choice that they will remember as being the right one for them. Integrating the palliative care principles of attending to the newborn's quality of life, family emotional and spiritual needs, and pain and symptom management[2] helps to ensure a memorable and relatively atraumatic experience.

Relieve Often

For many years, it was thought that newborns did not experience discomfort or pain due to an immature central nervous system. Procedures were performed without regard to the newborn's comfort or level of pain. Current evidence-based practice mandates vigilant nursing assessment and management to prevent and relieve unnecessary infant pain or discomfort.

Hunger

Some infants with life-limiting conditions may still express signs of what we believe to be hunger. Allowing sucking or feeding (orally or by nasogastric tube) may bring about a sense of satiation or fullness to the infant and thus comfort to both infant and family. Although the goals of feeding an infant who is very near death are not the same as for those whose growth and development are considerations, feeding a baby is a fundamental act of nurturing in which many families need, and choose, to participate. It will be important to teach family members to monitor signs of feeding intolerance, which will likely increase as the baby approaches the end of life, and can contribute to potentially severe discomfort for the infant. Frequent regurgitation of formula, choking, and lack of hunger cues may all be indications that the frequency, quantity, route, and/or viability of feedings needs to be reevaluated. In the face of feeding intolerance, but continued agitation/restlessness, comfort feedings via a syringe, eyedropper, or perhaps the sucking of a pacifier or finger may provide family with additional opportunities for memory making.[3] Conversely, the decision to withhold feedings in an infant who will not survive is also to be acknowledged and respected, after appropriate communications between family and the care team.

Mouth Care

For those infants not feeding, periodic moistening of the lips and tongue may be helpful. Use moist gauze wrapped around a finger or moistened small cotton swabs to gently wipe around the mouth area.

Skin Care

Although bathing is not necessary, it may be the parents' desire to either have this done or participate in grooming their baby. Wiping with a warm, moist washcloth or applying nonperfumed lotion may be satisfactory. Provide routine care for diaper changes.

Eye Care

In the event of eyelid non-closure, artificial tears may be helpful.

Symptom Management

As an infant nears death, there may be physiologic clues that, when recognized, can provide valuable opportunities to assist families in caring for their baby and to attend to symptoms that may need to be treated, ameliorated, or palliated.

Symptoms that may occur include the following:
- Bluish discoloration of skin, particularly around the mouth
- Breathing becomes irregular, may be labored, "gasping," or noisy
- Temperature instability
- Lethargy
- Agitation/restlessness/irritability

Management:
- Swaddling, positioning
- Pharmacologic methods—After attempts to otherwise comfort, medication may be necessary to relieve restlessness or discomfort. Commonly ordered sedatives for neonates include (dosage based on weight)
  - midazolam (IV or nasal drops)
  - lorazepam (IV or PO)
  - phenobarbital (IV or PO)
- Commonly ordered analgesics for neonates
  - morphine (IV or PO)
  - fentanyl (IV)
- Seizures may be treated with diazepam, lorazepam, or phenobarbital

Comfort Always

Comfort care, a component of palliative care, ensures that the highest possible quality of life is maintained.[4] Palliative care improves the quality of life of patients and families who face life-threatening illness by providing pain and symptom relief and spiritual and psychosocial support from diagnosis to the end of life and bereavement (Displays C.1, C.2, and C.3).[5]

DISPLAY C.1 COMFORT CARE FOR INFANTS	
INFANT COMFORT NEEDS	**CAREGIVER RESPONSE**
To be free from pain and suffering To feel loved	Assume that whatever would make an adult uncomfortable would also impact a newborn in a similar way. Treat accordingly. Enhance the newborn's life experiences through soft music, reduced environmental noise and light. Provide clustered care with minimal disturbance to the baby, allowing for maximal sleep and positive developmental stimulation. Utilize current evidence-based practice guidelines for pain and symptom management.[6] Encourage families to care for their babies as they are able through bathing rituals, gentle rocking, tender touching, and voice as they contribute to basic needs.

DISPLAY C.2	COMFORT CARE FOR FAMILIES
FAMILY COMFORT NEEDS	**CAREGIVER RESPONSE**
To make informed decisions To feel supported and respected	Facilitate conversations as needed between family and care team members regarding expected outcomes and processes. A translator must be included if family has difficulty with English. Some parents may have known their baby had a life-threatening condition while the baby was in utero and they may have had time to consider options. However, for many, time does not help in making these very difficult decisions. Care needs to be taken to offer respect for values and decisions that may differ from those of the health care team. Family conferences are helpful for the family to hear from various disciplines and perspectives. Meetings with staff from a palliative care program on a regular basis can ensure families receive support and answers to their questions, as information is available. Arrange for other support services as requested/needed: social worker, spiritual support, medical team, photography services for memory making, palliative care team. Provide quiet, private spaces for conversations and interactions with family, care team, and infant. Use lay language, visual aids, and printed material or notes. Solicit desire for "breaks"; assist mother with medical support from her provider, if needed; consider lactation support regarding preventing/treating breast engorgement. Allow time for remembering service conducted on annual basis as part of bereavement follow-up.

DISPLAY C.3	COMFORT CARE FOR HEALTH CARE PROVIDERS
HEALTH CARE PROVIDER COMFORT NEEDS	**ORGANIZATIONAL/LEADERSHIP RESPONSE**
Care for the caregiver	Arrange for support services as requested/needed. Shortly after the death of an infant, the staff may benefit from taking a few minutes to take their emotional "pulses."[7] • _P_ause–Take a minute to mourn • _U_nderstand and _U_tilize–Cognitively process the event and use your strengths to support one another • _L_isten to your emotional reactions • _S_tress–Determine how you need to deal with this loss (e.g., go home or take another admission) • _E_xperience–Grieve, reflect on the meaning this loss has to you. Compassion cart: A cart with tea pot, herbal teas and mugs; CD player with soft music, fragrant lotions, and books of poetry may be wheeled to the unit for staff. Debriefings may involve longer meetings to process events when cumulative stress or specific events are emotionally charged.

Summary

Unprecedented technology has enabled seriously ill neonates to live longer, but cure continues to be elusive at times. It is crucial that nurses respond with efforts to relieve physical and emotional pain and suffering of the baby and family. Caregivers continue to have much to learn about management of pain and discomfort in newborns. Nurses can promote the effort through use of current evidence-based practice and participation in research as clinicians work to learn more about neonatal comfort care.

Answers to Quiz

F, T, F, F, T, F, F

REFERENCES

1. Emanuel, L., Ferris, F., von Gunten, C. F., & Von Roenn, J. H. (2004). The last hours of living: Practical advice for clinicians. *Medscape,* Available at: www.medscape.com/viewprogram/5808_pnt. Accessed June 1, 2007.
2. Stowkowski, L. A. (2004). Palliative care and neonatal loss. *Medscape.* Available at: www.medscape.com/viewarticle/494959.
3. Carter, B. S., & Leuthner, S. R. (2003). The ethics of withholding/withdrawing nutrition in the newborn. *Seminars in Perinatology,* 27(6), 480–487.
4. Foster, T. (2007). Pediatric palliative care revisited: A vision to add life. *Journal of Hospice and Palliative Nursing, 9*(4), 212–219.
5. World Health Organization. (N.D.). WHO definition of palliative care. Available at: www.who.int/cancer/pallaitive/definition/en/. Accessed June 1, 2007.
6. Carter, B. S. (2004). Providing palliative care for newborns. *Pediatric Annals, 33*(11), 770–777.
7. Kendall, J. (2007). *PULSE protocol following the death of a patient.* Unpublished manuscript.

SUGGESTED READING

Gale, G., & Brooks, A. (2006). Implementing a palliative care program in a newborn intensive care unit. *Advances in Neonatal Care, 6*(1), 37.e1–37.

Ewing, A., & Carter, B. (2004). Once again, Vanderbilt NICU leads the way in nurses emotional support. *Pediatric Nursing, 30*(6), 471–472.

RESOURCES

Agency for Healthcare Research and Quality: www.ahrq.gov
Includes Evidence-Based Practice Centers (EBC), which review all relevant scientific literature on clinical, behavioral, and organization and financing topics to produce evidence reports and technology assessments.

American Academy of Hospice and Palliative Care: www.aahpm.org
Prevention and relief of patient and family suffering by providing education and clinical practice standards, fostering research, facilitating personal and professional development, and by public policy advocacy

ELNEC: End-of-Life Nursing Education Consortium: www.aacn.nche.edu/elnec
The End-of-Life Nursing Education Consortium (ELNEC) project is a national education initiative to improve end-of-life care in the United States.

Children's Hospice International: www.chionline.org
Provides resources and referrals to children with life-threatening conditions and their families

Bereavement services: www.bereavement.net
Offers support groups, private counseling, educational seminars, and workshops tailored to meet the needs of the bereaved and those wishing to learn more about the grief process.

Growth House, Inc.: www.growthhouse.org
Strives to improve the quality of compassionate care through public education and global professional collaboration from people who are dying.

International Journal and Online Forum of Leaders in End-of-Life Care: www.edc.org/lastacts
Features peer-reviewed articles striving to enhance comfort and dignity of dying persons and their families.

National Hospice and Palliative Care Organization: www.nhpco.org
Committed to improving end-of-life care and expanding hospice care with the goal of profoundly enhancing quality of life of people dying in America.

Guidelines for Implementing a Perinatal Education Program

Julie Martin Arafeh ■ Kimberly Yeager

Overview

The learning needs of staff in intrapartum units are varied from new graduates to experienced nurses. Intrapartum units require different types of programs to meet the educational needs of the staff. This text has been designed to address different educational levels in a variety of formats.

- Self-directed continuing education for the experienced nurse
- Orientation program for nurses new to intrapartum nursing
- Education program in a facility to promote continuity in cognitive and technical skills among staff
- Perinatal outreach program
- Adjunct text in nursing education program

This appendix reviews the basic concepts of adult learning theory including characteristics of the adult learner, application of theories in practice, and how the text can be used to support the development of cognitive, technical, and behavioral skills in intrapartum staff.

Adult Learning Theory

In the development of any educational program, the needs of adult learners should be considered and concepts of adult learning theory utilized in designing the program. The characteristics of the adult learner reflect a group that is internally motivated, is self-directed, and seeks new knowledge for immediate application.[1] It is important to be cognizant of the need to develop critical thinking skills through the use of this text. The cognitive domain can be broken into two levels: the primary and most basic level consisting of knowledge, comprehension, and application; and the higher level consisting of analysis, synthesis, and evaluation.[2] Traditionally, the bulk of education has concentrated on the lower level despite the fact that practitioners operate at the higher level during patient care. It is important to challenge the learners with an opportunity to put the new knowledge gained from reading this text into practice either through case review, in situ drills, or simulation. Much of the literature in adult education reflects the importance of hands on experience as a means to acquire and refine new knowledge. Experiential learning also leads to longer retention of new skills for a longer period of time when compared with traditional didactic presentations.[3–8]

Development of Cognitive Skills

The modules in the text are designed for either self directed review for the motivated learner or as an adjunct to didactic educational offerings. Review/practice questions can be found in each module to provide self assessment of the concepts presented in that module. Continuing educational credits can be awarded for review to those staff who are eligible.

The modules can also be used to augment the learners existing knowledge base to support development of a technical skill set specific to intrapartum nursing. Knowledge and cognitive skills are the basis for decision making in training sessions and ultimately at the bedside.

Development of Technical Skills

For staff new to intrapartum skills, review of the Skill Units in the text in conjunction with a technical skills presentation/demonstration will engage both visual and auditory learners.

Perinatal outreach programs can utilize a technical skills conference in two ways.

- Preceptors in hospitals served by the outreach program can be taught effective ways to teach these skills to new staff including the use of task trainers such as an artificial pelvis to demonstrate fetal positions or a fetal manikin to allow for practice of fetal scalp electrode placement.
- New staff in hospitals served by the outreach program or nurses in the region who want to acquire these skills may attend the conference.

A sample agenda for a technical skills conference can be found below.

Day One

8:30 to 9:00 AM	Introduction to Technical Skills Course
9:00 to 10:00 AM	Physical Examination of the Laboring Woman
	Discussion and Demonstration
10:00 to 10:15 AM	Break
10:15 to 11:15 AM	Testing for Ruptured Membranes
	Discussion and Demonstration
11:15 to 12:00 PM	Fern Testing for Ruptured Membranes
	Discussion and Demonstration
12:00 to 12:30 PM	Lunch Break
12:30 to 1:30 PM	Vaginal Examination
	Discussion and Demonstration
1:30 to 2:30 PM	Measuring Fundal Height
	Discussion and Demonstration
2:30 to 2:45 PM	Break
2:45 to 3:45 PM	Evaluating Fetal Lie, Presentation, and Position Using Leopold's Maneuvers
	Discussion and Demonstration
3:45 to 4:45 PM	Auscultation of Fetal Heart Tones
	Discussion and Demonstration
4:45 to 5:00 PM	Evaluations and Adjourn

Day Two

8:30 to 9:00 AM	Introduction
9:00 to 10:00 AM	Friedman Graph: Plotting and Analysis Discussion and Demonstration
10:00 to 10:15 AM	Break
10:15 to 11:15 AM	Techniques for Breathing and Effleurage Discussion and Demonstration
11:15 to 12:30 PM	Techniques for Second Stage and Birth Discussion and Demonstration
12:30 to 1:00 PM	Lunch Break
1:00 to 2:30 PM	Oxytocin Labor Induction/Augmentation Discussion and Demonstration
2:30 to 2:45 PM	Break
2:45 to 4:00 PM	Managing an Unexpected Birth Discussion and Demonstration
4:00 to 4:45 PM	Procedure for Obtaining Umbilical Cord Blood Sampling Discussion and Demonstration
4:45 to 5:00 PM	Evaluation and Adjourn

Supplies needed for demonstrations:

Fetal manikin and pelvis
Draw sheets (2)
K-Y lubricating jelly
Measuring tape
Speculums (variety of types and sizes)
Nitrazine paper
Lamp (gooseneck)
Gloves
Fetoscope and Doptone
Microscope and slides
Cotton-tipped applicators
Cotton balls and ring forceps
Delivery pack
Emesis basin
Bottle of water for pouring
Peribottle
Friedman graph paper (approximately five sheets per participant)
Case reviews (two or three) of oxytocin (Pitocin) induction or augmentation
Amniotic fluid (can use salt water solution—will give ferning effect when dried)

Consider employing a low-risk pregnant woman who is at 32 to 38 weeks gestation to enable limited numbers of workshop participants to demonstrate fundal height measurement, Leopold's maneuvers, and fetal heart rate assessment.

Simulation-Based Training

Experts in human performance training have suggested that 10 behaviors are critical to effective, efficient, and safe team performance. These skills can best be taught in either in-situ drills or simulation-based training sessions. Behavioral skills identified as important include:

- Know your environment
- Anticipate and plan
- Assume the leadership role
- Communicate effectively
- Distribute work load optimally
- Allocate attention wisely
- Utilize all available information
- Utilize all available resources
- Call for help early enough
- Maintain professional behavior

In-situ drills and/or simulation-based training are uniquely able to combine cognitive, technical, and behavioral skill practice. The addition of videotaping of training scenarios allows all participants to constructively review the session and discuss actions of the team. These sessions can advance individual performance and performance of the team as a whole. Topics for intrapartum scenarios can include shoulder dystocia, emergency cesarean birth, eclamptic seizure, hemorrhage, maternal hypotension, fetal bradycardia, neonatal resuscitation, and maternal arrest. A sample scenario can be found below.

Scenario: Managing an Unexpected Birth

Scene

A 32-year-old G3 P2 presents to labor and delivery in term labor with intact bulging bag of waters. VS and FHR within normal limits and are reassuring. Woman states urge to push. During vaginal exam ROM occurs and infant is born precipitously.

Level of Difficulty

It is important to be aware of the experience level of the learner. For experienced learners, consider increasing the intensity of the scenario through the following options:

- Family member present
- Hemorrhage at birth
- Equipment malfunction

Learning Objectives

Cognitive
- Awareness of situations that can result in a precipitous birth, including differences in labor patterns between nulliparous and multiparous women
- Signs of precipitous birth including vaginal exam and appearance of bulging perineum
- Cardinal movements of the fetus before and during birth
- Awareness of complications that can occur, for example shoulder dystocia or meconium-stained fluid

Technical
- Assembly of supplies at the bedside for a precipitous birth
- Assistance of the mother with the birth
- Creation of a safe environment for mother and infant during birth, including calling for help
- Care of the mother and infant immediately after birth

Behavioral
- Clear, concise communication among team during crisis
- Assumption of leadership role
- Ability to delegate tasks based on skill sets

Expected Critical Actions
- Call for help
- Woman positioned for birth in a manner that is safe and comfortable for her

- Perineum cleansed
- Gloves and necessary drapes placed for birth
- Determine position of fetus
- Support the perineum with nondominant hand
- Instruct the woman in clear, concise manner
- After birth of the head, check for nuchal cord
- Clamp and cut nuchal cord
- Support fetal head during restitution
- Support the fetal body during birth
- After birth, secures infant in an arm hold with head slightly down
- Cord clamped
- Warm, dry, and stimulate infant
- Control delivery of the placenta with steady downward traction with one hand and support of the fundus with the other hand
- Evaluate for perineal tears
- Evaluate bleeding

Consider the use of videotape to record the drill in order to review learners' performances. This provides the learners with the unique opportunity to see themselves in action and gain insight into their strengths and weaknesses. Reflection on performance followed by additional practice allows the learner to process new information leading to the ultimate goal of this manual: acquisition and *retention* of new skills and improved critical thinking.[9]

Evaluation for Skills Conference and/or Simulation-Based Training

The questions on the form on the next page will assist in evaluating the relevancy of the skills/simulation in enhancing your clinical knowledge and skills. Your answers will provide a basis for evaluating the effectiveness of this format for intrapartum education. In addition, this survey offers regional centers or agencies a means of determining the degree of participant satisfaction. You may duplicate this form as needed.

Conclusion

The ultimate goal of this text is to improve patient safety through increased content knowledge, acquisition of new skills and the eventual transfer to the clinical environment. The Joint Commission for Accreditation of Healthcare Organizations (JCAHO) conducted a root cause analysis of 71 cases of perinatal morbidity and mortality.[10] Causes topping the list included communication, staff competency, and training. This text directly addresses these issues through up to date information related to best practices as well as

recommendations for interactive teaching modules within this appendix. Team training through multidisciplinary drills on scenarios such as the ones listed above will assist teams in meeting JCAHO's recommendations to improve perinatal outcomes.[11]

REFERENCES

1. Knowles, M. S. (1984). *Andragogy in action.* San Francisco: Jossey-Bass.
2. Bloom, B. S., & Krathwohl, D. R. (1956). *Taxonomy of educational objectives: The classification of educational goals, by a committee of college and university examiners. Handbook 1: Cognitive domain.* New York: Longmans.
3. Ziv, A., Wolpe, P. R., Small, S. D., & Glick, S. (2006). Simulation-based medical education: An ethical imperative. *Simulation in Healthcare, 1,* 252–255.
4. Kneebone, R. L. (2006). Crossing the line: Simulation and boundary areas. *Simulation in Healthcare, 1,* 160–163.
5. Miettinen, R. (2000). The concept of experiential learning and John Dewey's theory of reflective thought and action. *International Journal of Lifelong Education, 19,* 54–72.
6. Weinstock, P. H., Kappus, L. J., Kleinman, M. E., Grenier, B., Hickey, P., & Burns, J. P. (2005). Toward a new paradigm in hospital-based pediatric education: The development of an onsite simulator program. *Pediatric Critical Care Medicine, 6,* 635–641.
7. Issenberg, S. B., McHaghie, W. C., Bart, I. R., Mayer, J. W., Felner, J. M., Petrusa, E. R., Waugh, R. A., et al. (1999). Simulation technology for health care professional skills training and assessment. *Journal of the American Medical Association, 282,* 861–866.
8. Epstein, R. M., & Hundert, E. M. (2002). Defining and assessing professional competence. *Journal of the American Medical Association, 287,* 226–235.
9. Kolb, D. (1984). *Experiential learning. Experience as the source of learning and development.* Englewood Cliffs, NJ: Prentice-Hall.
10. JCAHO. (2004). Sentinel event alert, Issue 30, July 21, 2004. Available at: www.jcaho.org/about+us/news+letters/ sentinel+event+alert/sea_30.htm. Retrieved July 3, 2007.
11. Miller, L. A. (2005). Patient safety and teamwork in perinatal care, resources for clinicians. *Journal of Perinatal & Neonatal Nursing, 19,* 46–51.

MANIKIN COMPANY CONTACTS

- Limbs and things: www.golimbs.com
- Simulaids: www.simulaids.com/
- Laerdal: www.laerdal.com/
- METI: www.meti.com/
- Gaumard: www.gaumard.com

Evaluation for Skills Conference and/or Simulation-Based Training

Program Title: _____

Date: _____ Participant name: _____

KEY:
  5 Strongly agree
  4 Agree
  3 Neither agree nor disagree
  2 Disagree
  1 Strongly disagree

1. The skills and content presented are relevant to my practice.

   1   2   3   4   5

   Comments: _____
   _____
   _____

2. This format was helpful with learning and retention of skills.

   1   2   3   4   5

   Comments: _____
   _____
   _____

3. The discussion/debriefing sessions were a valuable component of the conference/simulation.

   1   2   3   4   5

   Comments: _____
   _____
   _____

4. Review of skills/use of videotape was helpful in incorporating new behaviors.

   1   2   3   4   5

   Comments: _____
   _____
   _____

5. This conference/simulation will assist me in providing better care to intrapartum patients.

   1   2   3   4   5

   Comments: _____
   _____
   _____

6. I prefer reviewing skills in a conference/simulation format over receiving information in a lecture format.

   1   2   3   4   5

   Comments: _____
   _____
   _____

7. It is helpful to review skills with other intrapartum colleagues.

   1   2   3   4   5

   Comments: _____
   _____
   _____

8. The faculty facilitated the learning process and skill retention.

   1   2   3   4   5

   Comments: _____
   _____
   _____

Group B Streptococcus Infections in Pregnancy

Betsy B. Kennedy

ing the birth process. Medical management of the mother aims at reducing infection risks for both mother and neonate.

▶ **What is group B streptococcus?**

Group B streptococcus (GBS) is a naturally occurring Gram-positive bacteria with several different serotypes. The predominant types causing disease are Ia, Ib, II, III, and V.[1] It is one of the leading causes of morbidity and mortality among newborns when clinical signs and symptoms appear on the day of birth to within the first week of life, referred to as *early-onset disease,* or when signs and symptoms present after 1 week, usually evident in the first 3 months of life, and referred to as *late-onset disease.* Although recent screening and treatment recommendations have reduced the incidence of **early-onset** disease, no strategies exist to prevent **late-onset** disease. Careful monitoring of the infection remains a priority.[2]

Terminology

- **Colonization**—The presence of microorganisms in an organ or tissue of the body with or without any pathology. The presence of the organism is determined by culture. A positive culture does not indicate infection, but rather that the individual harbors or carries the organism without adverse consequences. For example, if the organism is obtained from surfaces such as skin, ears, or umbilical cord or from gastric contents in a healthy individual, exposure to the organism and colonization are documented. However, infection is not necessarily present.
- **Infection**—The invasion by microorganisms of a body site that is normally considered sterile (e.g., bladder, amniotic fluid, blood, lungs, cerebrospinal fluid), causing disease by local cellular injury, secretion of toxins, and other pathologic mechanisms.
- **Invasive disease**—High bacterial load affecting major body systems and inducing serious pathologic events, such as meningitis and respiratory distress.

NOTE: GBS resides in the gastrointestinal tract of many individuals (men and women) without causing any complications. However, close approximation of the anus to the introitus and urethra facilitates colonization of the vagina and urinary tract with GBS. Antibiotic treatment sufficient to eliminate GBS in the gastrointestinal tract of a colonized individual is not possible. Treatment eradicates the organism or, in instances of heavy colonization, lowers the colony count, for locally colonized or infected sites such as the cervix, vagina, or bladder. Colonization can be (1) transient, (2) intermittent, or (3) chronic. GBS colonization of the maternal genital tract involves the most risk to the newborn because of exposure dur-

Historical Perspective: Evolution of National Guidelines[1,3]

1970s	→	GBS emerges as a leading cause of neonatal morbidity and mortality, with up to a 50% fatality rate.
1980's	→	Clinical trials reveal that effective treatment of GBS colonized women with antibiotics in labor could dramatically reduce the rate of invasive neonatal disease.
1996	→	Preventive strategies, including recommendations for screening (risk-based or culture-based approach), to identify candidates for intrapartum antibiotic prophylaxis are issued by the CDC, ACOG, and AAP.
2002	→	Based on evaluation of data, a revision of the recommendations is issued reflecting the effectiveness of routine prenatal screening in active prevention of neonatal GBS disease, identifying a single prevention strategy.

Epidemiology[1-5]

- It is estimated that 20% to 30% of all pregnant women are GBS carriers.[1,4]
- GBS is a common cause of sepsis, pneumonia, and meningitis in neonates and young infants, affecting 0.5 cases per 1,000 live births.[1,2]
- Most neonatal infections occur in the first few days of life (**early onset**).[3]
- Reinfection can occur in a small percentage of neonates, and often this is at a new site.
- The lower female genital tract, that is, the lower third of the vagina, the vaginal introitus, and the rectum are the most common sites of colonization. The upper third of the vagina and cervix are less commonly colonized. The urethra can be colonized, leading to urinary tract involvement. The biologic

mechanism of colonization is not well understood, which limits the interpretation of epidemiology. Because the usual reservoir for the bacteria is in the GI tract, genitourinary colonization may occur as a function of poor hygiene, sexual practice, or underlying immune system issues that reduce the body's ability to eliminate the GBS.[5]

- Colonization of the lower maternal genital tract can lead to chorioamnionitis, postpartum endometritis, and neonatal infection.
- African-American race, high body mass index (BMI), higher income, higher educational level, and access to prenatal care have been associated with increased odds of GBS colonization.[5]
- GBS is a common cause of bacteremia (urinary tract infection) in pregnant women. This can be asymptomatic in a small percentage of women and can lead to pyelonephritis if untreated.
- It is the most common cause of intrapartal acute chorioamnionitis.

Clinical Features[1,4,6]

▶ How is GBS transmitted?

- Early-onset GBS infection is caused by vertical transmission whereby the organism invades the amniotic membranes and infects the fetus in utero. Many newborns are infected before birth.
- Although perhaps half of newborns are exposed to GBS when membranes rupture or during the birth process, only a small percentage (1% to 2%) develop the *disease*.[6]

▶ What are the risk factors for GBS?

- Maternal risk factors associated with *early-onset* newborn disease include a positive vaginal/rectal culture, rupture of membranes 12 hours or more before delivery, delivery before 37 weeks' gestation, maternal fever, GBS-positive urine culture during pregnancy, and having a GBS-affected infant previously.[4]
- Maternal risk factors associated with *late-onset* neonatal infection are thought to be vertical transmission and hospital-acquired infection.[4]

NOTE: When a GBS-positive infant has been identified, isolation of the infant is not recommended. Outbreaks in nurseries do not occur.[6]

- Intrapartal risk factors for GBS infection include the following[4]:
  - Prolonged rupture of membranes of 12 hours or more
  - Premature rupture of membranes (i.e., at less than 37 weeks' gestation)
  - History of a previous infant with GBS disease
  - Preterm labor

Perinatal Consequences[1,3,4,7]

▶ What are the effects of GBS on the mother and baby?

- Colonization in women can lead to spontaneous abortion, sepsis, stillbirth, premature rupture of membranes, preterm birth, and postpartum endometritis.

- Most newborns who develop *early-onset* invasive GBS disease are term infants.
- Preterm infants are more susceptible to *early-onset* infection.
- Signs and symptoms of *early-onset* infection are seen within the first 24 hours of life (even within the first hour) and include septicemia, pneumonia, and meningitis. Respiratory distress is the most common sign. Infants may be lethargic, have labile temperatures, exhibit poor feeding, and have glucose intolerance.
- *Signs of severe infection include fetal asphyxia (indicating in utero infection), newborn hypotension, accelerating signs of respiratory distress, and persistent pulmonary hypertension. This requires immediate attention.*
- Infants with GBS sepsis at more than 37 weeks' gestation have a survival rate of 98%, but for preterm infants, survival is lower: 90% for those at 34 to 36 weeks gestations and 70% for those less than 33 weeks gestation.[1]
- The clinical presentations of early and late onset disease may overlap; however, **late-onset** disease is more often associated with signs of neurologic involvement.[7]
- The ratio of **early-** to **late-onset** disease is now 1:1.[4]

Screening[1,4,8,9]

Previous recommendations described a variety of approaches to screening for GBS. In 2002, national prevention guidelines were adopted by the American College of Obstetricians and Gynecologists (ACOG), American Academy of Pediatrics (AAP), ACNM, and the CDC. These guidelines recommend a single strategy which is administering a *universal antenatal culture based screening at 35 to 37 weeks' gestation.*

1. **Culture-based screening**
   - Vaginal and rectal cultures should be performed at 35 to 37 weeks' gestation on all pregnant women.
   - Cultures done earlier in pregnancy do not predict that colonization will be present at birth. All culture-positive women are treated in the intrapartum period. It is NOT recommended to treat antepartum.[1]
   - Cervical cultures are not recommended and speculums should not be used for specimen collection.
   - Specimens may be collected by health care providers or self-collected by the woman.

NOTE: A GBS-positive urine culture (in any concentration) in the prenatal period indicates heavy colonization and an increased risk for infection or invasive disease. This requires immediate antibiotic treatment.[1]

▶ What if the mother's GBS status is unknown at admission?

2. **Risk based approach**—*When culture results are unknown in the intrapartum period, treat all women with a known risk factor.*
   Any woman with one or more of the following risk factors in the intrapartum period should be considered for antibiotic treatment.
   - A history of a previous newborn with invasive GBS infection

- A history of GBS bacteriuria during the current pregnancy
- Delivery predicted to occur before 37 weeks' gestation
- Rupture of membranes for 18 hours or more
- Presence of maternal fever of 38°C or higher

NOTE: Recently there has been interest in rapid testing for identification of GBS. Most are not sufficiently sensitive in positive predictive value from genital specimens; however, a polymerase chain reaction (PCR) test has received FDA approval. Rapid testing may be a viable option provided there is sufficient time before delivery to complete and receive the results of the test and for the woman to receive intrapartum antibiotic prophylaxis.[1]

Maternal Treatment[1,4,8]

▶ How is the mother treated in labor?

- Intrapartal treatment is targeted for women documented as being GBS positive (by history or antenatal culture) or for women with intrapartal risk factors.
- *The CDC recommends treatment must be completed at least 4 hours before the birth so that adequate antibiotic levels are reached in serum and amniotic fluid, thus reducing the risk of infant colonization.[4] As many as 50% of women who are identified as GBS carriers may not be able to meet this criteria due to rapid labors or other circumstances.[8]*

▶ What if the mother will deliver before 4 hours of treatment are completed?

- *The antibiotics used in treatment (bactericidal) are known to rapidly reach effective levels in amniotic fluid. Therefore, treatment given less than 4 hours before birth is beneficial. Recent studies have reported that as little as 1 to 2 hours of prophylaxis may be effective.[8]*

▶ What if the mother is allergic to penicillin?[4]

- Intrapartum chemoprophylaxis includes penicillin G with clindamycin, ampicillin, or erythromycin as alternatives for women with penicillin allergy.

Recommended regimen	→ Penicillin G	first dose 5 million units IV, subsequent doses 2.5 million units q4h until delivery
Alternative (Penicillin not available)	→ Ampicillin	first dose 2 g IV, subsequent doses 1 g q4h until delivery

Penicillin allergic (high risk for anaphylaxis)	→ Clindamycin	900 mg IV q8h until delivery or
	Erythromycin	500 mg IV q6h until delivery
Penicillin-allergic (high risk for anaphylaxis, susceptibility unknown)	→ Vancomycin	1 g IV q12h until delivery
Penicillin-allergic (low risk for anaphylaxis)	→ Cefazolin	first dose 2 g IV, subsequent doses 1 g q8h until delivery

▶ What if the mother is having a cesarean section?[4]

- Antibiotic prophylaxis is not indicated in women undergoing a planned cesarean delivery in the absence of labor or ruptured membranes due to the low incidence of acquiring disease.

▶ What if the mother doesn't have or want an IV?

- *There is currently no alternative oral or intramuscular regimen that is recommended for prophylaxis.[1,4]*
- Some studies have shown the use of chlorhexidine to cleanse the birth canal or to wipe the newborn can reduce the vertical transmission. This intervention is being evaluated for use in undeveloped countries where intravenous antibiotics are unavailable, unaffordable, and unfeasible.[1,9]

▶ Should vaginal examinations be limited on mothers who are GBS positive?

- *Obstetric procedures such as vaginal exams and internal electronic fetal monitoring should not be avoided solely on the basis of positive GBS status.[1,4]*

Onset of Labor or ROM before 37 Weeks' Gestation[4]

▶ What if the mother is preterm?

- Because the preterm infant is at significantly higher risk for GBS sepsis, the CDC Guidelines (2002) include a sample algorithm for management.
- If maternal GBS status is negative (in the last 6 weeks) no antibiotic prophylaxis is needed.
- If maternal GBS status is positive, antibiotic prophylaxis should be started and continued for at least 48 hours during tocolysis and during labor.

- If maternal GBS status is unknown or there has been no culture in the last 6 weeks, a rectovaginal culture should be obtained. Antibiotic prophylaxis should be started, but may be discontinued when negative results are confirmed.
- If amnionitis is suspected, then GBS prophylaxis should be replaced with broad spectrum antibiotic therapy (that includes an agent known to be effective against GBS).

Neonatal Treatment[1]

▶ How is the baby treated?

- Newborns with suspected sepsis are treated with a combination of IV antibiotics for 48 to 72 hours or until culture results are available.
- If GBS is isolated, IV penicillin G is administered for a 10-day course.
- If meningitis is diagnosed, treatment includes ampicillin, gentamicin, and a longer course of penicillin G.
- Some centers provide IM penicillin within an hour of birth to at-risk newborns.
- Any symptomatic newborn, whether term or preterm, should have a sepsis workup to rule out or identify the causative organism.

REFERENCES

1. Gibbs, R. S., Schrag, S., & Schuchat, A. (2004). Perinatal infections due to group B streptococci. *Obstetrics and Gynecology, 104*(5), 1062–1076.
2. Centers for Disease Control and Prevention. (2005). Early-onset group B streptococcal disease: United States, 2000–2004. *MMWR Morbidity and Mortality Weekly Report, 54,* 1205–1208.
3. Apgar, B. S., Greenberg, G., & Yen, G. (2005). Prevention of group B streptococcal disease in the newborn. *American Family Physician, 71*(5), 903–910.
4. Centers for Disease Control and Prevention. (2002). Prevention of perinatal group B streptococcal diseases: Revised guidelines from CDC. *MMWR Morbidity and Mortality Weekly Report, 51,* RR-11.
5. Stapleton, R. D., Kahn, J. M., Evans, L. E., Critchlow, C. W., & Gardella, C. M. (2005). Risk factors for group B streptococcal genitourinary tract colonization in pregnant women. *Obstetrics and Gynecology, 106*(6), 1246–1252.
6. Mullaney, D. M. (2001). Group B streptococcal infections in newborns. *Journal of Obstetric, Gynecologic, and Neonatal Nursing, 30*(6), 649–658.
7. Lott, J. W. (2006). State of the science: Neonatal bacterial infections in the early 21st century. *The Journal of Perinatal and Neonatal Nursing, 20*(1), 62–70.
8. Illuzzi, J. L., & Bracken, M. B. (2006). Duration of intrapartum prophylaxis for neonatal group B strep disease. *Obstetrics and Gynecology, 108*(5), 1254–1265.
9. Goldenberg, R. L., McClure, E. M., Saleem, S., Rouse, D., & Vermund, S. (2006). Use of vaginally administered chlorhexidine during labor to improve pregnancy outcomes. *Obstetrics and Gynecology, 107*(5), 1139–1146.

Caring for the Woman With Special Concerns

Donna Jean Ruth

Some women who present for care during pregnancy do not fit the "typical" picture associated with pregnant women—young, healthy, and married. They may require special consideration owing to a variety of circumstances they could be adolescents, women older than 40 having their first baby, women with disabilities, women who are obese, and women with substance abuse problems. These women present unique challenges — but also unique opportunities for health care providers to assist them in having a positive birth experience.

Adolescents

Adolescent pregnancy is a multifactorial issue that is not, unfortunately, a new phenomenon. Many factors contribute to the rate of adolescent pregnancy, and the challenge for health care providers is to optimize the health of both the mother and her baby. Adolescents are particularly vulnerable both psychologically and physiologically.

Growth and Development

The adolescent who becomes pregnant must accomplish both the developmental tasks of adolescence as well as the developmental tasks of pregnancy. Assuming adult roles (having a baby) before completing the work of adolescence can and does have significant long-term consequences that include:

- prolonged dependence on parents/family/society
- lack of education (these teens frequently drop out of high school)
- higher rates of depression and low self-esteem
- children of teens are less well socialized and are more likely to become teen parents themselves (repeating the cycle)

Prenatal Care

Adolescents often begin prenatal care late in the pregnancy or not at all. There are multiple reasons for this and some of them include:

- denial of the pregnancy (I can't be pregnant, therefore I'm not)
- fear of telling their parents
- lack of knowledge of how to access the health care system
- transportation issues
- lack of understanding of the importance of prenatal care

The goal of the health care provider in the prenatal period is to assist the adolescent in accessing and navigating the health care system, provide information and education related to her pregnancy, and help her to understand the importance of prenatal care.

Adolescents may benefit from a single provider to establish a trusting relationship and minimize the number of unfamiliar adults she must interact with during her care. Comprehensive prenatal care should include[1]:

- a complete health history
- nutritional assessment (teens may be reluctant to gain weight, so anticipatory teaching regarding weight gain and the benefit to the baby are important)
- a physical examination (including a pelvic examination, which may be her first)
- prenatal education (ideally provided in a one-to-one manner or a class with other teens; prenatal classes full of adults may be intimidating for many teens)
- plans for the baby (does she plan to keep the baby or is she considering adoption?)

Common Complications of Adolescent Pregnancy[2]

- Iron deficiency anemia—common in young women and will be exacerbated in pregnancy. It is important to take prenatal vitamins and increase intake of iron-rich foods.
- Preterm labor and delivery—very common in teen mothers. It is very important during prenatal care to discuss the subtle signs and symptoms of preterm labor and what to do if an adolescent experiences preterm labor.
- Low birth weight infants—closely tied to preterm delivery and also maternal weight gain.
- Pregnancy-induced hypertension—one of the most common complications of teen pregnancy. It may require hospitalization and early delivery.
- Higher rates of cephalopelvic disproportion—more common in younger teens who have not completed their physical growth. The result is cesarean delivery.

Intrapartum and Postpartum Care

Physical care for the adolescent during labor does not differ from care of other labor patients. However, the adolescent may require additional support from the health care provider; it is not unusual for the teen to become very dependent on her health care provider.

After delivery, careful assessment of the teen mother should be done to assess her knowledge regarding infant care. The health care provider may need to spend additional time observing the mother's interactions with her infant. Teens may have unrealistic views of the reactions of their infants, and get frustrated easily. Referrals to well-baby clinics, programs for school-aged mothers, community organizations, and state social service organizations may provide needed support.

Women Over 40

The number of women over age 40 who are giving birth for the first time is increasing. In fact, 2% to 3% of the births in the United States today are to women over 40.[3] There are many factors that have contributed to this trend, such as:

- availability of effective birth control options
- increased number of women pursuing advanced education and delaying parenthood until they are professionally established
- the increase in later marriage and second marriages
- the increased availability of assisted reproductive techniques that allow women who may have previously been considered infertile to have a baby

Common Complications in Women Over 40

- Increased risk for genetic abnormalities in the baby
- Increased risk for stillbirth[4]
- Increased rates of maternal mortality[5]
- Increased likelihood of a preexisting medical condition, such as chronic hypertension or diabetes
- Increased incidence of low birth weight babies[6]
- Increased rate of cesarean deliveries[7]
- Increased rates of pregnancy-induced hypertension and gestational diabetes[8,9]

Special Considerations: Genetic Testing

Because the increased risk of fetal chromosomal abnormalities is well documented, women who conceive after age 40 will be offered genetic testing. These tests range from simple blood tests to more invasive procedures. Participation in testing is elective, but all women should be informed regarding available tests and options. This information should include the purpose of the test (diagnostic or screening), any risk associated with the test, the information that will be obtained, and what follow-up tests, if any, may be needed to gain the information desired. Many health care providers assume that women who undergo genetic testing will choose to terminate a pregnancy if an abnormality is detected. However, many women undergo testing because they want all available information before making any decision to either terminate or continue a pregnancy. A referral to a genetic counselor should occur early in prenatal care.

Prenatal Care

Just as for any pregnant woman, prenatal care should begin early. In this age group, early prenatal care is more common. The health care provider should identify and discuss any concerns the woman may have related to her age, especially if a preexisting medical condition may complicate her care.

Intrapartum and Postpartum Care

Care of the woman over 40 in labor does not differ physically from care of other laboring women. If the woman has other medical conditions, such as diabetes or hypertension, care needs to be modified to include interventions related to these conditions. The woman with diabetes in labor should have her blood sugar monitored during labor; the goal of treatment will be to keep her blood sugar levels within normal range. If the woman has chronic hypertension, the provider should be very alert to signs and symptoms that indicate she is developing pregnancy-induced hypertension as well.

In the postpartum period, the provider should be aware that the older woman may find the childbirth experience and care of a newborn more exhausting than anticipated. Assist her in identifying sources of help and support. The postpartum period may be a time of social isolation as well. The woman who gives birth after age 40 may find that her peers are more likely to be the parents of adolescents and young adults and removed from the concerns of a new mother. Another concern for the older woman who gives birth is that she may be part of the "sandwich generation." These are women who are caring for elderly parents as well as children. Caring for both parents and a newborn may be emotionally, physically, and financially draining.

Women With a Physical Disability

The woman with a physical disability who presents for care during pregnancy may need specific modifications to care related to her condition. Care during pregnancy should be designed so that any needs, modifications, and potential problems are addressed.[10] Prejudices may exist regarding the ability of the disabled to give birth and parent successfully, and the care provided should be positive and supportive. Care for the woman with a disability needs to be comprehensive and multidisciplinary. When the needs related to the pregnancy and the needs related to her disability are fully met, her ability to have a positive birth experience is facilitated.

Modifications for Pregnancy

Women with disabilities may need some degree of modification to the usual routine care. At the first prenatal visit, it is important to explore with her any support, assistance, or modifications she feels are necessary. A complete and open discussion is essential so that any requests can be initiated. It is also important to discuss any assistance she feels she will need to care for her infant after delivery.

The provider should be careful not to convey the message that because she is disabled she is not competent. However, if assistance will be required, it is best to know ahead of time and make plans for this. Some women require assistance, some may require modifications to their homes, some require adaptive equipment, and some do not require anything different from every other new mother.

Prenatal Care

Modifications during prenatal care will be related to both the type and severity of the disability. The health care provider should collaborate with the primary care provider and/or the disability specialist to build a comprehensive plan of care. The disability may or may not affect the mother's risk status during pregnancy. The following information should be obtained at the first prenatal visit[12]:

- the general health state of the woman
- the nature of the disability
- any medications used to treat the disability
- any secondary conditions related to her disability
- any concerns she has related to her pregnancy and her condition

The physical examination may also need to be modified. Although women with disabilities may have been seen by health care providers in the past, it is not unusual to find that their reproductive health has been ignored. If she has not had a pelvic examination before, it is important for the provider to discuss all aspects of the examination—the purpose of the examination, what she can expect during the examination, and what information will be obtained. Some physical disabilities may limit the ability of the provider to perform the examination due to the limitation of the regular equipment. Obstetric examination tables are often too high to allow easy transfer from a wheelchair. Alternatives should be explored. For example, the physical and occupational departments may be of assistance in providing equipment that can accommodate transfers from one height to another. Positioning during the examination may also need modifications. The provider must listen and respond to any pain or discomfort reported during the pelvic examination. Some disabled women have reported being told that they could not possibly feel any pain because of their disability.[11]

Other aspects of routine prenatal care that may need modifications include obtaining weights, urine specimens, and fundal height assessments. Disabled women in wheelchairs have reported that they have gone through their whole pregnancies without ever being weighed.[10] Explore the hospital or clinic to see if a scale is available that will accommodate a wheelchair. Ask the woman how and where she is generally weighed; perhaps she can have her weight checked at that location and report it to the provider. If obtaining a urine specimen during a prenatal visit is a challenge, the woman may bring in a sample from home, especially if she is performing self-catheterizations.

Fundal height assessments may be waived and ultrasound used to assess fetal growth.

It is important that adjustments be made so that the disabled woman has the same level of monitoring and assessment as all other pregnant women.[13]

Intrapartum and Postpartum Care

The decisions regarding mode of delivery should be made based on obstetric indications. The woman, her provider, and her disability specialist should collaborate to discuss any issues that might impact the mode of delivery. Vaginal delivery is possible for many disabled women. This is the preferred mode for delivery whenever possible. *Cesarean section delivery should never be done arbitrarily because of a disability.* Anesthesia may be a concern, especially in women with spinal cord injuries and neurologic problems. A consultation with an anesthetic provider before labor is suggested so that a comprehensive plan for pain management can be developed.

Needs during the postpartum period vary based on changes that may have occurred during pregnancy and delivery. A more prolonged recovery and hospitalization may be necessary and should be assessed on a case-by-case basis.[11]

Breastfeeding should be encouraged, although some modification and adaptive equipment may be required, especially if the disability involves the upper extremities. Lactation consultants may be very helpful in identifying positions and adaptive equipment that will facilitate successful breastfeeding. Consider consultation with an occupational therapist for a home visit to identify equipment that can be used in the home environment for infant care. Such equipment may include cribs that are low or that

attach to wheelchairs like a side car on a motorcycle. Also consider the need for home health follow-up and make the referral if needed. Include the woman and her family in all discussions.

Women Who Are Obese

Obesity is at epidemic proportions in the United States. The number of obese women who present for care during pregnancy will continue to grow. Obese women are at increased risk for significant complications during pregnancy. Health care providers must be prepared to manage the needs of these pregnant women.

Prenatal Care

Early, comprehensive prenatal care is very important for obese women, as it is for all pregnant women. Obese women often enter pregnancy with conditions that coexist with obesity, such as chronic hypertension and diabetes, which may complicate their care.[14] In fact, as many as 40% of obese women have chronic hypertension and many also develop pregnancy-induced hypertension.[15,16]

Many obese women who present for care may also have type 2 diabetes mellitus. Pregestational diabetes is a concern because it increases the risk for birth defects, particularly if the diabetes has been poorly controlled. Many of these women develop gestational diabetes. Gestational diabetes is associated with an increase in large-for-gestational-age babies and macrosomia. This increases the risk for dysfunctional labor patterns, prolonged labors, birth trauma, perineal trauma, and increased rates of both operative vaginal deliveries and cesarean delivery. If the woman presents with pregestational diabetes or develops gestational diabetes, consultation with a diabetic educator in the prenatal period may facilitate better glucose control and minimize the complications associated with poorly controlled diabetes.[17] (See Module 12 for a full discussion of care of the diabetic woman.)

Prenatal visits should include a full and complete assessment. Close surveillance may help with early identification of the development of diabetes or hypertension. Make sure that when blood pressure measurements are done the appropriate size cuff is used. A cuff that is too small gives a falsely elevated reading.

Another important component of prenatal care is screening for fetal anomalies. Obese patients require only the standard screening assessments. Because obesity is often accompanied by irregular menstrual cycles, early ultrasound examination may be done for accurate dating of the pregnancy. Serial ultrasound examinations may be done to follow fetal growth patterns.

Weight loss in pregnancy is not recommended and should not be attempted; weight loss and the resulting catabolism may interfere with fetal growth and development. Some obese women will lose weight or have no weight gain during pregnancy.[18] Weight should be assessed at each prenatal visit. This may require finding scales that are appropriate for the obese patient. The amount of weight gain recommended by the Institute of Medicine for women with a body mass index (BMI) of greater than 29 is 15 pounds.[19] Obese women may benefit from a consultation with a dietician, especially if weight gain is either too little or excessive.

During the course of prenatal care, evaluation by an anesthetic provider is recommended.[20] If a consultation cannot be accomplished during prenatal care, it should be done as soon as possible after admission to the labor and delivery unit. Obesity increases the risks of anesthesia. Early consultation allows for a comprehensive plan of care to be developed. Obese women are at increased risk for cesarean delivery, so early assessment allows for early identification and intervention if anesthesia difficulties are anticipated.

Intrapartum and Postpartum Care

Obese women are also at increased risk for late stillbirth.[14,21,22] Any complaints of decreased fetal movement should be fully assessed. Antepartum and intrapartum fetal monitoring may be very challenging in these women due to maternal body habitus. External fetal monitoring may be very difficult or impossible. It may require that a nurse remain at the bedside to hold the transducer in place. Evaluation of uterine activity by palpation may also be difficult or impossible due to maternal adipose tissue. Internal monitoring, when possible, may give the most accurate information regarding fetal heart rate and uterine activity. Because obese women are at increased risk for labor dystocia and prolonged labor, accurate assessment is very important. The benefit of internal monitoring may outweigh the increased risk.

When obese women are admitted for delivery, it may be necessary to use special bariatric equipment that is designed for use with these patients. Such equipment may include special beds, wheelchairs, bedside commodes, and lifts. These accommodations make care safer for both the woman and her providers.

Keep maternal positioning in mind during the course of the labor. An upright or semi-Fowler's position facilitates lung expansion and maternal comfort. Make sure to avoid a supine position to avoid venacaval syndrome. The use of a pulse oximeter may be helpful to alert the provider to any signs of maternal hypoxemia, especially in women with sleep apnea or those who have received medications associated with respiratory depression.[23]

Progress of labor should be carefully monitored, as obese women may have prolonged labor, a dysfunctional labor pattern, and failure of descent. This increases the risk of a cesarean delivery. Be prepared and prepare the woman for this potential outcome.

Common Postpartum Complications

- Increased risk of wound infections
- Increased risk for wound dehiscence
- Increased risk for postpartum hemorrhage
- Increased risk for venous thrombus formation
- Increased risk for peripartum heart failure if hypertension is present[24]

The use of sequential compression devices and early ambulation may help decrease the risk of venous thrombus formation. Obese women are less likely to breastfeed.[25] Any interest in breastfeeding should be nurtured and encouraged. Any attempts at weight reduction should be delayed until at least 3 to 4 weeks after delivery, when the woman is sufficiently recovered from the birth experience and maternal healing has occurred. Many women find childbirth a time when they are motivated to make healthy life

changes. Weight loss strategies include behavioral, pharmacologic, and surgical options. A referral to a provider specializing in obesity may be beneficial.

Women With Substance Abuse Problems

Substance abuse has become a more prevalent issue in women who are pregnant. As many as 10% to 20% of pregnant women use illicit drugs.[3] Illicit drug use increases the risk for complications in both the mother and the baby. Health care providers should screen all women who present for care for substance abuse.

Assessment

Substance abuse is prevalent in all populations so providers should never make assumptions based on age, race, or socioeconomic status. There are many screening tools available and substance use screening should take place at the first prenatal visit.

Common Signs of Maternal Substance Abuse

- Late entry to prenatal care or does not seek prenatal care
- Failure to keep appointments or leaving without being seen
- Noncompliance with recommended treatments
- Inadequate weight gain and/or malnourished appearance
- Defensive or hostile behavior
- Frequent accidents or falls
- Signs of depression
- Signs of agitation or euphoria
- Dilated or constricted pupils
- Needle marks, thrombosed veins, and cellulitis

Table F.1 shows the effects on the mother, the fetus, and the infant of commonly abused drugs.

Management

Management of the woman with substance abuse must be comprehensive and should include social workers, nurses, and addiction specialists. To provide effective care, the provider should be nonjudgmental and nonpunative. Discussions regarding treatment options should be explored. Pregnancy may represent a period when the woman recognizes the need for care and intervention. Referrals to addiction specialists, inpatient treatment programs, 12-step programs, and individual counseling may be considered. The management of substance abuse may require hospitalization, as "cold turkey" withdrawal may have negative effects on both maternal and fetal health.

Pain Management

Pain control during labor and delivery may be challenging for some addicted women, particularly those who are addicted to narcotics and opiates. If they present in labor while they are still using drugs, determining the type, amount, or combination of drugs used before arrival is important, as the illicit drugs used may make the administration of additional medications dangerous.

Nonpharmacologic methods of pain management should be explored, including such interventions as back rubs, hot or cold compress, sacral pressure, deep breathing and relaxation, guided

| **TABLE F.1** | EFFECT ON THE MOTHER, FETUS, AND INFANT OF COMMONLY ABUSED DRUGS |

DRUG	EFFECT ON MOTHER	EFFECT ON FETUS/INFANT
1. Cocaine and crack: may be smoked, inhaled or injected	Increased heart rate, increased respiratory rate, vasoconstriction, decreased blood flow to placenta, increased number of abruptio placentae, increased number of first trimester miscarriages	Increased number of babies with IUGR, more preterm births, increased number of stillbirths, increased rate of SIDS, failure of infant to respond to consoling, irritable; ? long term–learning disabilities
2. Marijuana: smoked (Mothers who smoke pot very commonly abuse other drugs, so the effects of marijuana alone have not been well studied.)	Increased number of mothers with anemia Loss of short-term memory Increased maternal heart rate	Increased fine tremors Irritablility Sleep disturbances Unknown long-term effects
3. Amphetamines and methamphetamines: smoked	Increased heart rate, increased respiratory rate, vasoconstriction, and decreased blood flow to the placenta; increased numbers of abruptio placentae	Irritability Poor feeding ? Long-term effects
4. Narcotics and opiates: oral, smoked, and injected	Poor nutritional status Increased rate of preterm labor and birth If mother is IV user, may be HIV, hepatitis B positive and at risk for subacute bacterial endocarditis and STDs	Increased rates of IUGR Withdrawal symptoms in the newborn (usually within 72 hours) Restless, high-pitched shrill cry, inconsolable, seizures

Abbreviations: HIV, human immunodeficiency virus; IV, intravenous; IUGR, intrauterine growth restriction; SIDS, sudden infant death syndrome; STD, sexually transmitted disease.

imagery, and the support and encouragement of the health care providers. Support and encouragement from the provider may help to decrease the fear and anxiety that can heighten the perception of pain. If it is safe to administer medications, they should never be withheld because of concerns they may contribute to further addiction. This is incorrect. Regional and local anesthetics may be good options for these mothers.

Postpartum Care

If the mother is actively using drugs at the time of her delivery, it may be a good time to consider addiction treatment options. The postpartum period is a time when many mothers are very highly motivated to make healthy life changes. Some states require reporting a drug-addicted mother to child protective services. Providers need to be familiar with policies and laws in the state where they practice.

REFERENCES

1. Pilliteri, A. (2003). *Maternal and child health nursing: Care of the childbearing and childrearing family*. (4th ed.). Philadelphia: Lippincott Williams & Wilkins.
2. Phipps, M. G., & Sowers, M. (2002). Defining early adolescent childbearing. *American Journal of Public Health, 92*(1), 125–128.
3. Department of Health and Human Service. (2000). *Healthy people 2010*. Washington, DC: Author.
4. National Center for Health Statistics. (2002). Births: Preliminary data for 2001. *National Vital Statistics Report, 50*(10), 1–20.
5. Hoyert, D. L., Danel, I., & Tully, P. (2000). Maternal mortality, United States and Canada. *Birth, 27*(1), 4–11.
6. Tough, S. C., Newburn-Cook, C., Johnston, D. W., Svenson, L. W., Rose, S., & Belitok, J. (2002). Delayed childbearing and its impact on population rate changes in lower birth weight, multiple birth, and preterm delivery. *Pediatrics, 109*(3), 399–403.
7. Kirchengast, S. (2007). Maternal age and pregnancy outcome—An anthropological approach. *Anthropology, 65*(2), 181–191.
8. Parsons, M. T., & Spellacy, W. N. (2000). Preterm labor. In Scott, J. R. (Ed.), *Danforth's obstetrics and gynecology* (8th ed.). Philadelphia: Lippincott Williams & Wilkins.
9. Abu-Heija, A. T., Jallad, M. F., & Abukteish, F. (2000). Maternal and perinatal outcomes of pregnancy after the age of 45. *Journal of Obstetrics and Gynecology Research, 26*(1), 27–30.
10. Lipson, J. G., & Rogers, J. G. (2000). Pregnancy, birth and disability: Women's health care experiences. *Health Care for Women International, 21*(1), 11–26.
11. Smletzer, S. (2007). Pregnancy in women with physical disabilities. *Journal of Obstetric, Gynecologic and Neonatal Nursing, 36*(1), 88–96.
12. Welner, S. (2000). Pregnancy in women with disabilities. In Cohen, W. R. (Ed.), *Complications of pregnancy* (5th ed.). Philadelphia: Lippincott Williams & Wilkins.
13. Rogers, J. (2006). *The disabled woman's guide to pregnancy and birth*. New York: Demos.
14. Stephansson, O., Dickman, P. W., & Johansson, A. (2001). Maternal weight, pregnancy weight gain, and the risk of antepartum stillbirth. *American Journal of Obstetrics & Gynecology, 184*(2), 463–470.
15. Weiss, J., & Malone, F. (2001). Caring for the obese obstetrics patient. *Contemporary Obstetrics and Gynecology, 46*(6), 12–26.
16. Rossner, S. (1998). Obesity and pregnancy. In Bray, G., Bouchard, C., & James, E. (Eds.), *Handbook of obesity* (pp. 775–790). New York: Marcel Dekker.
17. Cesario, S. K. (2003). Obesity in pregnancy: What every nurse needs to know. *AWHONN Lifelines, 7*(2), 118–125.

18. Lederman, S. (2001). Pregnancy weight gain and postpartum loss: Avoiding obesity while optimizing the growth and development of the fetus. *Journal of the American Medical Women's Association, 56*(2), 53–58.

19. Institute of Medicine. (1990). *Nutrition during pregnancy: 1. Weight gain 2. Nutrient supplements*. Washington, DC: National Academy Press.

20. American College of Obstetrics and Gynecology (ACOG). (2002). *Obstetric analgesia and anesthesia* [Practice Bulletin Number 36]. Washington, DC: Author.

21. Cnattingius, S., Bergstrom, R., & Lipworth, L. (1998). Prepregnancy weight and the risk of adverse pregnancy outcomes. *New England Journal of Medicine, 338*(3), 147.

22. Baydock, S., & Chari, R. (2002). Prepregnancy obesity as an independent risk factor for unexplained stillbirth. *Obstetrics and Gynecology, 99,* 74S.

23. Sauer, A. (1992). Morbid obesity. In Angelini, D. & Knapp, C. (Eds.), *Case studies in perinatal nursing* (pp. 57–67). Gaithersburg, MD: Aspen.

24. Cunningham, F. G., Pritchard, J. A., & Hankins, G. D. (1986). Idiopathic cardiomyopathy or compounding cardiovascular events? *Obstetrics and Gynecology, 67*(3), 157–162.

25. Li, R., Jewell, S., & Grummer-Strawn, L. (2003). Maternal obesity and breastfeeding practices. *American Journal of Clinical Nutrition, 77*(3), 101–106.

POSTTESTS

Posttest: Module 1. Overview of Labor

Answer the following questions without referring back to the information in the module. Select the ONE BEST answer for each question.

1. Which theory can explain the beginning of labor?
   A. Increase in gap junctions near term
   B. Fetal membrane production of arachidonic acid
   C. Efficient flow of calcium into myometrial cells
   D. All of these can play a part in the explanation

2. The first stage of labor is:
   A. Expulsion
   B. Dilatation
   C. Recovery
   D. Placental separation

3. Which tissue layer is responsible for the expulsion efforts during the birth process?
   A. Myometrium
   B. Perimetrium
   C. Endometrium

4. Which characteristic *best* describes the uterus during labor?
   A. Undergoes sporadic contractions
   B. Becomes thicker in all areas
   C. Never relaxes
   D. Differentiates into two separate areas

5. Effacement of the cervix takes place as a result of:
   A. Passive relaxation of the lower uterine segment
   B. Pressure of the presenting part of the baby
   C. Active contractions of the uterus
   D. All of these

6. Which characteristic of a uterine contraction best describes the *increment phase*?
   A. Occurs at the middle of the contraction
   B. Is approximately the same length as the decrement phase
   C. Is approximately the same length as the acme phase
   D. Is longer than either the acme or the decrement phase

7. The duration of a contraction is the time from the beginning of the:
   A. Increment to the end of the decrement
   B. Increment to the beginning of the decrement
   C. Acme to the beginning of the next acme
   D. Increment to the end of the acme

8. Which explanation is the *best* reason why the fingers are placed lightly on the fundus of the uterus when timing contractions?
   A. This is the least painful area for the mother.
   B. The fundus cannot be indented with light pressure.
   C. This is where the contraction usually begins.
   D. The mother is likely to feel the contraction here.

9. To time contractions efficiently, it is best to:
   A. Ask the mother to let you know when they begin and end.
   B. Palpate the fundal area of the uterus.
   C. Observe the mother's abdomen rise and fall with the contraction.
   D. Use internal electronic fetal monitoring.

10. The intensity of a contraction:
    A. Cannot be accurately measured
    B. Can be described as strong if the palpating fingers cannot indent the uterus at the peak of a contraction
    C. Cannot be accurately measured by an internal fetal monitor
    D. Can be accurately measured only by an external monitor

11. To make an accurate assessment of cervical dilatation, a vaginal examination should be performed:
    A. As the contraction is beginning
    B. Throughout the contraction
    C. Between contractions
    D. As the contraction is ending

12. Which situation can be characterized as *normal* labor?
    A. Intensity of contractions is 35 mmHg with a frequency of every 10 minutes.
    B. Intensity of contractions is 12 mmHg with a frequency of every 5 minutes.
    C. Intensity of contractions is 20 mmHg with a frequency of every 8 minutes.
    D. Intensity of contractions approaches 50 mmHg with a frequency of every 5 minutes.

13. The most effective support for the laboring woman includes:
    A. Reducing the number of decisions she is required to make by eliminating any choices she might make in her labor and birth
    B. Allowing a family member to visit at selected periods of time throughout labor
    C. Telling her that "it will make the pain easier to bear" as you administer a sedative
    D. Keeping her informed of her progress

14. Which action provides the most effective support for the laboring woman?
    A. Including her in conversations that you are having with others in her presence
    B. When leaving the room, informing her of the reason and when to expect your return
    C. Telling her in advance of examinations or special procedures
    D. All of these

15. Under the influence of labor contractions, the muscle fibers in the fundal portion of the uterus shorten as the fibers in the lower uterine segment lengthen.
    A. True
    B. False

16. *Effacement* refers to the process in which the cervix becomes shortened or thinned out.
    A. True
    B. False

17. The process of labor has been divided into four stages according to the changes in the mother's body brought about through the process of birthing.
    A. True
    B. False

18. The end of the first stage of labor is defined by:
    A. Rupture of membranes
    B. 5 cm of dilatation
    C. Complete effacement of the cervix
    D. Complete dilatation of the cervix

19. To determine the onset of true labor, it is necessary to identify:
    A. Onset of regular uterine contractions
    B. Complete cervical effacement
    C. Rupture of membranes
    D. Occurrence of bloody show

The patterns of contractions below was repeated over a 2- to 7-hour time segment. Answer questions 20–23 based on this pattern.

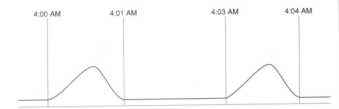

20. It is probably fair to conclude that the expectant woman is in labor.
    A. True
    B. False

21. Contractions are 60 seconds in duration.
    A. True
    B. False

22. The frequency of contractions is every 4 minutes.
    A. True
    B. False

23. The interval between contractions is 5 minutes.
    A. True
    B. False

24. Match the stage of labor in Column B with the appropriate description in Column A. Place the letter of your choice beside the appropriate number. You may use the choices more than once.

Column A
_____ 1. Is a 1-hour period of stabilizing of vital signs and body changes
_____ 2. Ends with the expulsion of the placenta
_____ 3. Includes a latent phase, which lasts several hours
_____ 4. Begins with the onset of fairly regular contractions
_____ 5. Begins with full dilatation of the cervix

Column B
A. Stage I
B. Stage II
C. Stage III
D. Stage IV

25. Evidence-based findings show that the continuous presence of a supportive person for the laboring woman is associated with all of the following *except:*
    A. A reduction in the need for cesarean birth
    B. Less likelihood for an Apgar score below 7 at 5 minutes
    C. Avoidance of medication use
    D. Less likelihood of the need for operative vaginal delivery (e.g., forceps, vacuum extraction)

26. A culturally competent nurse reflects all of the following characteristics *except:*
    A. Retains a sense of humor to keep a balanced perspective
    B. Moves beyond simply tolerating cultural differences to becoming comfortable with differences that exist between himself or herself and the patient
    C. Ignores his or her personal values and biases to interact effectively with a patient
    D. Becomes familiar with the unique needs of patients from different communities

Check your answers with the Module 1 Posttest Answer Key.

Posttest: Module 2. Maternal and Fetal Response to Labor

Answer the following questions without referring back to the information in the module. ONE OR MORE THAN ONE of the choices may be correct.

1. Which aspect of the fetal passenger is described by the following statement: "The fetal head is entering the pelvis first"?
   A. Presentation
   B. Attitude
   C. Position
   D. Lie

2. During an abdominal examination, you determine that Mrs. Hall's baby is lying in a transverse position. What aspect of the fetal passenger are you describing, and is it normal or abnormal?
   A. Attitude; abnormal
   B. Lie; abnormal
   C. Position; normal
   D. Lie; normal

3. The female pelvis has a predominant shape called:
   A. Platypelloid
   B. Android
   C. Anthropoid
   D. Gynecoid

4. The true pelvis is located:
   A. Above the inlet and has narrow dimensions
   B. At the pelvic outlet and has ample room
   C. Below the false pelvis and has narrow dimensions
   D. Above the false pelvis and has narrow dimensions

5. The descent of the fetus is sometimes stopped by the narrowest diameter of the true pelvis, which is called the
   A. Pelvic plane
   B. Inlet
   C. Plane of great dimensions
   D. Plane of least dimensions

6. An adaptation that permits the fetus to descend during birth is:
   A. Widening of the pelvic joints
   B. Change in size of the pelvic outlet
   C. Softening of the bony pelvis
   D. Molding of the fetal skull

7. During a vaginal examination, the posterior fontanelle is felt. Which part of the fetus is coming first?
   A. Breech
   B. Head
   C. Shoulder
   D. Foot

8. If you find that the fetal head is well flexed during a vaginal examination, you would expect to feel the:
   A. Sinciput
   B. Sagittal suture
   C. Mentum
   D. Vertex

9. While examining a laboring woman for admission, you discover that the fetus is in a transverse lie. You should know that (choose all answers that apply):
   A. This mother will not deliver vaginally
   B. This condition is associated with placenta previa
   C. There is something wrong with the baby
   D. This happens frequently and there is no reason for concern

10. Normally, the fetus assumes a flexed position because it:
    A. Is more comfortable
    B. Allows for better fetal circulation
    C. Permits the smallest fetal head measurements in relation to the pelvis
    D. Is easier for respirations to occur while labor is in progress

11. When the buttocks or feet enter the pelvis first, the denominator is the:
    A. Vertex
    B. Occiput
    C. Sacrum
    D. Mentum

12. If the occiput is in the left anterior portion of the mother's pelvis, which set of letters accurately describes the fetal position?
    A. ROA
    B. LOA
    C. ROP
    D. LOP

13. If the sacrum of the fetus is in the right posterior area of the mother's pelvis, which set of letters accurately describes the position?
    A. LSP
    B. LST
    C. LSA
    D. RSP

14. The fetal position of ROP describes the position of the fetus in which of the following diagrams?
    A. Diagram A
    B. Diagram B
    C. Diagram C

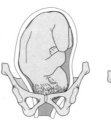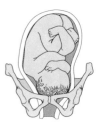

Diagram A   Diagram B   Diagram C

15. The fetal position of LSA describes the position of the fetus in which of the following diagrams?
    A. Diagram A
    B. Diagram B
    C. Diagram C

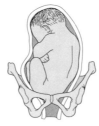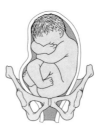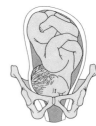

Diagram A   Diagram B   Diagram C

16. If the fetus is at a −1 station, it means that the presenting part is:
    A. At the pelvic outlet
    B. Engaged
    C. Above the ischial spines
    D. Below the ischial spines

17. The caput succedaneum is (more than one selection is possible):
    A. A result of the molding of the fetal skull
    B. A soft, swollen layer under the fetal scalp
    C. A cap of fetal hair
    D. Sometimes misleading to the examiner in evaluating fetal descent

18. An abdominal examination determines that the fetal head is "dipping," which means that the:
    A. Fetal head, although not easily moved, is not yet at station 0
    B. Fetal head is easily moved and is still not into the true pelvis
    C. Fetal presenting part is engaged
    D. Fetal presenting part is at station +2

19. Upon examining the newly admitted woman to labor and delivery, you find that the fetal position is LSA. This describes:
    A. Degree of fetal descent
    B. A malpresentation
    C. A fetal attitude
    D. A transverse lie

20. Which two clinical situations are associated with an abnormal lie?
    A. Hydramnios
    B. A fast labor
    C. A multiple pregnancy
    D. A gynecoid pelvis

21. A young primigravida with a fetus in a breech position is in early labor. You know that there is a better-than-average chance that (choose all answers that apply):
    A. The baby will turn.
    B. The presenting part will descend quickly.
    C. A prolapsed cord might occur.
    D. The baby might be delivered by cesarean birth.

22. The most appropriate action to take when the membranes rupture in a laboring mother with an unengaged fetal presenting part is to:
    A. Take fetal heart tones.
    B. Alert the primary care provider immediately.
    C. Do a vaginal examination.
    D. Give the mother some privacy.

23. A previous difficult and unpleasant labor will have little influence on the progress of a woman's next labor.
    A. True
    B. False

24. The progress of labor usually depends on the adaptations between the fetus and the bony pelvis.
    A. True
    B. False

Check your answers with the Module 2 Posttest Answer Key.

Posttest: Module 3. Admission Assessment of the Laboring Woman (Includes Content from Appendix A)

Answer the following questions without referring back to the information in the module. ONE OR MORE THAN ONE of the choices may be correct.

1. Which statement is *not* an example of an open-ended question?
   A. "What is it that brings you into the hospital?"
   B. "Are you in labor?"
   C. "What did you eat last?"
   D. "How much weight have you gained during this pregnancy?"

2. All of the following questions are important to ask the laboring woman. Which two questions should be asked before performing a vaginal examination?
   A. "How far apart are the contractions now?"
   B. "Have you had any problems during your pregnancy?"
   C. "Have you had any bleeding problems during your pregnancy?"
   D. "Has the bag of waters broken?"

3. Which of the following should *not* be done while taking a history on the woman being admitted for labor?
   A. Directing your questions to the person who comes with the laboring woman.
   B. Following open-ended questions with more specific ones.
   C. Maintaining good eye contact.
   D. Avoiding asking questions during contractions.

4. You admit a woman in advanced labor who cannot answer many questions. She is accompanied by her 16-year-old daughter. The method you select to obtain the *best* history on this mother before she delivers is to:
   A. Ask the daughter about her mother's pregnancy.
   B. Quickly review the woman's prenatal record.
   C. Have the medical records department find the delivery chart of the daughter from 16 years ago.
   D. None of these methods.

5. Which of the following women are *not* at risk for developing problems during labor? The woman who:
   A. Gained a total of 2 pounds with this pregnancy
   B. Has had no prenatal care
   C. Had preeclampsia with her last pregnancy
   D. Is 32 years old and having her first baby

6. A woman is expecting her fourth childbirth and is admitted in labor at 35 weeks' gestation. Compared with a term fetus at 40 weeks, this infant will:
   A. Weigh less and therefore be at risk for problems
   B. Be premature and therefore deliver more quickly
   C. Probably have little difficulty after birth
   D. Be preterm and therefore be at risk for problems

7. You are planning care for four laboring women. As you review the information, which woman needs continuous fetal monitoring?
   A. A 29-year-old woman expecting her fifth childbirth and who is in the early phase of labor.
   B. A 21-year-old woman who is in premature labor with her first baby.
   C. A 15-year-old who is in false labor.
   D. A 34-year-old woman expecting her second child and is progressing well.

8. Which assessment indicates that true labor is in progress?
   A. Contractions are felt in the back and are regular; bloody show is present; walking causes the contractions to intensify.
   B. Bloody show occurred 3 days ago; contractions are irregular and disappear when the woman lies down.
   C. Fatigue is present; diarrhea and low backache have been present for the past 12 hours.
   D. Woman cleans house over a 2-day period; low backache and bloody show are present.

9. Characteristics of normal amniotic fluid are:
   A. Greenish color and composed of salts, fetal hair, and cells.
   B. Highly alkaline and able to turn Nitrazine paper gray.
   C. Clear or straw colored with no foul odor.
   D. Greenish-brown color from fetal stool.

10. Fresh meconium staining in any laboring woman requires careful assessment of the fetus through continuous fetal monitoring.
    A. True
    B. False

11. Match the terms in Column B with the appropriate amniotic fluid conditions in Column A.

Column A	Column B
1. _____ Greenish-brown color	A. Oligohydramnios
2. _____ Less than 500 mL	B. Abruptio placentae
3. _____ Foul smelling	C. Fresh meconium
4. _____ Yellow color	D. Old meconium
5. _____ More than 2,000 mL	E. Infection
6. _____ Port wine color	F. Hydramnios
	G. Eclampsia

12. Hydramnios is associated with:
    A. Problems in the mother
    B. Problems in the fetus
    C. Problems in both mother and fetus
    D. No problems in the mother or fetus

13. A full bladder can make physical examination of the maternal abdomen:
    A. Inaccurate
    B. Difficult to do
    C. Uncomfortable for the woman
    D. More accurate

14. In conducting a physical examination on a woman who you are admitting to labor and delivery, you note that her blood pressure is elevated to 148/94 mmHg. It is also important to look for:
    A. An elevated temperature of greater than 99.6°F
    B. A glistening, rigid abdomen
    C. Bloody show
    D. Protein in the urine

15. To obtain an accurate blood pressure reading in a pregnant woman, which two positions are recommended?
    A. Lying supine
    B. Standing
    C. Sitting up
    D. On her left side

16. To determine whether a blood pressure of 138/88 mmHg is elevated in a pregnant woman, you need to:
    A. Note whether she is extremely anxious.
    B. Check her baseline blood pressure on her prenatal record.
    C. Watch her carefully over the next 3 hours.
    D. Determine whether she has a history of hypertension.

17. A brisk reflex is characterized as (choose all answers that apply):
    A. +1
    B. +2
    C. +3
    D. +4

18. Clonus in a laboring woman with brisk reflexes can be related to:
    A. Anxiety
    B. Central nervous system irritability
    C. The presence of preeclampsia
    D. All of these

19. The difference between the Graves and Pedersen speculum is that:
    A. The Graves speculum is used more often in women who are tense.
    B. The Pedersen speculum is narrower and flatter than the Graves.
    C. The Pedersen speculum is used for examining adult women.
    D. There is no marked difference.

20. To assist a woman in a vaginal examination, which action would *not* be helpful?
    A. Having her fold her arms across her abdomen
    B. Placing a pillow under her head
    C. Telling her to take slow deep breaths throughout the examination
    D. Using your hands to help her separate her legs

21. If the woman becomes upset during a speculum or vaginal examination, the first thing you should do is:
    A. Tell her to let herself relax like a rag doll.
    B. Tell her what you are going to do next.
    C. Stop what you are doing.
    D. Remove the speculum or examining hand.

22. To prevent discomfort to the sensitive bladder as the speculum is introduced into the vagina, you:
    A. Use a moderate downward pressure on the blades
    B. Warm the blades under the light
    C. Use a lubricant
    D. Tell the woman she might feel pressure

23. The *two* best methods of determining that the membranes have ruptured are:
    A. Viewing the leaking fluid as it escapes through the cervical opening
    B. Obtaining a blue-gray color using Nitrazine paper
    C. Obtaining a positive fern test
    D. Noting the smell of the amniotic fluid

24. In carrying out the fern test, how long must the slide be allowed to dry?
    A. 1 minute
    B. 15 minutes
    C. 5 to 7 minutes
    D. No drying period is necessary.

25. An abdominal examination should always precede an *initial* vaginal examination.
    A. True
    B. False

26. When ruptured membranes are suspected, it is acceptable to use clean instead of sterile gloves in a vaginal examination.
    A. True
    B. False

27. A cervix that feels at least 1 inch thick is probably:
    A. 10% effaced
    B. 50% effaced
    C. 100% effaced
    D. Uneffaced

28. When the sagittal suture and posterior fontanelle are felt through the cervical opening during a vaginal examination, the fetal presentation is:
    A. Breech
    B. Face
    C. Cephalic
    D. Shoulder

29. Performing a vaginal examination between contractions gives you the most accurate assessment of cervical dilatation.
    A. True
    B. False

30. Which *two* statements reflect current knowledge about HSV type 1 and type 2?
    A. Asymptomatic infections can occur with either HSV type 1 or type 2.
    B. There is a high correlation between antepartum HSV infection and cervical shedding of the virus at the time of delivery.
    C. Cesarean birth is recommended for all pregnant women with recurrent HSV infection during early pregnancy.
    D. Cesarean birth is recommended only for women who have an active herpes virus lesion at time of delivery, regardless of whether membranes have ruptured.

31. A woman presenting for admission to the labor unit is having contractions every 6 to 8 minutes and is dilated 3 cm. Membranes ruptured 30 minutes ago. She tells you that she has a history of genital herpes infection and that she just noticed this morning that she is developing a painful blister on her right labia. You confirm by inspection that the blister is there. Your next step depends on the fact that you anticipate:
    A. Admission with expected vaginal delivery.
    B. Eventual admission after patient reaches 4 cm dilatation.
    C. Admission with preparations begun for cesarean birth.
    D. Admission with pitocin augmentation of labor.

32. A presenting fetal part felt at 1 cm below the ischial spines is described as at station:
    A. +1
    B. 0
    C. +2
    D. −1

33. You are evaluating a young primigravida who is at 35 weeks' gestation and presents with a complaint of "leaking fluid." She denies having any contractions. The initial step in determining her intrapartum risk status would be to:
    A. Perform a sterile speculum examination.
    B. Perform a vaginal examination to rule out preterm labor.
    C. Carry out 1 hour of electronic fetal monitoring.
    D. Do a Nitrazine test.

34. For which of the following women is it appropriate to perform a vaginal examination?
    A. A multiparous woman presenting at 30 weeks' gestation in early labor with ruptured membranes
    B. A primigravida at 38 weeks' gestation who has leaking membranes and is not in labor
    C. A multiparous woman with ruptured membranes presenting at 39 weeks' gestation, not in labor, but with a cervix dilated to approximately 3 cm as judged by sterile speculum examination
    D. A primigravida at 37 completed weeks' gestation with ruptured membranes, 90-second contractions every 2 minutes, and pronounced bloody show.

35. Which of the women in question 35 has preterm premature rupture of membranes?
    A. A   C. C
    B. B   D. D

36. Fresh meconium staining in the absence of an abnormal fetal heart rate pattern:
    A. Indicates severe distress
    B. Can indicate that the fetus is not in distress
    C. Does not require continuous fetal heart rate auscultation
    D. Indicates fetal hypoxia

37. A mother who is at 43 weeks' gestation is admitted to the labor unit in advanced labor. Membranes are diagnosed as ruptured even though no amniotic fluid is seen. You anticipate that preparations for her delivery include (choose all answers that apply):
    A. Having a pediatrician or neonatal nurse practitioner present at delivery
    B. Setting up for a cesarean delivery
    C. No need for endotracheal suctioning because no meconium is visualized in the amniotic fluid
    D. The possible need for endotracheal suctioning

Check your answers with the Module 3 Posttest Answer Key.

Posttest: Module 4. Admission Assessment of the Fetus

Answer the following questions without referring back to the information in the module. ONE OR MORE THAN ONE of the choices may be correct.

1. Ms. T. tells you that her last normal menstrual period was October 1, 2008. According to Naegele's rule, the EDC would be:
   A. July 1, 2009
   B. August 8, 2009
   C. July 8, 2009
   D. August 1, 2009

2. To estimate an accurate gestational age you know that fetal heart tones are first heard during the:
   A. Tenth to 12th week with a Doptone
   B. Thirteenth to 15th week with a fetoscope
   C. Eighteenth to 20th week with a fetoscope

3. The correct order in the physical assessment of the fetus involves:
   A. Performing fundal height measurement after Leopold's maneuvers
   B. Obtaining fetal heart tones and rate before performing Leopold's maneuvers
   C. Obtaining fetal heart tones after fundal height assessment, fetal position, and fetal presentation are determined
   D. Determining fetal lie, position, and presentation before fundal height is measured

4. What steps are necessary to obtain an accurate fundal height measurement?
   A. Bring the measuring tape to the top of the fundus but not over the curve.
   B. Ask the woman to empty her bladder before the measurement is taken.
   C. Carefully identify the border of the symphysis pubis.
   D. Have the same person do the measuring each time.

5. At the 24th week of pregnancy, the fundal height is expected to range from 20 to 22 cm.
   A. True
   B. False

6. At 40 weeks, the fundal height usually approaches 38 cm.
   A. True
   B. False

7. You obtain a fundal height measurement of 34 cm in an actively laboring woman who is at term according to her EDC. Which of the following could be possibilities for the discrepancy in EDC and fundal height measurement?
   A. A multiple gestation
   B. A growth-restricted infant
   C. An inaccurate EDC
   D. A transverse lie

8. You obtain a fundal height measurement of 44 cm in a woman who is being admitted in early labor. Select the activity that could be omitted from your *immediate* care.
   A. Confirm the expected date of confinement.
   B. Palpate for the presence of twins or polyhydramnios.
   C. Review the mother's prenatal record for a history of diabetes.
   D. Begin an IV.

9. Referring to the situation in question 7, if the increased fundal height is caused by hydramnios, which of the following situations is *not* usually associated with that condition?
   A. Tuberculosis
   B. Syphilis
   C. Twin gestation
   D. A blood incompatibility

10. It is determined that a fetus is severely growth restricted in a mother who is just admitted in advanced labor. If you are in a small community hospital, which of the following are priorities for your nursing interventions?
    A. Monitor the fetus electronically.
    B. Prepare for the delivery of a high-risk infant in the event delivery is imminent.
    C. Anticipate that the mother will be transferred to the nearest regional hospital if she is stable.
    D. Do a complete history and careful physical examination on the mother to determine the cause.

11. One of the reasons that Leopold's maneuvers is performed is to assess where to begin listening for fetal heart tones. If the baby's sacrum is pointing to the mother's lower right side and toward her back, what is the baby's position?
    A. LSP
    B. LSA
    C. RSP
    D. RSA

12. When the fetus is in an ROA position, the fetal heart tones are best heard in the:
    A. Right lower quadrant
    B. Right upper quadrant
    C. Left lower quadrant
    D. Left upper quadrant

13. During the examination of a woman who is approximately 39 weeks pregnant, you use Leopold's maneuvers to determine that the lowest level of the fetal head has moved deep into the pelvis. It is immovable. You *estimate* that the fetal head may be:
    A. Hyperextended
    B. Floating
    C. Dipping
    D. Engaged

14. Baseline FHR refers to the fetal heart rate when the woman is either not in labor or is between uterine contractions.
    A. True
    B. False

15. The best time to begin listening to a fetal heart rate is between contractions.
    A. True
    B. False

16. Fetal tachycardia is a sustained baseline rate above 160 bpm.
    A. True
    B. False

17. Intermittent auscultation during labor has been found to be equivalent to EFM as a method of fetal surveillance in which of the following situations?
    A. In low-risk intrapartum situations
    B. When the laboring woman is at high risk
    C. When there is a 1:1 nurse:patient ratio
    D. When the nurse is experienced and skilled in the method and interpretation

18. In ensuring safe and sound clinical practice, decisions to use intermittent auscultation or EFM in laboring women will need to be guided by which combination of the following?
    1. Degree of risk in each clinical situation
    2. Staffing on the unit
    3. Expertise of the staff
    4. Preference of the laboring woman and her provider
    A. 1, 2, 3
    B. 1, 3, 4
    C. 1, 2, 4
    D. 1, 2, 3, 4

19. Current research supports findings that the skilled and experienced nurse or provider can use intermittent auscultation to identify:
    A. FHR baseline, rhythm, and audible accelerations and decelerations from baseline
    B. Early and late decelerations
    C. Short-term variability
    D. Long-term variability

20. Select the one guideline given when using the EFM Doppler *for the purpose of fetal heart rate auscultation.*
    A. The paper recorder can be running, and the tracing must be interpreted.
    B. The paper recorder must not be running.
    C. The paper recorder can be running, but no interpretation of the tracing should be recorded.
    D. None of the above apply.

21. Electronic fetal monitoring for high-risk laboring women results in better neonatal outcomes than when the auscultation method is used.
    A. True
    B. False

22. In caring for a low-risk, actively laboring woman at 40 weeks' gestation, you auscultate fetal heart sounds for 2 full minutes on three separate occasions over a 10-minute period. The rate on each occasion is 100 bpm. Having assisted the mother to side-lying position, your next step(s) are to:
    A. Begin oxygen, and continue auscultation for at least 30 minutes to assess the true heart rate
    B. Request that another nurse validate the fetal heart rate by auscultation
    C. Change to electronic fetal monitoring
    D. Continue auscultation because 100 bpm is within an acceptable fetal heart rate range

23. Which of the following two choices explain the rationale for the step taken in question 22?
    A. Intermittent auscultation for fetal heart rate is not able to discriminate among types of fetal heart rate changes such as late decelerations or short-term variability.
    B. Continuous electronic fetal monitoring is effective in predicting the extent of fetal distress in utero.
    C. Auscultation by an experienced clinician can identify mild, as well as severe, fetal distress.
    D. Bradycardia accompanied by moderate baseline variability indicates that the fetus is tolerating a stressful event, but only electronic fetal monitoring will reveal these variability patterns.

24. Using the auscultation method to establish the baseline fetal heart rate in a woman, you would:
    A. Begin listening immediately after a contraction ends and count for a minimum of 30 seconds
    B. Listen and count throughout the contraction and for a minimum of 30 seconds after
    C. Begin listening as the contraction begins and listen for 30 seconds; then multiply by 2
    D. Listen at least every 60 minutes during early labor

25. A multiparous woman seen in the labor unit is reportedly at 38 weeks' gestation. As you review her prenatal record, which of the following is the most reliable criterion for confirming her gestational age?
    A. Reported LMP consisting of only 3 days of spotting
    B. Serum hCG levels less than 10,000 that decrease between 5 and 8 weeks
    C. An ultrasound that revealed a fetal crown–rump length correlating with 9 weeks' gestation
    D. Quickening reported at 20 weeks' gestation

26. Which of the following situations has the greatest risk for the fetus?
    A. A fundal height of 25 cm at 30 weeks' gestation
    B. A fetal heart rate of 170 bpm with fetal movements
    C. A breech lie
    D. A gestational age of 41 weeks

27. A young, expectant woman calls at 6 PM, stating that this is her first pregnancy and that she is due in 3 weeks. Having just completed an hour of "fetal kick counting," her concern is that only six movements were experienced. Further questioning confirms that she has had a normal pregnancy. You:
    A. Instruct her to come in immediately for further evaluation
    B. Tell her to drink two glasses of water or juice, continue counting for 1 more hour, and call back with the results
    C. Explain that this is normal and that she does not need to count anymore today
    D. Praise the mother and tell her to call her primary care provider in the morning for evaluation

28. Which of the following are examples of a fetal adaptive response?
    A. A significant reduction in breathing movements for a few hours in the presence of maternal ingestion of alcohol
    B. A significant reduction in gross body movements before the beginning of labor
    C. A decrease in fetal breathing movements during active labor
    D. Decreased activity in the presence of hypoxia

29. During an early morning admission to the labor unit for a scheduled induction for postdates, the mother tells you that she has not felt any fetal movement since eating dinner last evening. An appropriate response to this would be to:
    A. Quickly finish the admission process and inform her primary care provider
    B. Auscultate for fetal heart tones as soon as the admission process is completed
    C. Alter your admission process and immediately place an external electronic fetal monitor on the mother
    D. Question the mother about her method of fetal movement assessment and about occurrences of contraction or bleeding activity

30. The rationale for your response to the situation in question 29 is:
    A. The primary care provider might alter the plan of management
    B. Completing the admission process will provide you with important information you need to complete a management plan
    C. Absence of fetal movement for more than 12 hours but with fetal heart tones present may indicate a severely distressed fetus and a need for immediate intervention
    D. Maternal perceptions of fetal movement may not always correlate with actual fetal activity, so confirming the presence or absence of fetal heart tones is critical

31. Many expectant women do not seek care concerning possible labor because they:
    A. Do not trust what they feel
    B. Have no prior experience on which to base a judgment
    C. Are fearful of advanced technology
    D. Fear being perceived as bothersome or overreacting

32. When an expectant woman in the third trimester of pregnancy calls to report decreased fetal movement, evaluation usually reveals:
    A. A normal fetal heart rate and activity pattern
    B. An overanxious expectant mother
    C. A fetal demise
    D. A fetus in some distress

Check your answers with the Module 4 Posttest Answer Key.

Posttest: Module 5. Caring for the Laboring Woman

Answer the following questions without referring back to the information in the module. ONE OR MORE THAN ONE of the choices may be correct.

1. Reducing a low-risk expectant mother's anxiety during labor can be accomplished by:
   A. Providing comfort measures, such as offering fluid and food choices throughout the first 12 hours of labor
   B. Giving her choices of resting in bed, ambulating, or using a rocking chair
   C. Looking at her and explaining in some detail what you are assessing during a vaginal examination
   D. Anticipating with her how long pushing might take to birth the baby

2. A supportive caregiver behavior(s) is (are):
   A. Nonverbal behaviors that enhance a woman's ability to cope
   B. Vital sign monitoring practices that adhere to standards for maternal and fetal assessments
   C. The provision of assistance with epidural administration
   D. Regulation of IV fluid administration to ensure adequate hydration

3. Maternal NPO (nothing by mouth) practices in labor and delivery units are associated with:
   A. Valid research to support its continuing practice
   B. Risk of fetal hyperglycemia
   C. High acidic gastric contents
   D. An assurance of little maternal stomach contents

4. You are admitting a nulliparous patient who is 5 cm dilated with ruptured membranes and bloody show. She tells you that her contractions began today at approximately 8 AM. Which question is most likely to assist you in estimating the onset of true labor?
   A. When did the contractions begin to last more than 1 minute?
   B. When did the bag of waters rupture?
   C. When did you begin to have bloody show?
   D. When did the contractions begin to come fairly regularly?

5. A nulliparous woman who is having a normal pattern of labor will:
   A. Reach full dilatation in approximately 10 hours of labor
   B. Dilate at a rate of approximately 1 cm per hour in the active phase
   C. Have a pattern of descent at approximately 2 cm per hour in the active phase
   D. Not have a predictable pattern of labor

6. A woman laboring with her third birth remains at 2 cm of dilatation for the first 10 hours. This is:
   A. A normal latent phase
   B. A protracted active phase
   C. Best treated with oxytocin stimulation
   D. An indication that labor will be lengthy

7. Assuming that contractions became fairly regular at approximately 1 PM and using the data given, graph the following labor.

Time	Cervical Dilatation (cm)	Station
1:00 PM	2	−2
2:00 PM	1	−1
3:00 PM	3	−1
4:00 PM	5	0
5:00 PM	9	+1
6:00 PM	10	+3

8. The labor in question 7 is most likely a multiparous labor.
   A. True   B. False

9. The descent pattern in question 11 is protracted.
   A. True   B. False

10. According to Friedman's recommendations, treatment at this time for the woman laboring in question 7 would include:
    A. Initiation of oxytocin stimulation
    B. A forceps delivery
    C. Continued observation
    D. A cesarean section

11. Which of the following steps ensures an effective but sensitive vaginal examination?
    A. Acknowledging the woman's pain if she indicates discomfort
    B. Performing the examination between contractions
    C. Waiting until the woman gives you consent to begin
    D. Because women will not usually give consent, beginning the examination gently without asking permission

12. A supportive companion (e.g., nurse, father, coach) can increase the laboring woman's chance to:
    A. Have a vaginal delivery
    B. Require less pain medication
    C. Deliver without the complication of meconium-stained amniotic fluid
    D. Experience a shorter labor than she might otherwise have had

The following two questions are about a nulliparous woman who has been admitted to the labor and delivery unit. Her labor curve has been plotted on a Friedman graph and appears in the following figure.

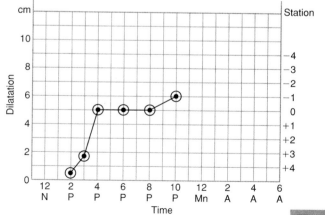

13. The endpoint (4 to 10 PM) of the curve shows:
    A. A prolonged latent phase
    B. Normal labor
    C. Arrested dilatation
    D. A protracted active phase

14. If cephalopelvic disproportion and malpresentation have been ruled out, which of the following treatments is *not likely* to improve the pattern, according to Friedman's recommendations?
    A. Sedation and rest
    B. Oxytocin stimulation
    C. Intravenous fluid
    D. Artificial rupture of membranes

15. A woman in active labor is dilating at an average rate of 1.5 cm per hour. Which of the following describes the woman's progress in labor?
    A. A protracted labor pattern for the multipara
    B. A precipitous labor pattern in the nullipara
    C. Normal rate of dilatation for the multipara
    D. A precipitous labor pattern in the multipara

16. A 28-year-old gravida 10, para 9, is 8 cm dilated but remains at 0 station for 2 hours. She is having labor induction for preeclampsia. Which of the following is *not* effective in treating arrest of descent?
    A. Allowing excessive sedation to wear off
    B. Providing therapeutic rest
    C. Continuing the oxytocin stimulation
    D. Encouraging a family member to remain in the room for support

17. A protracted descent pattern might be caused by an occiput posterior position of the fetus.
    A. True
    B. False

18. A woman you are caring for is experiencing a protracted active phase. Select the statement or statements that identify appropriate treatment for this situation.
    A. Amniotomy
    B. Increasing the rate of IV fluid intake if it is running at a rate of less than 1,000 mL every 8 hours
    C. Oxytocin stimulation
    D. Offering constant support to reduce the need for added sedation

19. You are caring for M.J., a 22-year-old low-risk laboring woman who is 7 cm dilated and at +1 cm. She does not have an electronic fetal monitor. Which of the following nursing actions are appropriate?
    A. Performing a vaginal examination every 15 minutes, as should be done on all laboring women who are dilated 7 cm or more
    B. When auscultating for fetal heart tones, counting the FHR throughout a contraction and for 30 seconds after the contraction
    C. Encouraging the mother to lie on either side during much of her remaining labor
    D. Discouraging any family members from remaining with M.J. during this difficult phase of labor

20. You auscultated M.J.'s fetal heart rate at 1:15 PM. The next time it should be evaluated is at:
    A. 1:20 PM   B. 1:25 PM
    C. 1:30 PM   D. 1:45 PM

21. M.J.'s blood pressure at 1:15 PM was 128/80 mmHg. Her blood pressure has been fairly stable throughout labor. If her status remains basically stable, you will evaluate her blood pressure again at:
    A. 1:30 PM   B. 1:45 PM
    C. 2:00 PM   D. 2:15 PM

22. A young woman at 39 weeks' gestation is admitted to the hospital; she is having uterine contractions every 5 minutes, and they last for 40 seconds. The cervix is well effaced and dilated 2 cm. There is no change in the findings after 1 hour. This patient exhibits:
    A. Active labor
    B. False labor or latent-phase labor
    C. Abruptio placentae
    D. Precipitous labor

23. A woman presents with questionable ruptured membranes. The most accurate method for determining whether membranes have ruptured is:
    A. The Nitrazine test
    B. A careful history obtained from the mother
    C. An ultrasound examination
    D. A sterile speculum examination and fern test

24. Pressure, traction, and stretching of body tissues cause labor pain, making it impossible to reduce the mother's discomfort.
    A. True
    B. False

25. Pain experienced by the laboring woman can ultimately make the brain cells of the fetus more susceptible to damage during a hypoxic period.
    A. True
    B. False

26. Rapid breathing in the laboring mother can lead to a decreased blood supply to the uterus.
    A. True
    B. False

27. You have just come on duty and have not yet made rounds in the labor unit. An order for pain medication has been received for a young nullipara who is restless and calling out. Which of the following will you do before giving the pain medication?
    A. Quickly review her prenatal record
    B. Take her blood pressure and FHR
    C. Note the size and maturity of the fetus according to gestational age
    D. Determine what progress she has made in labor

28. Slow chest breathing:
    A. Involves taking deep breaths in through the nose and exhaling through the mouth or nose
    B. Is used during stage II of labor
    C. Is done with the eyes closed
    D. Begins and ends with a cleansing breath

29. Effleurage is:
    A. A big deep sigh that begins and ends each contraction
    B. A massage technique that can be done by the mother, nurse, or support person
    C. Used between contractions
    D. Sometimes done by the coach

30. Which position for pushing does not make use of the effects of gravity or result in good circulation for the woman and fetus?
    A. Squatting
    B. Semi-Fowler's
    C. Sims
    D. Lithotomy

31. Select the statement that represents current recommendations for nursing assessment of maternal and fetal status during stage II of labor.
    A. Fetal heart rate is checked before and during each contraction, and maternal blood pressure is taken every 5 minutes.
    B. Fetal heart rate is checked after each contraction, and maternal blood pressure is taken every 30 minutes.
    C. Fetal heart rate and maternal blood pressure are checked every 15 minutes.
    D. Fetal heart rate and maternal blood pressure are checked after each contraction.

32. When you begin your evening shift at 4 PM, you receive a report on an 18-year-old gravida 1 who is in active labor. At 2 PM, she was 5 cm dilated and 100% effaced, with the vertex at 0 station. Membranes ruptured at 11 AM. You evaluate her and note that she is on her back, restless, and requesting pain medication. Contractions are occurring every 3 minutes, are of 70 seconds' duration, and are strong on palpation. Her physician plans to perform an emergency cesarean section. Which sequence of steps will you take next?
    A. Take vital signs, including temperature; perform an abdominal palpation for fetal position; check fetal heart rate; perform a vaginal examination; inform the woman of progress made; assist her to a side-lying position.
    B. Perform a vaginal examination; perform an abdominal palpation for fetal position; check fetal heart rate; inform the woman of progress made; take vital signs, including temperature; assist her to a side-lying position.
    C. Assist the woman to the bathroom for voiding; take vital signs, including temperature; perform a vaginal examination; check fetal heart rate; assist her to a side-lying position.
    D. Perform an abdominal palpation for fetal position; check fetal heart rate; perform a vaginal examination; inform the woman of progress made; take vital signs, including temperature; assist her to a side-lying position.

33. When you administer IV pain medication to the laboring woman you should:
    A. Use a filter needle when drawing the medication from a glass ampule
    B. Always position the mother on her side
    C. Give the medication at the beginning of a contraction and over a period of a few minutes, if possible
    D. Give the medication at the end of a contraction and over a period of a few minutes, if possible

34. Which of the following situations is (are) more likely to result in a depressed infant?
    A. Protracted labor treated with oxytocin augmentation
    B. Secondary arrest of labor with subsequent vaginal delivery
    C. Secondary arrest of labor with subsequent cesarean delivery
    D. Arrest of descent treated with oxytocin augmentation and forceps delivery

35. Nursing measures carried out in preparation for and during the test dosing for epidural anesthesia include all of the following *except:*
    A. Noting maternal blood pressure and pulse rate before and after administration of the test dose and at least every 5 minutes throughout the administration
    B. Ensuring that the woman's bladder is not full
    C. Explaining potential complications to the woman
    D. Confirming a reassuring fetal heart rate tracing before the procedure.

36. Select two statements that reflect what is currently appreciated about epidural anesthesia nursing care in the laboring woman.
    A. There are reliable, statistically significant data showing a cause-and-effect relationship between the use of epidural anesthesia and adverse effects.
    B. AWHONN guidelines for nursing care of women receiving epidural analgesia/anesthesia draw from considerable nursing research.
    C. Although concern exists that epidural anesthesia may be associated with prolonged stages of labor, increased use of vacuum extractions and forceps, and higher rates of cesarean births, some clinicians believe the individual styles of obstetric management may play a significant role as well.
    D. Administration of bolus medications for an epidural anesthesia by the nurse is not supported in AWHONN guidelines.

Check your answers with the Module 5 Posttest Answer Key.

Posttest: Module 6. Intrapartum Fetal Monitoring

Answer the following questions without referring back to the information in the module. ONE OR MORE THAN ONE of the choices may be correct.

1. For each of the following statements, indicate whether the statement refers to external fetal monitoring (E), internal fetal monitoring (I), or both (B).
   a. _____ Procedure is noninvasive.
   b. _____ Decelerations can be detected in the fetal heart rate.
   c. _____ Intensity of the uterine contractions can be assessed.
   d. _____ Procedure is associated with no fetal or maternal morbidity.
   e. _____ Procedure requires partial dilatation of the cervix.
   f. _____ Frequency of the uterine contractions can be determined.
   g. _____ Variability of the fetal heart rate can be assessed during labor.

2. The baseline fetal heart rate:
   A. Is between 110 and 160 bpm
   B. Is determined between contractions
   C. Can be influenced by maternal hyperthermia and hypoxia
   D. All of the above
   E. None of the above

3. Which of the following statements are *true* regarding baseline uterine tonus?
   A. Defined as the amount of tone in the uterus during a contraction
   B. Usually ranges between 5 and 15 mmHg, but is not greater than 30 mmHg
   C. Can be determined using an external or internal fetal monitor
   D. Can be increased with the use of oxytocin

4. Which of the following statements are *true* concerning fetal heart rate bradycardia?
   A. It is often defined as a decrease in the fetal heart rate to less than 110 bpm, lasting longer than 10 minutes.
   B. It can reflect prolonged fetal hypoxia.
   C. Oxygen therapy should be used in the treatment.
   D. All of the above are correct.

5. Uterine contractions can alter fetal heart rate via compression of the myometrial vessels, compression of the fetal head, and compression of the umbilical cord.
   A. True
   B. False

6. Indicate the appropriate type of periodic heart rate change using the following key. There may be more than one answer.

   Key
   A = accelerations
   ED = early decelerations
   VD = variable decelerations
   LD = late decelerations
   PD = prolonged decelerations

Characteristics of Periodic Heart Rate Changes
   a. _____ Rarely falls below 110 bpm
   b. _____ Most common type of periodic change
   c. _____ Not a sign of fetal stress
   d. _____ Usually associated with good fetal outcome
   e. _____ Reflect(s) fetal hypoxia
   f. _____ Has (have) no consistent onset in relation to the contraction pattern
   g. _____ Uniform in shape and always last longer than the contraction
   h. _____ Often associated with decreased variability
   i. _____ Usually associated with moderate variability
   j. _____ Should be treated with oxygen therapy
   k. _____ Caused by uteroplacental insufficiency
   l. _____ Caused by umbilical cord compression
   m. _____ Caused by fetal head compression

7. You are caring for a laboring patient who is being monitored. You notice several early decelerations. You should (more than one answer may be correct; list all):
   A. Continue to watch the monitor closely and perform a vaginal examination
   B. Begin oxygen therapy
   C. Notify the primary care provider immediately
   D. Change the patient's position

8. You are caring for a laboring patient who is being monitored. You notice a decrease in variability along with two subtle late decelerations in a 15-minute period. You should:
   A. Begin oxygen therapy
   B. Notify the primary care provider
   C. Change the patient's position to lateral
   D. Do the above *only* if the late decelerations begin to occur more frequently

9. Oxytocin infusion should be stopped in the following situation(s):
   A. Occurrence of repetitive late decelerations with loss of variability
   B. Occurrence of severe and prolonged variable decelerations
   C. Occurrence of early decelerations
   D. All of the above

Questions 10 through 16 refer to the following strip graph. Use this strip to answer these questions. (This is an internal fetal monitor strip.)

10. What type of periodic heart rate change is present?
    A. Acceleration
    B. Early deceleration
    C. Variable deceleration
    D. Late deceleration

11. The fetal heart rate short-term variability is:
    A. Absent
    B. Minimal
    C. Moderate
    D. Marked

12. The baseline fetal heart rate is:
    A. 165 bpm   B. 140 bpm   C. 150 bpm   D. 145 bpm

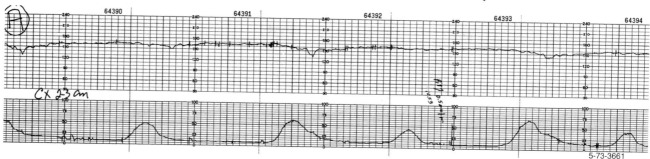

13. The cause of this periodic heart rate change is:
    A. Head compression
    B. Umbilical cord compression
    C. Uteroplacental insufficiency

14. The baseline uterine tone is:
    A. Within normal range
    B. Indeterminable with this type of monitoring
    C. Increased
    D. Decreased

15. The intensity of the uterine contractions is:
    A. 45 to 70 mmHg
    B. 75 to 85 mmHg
    C. Indeterminable with this type of monitoring
    D. Indicative of a moderate contraction

16. From the following list, determine the appropriate nursing action(s) for this type of periodic heart rate change. If the action is considered appropriate, write an "A" before the action. If the action is *not* considered appropriate, write an "N" before the action.
    a. _____ Turn the patient to her left side.
    b. _____ Continue watching the monitor closely.
    c. _____ Begin oxygen therapy.
    d. _____ Decrease the IV rate.
    e. _____ Place the patient on her back.
    f. _____ Turn off oxytocin (if infusing).
    g. _____ Notify the primary care provider immediately.

17. Mrs. S., a 35-year-old hypertensive patient at 38 weeks' gestation, is admitted in labor, and a fetal monitor is applied. Considering this patient's history, you must watch closely for:
    A. Early decelerations
    B. Late decelerations
    C. Variable decelerations

18. Hypoxia can be indicated by all of the following *except:*
    A. Late decelerations
    B. Decreased variability
    C. Early decelerations
    D. Fetal heart rate tachycardia

19. Complications of excessive oxytocin administration are:
    A. Uterine hypertonus
    B. Uterine rupture
    C. Fetal hypoxia
    D. All of the above
    E. None of the above

20. Variable decelerations:
    A. Start as a gradual drop from the baseline
    B. Must occur with contractions
    C. Are usually responsive to maternal position changes
    D. Rarely occur with shoulders

21. After administration of epidural anesthesia, late decelerations are observed. All of the following are appropriate interventions *except:*
    A. Increasing IV fluids
    B. Keeping the patient on her back
    C. Administering oxygen
    D. Discontinuing oxytocin infusion

22. Indications for internal FHR monitoring include all of the following *except:*
    A. Late decelerations with moderate variability
    B. A fetus with an irregular heartbeat
    C. Obese patient unable to trace externally
    D. An active fetus that is difficult to monitor externally

23. All of the following can cause prolonged FHR decelerations *except:*
    A. Cord prolapse
    B. Epidural anesthesia
    C. Hypertonic uterus
    D. Tetanic contractions
    E. Maternal fever

24. Which of the following is recommended *before* the initiation of electronic fetal monitoring?
    A. Auscultating the FHR
    B. Performing Leopold's maneuvers
    C. Starting IV fluids
    D. A and B
    E. B and C

25. In the presence of an intrauterine fetal death, the fetal electrode:
    A. Occasionally picks up the maternal ECG signal
    B. Always picks up the maternal ECG signal
    C. Will generate no signal
    D. Never picks up the maternal ECG signal

26. The spiral electrode permits accurate recording of:
    A. Variability
    B. Decelerations
    C. Accelerations
    D. All of the above

27. Ominous signs on the fetal heart rate tracing include all of the following *except:*
    A. Absent FHR variability
    B. Accelerations of the FHR
    C. Late decelerations
    D. Sinusoidal pattern

28. Variable decelerations probably indicate:
    A. Severe fetal distress
    B. The need for preparation for an aggressive resuscitation of the newborn
    C. Increasing placental dysfunction
    D. Respiratory acidosis
    E. A and D
    F. B and C

29. Absent variability can be indicative of:
    A. Metabolic acidosis
    B. Fetal hypoxia
    C. Respiratory acidosis
    D. Mixed acidosis
    E. A and B
    F. B and C
    G. C and D

30. Characteristic(s) of an abruptio placentae seen on the fetal monitor strip might include:
    A. A wavelike contraction pattern
    B. Increased baseline tone
    C. Frequent contractions
    D. Fetal tachycardia
    E. B and C
    F. A, B, and C
    G. All of the above

Label the statements in questions 31 through 72 as:
    A. True
    B. False

31. _____ Variable decelerations indicate maternal hypotension.

32. _____ Early decelerations are uniform in shape.

33. _____ Some deceleration patterns may be corrected by giving terbutaline.

34. _____ The presence of variability and periodic changes can usually be detected accurately with both internal and external monitoring.

35. _____ Fetal tachycardia, if untreated, can proceed to bradycardia and finally death.

36. _____ When fetal stress is suspected, it is appropriate to turn the patient on her side; discontinue the oxytocin, if it is infusing; administer a bolus of IV fluids; and perform a vaginal examination.

37. _____ Late decelerations are uniform in shape, last beyond the contraction, and often are associated with acidosis and hypoxia.

38. _____ The fetal heart rate baseline is determined in beats per minute during a contraction.

39. _____ Variable decelerations are believed to be a result of cord compression.

40. _____ Everything pertaining to the care of a patient should be on the tracing except the diagnosis or identification of periodic changes.

41. _____ Anything that affects maternal blood flow can affect the blood flow through the placenta.

42. _____ Chronic maternal diseases such as hypertension, diabetes mellitus, and collagen vascular disease can all compromise placental gas exchange.

43. _____ A persistent sinusoidal pattern can be associated with fetal asphyxia.

44. _____ Variability is a sensitive indicator of adequate fetal oxygenation and reserve.

45. _____ A true sinusoidal pattern is uncommon.

46. _____ Early decelerations do not require intervention.

47. _____ Tachycardia usually proceeds bradycardia.

48. _____ The FSE can pick up the maternal heart rate if the fetus dies.

49. _____ Events such as blood pressure, VE, and medications should be accurately noted on the tracing. Therefore, tracings are replacements for conventional notes.

50. _____ Baroreceptors are stimulated by changes in the arterial blood pressure.

51. _____ Periodic changes should be marked and identified on all tracings.

52. _____ During cord compression, the arteries are the first vessels to be compressed.

53. _____ Late decelerations always begin at the peak of the contraction.

54. _____ Maturation of the parasympathetic nervous system is usually complete by week 28 to 32 of gestation.

55. _____ The fetal heart rate can stay within the normal range and still show signs of stress.

56. _____ A FHR baseline above 100 bpm with good variability is almost always benign.

57. _____ Variable decelerations can vary in shape and onset and are caused by placental dysfunction.

58. _____ Late decelerations usually remain within the normal FHR range.

59. _____ When determining whether the FHR pattern is reassuring or nonreassuring, one must assess variability.

60. _____ FHR accelerations can be a response to contractions, fetal movement, or abdominal palpation.

61. _____ Variable decelerations are thought to be caused by cord compression.

62. _____ The gradual decrease in FHR that occurs with increasing gestational age can be explained as increased maturation of the parasympathetic nervous system.

63. _____ In the presence of persistent late decelerations, there is nothing that the caregiver can do to improve the FHR pattern.

64. _____ FHR accelerations are almost always a sign of fetal well-being.

65. _____ When variability is absent, late decelerations, regardless of depth, should always be considered nonreassuring.

66. _____ Variables are uniform decelerations.

67. _____ Patients in labor should always lie on their backs so that the monitor can function properly.

68. _____ The fetal baseline heart rate is usually the best indicator of fetal oxygenation.

69. _____ FHR variability is determined exclusively by the sympathetic nervous system.

70. _____ The characteristic that distinguishes a variable deceleration from late and early decelerations is the abrupt drop from baseline.

71. _____ Periodic and nonperiodic changes (accelerations and decelerations) should be *marked* on all tracings.

72. _____ A sign on the monitor strip that might indicate *early* fetal hypoxia is bradycardia.

73. Select the appropriate interpretation of the following umbilical cord blood gas values. Choose from the following:
1. Normal
2. Normal with a shift toward metabolic acidosis
3. Normal with a shift toward respiratory acidosis
4. Metabolic acidosis
5. Respiratory acidosis
6. Metabolic and respiratory acidosis (mixed acidosis)

a. _____ pH 7.12
   P_{CO_2} 69 mmHg
   P_{O_2} 22 mmHg
   BD 4.4

b. _____ pH 7.25
   P_{CO_2} 50 mmHg
   P_{O_2} 24 mmHg
   BD 4.5

c. _____ pH 7.16
   P_{CO_2} 36 mmHg
   P_{O_2} 16 mmHg
   BD 12.0

Check your answers with the Module 6 Posttest Answer Key.

Posttest: Module 7. Induction and Augmentation of Labor

Answer the following questions without referring back to the information in the module. Select the ONE BEST answer for each question.

Mrs. Lea K. Waters is a 27-year-old woman admitted to the labor unit. She is at term with her second pregnancy. Her membranes ruptured 10 hours ago, and she has no palpable uterine contractions. Upon abdominal examination, you estimate fetal weight at 8 to 8.5 pounds and determine that the fetus is vertex presentation, ROA, and not engaged. Sterile vaginal examination reveals a roomy pelvis with presenting part at −2 station and cervix anterior soft, 80% effaced, and 3 cm dilated. The fluid is clear; vital signs and fetal heart rate are normal.

Mrs. Waters' first pregnancy was uneventful, and she delivered her 8-pound, 2-ounce son over an intact perineum. This pregnancy has been a good one for her. Family history; past medical, surgical, and gynecologic history; and current laboratory work are all normal. She and her husband plan to use their prepared childbirth techniques. Mrs. Waters will breastfeed this baby.

1. On the basis of this information, Mrs. Waters is a good candidate for oxytocin stimulation.
   A. True
   B. False

2. Her Bishop's score is:
   A. 6
   B. 8
   C. 10

You call Mrs. Waters' health care provider to give him your assessment. He informs you that he saw her several days ago in the office and that your vaginal examination findings are the same as his were at the time. He then directs you to start electronic fetal heart rate monitoring and to insert an intrauterine pressure catheter. After you have obtained a normal baseline evaluation, he wants you to start an oxytocin induction. He is readily available in his office next door and will be in to evaluate Mrs. Waters in an hour or two. You have his approved induction/augmentation protocols on file, and you are properly credentialed to initiate and conduct internal electronic monitoring, insert an intrauterine pressure catheter, and administer oxytocin per protocol.

3. The nurse should begin the oxytocin administration after a baseline evaluation to prevent delay and possible infection.
   A. True
   B. False

4. Before oxytocin is administered, the:
   A. Nurse must sedate the anxious woman if she refuses induction/augmentation
   B. Woman should be examined and a physician credentialed to perform a cesarean section must be readily available
   C. Woman's health care provider must write the order for the oxytocin administration rate that will dilate the woman's cervix most rapidly
   D. Nurse knows that if the woman is parous, her Bishop's score must be more than 5

5. Match the terms in Column A with the appropriate definition in Column B.

Column A	Column B
1. _____ Tetanic contractions	a. Trade name for a synthetic hormone that makes the uterus contract
2. _____ Fetal hypoxia	b. Stimulating uterine contractions to become more powerful
3. _____ Water intoxication	c. Retention of water, low serum levels of salt, and poor urinary output
4. _____ Fetal bradycardia	d. Powerful contractions without adequate rest periods
5. _____ Uterine dystocia	e. Poor-quality contractions
6. _____ Pitocin	f. Slow heartbeat
7. _____ Secreted by the posterior pituitary	g. Decreased oxygen
8. _____ Augmentation of labor	h. Oxytocin

6. For safe administration of oxytocin, the following is recommended.
   A. Piggyback setup, electronic fetal/uterine monitoring, and nasal oxygen
   B. Two-bottle IV administration setup, fluid administration setup, and fetal/uterine electronic monitoring
   C. IV fluid administration pump, piggyback setup, and electronic fetal/uterine monitoring
   D. Infusion control pump with filter needle attached, two-bottle setup, and fetal/uterine electronic monitoring.

7. If sustained fetal bradycardia, tachycardia, or loss of variability is observed during the administration of an oxytocin infusion, the first thing the nurse must do is:
   A. Call the woman's health care provider
   B. Change the woman's position and reassure her
   C. Keep the rate of oxytocin administration at the same setting until the fetal heart rate improves
   D. Discontinue the administration of the oxytocin

8. When administering oxytocin for augmentation of labor, the nurse must be aware that it will:
   A. Usually cause tetanic contractions, which dilate the cervix quickly
   B. Cause a forceful and rapid birth of the baby
   C. Be safe when the woman is evaluated before the administration of the drug and the guidelines for administration are followed
   D. Be safe for any woman with a large pelvis who is at term

9. At least every 30 minutes, the nurse should take and record blood pressure, pulse, respiration, fetal heart tones, frequency and quality of contractions, and resting uterine tone.
   A. True
   B. False

10. Rate of fluid administration and dosage should be recorded every hour.
    A. True
    B. False

11. Noting maternal response to augmented labor contractions is more important than noting fetal response.
    A. True
    B. False

12. Elective induction/augmentation with oxytocin is not recommended.
    A. True
    B. False

13. Preinduction cervical ripening with Prepidil Gel (PGE2) should be performed in the hospital. The Prepidil Gel:
    A. Should be carefully introduced into the extra-amniotic space if the membranes have ruptured
    B. Should be warmed to 96.8°F before use and liberally applied to the cervix
    C. Should be inserted into the endocervical canal, below the level of the interval os
    D. Can be repeated every 4 hours until cervical changes occur or oxytocin induction is initiated

14. Cervidil Vaginal Insert dosing may be repeated as long as each insert is changed every 12 hours.
    A. True
    B. False

15. When misoprostol is used for safety and best outcomes, the 100-μg tablet should be cut by the pharmacist and placed in the posterior vaginal fornix with a small amount of lubricant.
    A. True
    B. False

16. All of the following are elements of active management of labor *except:*
    A. Is an attempt to reduce cesarean births resulting from dystocia
    B. Involves vigorous management of labor, often by using oxytocin induction and amniotomy
    C. Is carried out for nulliparas with a term single fetus in no distress who are in active labor, have ruptured membranes, and are progressing at less than 1 cm per hour
    D. Often uses higher starting dosages of oxytocin and increases at greater increments than does labor induction

Check your answers with the Module 7 Posttest Answer Key.

Posttest: Module 8. Caring for the Woman at Risk for Preterm Labor or With Premature Rupture of Membranes

Answer the following questions without referring back to the information in the module. Select the ONE BEST answer for each question.

1. When you admit a woman with ruptured membranes at 32 weeks of gestation, the greatest risk results from:
   A. Chorioamnionitis
   B. Spontaneous labor
   C. Immature fetus
   D. Impending cesarean birth

2. Mrs. A.M. is admitted to the labor unit at 38 weeks' gestation with leaking membranes. Labor has not begun and she tested group B strep negative last week. The plan of management probably will include:
   A. Beginning oxytocin induction of labor immediately
   B. Evaluating Mrs. A.M.'s white blood cell count to see if it is elevated
   C. Waiting until labor begins spontaneously unless signs of infection develop
   D. Starting antibiotics immediately

3. Treatment of premature ruptured membranes depends on:
   A. The gestational age of the fetus at the time of ruptured membranes
   B. The presence or absence of an infection
   C. Whether the fetus is assessed as mature or immature
   D. All of the above

4. A young primigravida comes to a small community hospital stating that her "bag of waters" has broken. She is at 29 weeks' gestation by dates and size. Labor has not begun. The nurse can anticipate that he or she will need to:
   A. Prepare the woman for transfer to a Level III regional center
   B. Prepare for a high-risk delivery
   C. Admit the woman to the labor unit and wait for labor to begin spontaneously
   D. Admit the woman to the labor unit for expectant management

5. A sterile speculum examination is recommended for the woman being seen at term or preterm for the first time after membranes have ruptured *prematurely* regardless of whether the woman is in labor. The main reason(s) for this is (are) to:
   A. Assess for infection
   B. Note whether a prolapsed cord is present
   C. Determine the extent of cervical dilatation
   D. Confirm rupture of membranes
   E. B, C, and D

6. A *newly admitted* laboring woman with premature rupture of membranes at 37 weeks is 3 cm dilated. Which of the following are the three correct priorities for nursing intervention?
   1. Obtain a culture of the amniotic fluid.
   2. Attach the external fetal monitor.
   3. Take and record her temperature.
   4. Note the color and odor of the amniotic fluid.
   5. Time the contractions.
   6. Ensure that resuscitation equipment in the delivery room is in good working order.

A. 2, 3, 4
B. 2, 5, 6
C. 1, 4, 6
D. 3, 5, 6

7. The diagnosis of preterm labor can be made if:
   A. The cervix is 20% effaced and 2 cm dilated
   B. The cervix is dilated 4 cm on admission
   C. Contractions are lasting 45 seconds and are 18 minutes apart
   D. Contractions are 30 seconds long and are occurring 10 to 15 minutes apart

8. The primary action of terbutaline is to:
   A. Cause fetal lungs to mature
   B. Quiet the myometrium of the uterus and stop contractions
   C. Lower the possibility of convulsion
   D. Reduce fluid retention in the preeclamptic woman

9. Using the criteria given in each brief situation following, state whether the woman is a good candidate for terbutaline tocolysis.
   A. Melinda is at 18 weeks' gestation with her third child. Contractions are occurring every 3 minutes and lasting 60 seconds. _____
   B. Susan is at 25 weeks' gestation with contractions occurring every 6 minutes and lasting 45 seconds.
      _____
   C. Mary is an uncontrolled diabetic who is now 32 weeks pregnant. She has just started having 60-second contractions every 5 minutes. _____
   D. Yvonne is admitted to the labor unit at 37 weeks' gestation with heavy vaginal bleeding and 30-second contractions occurring every 4 minutes.
      _____
   E. Lou Ella is 32 weeks pregnant with ruptured membranes. Chorioamnionitis has just been diagnosed. Two hours ago she began having contractions of approximately 30 seconds' duration. 5 minutes apart.
      _____

10. Select the one most critical nursing action to be initiated during the administration of terbutaline:
    A. Allow the patient to assume any comfortable position.
    B. Assess patient's deep tendon reflexes.
    C. Allow clear liquids for nourishment.
    D. Monitor maternal pulse.

11. The standard initial IV bolus of magnesium sulfate is:
    A. 4–6 g
    B. 2–3 g
    C. 6–8 g
    D. 4–8 g

12. Which of the following complications might result from bed rest prescribed for preterm labor?
    A. A deep vein thrombosis
    B. Muscle weakness
    C. Dizziness when standing
    D. All of the above

13. A patient at 34 weeks' gestation presents in labor and delivery with preterm labor. Her cervix is 4 cm dilated. At 32 weeks' gestation, she received a course of corticosteroids and 2 days of magnesium sulfate given intravenously. This is a hospital with a Level III nursery. What should the nurse anticipate and prepare for in her care of the patient?
    A. Magnesium sulfate administration
    B. Delivery of 34-week-old infant if patient continues to labor
    C. Additional course of corticosteroids
    D. Fetal fibronectin testing

14. A patient has been receiving a maintenance dose of magnesium sulfate at 2 g/h for 24 hours. The nurse notes on her assessment that the patient is lethargic. Her respiratory rate is 11 breaths per minute and patellar deep tendon reflexes are absent. The nurse should plan to do all of the following except:
    A. Stop the administration of magnesium sulfate
    B. Draw a blood sample for a magnesium sulfate level
    C. Prepare for a fluid bolus of 500 mL normal saline
    D. Notify the physician
    E. Have calcium gluconate present at the patient's bedside.

15. The major obstetric complication associated with perinatal mortality and morbidity is:
    A. Preeclampsia/eclampsia
    B. Premature delivery
    C. Maternal malnutrition
    D. Breech delivery

16. A pregnant woman presents to the delivery suite at 34 weeks' gestation. Her contractions are regular, occurring every 6 minutes, and are 50 seconds in duration. Progressive cervical changes occur with time. The diagnosis is:
    A. Braxton-Hicks contractions
    B. Preterm labor
    C. False labor
    D. Irritable uterus

17. Attempts to stop preterm labor should be minimized if there is also associated:
    A. Placental separation
    B. Severe preeclampsia
    C. Intrauterine fetal demise
    D. All of the above

18. Antibiotic administration should be anticipated in all of the following patients except:
    A. Patient at 38 weeks' gestation with PROM, positive GBS culture
    B. Patient at 32 weeks' gestation with preterm PROM, not laboring
    C. Patient at 25 weeks' gestation, 8 cm dilated, contracting, intact membranes, unknown GBS status
    D. Patient at 33 weeks' gestation, 3 cm dilated, intact membranes, no contractions at this time

19. In which position is cardiac output and renal blood flow highest?
    A. Left lateral decubitus
    B. Lithotomy
    C. Standing
    D. Trendelenburg

20. The number of vaginal examinations should be minimized in patients with premature rupture of membranes because:
    A. The risk of infection is increased
    B. Plasma concentrations of oxytocin increase
    C. The risk of rupturing the membranes is increased
    D. Plasma concentrations of prostaglandins decrease

21. During the initial treatment of a patient in preterm labor, the most important intervention from the following list is:
    A. Barbiturate sedation
    B. X-ray examination of the abdomen for fetal position
    C. Oral liquid diet
    D. Urine analysis

22. Signs and symptoms of premature labor that the patient may report include all of the following *except:*
    A. Backache
    B. Change in vaginal discharge
    C. Constipation
    D. Pelvic pressure

23. Which of the following actions is most likely to minimize the risk of pulmonary edema during tocolytic therapy?
    A. Avoidance of glucocorticoid therapy
    B. Meticulous monitoring of intake and output
    C. Bed rest
    D. Nothing by mouth

24. A woman who is 32 weeks pregnant with her first baby and who has no significant risk factors for preterm labor calls the office and states she has felt Braxton-Hicks contractions all day long. A friend told her "she probably just overdid it." She has been lying down for an hour with no change in symptoms. An appropriate response would be to:
    A. Reassure her that what she is experiencing is normal
    B. Review signs and symptoms of labor
    C. Tell her to keep her appointment the next day
    D. Have her come in for immediate evaluation

25. Risk appraisal systems for identifying women at risk for preterm labor have been shown to be:
    A. More effective in identifying primigravidas at risk for preterm labor
    B. Effective in identifying most women at risk for preterm labor
    C. Ineffective in identifying 50% of women who enter preterm labor with no risk factors
    D. Ineffective in identifying any women at risk for preterm labor

26. Reports about care-seeking behaviors of pregnant women emphasize that:
    A. Pregnancy motivates women to seek help for discomforts quickly
    B. Having previous experience with contractions (a previous labor and delivery) ensures early recognition of preterm labor symptoms
    C. Most women are aware of the difference between symptoms of common discomforts of pregnancy and preterm labor
    D. Denial of significance of symptoms and seeking advice from family or friends often precedes obtaining medical assistance for preterm labor symptoms and results in delayed treatment

27. In the United States, the rate of preterm labor resulting in low-birth-weight infants:
    A. Contributes to the majority of all perinatal deaths
    B. Has improved significantly in the past 10 years because of widespread use of tocolysis
    C. Is a problem only in women of lower socioeconomic status
    D. Has been significantly lowered by risk assessment and preterm birth prevention programs.

28. The NIH consensus statement on the antenatal use of corticosteroids concludes that which of the following statements is/are true?
    1. Antenatal corticosteroid therapy for fetal maturation reduces mortality, respiratory distress syndrome, and intraventricular hemorrhage in preterm infants
    2. All fetuses between 24 and 34 weeks' gestation at risk of preterm delivery should be considered candidates for antenatal treatment with corticosteroids
    3. The benefits of antenatal corticosteroids are additive to those derived from surfactant therapy
    4. There is no advantage in treating with antenatal corticosteroids if preterm delivery is anticipated in less than 24 hours
    A. 1
    B. 1, 2
    C. 1, 2, 3
    D. 1, 2, 3, 4

29. Select the correct completion(s) of the sentence: Risk factors for preterm labor
    1. Have been clearly defined in multiparas
    2. Can vary in different populations
    3. Include psychosocial and physical factors
    4. Are multifactorial and need further research
    A. 1, 2, 4
    B. 2, 3, 4
    C. 1, 2, 4
    D. 1, 2, 3, 4

30. Which set of the following signs are signs of chorioamnionitis?
    1. Abdominal tenderness
    2. Maternal heart rate of 124 beats per minute
    3. FHR tracing with baseline of 175, minimal variability, no decelerations
    4. Maternal temperature of 98.8°F
    A. 2, 3, 4
    B. 1, 3, 4
    C. 1, 2, 3
    D. 1, 2, 3, 4

Check your answers with the Module 8 Posttest Answer Key.

Posttest: Module 9. Caring for the Laboring Woman With Hypertensive Disorders Complicating Pregnancy (Includes Content from Appendix B)

Answer the following questions without referring back to the information in the module. ONE OR MORE THAN ONE of the choices may be correct.

1. The primary goal of management in severe preeclampsia is to:
   A. Prevent nausea and vomiting
   B. Prevent convulsions and deliver the baby
   C. Ensure a mature fetus
   D. Prevent the premature onset of labor

2. Magnesium sulfate is a drug effective in treating preeclampsia. The drug:
   A. Causes blood vessels to constrict and therefore increases circulation to the placenta
   B. Aids in maturation of the fetus
   C. Lowers blood pressure
   D. Depresses central nervous system activity and reduces the chances of convulsions

3. Which of the following pregnant women are at increased risk for developing preeclampsia?
   A. A teenaged girl who is pregnant for the first time
   B. A 30-year-old woman who is pregnant for the first time and who has a twin gestation
   C. A multipara who is also a diabetic
   D. All of the above

4. A 35-year-old woman expecting her third child presents at the labor unit with a blood pressure of 160/100 mmHg and 2+ proteinuria. You note in her prenatal record that she has had a history of elevated blood pressure (approximate range of 140/90 mmHg) since age 30. According to the classification system given in Module 9, she has:
   A. Eclampsia
   B. Chronic hypertension with superimposed preeclampsia
   C. Superimposed eclampsia
   D. Gestational hypertension

5. According to the classification system used in Module 9, when pregnancy occurs with developing hypertension and proteinuria after 20 weeks' gestation, it is called:
   A. Gestational hypertension
   B. HELLP syndrome
   C. Preeclampsia
   D. Chronic hypertension

6. A 20-year-old gravida 1 had a blood pressure range of 90/60 to 98/64 mmHg at 6 through 28 weeks' gestation. At 39 weeks' gestation, she presents on the labor unit with a complaint of headaches and a total weight gain of 50 pounds—8 pounds were gained in the previous 2 weeks. Her blood pressure today is 134/86 mmHg with 2+ proteinuria. You determine that she is not in true labor. Your next step will be to:
   A. Call her primary care provider
   B. Discuss signs and symptoms of preeclampsia and send her home

C. Ask her to walk for 2 hours and return for a blood pressure recheck
D. Send her home with strict bed rest orders

7. Which of the following are acceptable screening procedures for predicting preeclampsia?
   A. The roll-over test
   B. Absence of a decline in blood pressure late in the second trimester
   C. Calculation of mean arterial pressure in the second trimester
   D. None of the above

8. A 27-year-old gravida 2 at 40 weeks' gestation experienced a normal labor and birth. During the third blood pressure check in the recovery room, you note that her blood pressure has risen from approximately 118/68 to 128/74 mmHg (baseline pressure during pregnancy and labor) to 150/100 mmHg. To determine whether this might be preeclampsia or late transient hypertension, you would:
   1. Review her prenatal record for any signs of preeclampsia
   2. Keep her in the recovery room for additional time to continue evaluation
   3. Evaluate her urine for proteinuria
   4. Question her regarding headaches or blurred vision
   A. 2, 3
   B. 1, 4
   C. 2, 4
   D. All of the above

9. You have been caring for a severely preeclamptic woman who is in labor. Laboratory tests indicate a hematocrit at 48 mg/dL, bilirubin at 2.1 mg/dL, ALT at 70 IU/L, LDH at 820 IU/L, and a platelet count of 70,000/mm^3. This is suggestive of:
   A. Severe diabetes
   B. Late, transient hypertension
   C. HELLP syndrome
   D. Eclampsia

10. In which of the following situations is maternal transport from a Level I hospital to a high-risk regional center indicated?
    A. 21-year-old gravida 3 who is at 33 weeks' gestation with mild preeclampsia and in early labor
    B. 14-year-old gravida 1 at 39 weeks' gestation with severe preeclampsia and in advanced labor
    C. 42-year-old gravida 2 at 40 weeks' gestation with mild preeclampsia
    D. 30-year-old gravida 4, twin gestation, at 38 weeks with mild preeclampsia and not in labor

11. Match the clinical signs and symptoms with the pathophysiologic alteration that occurs in preeclampsia. More than one sign or symptom may apply to a single pathophysiologic alteration and each sign or symptom may apply to more than one pathophysiologic alteration.

**Clinical Signs and
Symptoms**

a. Hyperreflexia/clonus
b. Proteinuria
c. Headaches
d. Fetal distress
e. Rise in blood pressure
f. Sudden weight gain
   and edema
g. Blurred vision/
   scotomata
h. Rising hematocrit
i. Epigastric pain

Pathophysiologic Alteration

1. _____ Decreased blood
   supply to the placenta
2. _____ Decreased intravascular
   volume with a shift of
   plasma to the tissues of
   the body
3. _____ Hemoconcentration
   within the circulatory
   system
4. _____ Loss of renal integrity
5. _____ Spasm of the blood
   vessels and edema in
   the optical bed of the
   eye
6. _____ Spasm of the blood
   vessels and edema in
   the brain
7. _____ Irritation of the central
   nervous system
8. _____ Spasm and hemorrhage
   in the liver capsule

12. To ensure that the woman receiving magnesium sulfate therapy is not at increasing risk for serum magnesium blood levels above the therapeutic range, the nurse should:
    A. Assess the hematocrit level every 4 hours
    B. Evaluate for proteinuria every hour
    C. Determine that urinary output is greater than 30 mL per hour
    D. Time the contractions

13. In which two situations should the physician be consulted for possible magnesium toxicity during magnesium sulfate therapy?
    1. Serum magnesium level is 7 mg/dL (or 8.4 mEq/L)
    2. Maternal respirations are 10 per minute and shallow
    3. The patellar reflex has disappeared
    4. Proteinuria is 3+
       A. 1, 4
       B. 2, 3
       C. 2, 4
       D. 3, 4

14. You are administering hydralazine (Apresoline) to a severely preeclamptic woman. The appropriate blood pressure evaluations should be done every:
    A. 2–5 minutes
    B. 10 minutes
    C. 15 minutes
    D. 20 minutes

15. The frequency of blood pressure evaluation by the nurse in a severely hypertensive woman who is receiving hydralazine (Apresoline) is critical because which two of the following considerations?
    1. The peak effect of hydralazine is reached in 15 to 20 minutes
    2. The woman might have an increased intravascular blood volume and have a stroke

3. The woman might have a decreased intravascular blood volume and become severely hypotensive
4. The woman might experience a seizure
   A. 1, 3
   B. 2, 4
   C. 1, 2
   D. 3, 4

16. Pregnant women with moderate hypertension might need which set of the following interventions?
    1. More frequent prenatal visits
    2. Antihypertensive medication
    3. Moderate salt restriction
    4. Careful fetal growth surveillance
       A. 1, 3
       B. 1, 2, 3
       C. 1, 4
       D. 1, 2, 3, 4

17. Sodium restriction in a moderately hypertensive woman during pregnancy:
    A. Reduces urinary output
    B. Can lead to lower plasma volume
    C. Promotes increased plasma volume
    D. Has been shown to benefit women with elevated diastolic blood pressure between 95 and 104 mmHg

18. Select the best steps and correct order in which the following should be carried out when taking blood pressure readings on the laboring woman with a pregnancy complicated by hypertension.
    1. Use the same arm throughout.
    2. Either arm may be used provided that blood pressure is essentially the same in each arm on admission.
    3. If pressures differ in each arm by more than 10 mmHg, use the arm with the lower pressure.
    4. If pressures differ in each arm by more than 10 mmHg, use the arm with the higher pressure.
    5. Perform blood pressure readings with the woman in a supine position.
    6. Perform blood pressure readings with the woman in essentially the same position each time.
    7. Record the diastolic pressure at the point of disappearance.
    8. Record the diastolic pressure at the point of muffled pulse sound.
       A. 1, 4, 5, 8
       B. 2, 3, 4, 7
       C. 1, 4, 6, 7
       D. 2, 4, 5, 7

19. Select the appropriate set of calculations to prepare and administer a 4-g *loading dose* of magnesium sulfate from available ampules of 50% $MgSO_4 \cdot 7H_2O$ containing 5 g each.
    A. 2 ampules of the $MgSO_4 \cdot 7H_2O$ solution added to 1,000 mL of 5% dextrose and water and run at 125 mL per hour
    B. 8 ampules of the $MgSO_4 \cdot 7H_2O$ solution added to 1,000 mL of 5% dextrose and water and run at 100 mL over 25 minutes (4 mL per minute)

C. 8 ampules of the $MgSO_4 \cdot 7H_2O$ solution added to 1,000 mL of 5% dextrose and water and run at 150 mL over 25 minutes (6 mL per minute)

D. 8 ampules of the $MgSO_4 \cdot 7H_2O$ solution added to 1,000 mL of 5% dextrose and water and run at 50 mL per hour

20. A 28-year-old gravida 2 para 1 at 35 weeks' estimated gestational age presents complaining of a sharp pain just below her sternum. During the intake process, she also tells you she has had the "flu" for the past 3 days. In addition to the sharp pain below her sternum, her complaints include nausea and vomiting, diarrhea, and feeling "down" and tired all the time. Her blood pressure is 134/82 mmHg, and she has 1+ proteinuria. She has gained 9 pounds since her last prenatal visit 5 days ago. You determine that she is not in true labor. After calling her primary care provider, the next steps you take are in anticipation of a differential diagnosis of:
    A. Gastroenteritis
    B. Gallbladder disease
    C. HELLP syndrome
    D. Eclampsia

21. You are caring for a woman at 35 weeks' estimated gestation who has HELLP syndrome. She is receiving magnesium sulfate therapy and undergoing induction of labor. While performing routine care, you notice that her IV site has begun oozing and that she has petechiae covering her extremities. Her urine is rose-colored, and she is complaining of pain in her right upper quadrant. Her last laboratory studies were taken 6 hours ago. Her blood has been typed and cross-matched. The physician is on the way to the hospital. You anticipate that a critical management step will be to:
    A. Draw a complete blood cell count with platelets and liver function tests
    B. Prepare for a cesarean delivery
    C. Keep the oxytocin infusion at its present rate
    D. Stop the magnesium sulfate therapy

22. The term *gestational hypertension* is applied to expectant women who:
    A. Have chronic hypertension before the 20th week of pregnancy
    B. Will go on to develop preeclampsia
    C. Are at minimal risk from hypertension
    D. Have elevated blood pressure after 20 weeks' gestation but without proteinuria or edema

23. Which of the following reflect what is known about perinatal mortality/morbidity rates in pregnancies complicated by hypertension? (Select more than one choice.)
    A. HELLP syndrome, a form of preeclampsia, places both the mother and fetus at considerable risk related to cerebrovascular cranial hemorrhage accidents.
    B. As maternal blood pressure increases, so does the perinatal mortality rate.
    C. Perinatal morbidity rates are similar for both chronic hypertension and preeclampsia.
    D. Perinatal mortality is significantly higher in superimposed preeclampsia than in preeclampsia.

24. A 26-year-old gravida 1 at 38 weeks' gestation is seen in her primary care provider's office. She has gained 3 pounds over the past week, has a blood pressure of 130/80 mmHg (first trimester blood pressure was 110/60 mmHg), and on a clean-catch urine test, is noted to have 3+ proteinuria. Which of the following statements reflect an appreciation for this mother's status? (Select more than one choice.)
    A. A clean-catch urine dipstick is not sufficient to determine significant proteinuria.
    B. The 3+ proteinuria is considered "significant."
    C. The blood pressure elevation is not worrisome.
    D. In light of the proteinuria and the elevated diastole, the prognosis for perinatal risk increases.
    E. The 3-pound weight gain will be seen with the presence of edema.

25. Protein in urine (select more than one choice):
    A. Is difficult to quantify
    B. Can be the most ominous sign of preeclampsia
    C. Is normally seen in a 24-hour urine specimen in amounts less than 300 g per L
    D. Is normally seen in a 24-hour specimen in amounts of approximately 5 g per L

26. An elevated hematocrit level in a preeclamptic woman might be reflecting:
    A. An increase in intravascular blood volume
    B. A loss of intravascular blood volume
    C. Enhanced uteroplacental perfusion
    D. Hemodilution

27. A rising LDH can reflect (select more than one choice):
    A. Microangiopathic hemolytic anemia
    B. Thrombocytopenia
    C. Increased blood glucose
    D. Liver tissue damage

28. When personnel on a labor and delivery unit follow protocols for taking blood pressures by using the Korotkoff IV sound, they:
    A. Run the risk of underdiagnosing preeclampsia
    B. Will have abnormally low diastolic measurements
    C. Run the risk of overdiagnosing preeclampsia
    D. Will accurately diagnose preeclampsia if they use the criteria of a 30/15 mmHg rise in blood pressure

29. A lateral recumbent position in an expectant woman receiving $MgSO_4 \cdot 7H_2O$ can (select more than one choice):
    A. Promote cardiac output
    B. Reduce the risk of magnesium toxicity
    C. Lower placental profusion
    D. Increase the likelihood of fetal hypoxia

30. Normal physiologic changes in renal blood flow and glomerular filtration during pregnancy are reflected in laboratory values that show a(n):
    A. Increase in both urine and blood creatinine levels
    B. Increase in urine creatinine levels and decrease in blood creatininie levels
    C. Decrease in urine creatinine levels and increase in blood creatininie levels
    D. Decrease in both urine and blood creatinine levels

31. A young mother with severe preeclampsia has been treated with magnesium sulfate throughout her labor induction and delivered a 5-pound, 12-ounce boy under epidural anesthesia. Besides a continued risk from hypertension immediately after delivery, what other serious maternal risks should be anticipated?

    A. Anemia

    B. Liver dysfunction

    C. Uterine atony

    D. Hypotension

32. In anticipation of delivery of a high-risk infant, the priority for preparation is to:

    A. Alert appropriate on-call neonatal resuscitation personnel

    B. Prepare the expectant parent

    C. Have cross-matched blood for the mother available on the labor and delivery unit

    D. Have appropriate neonatal resuscitation personnel in the delivery room

33. Which of the following statements reflects what is currently known regarding the immediate postpartum period for the woman recovering from severe preeclampsia or HELLP syndrome?

    A. The signs and symptoms of her disease will resolve quickly.

    B. Pulmonary edema is a serious potential risk.

    C. Oliguria is unlikely to occur.

    D. Her abnormal laboratory values will steadily improve.

Check your answers with the Module 9 Posttest Answer Key.

Posttest: Module 10. Caring for the Laboring Woman With HIV Infection or AIDS

Answer the following questions without referring back to the information in the module. ONE OR MORE THAN ONE of the choices may be correct.

1. A 30-year-old newly delivered mother has been diagnosed as HIV positive. She has no symptoms of the infection as yet. Which activities do not carry the risk of transmitting the infection?
   A. Breastfeeding her newborn
   B. Resuming sexual activity with her husband 6 weeks after delivery
   C. Kissing her other two children
   D. Donating blood at the local Red Cross

2. A registered nurse works in a labor and delivery unit in a busy metropolitan area. Select the following activities that are most likely to put her at risk of contracting HIV infection.
   A. Using universal precautions only when caring for patients who are at high risk for HIV infection.
   B. Recapping all needles carefully after use.
   C. Wearing gloves only while bathing those babies who have been born to intravenous drug users.
   D. Hugging an HIV-infected mother after the birth of her child.

3. A patient is admitted to the labor unit and has had two positive (reactive) EIA tests and one unequivocal positive Western blot test. You can reasonably conclude that the patient:
   A. Does not have HIV infection
   B. Has HIV infection
   C. Is an intravenous drug user
   D. Has AIDS

4. A pregnant nurse working on a labor and delivery, nursery, or postpartum unit should:
   A. Request a change to another hospital unit
   B. Be assigned to low-risk patients on those units
   C. Receive an HIV screen
   D. Use universal precautions

5. You are going to give a bath to an HIV-infected mother who has just delivered her baby. After the bath you need to begin an IV line. Which sequence of steps is recommended in universal precautions?
   A. No gloves are needed for the bath, but put gloves on when starting the IV line.
   B. Continue to use the same pair of gloves without interrupting for handwashing.
   C. Wash hands, put on gloves for the bath, remove gloves, wash hands, and put on the same pair of gloves if you see no tears.
   D. Remove gloves after the bath, wash hands immediately, and put on another pair of gloves before starting the IV line.

6. Measures that reduce the risk of HIV transmission to the newborn of an HIV-infected mother include:
   A. Using internal fetal monitoring for this high-risk infant
   B. Changing gloves after giving perineal care to the mother and before bathing the baby
   C. Bathing the baby before administering vitamin K
   D. Isolating the baby from the mother

7. What is seroconversion?
   A. When the patient has AIDS but blood tests are unable to isolate the virus
   B. The period of time before the patient developing full-blown AIDS
   C. The point when there are enough antibodies to HIV to make detection possible
   D. The period of time before there are enough antibodies to HIV to make detection possible

8. Name the two modes of transmission for HIV.
   A. Horizontal transmission
   B. Diagonal transmission
   C. Dominant transmission
   D. Vertical transmission

9. The drug currently recommended for pregnant women to prevent transmission of HIV to the newborn is:
   A. Zithromax
   B. Zovirax
   C. Zalcitabine
   D. Zidovudine

10. What is the current method of delivery recommended for the woman who is HIV positive with a viral load of 2,150 copies/mL?
    A. Low forceps vaginal delivery
    B. Cesarean delivery
    C. Spontaneous vaginal delivery
    D. Vacuum extraction vaginal delivery

11. The highest percentage of perinatal transmission of HIV occurs in:
    A. The first trimester
    B. The third trimester
    C. Postpartum
    D. Intrapartum

12. When is antiretroviral treatment recommended for the pregnant woman?
    A. It is clinically indicated by her HIV status.
    B. If already initiated, it is continued (during the first trimester) throughout pregnancy, labor, and delivery.
    C. It is given only to women who have AIDS.
    D. It is not recommended for women who have full-blown AIDS.

13. What is the primary adverse effect of ZDV?
    A. Bone marrow suppression
    B. Nausea and vomiting
    C. Loss of hair and skin eruption
    D. Diarrhea

14. Name two educational topics that should be presented to the expectant woman during the intrapartum period.
    A. Risks and benefits of drug therapy
    B. Pain management options and their risks and benefits
    C. Contraceptive options after delivery
    D. Bathing the newborn

15. Which psychosocial considerations should be promoted in caring for the HIV-positive mother and her family during labor or immediately after delivery?
    A. Maternal–child bonding
    B. Family bonding
    C. Psychological adjustment
    D. None of the above

16. Name key ethical issues in the treatment of the HIV-positive patient.
    A. Confidentiality
    B. Advance directives
    C. Right to medical care
    D. Consent

17. What measures can be taken to help protect the fetus/newborn from HIV infection?
    A. Avoid internal monitoring if possible.
    B. Dry the infant immediately after delivery.
    C. Wait until 2 hours after delivery before bathing the baby.
    D. Avoid aspiration of gastric contents.

18. The use of zidovudine therapy in HIV-infected pregnant women showed:
    A. No change in the risk of HIV vertical transmission
    B. A 8.3% increase in the risk of HIV vertical transmission
    C. A 25.5% decrease in the risk of HIV vertical transmission
    D. A 70% decrease in the risk of HIV vertical transmission

19. You are in an antepartum clinic providing care for an 18-year-old gravida 3 para 2 abortus 0 at 34 weeks' gestation. She was diagnosed as being HIV positive 1 year ago. She is presently receiving zidovudine therapy. Which of the following issues should be addressed in your education plans for this patient?
    A. The benefits and risks of zidovudine therapy during labor
    B. The benefits of breastfeeding
    C. The benefits and risks of zidovudine therapy for her newborn
    D. Pain management during labor

20. A 23-year-old gravida 4 para 1 abortus 2 at 38 4/7 weeks' gestation presents to the labor and delivery unit for evaluation of labor. She was diagnosed as being HIV positive 4 months ago when she began her prenatal care. Examination revealed that she was 5 cm, 75%, vertex −1 with intact membranes. Which of the following precautions should be taken to reduce her exposure to opportunistic organisms?
    A. Do not start an IV line.
    B. Insert a Foley catheter on admission.
    C. Limit vaginal examinations.
    D. Artificially rupture membranes and place helix and intrauterine pressure catheter to monitor her labor pattern.

Check your answers with the Module 10 Posttest Answer Key.

Posttest: Module 11. Hepatitis Infections

Answer the following questions without referring back to the information in the module. Select the BEST answer for each question.

1. Which form of hepatitis can result in the *highest* rate of chronic infection among infected individuals?
   A. Hepatitis A
   B. Hepatitis B
   C. Hepatitis C
   D. Hepatitis E

2. When maternal infection exists, which of the following poses the *highest* risk of vertical transmission?
   A. HIV
   B. Hepatitis A
   C. Hepatitis B
   D. Hepatitis C

3. The *highest* risk of infection transmission from bloodborne exposures occurs from which one of the following diseases?
   A. HIV
   B. Hepatitis B
   C. Hepatitis C

4. All of the following statements reflect what is known about hepatitis A infection *except:*
   A. Infection with the hepatitis A virus results in subsequent immunity to the infection
   B. When the infection occurs during pregnancy, the disease is generally worse and teratogenic effects are possible
   C. No carrier state exists for this disease
   D. Hepatitis A vaccination may be given to pregnant women

5. All of the following statements regarding hepatitis A are accurate *except:*
   A. It is usually transmitted by blood
   B. It can be prevented by immunization
   C. It was previously known as "infectious hepatitis"
   D. It causes no serious problems in the well-nourished, healthy pregnant woman

6. Which type of hepatitis, not seen in the United States, is characterized by mild illness but also by a fulminant form of illness causing a high mortality rate?
   A. Hepatitis A
   B. Hepatitis C
   C. Hepatitis D
   D. Hepatitis E

7. Elizabeth Manfred contracted hepatitis C virus infection 1 year ago. Recent serologic testing reveals the presence of anti-HCV. This can be interpreted to indicate that she:
   A. Is immune
   B. Is infected
   C. Has cleared her system of the virus
   D. Is not infectious

8. Hepatitis B infection:
   A. Was formerly known as "infectious hepatitis"
   B. Is diagnosed by excluding other hepatitis types
   C. Can occur without the individual having symptoms of an acute infection
   D. Does not carry with it any long-term risks

9. Individuals with chronic hepatitis B infection:
   A. Have the potential for being a carrier
   B. Are never infectious
   C. Have few long-term risks
   D. Always have serious symptoms, which aid in the diagnosis

10. Which of the following hepatitis B serologic markers is done to screen pregnant women?
    A. HBsAg
    B. anti-HBs
    C. anti-HBc
    D. All of the above

11. A high possibility exists that a pregnant woman can transmit hepatitis B to her infant if her blood serum reveals the presence of HBsAg and:
    A. anti-HBc
    B. anti-HBe
    C. HBeAg
    D. HBcAg

12. Transmission of hepatitis B infection from an acutely infected or carrier mother to her infant:
    A. Occurs in a few infants transplacentally before birth
    B. Is unlikely if the mother has no symptoms of the infection throughout her pregnancy
    C. Is unlikely during labor and delivery in the mother who has no symptoms of the infection
    D. Rarely occurs from the infant's contact with infected blood or amniotic fluid at birth

13. In a hepatitis B virus-infected mother who is HBsAg and HBeAg positive, the rate of transmitting infection to her newborn:
    A. Is estimated at 30%
    B. Is estimated at 90%
    C. Is not a concern
    D. Depends on whether the mother is symptomatic

14. A woman who has had two positive HBsAg tests 7 months apart is admitted to the labor unit. You can reasonably conclude that the woman:
    A. Does not have hepatitis B infection
    B. Has resolving hepatitis B infection
    C. Is a carrier
    D. Is susceptible to hepatitis B infection

15. Current recommendations for follow-up on a pregnant woman who tests positive for HBsAg include:
    A. Immediate immunization
    B. Liver function tests
    C. Hospitalization
    D. None of the above

16. Members in the household of a hepatitis B carrier are at risk for viral transmission through:
    A. Air contamination
    B. Water contamination
    C. Hugging and nonintimate kissing
    D. Shared toothbrushes and razor blades

17. The hepatitis B virus has been found in all body fluids of infected individuals. Which body fluid can be a source of transmission?
    A. Urine
    B. Tears
    C. Breast milk
    D. Vaginal secretions

18. Feces with gross contamination of blood is a source of hepatitis B virus transmission because:
    A. Hepatitis B virus is an enterically transmitted virus
    B. The blood contains concentrations of hepatitis B virus sufficient to cause disease
    C. Feces alone contains concentrations of hepatitis B virus sufficient to cause disease
    D. All of the above statements are correct

19. Pregnant women who contract hepatitis B usually experience:
    A. Severe jaundice, hepatic tenderness, and weight loss
    B. Special dietary needs
    C. No symptoms
    D. An aggravated course of the disease because of pregnancy

20. If an infant is born to a mother who has not been screened for hepatitis B virus but who belongs to one of the risk groups, the recommendation for treating the infant is to:
    A. Obtain a blood specimen from the infant for a hepatitis screen
    B. Isolate the infant until discharge
    C. Immunize the mother
    D. Give the baby HBIG and hepatitis B vaccine within 12 hours of birth

21. To confer passive immunity quickly to the newborn whose mother is a hepatitis B carrier, administer 0.5 mL of:
    A. Engerix-B, Pediatric/Adolescent, IM within 2 to 12 hours of birth
    B. HBIG IM within 2 to 12 hours of birth
    C. Recombivax HB, Pediatric, IM within 12 hours of birth
    D. HBIG IM within 1 week of birth

22. The treatment regimen used to confer active immunity on the newborn is:
    A. An initial 0.5-mL dose of Recombivax HB, Pediatric, IM within 12 hours of birth, followed by two additional immunizations at 1 to 4 months after the first dose and 6 to 18 months after the second dose
    B. An initial 0.5-mL dose of HBIG IM within 12 hours of birth, followed by immunization with Recombivax HB, Pediatric, at 1 month of age and 5 months of age
    C. A single immunization with Engerix-B, Pediatric/Adolescent, or Recombivax HB, Pediatric, within 12 hours of birth
    D. An initial 0.5-mL dose of HBIG within 12 hours of birth, followed by immunization with HBIG at 2 months of age and 6 months of age

23. As a member of a health care team working in areas where exposure to body fluids, including blood, is common, you are tested for immune status to hepatitis B. The plan is to begin the three-part Recombivax HB vaccine if appropriate.
    Test Report 1: HBsAg = positive
    Test Report 2: anti-HBc = positive
    Test Report 3: anti-HBs = positive
    Test Report 4: HBsAg = positive; HBeAg = positive
    Test Report 5: HBsAg = positive; IgM anti-HBc = negative; IgG anti-HBc = positive
    Test Report 6: antigens = negative; antibodies = negative
    ____ A. Which of the laboratory reports above (1–6) is preferable?
    ____ B. Which laboratory report indicates that you are susceptible to hepatitis B infection?
    ____ C. Select the laboratory report that indicates a high degree of infectivity.
    ____ D. Select the laboratory report that documents a carrier state.

24. Alice Scottie, a 22-year-old gravida 1 who admits to IV drug abuse, received an initial physical examination and laboratory workup at 13 weeks' gestation. Her hepatitis B screen 1 week later revealed that she was HBsAg positive. Unfortunately, the health department personnel were unable to locate her and she never returned for further care. Approximately 6 months later she presents at the hospital emergency room in active labor. Her prenatal record reflects only information obtained at the initial visit. Select the statement(s) that accurately reflect what can be assessed about Alice's hepatitis B status from the information known to date.
    A. She might have cleared her system of HBsAg by now.
    B. A highly infectious state is present.
    C. An immune state exists.
    D. She is now a carrier.

25. In admitting a laboring woman who has been identified as a hepatitis B carrier, you will:
    A. Put her in isolation
    B. Label all soiled linens from her with "blood precautions"
    C. Send her blood specimens under separate cover and clearly label "hepatitis B precautions"
    D. Treat her laboratory specimens and linens as you would all other patients' blood and body fluids

26. Measures that reduce the risk of hepatitis B transmission to the fetus of an infected mother include:
    A. Using external fetal monitoring or intermittent auscultation of fetal heart tones
    B. Isolating the mother throughout labor
    C. Performing frequent vaginal examinations to assess progress
    D. Initiating early artificial rupture of membranes during labor

27. The blood of an infant of a drug-abusing 30-year-old mother showed the presence of hepatitis B surface antibodies. From this you can definitely conclude that the:
    A. Infant has hepatitis B virus infection
    B. Infant does not have hepatitis B virus infection
    C. Mother had hepatitis B virus infection at one time
    D. Mother is currently infected

Posttest ▶ **MODULE 11**

28. What treatment is appropriate for the situation in question 27?
    A. Immunize the mother.
    B. Immunize the infant.
    C. Isolate the infant from the mother.
    D. No immunization is needed for the baby.

29. Carrier states:
    A. Are a key factor in the spread of hepatitis B worldwide
    B. Pose minimal problems for individual carriers themselves
    C. Are associated with high prevalence rates in most populations worldwide
    D. Are easily identified through symptoms of the disease

30. A hepatitis B carrier state never exists in an individual without the presence of _____ in his or her blood.
    A. HBsAg
    B. HBeAg
    C. HBcAg
    D. Anti-HBs

31. Gloves should be worn when:
    A. Giving a first bath to a newborn
    B. Changing the diaper of a newborn who received HBIG and the first hepatitis vaccine dose 2 days ago
    C. Bathing a 4-day-old infant who received HBIG only
    D. Changing diapers on all newborns

32. Postpartum education of the hepatitis B carrier mother includes all of the following *except:*
    A. The benefits of immunization for herself
    B. Handwashing procedures to reduce contamination
    C. The benefits of screening and immunization for members of her household
    D. Potential sources of contamination (e.g., saliva)

33. A mother diagnosed with acute infectious hepatitis B delivers and is discharged from the postpartum unit. The infant has received HBIG and his first vaccine dose. Plans regarding follow-up on the status of the mother's infection should include:
    A. Periodic breast milk testing for HBsAg
    B. Serologic testing for the continued presence of HBsAg or detection of anti-HBs
    C. Immunization with hepatitis B vaccine
    D. Serologic testing for HBcAg

34. What is the difference in the recommended schedule of immunoprophylaxis for an infant born to an HBsAg-positive mother and one who is known to be HBsAg negative and immune? (Select two answers.)
    A. The infant born to the HBsAg-negative mother need not receive HBIG at the time of birth.
    B. The infant born to the HBsAg-positive mother needs to have HBIG immediately and hepatitis B vaccine within the first 12 hours of life.
    C. There is no difference.
    D. The infant born to the HBsAg-negative mother needs no immunoprophylaxis.

35. Appropriate delivery plans for a laboring woman who has been identified as HBsAg positive include:
    A. Keeping the mother and baby separated until after the baby has been bathed
    B. Using an isolation room
    C. Obtaining consent for immunization of the newborn before delivery
    D. Assigning one nurse to attend to the baby after delivery

36. It is recommended that all newborns of hepatitis B carrier mothers have oropharyngeal and nasal suctioning because:
    A. All newborns of carrier mothers will have become infected with the hepatitis B virus
    B. Prompt removal of infectious fluids reduces the risk for newborns and caregivers for contracting the infection
    C. All newborns need suctioning regardless of the infection status of the mother
    D. This is an appropriate newborn stimulating intervention

37. Select the situation that typifies a nosocomial infection.
    A. A 26-year-old hepatitis B virus carrier mother was admitted and delivered at a community hospital.
    B. The infant of a hepatitis B virus carrier mother was diagnosed as HBsAg positive at 6 months of age.
    C. The HBsAg negative, anti-HBs negative nurse sustained a needlestick while caring for the hepatitis B carrier mother and her baby. She became acutely ill with hepatitis B 4 months later.

Read the following patient profiles and then answer questions 38 through 41 by matching the correct patient(s) with the statement.

Patient A: Mary is a 19-year-old who is expecting her second child in 7½ months. She contracted hepatitis B 8 months before becoming pregnant and now tests anti-HBs positive.

Patient B: Jane is a 21-year-old expecting her first child in approximately 4 weeks. A hepatitis B panel drawn last week reveals that she is HBsAg and HBeAg positive.

Patient C: Maria is 3 months pregnant. Her boyfriend has revealed that he is bisexual and a hepatitis carrier. Subsequently, Maria's hepatitis B workup indicates that she is HBsAg negative and possesses no antibodies for hepatitis B.

38. _____ Vertical transmission is a high risk.

39. _____ Vertical transmission is not a risk.

40. _____ Hepatitis B vaccine should be offered to this woman during her pregnancy.

41. _____ Hepatitis B immunization is not an appropriate intervention.

42. Which of the following newborns is *not* at risk for contracting hepatitis B virus infection?
    A. Baby A, born to a Vietnamese woman who has had no prenatal care
    B. Baby B, born to a mother whose hepatitis B panel has just been done because of late prenatal care
    C. Baby C, whose mother was immunized 6 months ago and now tests anti-HBs positive
    D. Baby D, whose mother cares for a father receiving renal dialysis and who tested anti-HBs negative 2 months ago

43. Indicate whether the following statements are true (T) or false (F).

    a. _____ The fetus of a hepatitis B virus carrier mother is presumed to be infected.

    b. _____ When caring for the fetus of a hepatitis B virus-infected mother, it is important to use fetal monitoring strategies that avoid inadvertent breaks in the skin barrier of the fetus.

    c. _____ Hepatitis B immunization is 100% effective.

    d. _____ A high rate of hepatitis B transmission occurs from infected health care personnel to newborns.

    e. _____ A high intrapartal morbidity rate is experienced by fetuses of hepatitis B virus carrier mothers.

    f. _____ The lowest risk of hepatitis B virus vertical transmission occurs during the second trimester.

    g. _____ Pregnant women in developing countries have a high fatality rate from fulminant hepatitis E.

    h. _____ Unvaccinated newborns have a higher likelihood of becoming chronically infected with hepatitis B than do exposed children.

44. The percentage of hepatitis B–infected health care workers who become chronically infected (i.e., a carrier state exists) is:

    A. 5%–10%

    B. 3%

    C. 1%

    D. Rare

45. A nonvaccinated health care worker who experiences a needlestick injury has what chance of developing clinical hepatitis B if the source person is both HBsAg positive and HBeAg positive?

    A. 22%–31%

    B. 10%

    C. 5%

    D. Little chance

46. When a health care worker experiences a blood exposure, OSHA's 1992 postexposure guidelines indicate that:

    A. Vaccination is mandatory

    B. Prescreening of the worker is not a requirement for receiving the vaccine

    C. Only a booster dose of the vaccine should be given

    D. It is not helpful to know the worker's serology status for hepatitis B

47. Postexposure prophylaxis for exposure to hepatitis B includes all of the following approaches *except:*

    A. Evaluating the nonresponder to determine whether he or she is HBsAg positive

    B. Giving one dose of HBIG and initiating revaccination if the nonresponder has not completed a second vaccine series

    C. Giving two doses of HBIG if the nonresponder has completed a second vaccine series but still fails to respond

    D. Giving a single booster injection

Check your answers with the Module 11 Posttest Answer Key.

Posttest: Module 12. Caring for the Pregnant Woman With Diabetes (Includes Content From Appendix B)

Answer the following questions without referring back to the information in the module. Select the ONE BEST answer for each question.

1. All the following metabolic changes occur during pregnancy *except:*
   A. Transplacental delivery of insulin to the fetus to promote growth
   B. Insulin resistance owing to human placental lactogen, prolactin, and cortisol levels
   C. Increased blood volume
   D. Thermoregulatory changes, including an increase in basal metabolic rate and an increase in heat production

2. Valsalva pushing during a vaginal delivery is contraindicated in a diabetic patient with:
   A. A macrosomic infant
   B. Neuropathy
   C. Elevated blood glucoses greater than 180 mg/dL
   D. Untreated proliferative retinopathy

3. Which of the following groups are at risk to have babies with congenital anomalies if their blood glucose is not in control?
   A. Gestational diabetic mothers
   B. Gestational diabetic and type 2 diabetic mothers
   C. Type 1 and type 2 diabetic mothers
   D. Gestational diabetic and type 1 diabetic mothers

4. Gestational diabetes can be diagnosed with which of the following tests?
   A. A fasting blood glucose and a 1-hour Glucola
   B. A 1-hour Glucola of 160 mg/dL and 1-hour glucose tolerance test
   C. A 1-hour Glucola of 146 mg/dL followed by a 3-hour glucose tolerance test with the following values: fasting, 101 mg/dL; 1-hour, 208 mg/dL; 2-hour, 155 mg/dL; and 3-hour, 150 mg/dL
   D. A 1-hour Glucola of 140 mg/dL followed by a 3-hour glucose tolerance test with the following values: fasting, 88 mg/dL; 1-hour, 185 mg/dL; 2-hour, 140 mg/dL; and 3-hour, 135 mg/dL

5. Pregestational diabetes can be diagnosed by all of the following tests if confirmed on a subsequent day *except:*
   A. Acute symptoms of diabetes plus a casual plasma glucose of 200 mg/dL or higher
   B. Fasting plasma glucose of 126 mg/dL or higher
   C. 2-hour plasma glucose of 200 mg/dL or higher during an oral glucose tolerance test
   D. Fasting plasma glucose of 105 mg/dL or higher plus a 2-hour glucose test of 195 mg/dL or higher

6. Pregnant women who need to be screened for gestational diabetes should be screened between:
   A. 20 and 24 weeks' gestation
   B. 24 and 28 weeks' gestation
   C. 28 and 32 weeks' gestation
   D. 32 and 36 weeks' gestation

7. In the general population, which type of diabetes is the most common?
   A. Type 1 diabetes
   B. Type 2 diabetes
   C. Gestational diabetes
   D. Secondary diabetes

8. The typical pattern of insulin requirements during pregnancy is:
   A. Decreased in first trimester, increased in second trimester, increased in third trimester, and increased during the postpartum period
   B. Decreased in first trimester, increased in second trimester, decreased in third trimester, and decreased during the postpartum period
   C. Increased in first trimester, increased in second trimester, increased in third trimester, and decreased during the postpartum period
   D. Decreased in first trimester, increased in second trimester, increased in third trimester, and decreased during the postpartum period

9. The American College of Obstetricians and Gynecologists recommends which of the following maternal glucose goals for type 1 and type 2 diabetic mothers?
   A. Fasting blood glucose between 60 and 90 mg/dL, 1-hour postprandial blood glucose between 100 and 120 mg/dL, and 2-hour postprandial blood glucose between 60 and 120 mg/dL
   B. Fasting blood glucose between 60 and 95 mg/dL, 1-hour postprandial blood glucose below 130 to 140 mg/dL, and 2-hour postprandial blood glucose below 120 mg/dL
   C. Fasting blood glucose between 60 and 90 mg/dL, premeal blood glucose between 60 and 105 mg/dL, 1-hour postprandial blood glucose between 60 and 140 mg/dL, and 2-hour postprandial blood glucose between 100 and 140 mg/dL
   D. Fasting blood glucose between 60 and 95 mg/dL, premeal blood glucose between 60 and 110 mg/dL, 1-hour postprandial blood glucose below 140 mg/dL, and 2-hour postprandial blood glucose below 130 mg/dL

10. Glucagon is:
    A. Intravenous glucose
    B. A hormone that can be given intramuscularly to stimulate hepatic glucose production from glycogen
    C. Glucose tablets that a patient can use during hypoglycemia
    D. The type of glucose produced by the liver

11. Which of the following methods of teaching for meal planning gives the patient the greatest flexibility?
    A. Carbohydrate counting
    B. Food pyramid
    C. Exchange list
    D. Calorie counting

12. Pregnancy causes which of the following physiologic changes?
    A. Cardiovascular, respiratory, mechanical, thermoregulatory, and metabolic
    B. Cardiovascular, respiratory, mechanical, thermoregulatory, and neurologic
    C. Cardiovascular, respiratory, immunologic, metabolic, and thermoregulatory
    D. Cardiovascular, immunologic, neurologic, thermoregulatory, and metabolic

13. A 37-year-old woman, gravida 3 para 2 abortus 0 with type 2 diabetes, presents at 6 weeks' gestation taking Glucophage. She is 5 feet, 6 inches tall and weighs 238 pounds. She has a hectic schedule and often misses lunch. Which is the best insulin regimen for her?
    A. Regular and NPH insulin
    B. Keep on Glucophage
    C. Switch to Gylburide
    D. Humalog and Glargine insulin

14. A pregnant women with type 2 diabetes presents at 6 weeks' gestation. Her weight is 238 pounds. Calculate her insulin dose for Regular and NPH.
    A. 30 minutes before breakfast, administer 20 units Regular + 38 units of NPH and 30 minutes before supper, administer 14 units Regular + 14 units of NPH
    B. 10 minutes before breakfast, administer 20 units Regular + 38 units of NPH and 10 minutes before supper, administer 14 units Regular + 14 units of NPH
    C. 30 minutes before breakfast, administer 38 units Regular + 20 units of NPH and 30 minutes before supper, administer 14 units Regular + 14 units of NPH
    D. 30 minutes before breakfast, administer 14 units Regular + 14 units of NPH and 30 minutes before supper, administer 20 units Regular + 38 units of NPH

15. The fetal pancreas begins to function at approximately:
    A. 13 weeks' gestation
    B. 20 weeks' gestation
    C. 28 weeks' gestation
    D. 35 weeks' gestation

16. The peak incidence of neonatal hypoglycemia is usually at:
    A. Immediate postpartum
    B. 2–6 hours postpartum
    C. 6–12 hours postpartum
    D. 24 hours postpartum

17. A type 1 diabetic mother presents for prenatal care at 14 weeks' gestation with a HbA_{1c} of 9.4%. What is her approximate risk of fetal congenital anomalies based on her HbA_{1c}?
    A. Her risk of fetal congenital anomalies is 2%–3%.
    B. Her risk of fetal congenital anomalies is the same as a woman with gestational diabetes.
    C. Her risk of fetal congenital anomalies is increased.
    D. Her risk of fetal congenital anomalies is decreased from the general population.

18. The hallmarks in the treatment of diabetes are:
    A. MNT (medical nutritional therapy)
    B. SMBG (self-management of blood glucose)
    C. Exercise
    D. Medication if indicated
    E. All of the above

19. Preconception health care should be offered to which of the following women?
    A. All women of childbearing age
    B. All women with a poor obstetric history
    C. All women older than 35 years of age
    D. All diabetic women

20. If the medical nutritional therapy plan indicates that a woman needs 50% of calories from carbohydrates, calculate the total number of daily carbohydrate grams required by her if she is at her ideal body weight of 139 pounds.
    A. 288 g each day
    B. 150 g each day
    C. 236 g each day
    D. 216 g each day

Check your answers with the Module 12 Posttest Answer Key.

Posttest: Module 13. Delivery in the Absence of a Primary Care Provider

Answer the following questions without referring back to the information in the module. Select the ONE BEST answer for each question.

1. Which of the following is a sign that the baby's birth is about to occur?
   A. The woman pushing at the peak of her contractions
   B. The woman's saying, "The baby is coming"
   C. An increasing fullness and pressure against the perineum
   D. A sudden gush of bright red blood

2. In the immediate care of the newborn, the nurse must *first:*
   A. Dry the baby thoroughly, especially the head
   B. Note and record the Apgar scores
   C. Weigh the baby and instill eye prophylaxis
   D. Maintain a clear airway

3. Excessive bright red bleeding from the vagina of a postpartum woman is a sign of:
   A. Uterine atony or retained placenta
   B. Lacerated cervix or retained placenta
   C. Lacerated cervix or lacerated vaginal wall
   D. Lacerated vaginal wall or uterine atony

4. When assisting the mother with the delivery of her baby, you must:
   A. Thoroughly wash your hands before gloving to prevent infection
   B. Wipe the baby's face, especially the nose and mouth, and check for a cord around the neck
   C. Suction the mouth and nose before pushing on the fundus to deliver the shoulders
   D. Wipe the baby's face and deeply suction the nose and mouth with the mucus trap

5. When the placenta is delivered:
   A. The cord should be pulled firmly in an upward direction to hasten its delivery
   B. The uterus should be vigorously rubbed to hasten its delivery
   C. Lengthening of the cord is a sign of placental separation
   D. A change in the shape of the uterus from globular to oval is a sign that the placenta has separated

6. Women at risk for excessive postpartum bleeding are those who have had:
   A. A gush of blood just before the delivery of the placenta
   B. Oxytocin administration and a long labor
   C. One or two babies previously
   D. Their placenta delivered in less than 5 minutes

7. Control of the delivering head is important to prevent damage to the head and the mother's tissues.
   A. True
   B. False

8. If the head is crowning and the primary care provider is on the way to the labor unit, the nurse should delay the birth by holding back the delivering head.
   A. True
   B. False

9. Pieces of the placenta can remain attached to the lining of the uterus or break off from the placenta.
   A. True
   B. False

10. If you know the mother's blood type, it is not necessary to obtain cord blood.
    A. True
    B. False

11. All umbilical cords should have two arteries and one vein.
    A. True
    B. False

12. By reviewing a woman's antepartum records, you will be able to eliminate shoulder dystocia as a concern.
    A. True
    B. False

13. Meconium-stained fluid may be associated with fetal hypoxia, uterine hyperstimulation, mature gastrointestinal tract, or a Biophysical Profile of less than 6.
    A. True
    B. False

14. Match the phrase in Column B with the item in Column A.

Column A	Column B
a. _____ McRoberts maneuver	1. Aids in controlling the urge to push
b. _____ Bonding	2. Sign of impending birth
c. _____ Feather blow	3. A rapid labor
d. _____ Side-lying position	4. Use a mucus trap
e. _____ Umbilical cord	5. Cord around the neck
f. _____ Placenta	6. Maintaining infant's body heat
g. _____ Breech	7. Promotes good parenting
h. _____ Bulging of perineum	8. Less strain on the perineum
i. _____ Nuchal cord	9. Three vessels
j. _____ Meconium-stained amniotic fluid	10. Inspect for missing pieces
k. _____ Thermoregulation	11. Avoid excessive handling
l. _____ Possibility of postpartum hemorrhage	12. Exaggerated flexion of maternal knees and hips
	13. Apgar score

Check your answers with the Module 13 Posttest Answer Key.

Answer the following questions without referring back to the information in the module. Select the ONE BEST answer for each question.

1. What is the Apgar score of Baby Smith?

Heart rate:	120 bpm
Respiratory effort:	Slow, irregular
Muscle tone:	Some extremity flexion
Reflex irritability:	Grimace
Color:	Blue extremities

   A. 4
   B. 6
   C. 8
   D. 3

2. Based on the score from question 1, Baby Smith needs:
   A. Immediate intubation
   B. Routine newborn care
   C. Assistance with resuscitation
   D. Further observation

3. Dr. Jones asks that umbilical cord gas samples be obtained on Baby Smith. The proper procedure includes:
   A. Collection of two specimens: one arterial and one venous
   B. Placement of needle through both vessels and specimen drawn
   C. Immediate analysis for accurate results
   D. Repetition of examination within 2 hours to ensure adequate treatment

4. The umbilical cord blood obtained on Baby Smith reveals the following arterial results:

pH:	7.23	HCO_3:	24.3
PCO_2:	60.5 mm Hg	Base excess:	28.4
PO_2:	9.8 mm Hg		

   The preceding values are:
   A. Normal
   B. Abnormal

5. Based on what is known about Baby Smith, it can be said that this baby's long-term outcome will be:
   A. Good, because all parameters are within normal limits
   B. Poor, because all parameters are abnormal
   C. Unknown, because not all variables have been examined
   D. Dependent on the care received before transport to the nursery

6. The most important factor to consider when evaluating the newborn at birth is:
   A. The baby's total clinical picture
   B. The baby's heart rate
   C. The Apgar score
   D. The baby's cord gases

7. Baby David has a 1-minute Apgar score of 3. Your first responsibility is to:
   A. Maintain an external heat source
   B. Conduct another Apgar assessment
   C. Initiate resuscitation
   D. Keep the parents informed of what is happening

8. The primary purpose of Apgar scoring is to:
   A. Clinically assess the newborn
   B. Predict long-term outcome
   C. Guide resuscitative efforts
   D. Determine the presence of hypoxia

9. Umbilical cord blood gas sampling allows identification of:
   A. Newborn response to oxygenation
   B. Intrapartum fetal distress
   C. Fetal maturity
   D. Undiagnosed congenital anomalies
   E. All of the above
   F. None of the above

10. Metabolic acidosis in the newborn is:
   A. Usually inconsequential and easily resolved
   B. Caused by the trauma of the vaginal birth process
   C. Potentially life threatening if uncorrected
   D. Readily diagnosed and responsive to treatment

11. For collection of the umbilical cord blood gas samples:
   A. Use at least a 10-mL syringe
   B. Flush the syringe with a heparinized solution
   C. Chill the syringe with ice before the sample is obtained
   D. Attach the syringe to an 18-gauge needle

12. The care of the newly delivered mother will be transferred from the nurse who followed the woman in labor to another nurse. What information will the new nurse need to care for this patient?
   A. Summary of antepartum events
   B. Plans for method of infant feeding
   C. Time of delivery
   D. Gender of the infant
   E. All of the above

13. During the immediate postpartum period, the fundus will be located:
   A. 2 fingerbreadths above the umbilicus, deviated to right of midline
   B. 3 fingerbreadths below the umbilicus
   C. At the level of the umbilicus or slightly below and in the midline

14. A 21-year-old woman delivers a 9-pound, 15-ounce infant after an 18-hour labor. The last 5 hours of labor required oxytocin augmentation and epidural anesthesia. During the immediate postpartum assessment, the single most critical element to be observant of is:
   A. A temperature elevation
   B. Pregnancy-related hypertension
   C. Uterine atony
   D. A full bladder

15. During the first hour postpartum, the newly delivered mother's temperature is 100.3°F. Which of the following may be the cause?
   A. Dehydration
   B. Infection
   C. Epidural anesthesia
   D. All of the above

16. Early signs of normal attachment to the newborn by the parent include:
    A. Asking the more experienced nurse to care for the infant
    B. Talking to the infant in a low-pitched voice
    C. Keeping the infant in a warmer to maintain temperature
    D. Calling the infant by name

17. A new mother plans to breastfeed. After a long labor, she asks that the infant be given a bottle for 24 hours so that she can rest. You:
    A. Respect the woman's wishes and bottle feed the infant
    B. Tell the woman that she has to either bottle feed or breastfeed and has to decide now
    C. Arrange for rest periods for the woman and wait to see if the lactation consultant can convince her to begin to nurse the baby
    D. Explain the advantages of early breastfeeding and plan with the woman ways to achieve adequate rest and initiate lactation

18. Normal findings after a cesarean delivery include:
    A. The woman is unable to move her legs after spinal anesthesia
    B. Bloody urine in the catheter bag
    C. A boggy uterus
    D. Elevated blood pressure

19. Before postpartum sterilization, a woman should:
    A. Be allowed to rest after a long labor
    B. Have documentation of informed consent
    C. Have a catheter inserted in her bladder
    D. Have at least two children

20. You have been assigned to care for a woman whose infant was stillborn. Which of the following behaviors are not supportive of this family's grief process?
    A. Allowing the family to see and hold the infant
    B. Asking the name of the infant
    C. Reminding the mother that she can have more children
    D. Offering to take pictures of the infant

21. Your patient will be discharged 8 hours after the birth of her infant. What information should she know before discharge?
    A. Who to call with questions or for help
    B. How to care for and feed her infant
    C. How to care for her episiotomy
    D. When to come for a postpartum examination
    E. All of the above

Check your answers with the Module 14 Posttest Answer Key.

Posttest: Module 15. Liability Issues in Intrapartum Nursing

Answer the following questions without referring back to the information in the module. Select the ONE BEST answer for each question.

1. As a nurse, you have been asked to obtain a patient's consent for a tubal ligation. Your response is to:
   A. Clearly explain the procedure to this woman
   B. Check the unit procedure/policy manual for the correct forms
   C. Refuse to obtain the consent
   D. Clearly explain the procedure and the risks to the woman

2. The difference between the professional and lay standards for the information part of a consent is:
   A. The language used to explain the procedure
   B. How the risk factors and outcomes are presented to the patient
   C. The length of the explanation about the procedure
   D. Only the professional standard requires a statement about the risks

3. Under what circumstances can a consent be invalid?
   A. When a 17-year-old gravida 2 para 1001 signs a consent for surgery
   B. When a patient's husband signs a consent for a cesarean birth
   C. When a procedure results in a negative outcome
   D. When the patient gives verbal consent for a nursing procedure

4. When you need to correct a charting error, the most appropriate action is to:
   A. Use correction fluid to cover the incorrect information and carefully write in the correct information
   B. Rewrite the whole page of notes
   C. With a single line, cross out the entry and write "error" above it with the date, time, and your initials
   D. Cross out the error and enter the correct information above it

5. Your initial assessment of the laboring patient should include all of the following *except:*
   A. Significant health problems
   B. The course of this pregnancy
   C. Facts about the onset of labor
   D. Your belief that the patient's husband is unsupportive of her plans for the birth

6. After instituting appropriate nursing interventions for a late deceleration in the fetal heart rate, you should document:
   A. The action taken
   B. Maternal and fetal response
   C. That the care provider was notified
   D. All of the above

7. According to current national standards of nursing practice, the person liable for an individual nurse's practice is the:
   A. Physician in charge of the case
   B. Individual professional nurse
   C. Hospital administration staff
   D. Nursing supervisor

8. When you are asked to chart a procedure for a co-worker, what should you do?
   A. Ask enough questions to be sure your notes are accurate.
   B. Have that person cosign your notes.
   C. Refuse to do the charting.
   D. Ask the person to dictate the information and both of you sign the entry.

9. When a patient refuses a medication, the most appropriate nursing action is to:
   A. Write a note documenting why the medication was not administered
   B. Try to talk the patient into accepting the medication
   C. Obtain assistance from a co-worker to administer the medication because it is in the best interest of the patient
   D. Write "withheld" on the medication record

10. A nurse can be held liable for malpractice in all of the following circumstances *except:*
    A. When it can be shown that the nurse did not meet a standard of care
    B. Whenever there is a poor outcome
    C. When in similar circumstances other nurses would have foreseen the possibility of a negative outcome for a particular action
    D. When the chart documents the patient's refusal of a nursing intervention that contributed to the negative outcome

11. You would expect a unit guideline delegating the responsibility for obtaining an informed consent for oxytocin augmentation to nursing personnel to include all of the following *except:*
    A. Criteria for patient selection
    B. Authorization for the protocol indicated by the medical director's signature
    C. Therapeutic goals for the augmentation
    D. Arguments to present if the patient refuses to sign the consent form

12. Documentation of a telephone triage contact should be determined by the:
    A. Patient's primary provider
    B. Seriousness of the problem
    C. Unit policy
    D. Person taking the call

13. You may discuss your preparation in a malpractice suit with:
    A. A nurse whose judgment you trust
    B. Counsel
    C. Other staff members present at the time of the incident
    D. Your spouse

14. Titration of oxytocin for labor augmentation or induction is based on all of the following except:
    A. Uterine activity
    B. Cervical change
    C. Friedman's labor curve
    D. Fetal response

15. You have just assisted with a vaginal delivery where a shoulder dystocia was encountered. To reduce liability risks, all of the following would be helpful except:
    A. Discussing the events with other members of the health care team present to provide adequate documentation.
    B. Document the timing and sequence of all maneuvers.
    C. Describe to the mother and family the difficulty in delivering a large-for-gestational-age baby.
    D. Document the presence of neonatal staff at delivery for newborn resuscitation.

16. If you have a disagreement with the attending CNM about the plan of care for your laboring patient, you should first:
    A. Discuss the issue with the attending CNM.
    B. Notify the Chief of Obstetrics.
    C. Tell the patient.
    D. Let the charge nurse handle it.

17. Which of the following represents the use of effective communication strategies?
    A. "Dr. Smith, I want you to come and assess Ms. B. in recovery. She is a gravida 6, para 5005 who delivered vaginally 30 minutes ago after a rapid labor. She is now having increased vaginal bleeding with large, fist-sized clots, and her heart rate has increased from 88 to 120. I think she may be having a postpartum hemorrhage. Please come now."
    B. "Dr. Jones, Ms. S. in Room 30 is having variable decelerations."
    C. "Susan, your patient in room 3 is requesting VBAC. I know you are probably too busy to come now, so I'll just find a resident."
    D. "Just giving you a quick report on Jane, she's fine. The baby looks fine."

18. Which of the following examples of documentation reflects the nurse's critical thinking and clinical decision making skills?
    A. "Physician notified. No new orders received."
    B. "Pt with repetitive late decelerations and decreased variability for last 30 minutes. Pt repositioned on L side, O_2 started per face mask at 10 L/min, IVF increased, oxytocin off. VE done, no cervical change. FSS attempted with no response. Dr. Smith notified of FHR tracing and interventions. Dr. Smith to come in now for assessment of fetal status."
    C. "EFM tracing difficult due to patient movement."
    D. "Patient agitated. Unable to trace SaO_2 after 2 machines used. Increased bleeding noted on c/sx dsg."

Check your answers with the Module 15 Posttest Answer Key.

Posttest: Module 16. Maternal Transport

Answer the following questions without referring back to the information in the module. ONE OR MORE THAN ONE of the choices may be correct.

1. A primary advantage of maternal transport to a regional center is that:
   A. The community hospital experiences less strain on its limited resources
   B. The hospital stay of the mother and baby is increased to ensure complete stabilization
   C. Total cost of care and delivery is reduced
   D. A more accurate assessment of when and how to deliver the baby can be made

2. In preparing a high-risk mother for transport to a regional center, it is important that:
   A. Arrangements be made for a family member to accompany the mother
   B. The mother be in labor
   C. The mother be brought directly to the admitting office of the regional hospital
   D. A copy of the mother's records be sent with her

3. In initiating the referral of the mother to the regional center, it is recommended that:
   A. The nurse in the referring hospital call the physician in the regional center
   B. The physician in the referring hospital call the physician in the regional center
   C. The nurse in the referring hospital call the nurse in the regional center
   D. The physician in the referring hospital call the nurse in the regional center

4. The regional (receiving) center has all of the following responsibilities in the maternal transport process *except:*
   A. A report by phone is given to the referring physician within 24 hours of an important change or outcome in the mother
   B. A discharge summary is sent to the referring hospital
   C. The consent for transport is obtained from the mother or a family member
   D. A physician sees the mother shortly after her arrival at the regional center

5. Which of the following conditions is characteristic of a high-risk transport situation?
   A. The mother's condition is stable.
   B. Time of delivery is not predictable.
   C. A skilled attendant may not need to accompany the mother.
   D. A transport incubator is unnecessary.

6. Which condition can require that a mother be transported from a small Level I community hospital to a regional center?
   A. A laboring woman with a breech baby
   B. A mother requiring a oxytocin induction
   C. A mother with poorly controlled diabetes mellitus
   D. A mother expecting her eighth child

7. A gravida 2 at 34 weeks' gestation is expecting twins. She is in early labor at a Level I hospital. The decision to transport her to a high-risk regional center is most likely because of the:
   A. Increased risk of the babies having birth weights below 2,000 g
   B. Increased risk that preeclampsia can occur in multiple gestations
   C. Increased risk of a cesarean birth
   D. Desire to stop her labor by tocolysis

8. During a high-risk transport situation, when either the mother's condition is unstable or the time of delivery is unpredictable, it is highly recommended that the mother be accompanied by a:
   A. Family member
   B. Certified registered nurse anesthetist
   C. Skilled medical attendant, such as an obstetrician
   D. Paramedic skilled in the delivery of the newborn

9. All of the following statements regarding maternal transport to a regional perinatal center are true *except:*
   A. A woman whose membranes have ruptured prematurely at any gestational age should be referred to a regional center
   B. Transport of the undelivered woman to a regional center should be considered if it is anticipated that the infant might require intensive care not available at the referring hospital
   C. Transfer of high-risk women in early labor is recommended if the transport will take less than 2 hours
   D. A woman with poorly controlled diabetes mellitus should be referred to a regional center

10. Select the nursing intervention most likely to assist the pregnant woman and her family in adjusting at the high-risk regional hospital.
    A. Delay orientation of the mother and family member to the unit until the mother has rested for a day or two.
    B. Limit the number of incoming and outgoing phone calls to and from family members to ensure adequate rest for the mother.
    C. To reduce the mother's anxiety about the pregnancy outcome, avoid paying too much attention to a fetus who might be greatly compromised.
    D. Assign one primary nurse to care for the mother for the first few days.

11. A nursing intervention critical to ensuring a safe maternal transport is to:
    A. Ensure the expectant woman's comfort in a supine position
    B. Make certain that the expectant woman knows what to expect during the transport
    C. Carefully label any bag of intravenous fluid
    D. Keep family members informed of the woman's status

12. All of the following statements reflect recommendations of the 2000 National Institutes of Health consensus conference on corticosteroid therapy for fetal maturation *except:*
    A. Corticosteroid therapy is strongly recommended for its effectiveness in decreasing RDS in infants born between 29 and 34 weeks' gestation
    B. Administration of a glucocorticoid to the mother is advised 24 to 48 hours before delivery
    C. Use of corticosteroids in infants born between 24 and 28 weeks' gestation decreases the severity of the disease but not the incidence
    D. No strong recommendations were made because research data remain inconclusive

13. The National Institutes of Health has released clinical recommendations on antenatal corticosteroid administration. Recommendations call for the administration of:
    A. Weekly doses
    B. Rescue therapy
    C. A single course
    D. Occasional doses

14. A single course of antenatal corticosteroid treatment using dexamethasone consists of:
    A. Two 12-mg doses given intramuscularly 6 hours apart
    B. Four 6-mg doses given intramuscularly 12 hours apart
    C. Four 12-mg doses given intramuscularly 24 hours apart
    D. Two 6-mg doses given intramuscularly 24 apart

15. Optimal benefits from antenatal corticosteroid treatment last:
    A. 1 day
    B. 2 days
    C. 5 days
    D. 7 days

16. Cyanosis resulting from a cardiac abnormality rather than peripheral cyanosis should be suspected when it occurs in a:
    A. Term baby who has had a normal delivery with little respiratory distress
    B. Baby who has radiologic evidence of lung disease
    C. Baby experiencing premature rupture of membranes and passage of meconium in utero
    D. Premature baby who is in marked respiratory distress

17. A critical management step in caring for a woman with preterm premature rupture of membranes is to:
    A. Perform a sterile-gloved vaginal examination
    B. Use a sterile cotton-tipped applicator to take a vaginal culture for group B streptococcus
    C. Keep the mother in a flat, supine position
    D. Insert an internal fetal monitor

18. Women presenting with premature rupture of membranes need to be observed for:
    A. Rising temperatures
    B. Ruptured uterus
    C. Any sign of abruptio placentae
    D. Eclampsia

19. In transporting a high-risk laboring mother who has the possibility of delivery before reaching the referral hospital, a transport incubator should be part of the equipment.
    A. True
    B. False

20. Liability issues for health care personnel involved in transport are:
    A. Failure to stabilize before transport
    B. Failure or delay by the receiving hospital to diagnose a problem more significant than what was relayed by the referring hospital
    C. Delay in making a decision to transfer
    D. Failure to use treatment protocols

Check your answers with the Module 16 Posttest Answer Key.

Posttest: Module 17. Intimate Partner Violence During Pregnancy

Answer the following questions without referring back to the information in the module. ONE OR MORE THAN ONE of the choices may be correct.

1. Intimate partner violence can only occur in opposite-sex couples.
   A. True
   B. False

2. The violence that characterizes IPV can be:
   A. Physical
   B. Emotional
   C. Sexual
   D. Threatened

3. IPV affects only a small amount of women and therefore should not be routinely screened for.
   A. True
   B. False

4. Factors associated with a higher prevalence of IPV during pregnancy include:
   A. Adolescence
   B. Alcohol and drug use
   C. STIs
   D. Desired pregnancy

5. What are the phases of the cycle of violence?
   A. Plateau
   B. Tension building
   C. Reconciliation
   D. Acute violence

6. Which of the following are effects of violence during pregnancy?
   A. Delayed prenatal care
   B. Preeclampsia
   C. Fetal fractures
   D. Miscarriage

7. Which of the following parameters should the nurse assess for manifestations of violence?
   A. Client behaviors
   B. Partner behaviors
   C. Physical indicators
   D. All of the above

8. Which of the following is NOT a reason why pregnancy is a unique opportunity for IPV screening?
   A. Most women seek prenatal care
   B. Trust in health care providers
   C. Pregnancy is a powerful motivator for change
   D. Violence is frequently decreased during pregnancy

9. To complete screening for IPV, the nurse would need to:
   A. Review the woman's medical and obstetric history
   B. Observe behaviors of the woman and her partner
   C. Direct questioning of mother with active listening to responses
   D. Accurate documentation of behaviors and responses

10. To create and environment of trust, the nurse should introduce screening questions for IPV with a statement such as:
    A. "I have to ask these questions, please bear with me."
    B. "I know this probably doesn't apply to you, but I have to ask about domestic violence."
    C. "Because violence against women is so common and because there is help available, I ask every patient about domestic abuse."

11. Which of the following statements would be an appropriate response from the nurse if the woman discloses abuse?
    A. "Why don't you leave?"
    B. "You don't deserve this, we can help."
    C. "What did you do to make your partner hurt you?"
    D. "I'm glad you told me, we see many women in similar situations."

12. In determining an immediate threat to the woman, the nurse would need to assess all of the following EXCEPT:
    A. The abuser's presence in the birth setting
    B. The severity of past injuries
    C. The presence of weapons in the household
    D. The need for immediate counseling

13. Why is accurate and appropriate nursing documentation of IPV screening and response essential?
    A. The chart may be used in future legal proceedings.
    B. The language of the documentation may be open for misinterpretation if recorded inappropriately.
    C. To ensure the nurse's judgments of the situation are recorded.

14. Patient history relevant to IPV would include which of the following?
    A. Past history of abuse
    B. Statements made by the woman about abuse
    C. Name and relationship of the abuser
    D. Witnesses to the abuse
    E. A body map

15. Mandatory reporting of IPV may cause women to be reluctant to disclose abuse due to fear of retaliation.
    A. True
    B. False

16. The best way to encourage nurses' comfort with IPV screening is:
    A. Continued efforts in educating nurses about proper screening techniques
    B. An increase in pamphlets, brochures, and other literature available in the birth setting
    C. The organization of support groups for nurses who are victims of abuse
    D. An increased availability of translators

Check your answers with the Module 17 Posttest Answer Key.

Posttest: Module 18. Intrapartum Emergencies

Answer the following questions without referring back to the information in the module. ONE OR MORE THAN ONE of the choices may be correct.

1. When you detect a prolapsed umbilical cord, you should:
   A. Reposition the mother
   B. Exert upward internal pressure on the cord
   C. Reposition the cord externally
   D. Exert downward external pressure on the presenting part

2. When a prolapsed cord extends outside the mother's vagina, you should:
   A. Clamp the cord
   B. Reposition the cord
   C. Cover the cord with saline-soaked gauze
   D. Reinsert the cord

3. Risk factors associated with prolapsed cord are:
   A. Artificial rupture of membranes
   B. Oligohydramnios
   C. Fetal malpresentation
   D. Nonengaged fetal presenting part

4. Even though shoulder dystocia is unpredictable and unpreventable, there are some risk factors that may increase the likelihood that shoulder dystocia may occur. Which of the following is *not* a risk factor?
   A. "Small-frame" build of mother
   B. Instrumented delivery (forceps and/or vacuum)
   C. Diabetes mellitus
   D. Asian ethnicity of mother

5. Maternal complications of shoulder dystocia may include:
   A. Postpartum hemorrhage
   B. Extensive perineal lacerations (third or fourth degree)
   C. Uterine inversion during the immediate postpartum period
   D. Uterine rupture

6. Newborn injury associated with shoulder dystocia may include
   A. Brachial plexus injury
   B. Fracture of the clavicle
   C. Hypoglycemia
   D. Hypoxia

7. Nursing interventions for shoulder dystocia are:
   A. Fundal pressure
   B. Suprapubic pressure
   C. Call for help
   D. McRoberts positioning

8. Documentation following a shoulder dystocia should include:
   A. Team members present
   B. How much pressure was applied with fundal pressure
   C. Time from delivery of head to delivery of body
   D. That suprapubic pressure was performed

9. According to the national registry data, the most common signs and symptoms of amniotic fluid embolism (AFE) are:
   A. Hypertension
   B. Hypotension
   C. Cardiopulmonary arrest
   D. Headache

10. All of the following are symptoms associated with a Class III hemorrhage (1,800 to 2,400 mL blood loss) *except*:
    A. Maternal hypotension
    B. Maternal tachycardia and tachypnea
    C. Bounding pulses
    D. Cool extremities

11. Symptoms of hypovolemic shock from a class IV hemorrhage include:
    A. Urine output >30 mL/h
    B. Hypotension
    C. Signs of decreased organ perfusion
    D. Oliguria

12. Choose all appropriate nursing actions related to the care of a patient experiencing an obstetric hemorrhage:
    A. Intake and output every 8 hours
    B. Vital signs every 4 hours
    C. Continuous electronic fetal monitoring
    D. Foley catheter to bedside drainage system measurements each hour

13. Symptoms of abruption include all of the following *except*:
    A. Painful uterine tenderness
    B. Frequent uterine contractions
    C. Fetal compromise
    D. Relaxed uterine resting tone

14. At 38 4/7 weeks EGA, a patient has a diagnosis of placental abruption. Symptoms of the abruption include a nonreassuring fetal status, moderate vaginal bleeding, a painful, tender uterus, with frequent uterine contractions, and increased uterine resting tone. As the nurse, you anticipate this placental abruption to be a grade
    A. I
    B. II
    C. III
    D. The nurse does not need to anticipate this diagnosis

15. Risk factors strongly associated with placental abruption include all of the following *except*:
    A. Previous instrumented vaginal delivery
    B. Cocaine use
    C. Preeclampsia
    D. Previous placental abruption

16. A patient at 40 EGA desires a vaginal birth after cesarean section (VBAC). Her physician discusses the risks of uterine rupture with the patient, which include:
    A. The use of prostaglandins
    B. Labor
    C. The use of pitocin or misoprostil for induction of labor
    D. All of the above

17. The symptom of uterine rupture that is most frequently seen is
    A. Vaginal bleeding
    B. Nonreassuring fetal status
    C. Abdominal pain
    D. A cessation of uterine contractions

18. Early cause(s) of postpartum hemorrhage is/are
    A. Vaginal side wall laceration
    B. Placenta accrete
    C. Uterine rupture
    D. Uterine subinvolution

19. Nursing actions for uterine atony include
    A. IV fluid bolus
    B. Notification of delivery attendant (MD and/or CNM)
    C. Uterine massage
    D. Assessment of blood loss every shift

20. Uterotonic medications may be ordered to prevent postpartum hemorrhage. Correct dosing regimes include:
    A. Oxytocin 20 U in 1,000 mL crystalloids
    B. Methergine 0.2 mg IM
    C. Misoprostil 400 μg per rectum
    D. Oxytocin 10 U IM

Check your answers with the Module 18 Posttest Answer Key.

Posttest: Module 19. Caring for the Woman Undergoing an Instrumented or Operative Delivery

Answer the following questions without referring back to the information in the module. ONE OR MORE THAN ONE of the choices may be correct.

1. Operative vaginal deliveries occur in what percentage of all deliveries?
   A. 25%–30%
   B. 50%
   C. 10%–15%
   D. 5%

2. Which of the following is a contraindication of vacuum use?
   A. Evidence of cephalopelvic disproportion
   B. Vertex presentation
   C. Ruptured membranes
   D. Cervix completely dilated

3. Which of the following complications is encountered more frequently with vacuum-assisted birth?
   A. Shoulder dystocia
   B. Cephalopelvic disproportion
   C. Preterm delivery

4. Which of the following describes the nurse's role in a vacuum-assisted birth?
   A. The nurse has no role in a vacuum-assisted birth
   B. To educate the mother and family and support the birth attendant
   C. To apply the vacuum and assist with delivery

5. The maximum total time of vacuum application on the fetal head should not exceed
   A. 10 minutes
   B. 20 minutes
   C. 30 minutes
   D. 40 minutes

6. During a vacuum-assisted birth, the time of maximum total pressure (0.8 kg/cm^2) should not exceed
   A. 5 minutes
   B. 10 minutes
   C. 15 minutes
   D. 20 minutes

7. The vacuum is generally preferred over the use of forceps for an operative vaginal delivery because
   A. There are no risks to the fetus
   B. A vacuum-assisted delivery is faster than a forceps delivery
   C. A vacuum-assisted delivery has a lower failure rate than a forceps delivery
   D. A vacuum is easier to apply than forceps

8. A forceps-assisted birth is considered safer than a vacuum-assisted birth in which of the following situations?
   A. A prolonged second stage of labor
   B. A preterm delivery
   C. Fetal compromise
   D. Poor pushing effort

9. During an operative vaginal delivery, if EFM is not used, how often should the fetal heart rate be auscultated and documented?
   A. Every 2 minutes
   B. Every 5 minutes
   C. Every 10 minutes
   D. Every 15 minutes

10. Facial palsy related to pressure on cranial nerve VII will most likely be observed after a
    A. Spontaneous vaginal birth
    B. Cesarean birth
    C. Vacuum-assisted birth
    D. Forceps-assisted birth

11. A third- or fourth-degree laceration is more likely to occur after a
    A. Spontaneous vaginal birth
    B. Cesarean birth
    C. Vacuum-assisted birth
    D. Forceps-assisted birth

12. In 2004, the cesarean birth rate was close to
    A. 15%
    B. 30%
    C. 45%
    D. 50%

13. All of the following factors contribute to the increase in the cesarean birth rate *except*:
    A. Increased number of labor inductions
    B. Increased use of regional anesthesia
    C. Increased number of high-risk pregnancies
    D. Increase in the attempt of forceps-assisted deliveries

14. General considerations for candidate selection for a VBAC include all of the following *except*:
    A. The patient has a previous classical fundal uterine incision
    B. The maternal pelvis is clinically adequate
    C. The appropriate surgical staff is available
    D. The patient has no more than two prior low-transverse cesarean births

15. Common indications for cesarean birth are all of the following *except*:
    A. CPD
    B. Labor dystocia
    C. Nonreassuring fetal status
    D. Inactive herpes lesions

16. A patient has a midline vertical incision on the upper portion of the uterus. As a nurse you know that
    A. This patient is a good candidate for a VBAC
    B. This patient must have a cesarean section with all pregnancies
    C. Incisions made in this area are less likely to rupture
    D. This is the most popular incision for mother's and physicians

17. A patient has a low-segment transverse incision. As a nurse you know that
    A. The incision that is visually apparent on the mother's skin may not be the incision on the uterus
    B. There is a greater risk that the uterus will rupture during a trial of labor
    C. The incision on the mother's skin always matches the incision on the uterus
    D. Incisions made in this area will be disfiguring to the patient

18. A cesarean hysterectomy may need to be performed in which of the following situations?
    A. Uterine hemorrhage
    B. Uterine rupture
    C. Placenta accreta
    D. All of the above

19. A patient with a history of four previous cesarean births is
    A. A candidate for VBAC
    B. At increased risk for placenta accreta
    C. Anticipating a shorter hospital stay
    D. All of the above

20. While caring for a mother attempting a TOL and VBAC, the intrapartum nurse is aware that
    A. This patient should be monitored (EFM) continuously
    B. This patient is not a candidate for an epidural
    C. Cervical ripening can be done in the outpatient setting
    D. This patient should have an intrauterine pressure catheter
    E. All of the above

21. Which of the following is a reason for a maternal choice cesarean birth?
    A. The ability to schedule the timing of the birth
    B. Decreased risk of future maternal pelvic floor problems
    C. Fear of labor
    D. Desire for control
    E. All of the above

22. Which of the following is a contraindication for a cesarean birth?
    A. CPD
    B. Labor dystocia
    C. Nonviable fetus
    D. Umbilical cord prolapse

23. An estimated birth weight of more than 4,000 g may suggest
    A. Fetal malpresentation
    B. Maternal hypertensive disorder
    C. Cephalopelvic disproportion
    D. A congenital fetal anomaly

24. Obtaining a 20- to 30-minute baseline fetal heart rate by EFM for a patient having a cesarean birth is an example of
    A. Preoperative care
    B. Intraoperative care
    C. Postoperative care

25. Ensuring that sponge, needle, and equipment counts are correct is a duty that should be done during the
    A. Preoperative period
    B. Intraoperative period
    C. Postoperative period

Check your answers with the Module 19 Posttest Answer Key.

POSTTEST ANSWER KEY

Module 1. Overview of Labor
1. D
2. B
3. A
4. D
5. D
6. D
7. A
8. C
9. B
10. B
11. B
12. D
13. D
14. D
15. A
16. A
17. A
18. D
19. A
20. A
21. A
22. B
23. B
24. 1. D
   2. C
   3. A
   4. A
   5. B
25. C
26. C

Module 2. Maternal and Fetal Response to Labor
1. A or D
2. B
3. D
4. C
5. D
6. D
7. B
8. D
9. A, B
10. C
11. C
12. B
13. D
14. C
15. A
16. C
17. B, D
18. A

19. B
20. A, C
21. C, D
22. C
23. B
24. A

Module 3. Admission Assessment of the Laboring Woman
1. B
2. C, D
3. A
4. B
5. D
6. D
7. B
8. A
9. C
10. A
11. 1. C
   2. A
   3. E
   4. D
   5. F
   6. B
12. C
13. C
14. D
15. C, D
16. B
17. C, D
18. D
19. B
20. D
21. C
22. A
23. A, C
24. C
25. A
26. B
27. D
28. C
29. B
30. A, D
31. C
32. A
33. A
34. D
35. A
36. B
37. A, D

Module 4. Admission Assessment of the Fetus

1. C
2. A, C
3. C
4. B, C, D
5. B
6. A
7. B, C, D
8. D
9. A
10. A, B
11. C
12. A
13. D
14. A
15. B
16. A
17. D
18. D
19. A
20. B
21. B
22. C
23. A, D
24. A
25. C
26. A
27. B
28. A, C, D
29. C
30. D
31. A, B, D
32. A

Module 5. Caring for the Laboring Woman

1. A, B, C, D
2. A
3. B, C
4. D
5. B
6. A
7.

8. A (keep in mind that it could be a nullipara)
9. A (4 cm in 4 hours [active phase] = 1.0 cm/hr = pro-tracted for a multiparous woman but a normal rate for a nullipara)
10. C
11. A, C
12. A, B, D
13. D
14. B, D
15. C
16. C
17. A
18. B, D
19. B, C
20. C
21. B
22. B
23. D
24. B
25. A
26. A
27. A, B, C, D
28. A, D
29. B, D
30. D
31. B
32. D
33. A, C
34. D
35. C
36. C, D

Module 6. Intrapartum Fetal Monitoring

1. a. E
   b. B
   c. I
   d. E
   e. I
   f. B
   g. I
2. D
3. B, D
4. D
5. A
6. a. ED, LD
   b. A
   c. A, ED
   d. A, ED, VD
   e. LD
   f. VD
   g. LD
   h. LD
   i. A, ED, VD
   j. VD, LD, PD

k. LD
l. VD
m. ED
7. A
8. A, B, C
9. A, B
10. D
11. A,B
12. A
13. C
14. A
15. A
16. a. A
b. A
c. A
d. N
e. N
f. A
g. A
17. B
18. C
19. D
20. C
21. B
22. C
23. E
24. D
25. A
26. D
27. B
28. D
29. E
30. G
31. B
32. A
33. A
34. A
35. A
36. A
37. A
38. B
39. A
40. B
41. A
42. A
43. A
44. A
45. A
46. A
47. A
48. A
49. B
50. A
51. B

52. B
53. B
54. A
55. A
56. A
57. B
58. A
59. A
60. A
61. A
62. A
63. B
64. A
65. A
66. B
67. B
68. B
69. B
70. A
71. B
72. B
73. a. 5
b. 1
c. 4

Module 7. Induction and Augmentation of Labor

1. A
2. C
3. A
4. B
5. 1. d
2. g
3. c
4. f
5. e
6. a
7 h
8. b
6. C
7. D
8. C
9. A
10. B
11. B
12. A
13. C
14. B
15. A
16. B

Module 8. Caring for the Woman at Risk for Preterm Labor or With Premature Rupture of Membranes

1. C
2. A
3. D
4. A
5. E
6. A
7. B
8. B
9. A. No, tocolysis is not indicated at gestations less than 20 weeks.
    B. Yes.
    C. No, terbutaline tocolysis is not indicated with uncontrolled diabetes. $MgSO_4$ may be used along with insulin drip.
    D. No, tocolysis is not indicated with heavy vaginal bleeding or at-term gestation.
    E. No, tocolysis is not indicated in the presence of chorioamnionitis.
10. D
11. A
12. D
13. B
14. C
15. B
16. B
17. D
18. D
19. A
20. A
21. D
22. C
23. B
24. D
25. C
26. D
27. A
28. C
29. B
30. C

Module 9. Caring for the Laboring Woman With Hypertensive Disorders Complicating Pregnancy

1. B
2. D
3. D
4. B
5. C
6. A
7. D
8. D
9. C
10. A
11. 1. d, e
    2. f, h
    3. h
    4. b
    5. g
    6. c
    7. a
    8. i
12. C
13. B
14. A
15. A
16. C
17. B
18. C
19. B
20. C
21. A
22. D
23. A, B, D
24. B, D
25. B, C
26. B
27. A, D
28. C
29. A, B
30. B
31. C
32. D
33. B

Module 10. Caring for the Laboring Woman With HIV Infection or AIDS

1. C
2. A, B, C
3. B
4. D
5. D (Initially, gloves are worn because of the presence of lochia.)
6. B, C
7. C
8. A, D
9. D
10. B
11. D
12. A, B
13. A
14. A, B
15. A, B, C
16. A, B, C, D
17. A, B

18. D
19. A, C, D
20. C

Module 11. Hepatitis Infections
1. C
2. C
3. B
4. B
5. A
6. D
7. B
8. C
9. A
10. A
11. C
12. A
13. B
14. C
15. B
16. D
17. D
18. B
19. C
20. D
21. B
22. A
23. A. Test Report 3—this means you are immune
    B. Test Report 6—no immunity developed that can be documented
    C. Test Report 4—due to the presence of HBeAg
    D. Test Report 5—when IgM anti-HBc is negative, an acute infection is not present, hence the carrier state
24. A
25. D
26. A
27. C
28. B
29. A
30. A
31. A
32. A
33. B
34. A, B
35. C, D
36. B
37. C
38. Patients B and C
39. Patient A
40. Patient C
41. Patients A and B
42. C

43. a. F
    b. T
    c. F
    d. F
    e. F
    f. F
    g. T
    h. T
44. A
45. A
46. B
47. D

Module 12. Caring for the Pregnant Woman With Diabetes
1. A
2. D
3. C
4. C
5. D
6. B
7. B
8. D
9. B
10. B
11. A
12. A
13. D
14. A
15. A
16. C
17. C
18. E
19. A
20. C

Module 13. Delivery in the Absence of a Primary Care Provider
1. C
2. D
3. C
4. B
5. C
6. B
7. A
8. B
9. A
10. B
11. A
12. B
13. A
14. a. 12
    b. 7

c. 1
d. 8
e. 9
f. 10
g. 11
h. 2
i. 5
j. 4
k. 6
l. 3

Module 14. Assessment of the Newborn and Newly Delivered Mother

1. B
2. C
3. A
4. A
5. C
6. A
7. C
8. C
9. F
10. C
11. B
12. E
13. C
14. C
15. D
16. D
17. D
18. A
19. B
20. C
21. E

Module 15. Liability Issues in Intrapartum Nursing

1. C
2. B
3. B
4. C
5. D
6. D
7. B
8. C
9. A
10. B
11. D
12. C
13. B (When opposition counsel learns that you have discussed the case with an individual, the person can be called as a witness for the opposition. The only exception is your counsel.)
14. C

15. C
16. A
17. A
18. B

Module 16. Maternal Transport

1. D
2. A, D
3. B
4. C
5. B
6. C
7. A
8. C
9. A
10. D
11. C
12. D
13. C
14. B
15. D
16. A
17. B
18. A
19. A
20. A, B, C, D

Module 17. Intimate Partner Violence During Pregnancy

1. B
2. A, B, C, D
3. B
4. A, B, C
5. B, C, D
6. A, C, D
7. D
8. D
9. A, B, C, D
10. C
11. B, D
12. B
13. A, B
14. A, B, C, D
15. A
16. A

Module 18. Intrapartum Emergencies

1. A
2. C
3. B
4. D
5. A, B, D
6. A, B, D
7. B, C, D

8. A, C, D
9. B, C
10. C
11. B, C, D
12. C, D
13. D
14. C
15. A
16. D
17. B
18. A, B, C
19. B, C
20. A, B, C, D

Module 19. Care of the Woman Undergoing an Operative or Instrumented Delivery

1. C
2. A
3. A
4. B
5. B

6. B
7. D
8. B
9. B
10. D
11. D
12. B
13. D
14. A
15. D
16. B
17. A
18. D
19. B
20. A
21. E
22. C
23. C
24. A
25. B

INDEX

Page numbers in *italics* denote figures; those followed by "t" denote tables.

INTRAPARTUM MANAGEMENT MODULES
MODULE 1
OVERVIEW OF LABOR

General Purpose: To provide registered professional nurses and other providers of women's health care with an overview of labor and interventions for supporting the laboring woman.

Objectives
After reading this module and taking this test you will be able to:
1. Describe the physiologic processes involved in initiating labor
2. Outline the stages of labor and the characteristics of uterine contractions
3. Discuss principles or factors helpful in planning interventions for the laboring woman

Directions
To earn continuing education credit, follow these instructions:
1. Read Module 1.
2. Complete the following posttest. Each question has only one answer. Choose the one that is best in each case and darken the corresponding box on the Enrollment Form (Section B).
3. Complete Section A and record your answers to the Evaluation Questions (Section C) on the Enrollment Form.
4. The passing score for this CE activity posttest is 7 correct answers (70%).
5. Registration deadline is May 25, 2010. After this date, please contact Lippincott Williams & Wilkins Continuing Education Department at 800-787-8985 for course renewal information.
6. Send the completed Enrollment Form with the appropriate fee (U.S. checks, money order, or Visa, Mastercard, or American Express credit card) to:

Lippincott Williams & Wilkins
Continuing Education Department
333 Seventh Avenue, 19th Floor
New York, NY 10001

1. The chemical substances that trigger smooth muscle contractions and help prepare the cervix for dilatation are synthesized by:
   A. Macrophages
   B. Calcium
   C. Cytokines
   D. Progesterone

2. In late pregnancy, muscle fibers in the uterine myometrium communicate with each other via:
   A. The decidua
   B. Calcium channels
   C. Gap junctions
   D. Cytokines

3. During which stage of labor does the cervix reach full dilatation?
   A. The latent phase of stage I
   B. The active phase of stage I
   C. Stage II
   D. Stage III

4. During labor, the upper portion of the uterus:
   A. Softens
   B. Recedes passively
   C. Becomes thicker
   D. Undergoes a lengthening of its muscle fibers

5. The strongest portion of a uterine contraction is represented on a waveform as the:
   A. Acme
   B. Increment
   C. Base
   D. Decrement

6. Prolonged labor is characterized by contractions:
   A. Less than 35 mmHg in intensity and less frequently than five in 10 minutes
   B. Less than 25 mmHg in intensity and less frequently than four in 10 minutes
   C. Less than 35 mmHg in intensity and less frequently than two in 10 minutes
   D. Less than 25 mmHg in intensity and less frequently than two in 10 minutes

7. The duration of a uterine contraction is the time that elapses from:
   A. One acme to the next
   B. The beginning of the increment to the end of the decrement
   C. The acme to the end of the decrement
   D. The beginning of one wave to the beginning of the next wave

8. While assessing a uterine contraction by the palpation method, you can indent the uterus only with firm fingertip pressure at the peak of a contraction. You would consider this contraction:
   A. Ineffective
   B. Mild
   C. Moderate
   D. Strong

9. Propagation of a uterine contraction begins at the:
   A. Cervix
   B. Pacemaker
   C. Decidua
   D. Pelvis

10. An appropriate intervention for the laboring woman is:
    A. Keeping her room darkened at all times to promote a soothing atmosphere
    B. Directing all progress reports to her and not to her coach because she is the focus of your care
    C. Avoiding the use of drapes and other coverings because they can create unnecessary pressure and inconvenience
    D. Encouraging a family member to remain with her because family can also provide comfort and reassurance

LIPPINCOTT WILLIAMS & WILKINS
CONTINUING EDUCATION ENROLLMENT FORM

Intrapartum Management Modules: A Perinatal Education Program
4th Edition

Module 1—Overview of Labor
Nursing CE contact hours: 3.0
Fee: $27.95 (For every four tests submitted, get the lowest priced test for free. Submit all tests for $299, a savings of more than 50%.)

A. Last Name _____ First Name _____ MI _____

    Address _____

    City _____ State _____ Zip _____

    Telephone _____ Fax number _____

    E-mail _____

    ☐ Please check here to have your certificate faxed

    State of Licensure #1 _____ License #1 Number _____

    ☐ LPN   ☐ RN   ☐ CNM   ☐ CNS   ☐ NP   ☐ Other _____

    State of Licensure #2 _____ License #2 Number _____

    ☐ LPN   ☐ RN   ☐ CNM   ☐ CNS   ☐ NP   ☐ Other _____

    State of Licensure #3 _____ License #3 Number _____

    ☐ LPN   ☐ RN   ☐ CNM   ☐ CNS   ☐ NP   ☐ Other _____

☐ From time to time, we make our mailing list available to outside organizations to announce special offers. Please check here if you do not wish us to release your name and address.

B. Test answers: Please record your answers by filling in the appropriate boxes.

	a	b	c	d
1.	☐	☐	☐	☐
2.	☐	☐	☐	☐
3.	☐	☐	☐	☐
4.	☐	☐	☐	☐
5.	☐	☐	☐	☐
6.	☐	☐	☐	☐
7.	☐	☐	☐	☐
8.	☐	☐	☐	☐
9.	☐	☐	☐	☐
10.	☐	☐	☐	☐

C. Course Evaluation
1. Did this CE activity's learning objectives relate to its general purpose? ☐ Yes ☐ No
2. Was this format an effective way to present the material? ☐ Yes ☐ No
3. Was the content relevant to your nursing practice? ☐ Yes ☐ No
4. How long did it take you to complete this CE activity? _____ Hours _____ Minutes
5. Suggestion for future topics_____

Continuing Education Posttests

■ ■ ■ ■

INTRAPARTUM MANAGEMENT MODULES
MODULE 2
MATERNAL AND FETAL RESPONSE TO LABOR

General Purpose: To present registered professional nurses and other providers of women's health care with a description of both the fetal and the maternal responses to labor and techniques for assessing fetal descent and fetal malpresentation.

Objectives

After reading this module and taking this test, you will be able to:

1. Outline the dimensional and relational parameters that help to predict the course of labor and delivery
2. Discuss assessment techniques used to help monitor the progress of labor
3. Plan interventions for evaluating and managing the laboring woman

Directions

To earn continuing education credit, follow these instructions:

1. Read Module 2.
2. Complete the following posttest. Each question has only one answer. Choose the one that is best in each case and darken the corresponding box on the Enrollment Form (Section B).
3. Complete Section A and record your answers to the Evaluation Questions (Section C) on the Enrollment Form.
4. The passing score for this CE activity posttest is 7 correct answers (70%).
5. Registration deadline is May 25, 2010. After this date, please contact Lippincott Williams & Wilkins Continuing Education Department at 800-787-8985 for course renewal information.
6. Send the completed Enrollment Form with the appropriate fee (U.S. checks, money order, or Visa, Mastercard, or American Express credit card) to:

Lippincott Williams & Wilkins
Continuing Education Department
333 Seventh Avenue, 19th Floor
New York, NY 10001

1. The relationship of the long axis of the fetus to the long axis of the mother is called the fetal:
   A. Position
   B. Lie
   C. Attitude
   D. Presentation

2. The pelvic cavity:
   A. Includes the true and the false pelvis
   B. Includes only one of the pelvic planes
   C. Extends from the pelvic inlet to the pelvic outlet
   D. Is another name for the false pelvis

3. Hyperextension of the fetal head results in which of the following presentations?
   A. Transverse
   B. Cephalic
   C. Shoulder
   D. Breech

4. The denominator in a vertex presentation is the:
   A. Occiput
   B. Mentum
   C. Sacrum
   D. Acromial process

5. When the level of the fetal presenting part is 3 cm past the mother's ischial spines and into the pelvic outlet, its station is:
   A. −1
   B. 0
   C. +1
   D. +3

6. When the fetal presenting part has entered the false pelvis but has yet to pass the pelvic inlet, the fetus is:
   A. Presenting
   B. Floating
   C. Molding
   D. Dipping

7. When it is possible to move the presenting part just above the symphysis pubis via abdominal examination, the fetus is:
   A. Presenting
   B. Floating
   C. Molding
   D. Dipping

8. When the station is high at the onset of labor:
   A. Labor tends to be short
   B. The cervix is likely to be considerably effaced
   C. Disproportion is a significant possibility
   D. Nonprogressive labor is unlikely

9. If the presenting part fails to fit the pelvic inlet closely, there is a danger of:
   A. Prolapsed cord
   B. Prolonged labor
   C. Fetal anoxia
   D. Caput succedaneum

10. If the nurse suspects fetal malpresentation during assessment, the first action would be to:
    A. Observe for prolonged labor
    B. Reposition the mother
    C. Alert the primary care provider immediately
    D. Perform a vaginal examination to check for a prolapsed cord

LIPPINCOTT WILLIAMS & WILKINS
CONTINUING EDUCATION ENROLLMENT FORM

Intrapartum Management Modules: A Perinatal Education Program
4th Edition

Module 2—Maternal and Fetal Response to Labor
Nursing CE contact hours: 1.5
Fee: $17.95 (For every four tests submitted, get the lowest priced test for free. Submit all tests for $299, a savings of more than 50%.)

A. Last Name _____ First Name _____ MI _____

Address _____

City _____ State _____ Zip _____

Telephone _____ Fax number _____

E-mail _____

☐ Please check here to have your certificate faxed

State of Licensure #1 _____ License #1 Number _____

☐ LPN ☐ RN ☐ CNM ☐ CNS ☐ NP ☐ Other _____

State of Licensure #2 _____ License #2 Number _____

☐ LPN ☐ RN ☐ CNM ☐ CNS ☐ NP ☐ Other _____

State of Licensure #3 _____ License #3 Number _____

☐ LPN ☐ RN ☐ CNM ☐ CNS ☐ NP ☐ Other _____

☐ From time to time, we make our mailing list available to outside organizations to announce special offers. Please check here if you do not wish us to release your name and address.

B. Test answers: Please record your answers by filling in the appropriate boxes.

	a	b	c	d
1.	☐	☐	☐	☐
2.	☐	☐	☐	☐
3.	☐	☐	☐	☐
4.	☐	☐	☐	☐
5.	☐	☐	☐	☐
6.	☐	☐	☐	☐
7.	☐	☐	☐	☐
8.	☐	☐	☐	☐
9.	☐	☐	☐	☐
10.	☐	☐	☐	☐

C. Course Evaluation
1. Did this CE activity's learning objectives relate to its general purpose? ☐ Yes ☐ No
2. Was this format an effective way to present the material? ☐ Yes ☐ No
3. Was the content relevant to your nursing practice? ☐ Yes ☐ No
4. How long did it take you to complete this CE activity? _____ Hours _____ Minutes
5. Suggestion for future topics_____

Continuing Education Posttests

■ ■ ■ ■

INTRAPARTUM MANAGEMENT MODULES
MODULE 3
ADMISSION ASSESSMENT OF THE LABORING WOMAN

General Purpose: To present registered professional nurses and other providers of women's health care with a detailed admission assessment procedure for the laboring woman, including the physical examination, testing for ruptured membranes, and the vaginal examination.

Objectives
After reading this module and taking this test, you will be able to:
1. List reasons why collecting an adequate admission history from a pregnant woman is vital for optimal perinatal outcomes
2. Discuss warning signs indicating perinatal compromise
3. Outline the essential actions and observations necessary for a thorough and appropriate vaginal examination of the laboring woman

Directions
To earn continuing education credit, follow these instructions:
1. Read Module 3.
2. Complete the following posttest. Each question has only one answer. Choose the one that is best in each case and darken the corresponding box on the Enrollment Form (Section B).
3. Complete Section A and record your answers to the Evaluation Questions (Section C) on the Enrollment Form.
4. The passing score for this CE activity posttest is 7 correct answers (70%).
5. Registration deadline is May 25, 2010. After this date, please contact Lippincott Williams & Wilkins Continuing Education Department at 800-787-8985 for course renewal information.
6. Send the completed Enrollment Form with the appropriate fee (U.S. checks, money order, or Visa, Mastercard, or American Express credit card) to:

Lippincott Williams & Wilkins
Continuing Education Department
333 Seventh Avenue, 19th Floor
New York, NY 10001

1. How many infants born to mothers who have experienced a primary genital herpes virus infection during the pregnancy acquire the virus?
   A. 1 in 2
   B. 1 in 3
   C. 1 in 50
   D. 1 in 100

2. Which of the following is a sign of false labor?
   A. Contractions that start at the back and spread to the front
   B. Loose bowel movements
   C. Contractions that intensify with walking
   D. A brownish "bloody show"

3. Which of the following is a sign of true labor?
   A. Brief increases in fetal movement
   B. No change in contractions after sedation is administered
   C. Contractions that diminish temporarily with increased maternal activity
   D. Moderate contractions felt only in the back

4. Meconium-stained amniotic fluid is a dangerous sign because:
   A. Of its high bacterial content
   B. It always indicates fetal distress
   C. It may be aspirated
   D. It is a sure marker of prematurity

5. Which of the following findings requires immediate surgical intervention?
   A. Too little amniotic fluid
   B. Too much amniotic fluid
   C. Meconium-stained amniotic fluid
   D. Port wine–colored amniotic fluid

6. You should forego the initial vaginal examination when admitting a pregnant woman who is:
   A. In labor and whose membranes have not yet ruptured
   B. Not in labor and whose membranes have ruptured
   C. In labor and whose membranes have ruptured
   D. Not in labor and whose membranes have not yet ruptured

7. When performing a vaginal examination on a woman in labor, you should:
   A. Have her empty her bladder before the examination
   B. Position her hands above her head for the examination
   C. Maintain a moderate upward pressure on the blades as you insert the speculum
   D. Apply a water-based lubricant to the speculum

8. Which of the following is a definitive sign of ruptured membranes?
   A. A glistening perineum
   B. A color change indicating alkalinity on Nitrazine paper
   C. Positive arborization
   D. Leakage of straw-colored fluid with a neutral odor

9. A cervix that is ¼-inch thick is:
   A. 25% effaced
   B. 50% effaced
   C. 75% effaced
   D. 100% effaced

10. During the vaginal examination of a laboring woman, you can fit the tips of three of your fingers inside the cervical opening. The cervix is approximately:
    A. 3 cm dilated
    B. 5 to 6 cm dilated
    C. 8 to 9 cm dilated
    D. Fully dilated

LIPPINCOTT WILLIAMS & WILKINS
CONTINUING EDUCATION ENROLLMENT FORM

Intrapartum Management Modules: A Perinatal Education Program
4th Edition

Module 3—Admission Assessment of the Laboring Woman
Nursing CE contact hours: 4.0
Fee: $32.95 (For every four tests submitted, get the lowest priced test for free. Submit all tests for $299, a savings of more than 50%.)

A. Last Name _____ First Name _____ MI _____

Address _____

City _____ State _____ Zip _____

Telephone _____ Fax number _____

E-mail _____

☐ Please check here to have your certificate faxed

State of Licensure #1 _____ License #1 Number _____

☐ LPN   ☐ RN   ☐ CNM   ☐ CNS   ☐ NP   ☐ Other _____

State of Licensure #2 _____ License #2 Number _____

☐ LPN   ☐ RN   ☐ CNM   ☐ CNS   ☐ NP   ☐ Other _____

State of Licensure #3 _____ License #3 Number _____

☐ LPN   ☐ RN   ☐ CNM   ☐ CNS   ☐ NP   ☐ Other _____

☐ From time to time, we make our mailing list available to outside organizations to announce special offers. Please check here if you do not wish us to release your name and address.

B. Test answers: Please record your answers by filling in the appropriate boxes.

	a	b	c	d
1.	☐	☐	☐	☐
2.	☐	☐	☐	☐
3.	☐	☐	☐	☐
4.	☐	☐	☐	☐
5.	☐	☐	☐	☐
6.	☐	☐	☐	☐
7.	☐	☐	☐	☐
8.	☐	☐	☐	☐
9.	☐	☐	☐	☐
10.	☐	☐	☐	☐

C. Course Evaluation
1. Did this CE activity's learning objectives relate to its general purpose? ☐ Yes ☐ No
2. Was this format an effective way to present the material? ☐ Yes ☐ No
3. Was the content relevant to your nursing practice? ☐ Yes ☐ No
4. How long did it take you to complete this CE activity? _____ Hours _____ Minutes
5. Suggestion for future topics_____

■ ■ ■ ■

Continuing Education Posttests

INTRAPARTUM MANAGEMENT MODULES
MODULE 4
ADMISSION ASSESSMENT OF THE FETUS

General Purpose: To present registered professional nurses and other providers of women's health care with information on the components of a thorough fetal assessment.

Objectives

After reading this module and taking this test, you will be able to:
1. Discuss the assessment techniques used to approximate gestation
2. Outline principles essential for evaluating fetal position and movement
3. Describe actions that will yield information about fetal heart tones

Directions

To earn continuing education credit, follow these instructions:
1. Read Module 4.
2. Complete the following posttest. Each question has only one answer. Choose the one that is best in each case and darken the box on the Enrollment Form (Section B).
3. Complete Section A and record your answers to the Evaluation Questions (Section C) on the Enrollment Form.
4. The passing score for this CE activity posttest is 7 correct answers (70%).
5. Registration deadline is May 25, 2010. After this date, please contact Lippincott Williams & Wilkins Continuing Education Department at 800-787-8985 for course renewal information.
6. Send the completed Enrollment Form with the appropriate fee (U.S. checks, money order, or Visa, Mastercard, or American Express credit card) to:

Lippincott Williams & Wilkins
Continuing Education Department
333 Seventh Avenue, 19th Floor
New York, NY 10001

1. Using Naegele's rule, a pregnant woman whose last normal menstrual period began on November 13 would have an estimated date of confinement of:
   A. August 6
   B. August 10
   C. August 13
   D. August 20

2. With a Doppler ultrasound, the earliest that fetal heart tones can typically be heard is between:
   A. 6 and 8 weeks
   B. 10 and 12 weeks
   C. 14 and 16 weeks
   D. 18 and 20 weeks

3. Which of the following is a true statement about the effects of maternal behavior on fetal body movements (FBMs)?
   A. Smoking increases FBMs.
   B. Drinking alcohol stops FBMs for at least 6 hours.
   C. Eating decreases FBMs for 2 to 3 hours.
   D. FBMs increase during active labor.

4. When evaluating fetal movement, it is important to remember that:
   A. Most women feel at least 10 distinct fetal movements in 2 hours
   B. Fetal movement has been known to cease completely for as long as 20 hours before fetal death
   C. Any woman who does not feel the appropriate number of movements in 2 hours should count them for another 2 hours
   D. Hiccups should be counted as fetal movements

5. When measuring fundal height, the zero point of the tape measure should be positioned at the:
   A. Midline of the umbilicus
   B. Top of the fundus
   C. Anterior border of the symphysis pubis
   D. Lowermost edge of the curved fundus

6. Approximately where should the fundus be at 28 weeks' gestation?
   A. Approximately three fingerbreadths below the xiphoid
   B. Approximately three fingerbreadths above the umbilicus
   C. Approximately one to two fingerbreadths above the umbilicus
   D. Approximately one to two fingerbreadths below the umbilicus

7. Using one hand to stabilize the gravid uterus on one side of the abdomen and the other hand to feel along the side of the abdomen, you are attempting to palpate the fetal:
   A. Head
   B. Chest
   C. Back
   D. Cephalic prominence

8. While facing the mother's feet and moving your hands down the sides of her abdomen toward the symphysis pubis, you are attempting to palpate the fetal:
   A. Head
   B. Chest
   C. Back
   D. Cephalic prominence

9. With a breech position, the best place to auscultate fetal heart tones is:
   A. Below the umbilicus on the right side
   B. Below the umbilicus on the left side
   C. Above the umbilicus on the right side
   D. Above the umbilicus on the left side

10. The best place to begin listening for fetal heart tones when the fetus is at 20 weeks' gestation is:
    A. In the right lower quadrant
    B. One fingerbreadth above the umbilicus
    C. Two fingerbreadths above the pubic hairline at the midline of the abdomen
    D. In the left lower quadrant at the upper border of the pubic hair

LIPPINCOTT WILLIAMS & WILKINS
CONTINUING EDUCATION ENROLLMENT FORM

Intrapartum Management Modules: A Perinatal Education Program
4th Edition

Module 4—Admission Assessment of the Fetus

Nursing CE contact hours: 3.0

Fee: $27.95 (For every four tests submitted, get the lowest priced test for free. Submit all tests for $299, a savings of more than 50%.)

A. Last Name _____ First Name _____ MI _____

Address _____

City _____ State _____ Zip _____

Telephone _____ Fax number _____

E-mail _____

☐ Please check here to have your certificate faxed

State of Licensure #1 _____ License #1 Number _____

☐ LPN   ☐ RN   ☐ CNM   ☐ CNS   ☐ NP   ☐ Other _____

State of Licensure #2 _____ License #2 Number _____

☐ LPN   ☐ RN   ☐ CNM   ☐ CNS   ☐ NP   ☐ Other _____

State of Licensure #3 _____ License #3 Number _____

☐ LPN   ☐ RN   ☐ CNM   ☐ CNS   ☐ NP   ☐ Other _____

☐ From time to time, we make our mailing list available to outside organizations to announce special offers. Please check here if you do not wish us to release your name and address.

B. Test answers: Please record your answers by filling in the appropriate boxes.

	a	b	c	d
1.	☐	☐	☐	☐
2.	☐	☐	☐	☐
3.	☐	☐	☐	☐
4.	☐	☐	☐	☐
5.	☐	☐	☐	☐
6.	☐	☐	☐	☐
7.	☐	☐	☐	☐
8.	☐	☐	☐	☐
9.	☐	☐	☐	☐
10.	☐	☐	☐	☐

C. Course Evaluation

1. Did this CE activity's learning objectives relate to its general purpose? ☐ Yes ☐ No
2. Was this format an effective way to present the material? ☐ Yes ☐ No
3. Was the content relevant to your nursing practice? ☐ Yes ☐ No
4. How long did it take you to complete this CE activity? _____ Hours _____ Minutes
5. Suggestion for future topics_____

■ ■ ■ ■

INTRAPARTUM MANAGEMENT MODULES
MODULE 5
CARING FOR THE LABORING WOMAN

General Purpose: To present registered professional nurses and other providers of women's health care with detailed guidelines for intrapartum care, including maternal and fetal assessment, hydration, and pain management strategies.

Objectives
After reading this module and taking this test, you will be able to:
1. Outline assessment parameters or techniques for monitoring the laboring woman and her fetus
2. Discuss the indications, rationale, and guidelines for appropriate maternal and fetal hydration
3. Plan pain control strategies for the laboring woman

Directions
To earn continuing education credit, follow these instructions:
1. Read Module 5.
2. Complete the following posttest. Each question has only one answer. Choose the one that is best in each case and darken the box on the Enrollment Form (Section B).
3. Complete Section A and record your answers to the Evaluation Questions (Section C) on the Enrollment Form.
4. The passing score for this CE activity posttest is 7 correct answers (70%).
5. Registration deadline is May 25, 2010. After this date, please contact Lippincott Williams & Wilkins Continuing Education Department at 800-787-8985 for course renewal information.
6. Send the completed Enrollment Form with the appropriate fee (U.S. checks, money order, or Visa, Mastercard, or American Express credit card) to:

Lippincott Williams & Wilkins
Continuing Education Department
333 Seventh Avenue, 19th Floor
New York, NY 10001

1. For a fetus in a normal position of flexion, the optimal location for auscultating the fetal heart tones is over the fetus':
   A. Chest
   B. Back
   C. Vertex
   D. Buttocks

2. For a high-risk woman in active labor, fetal heart sounds should be evaluated every:
   A. 5 minutes
   B. 10 minutes
   C. 15 minutes
   D. 30 minutes

3. A woman laboring with her first birth remains at 2 cm of dilation for the first 10 hours. This is:
   A. A normal latent phase
   B. A protracted active phase
   C. Best treated with oxytocin stimulation
   D. An indication for an immediate cesarean delivery

4. A nulliparous woman who is having a normal pattern of labor will:
   A. Reach full dilation in approximately 10 hours of labor
   B. Dilate at a rate of approximately 1 cm per hour in the active phase
   C. Have a pattern of descent at approximately 2 cm per hour in the active phase
   D. Not have a predictable course of labor

5. Which position for pushing in the second stage of labor does not make use of the effects of gravity or optimize circulation for the mother and fetus?
   A. Squatting
   B. Semi-Fowler's
   C. Sims
   D. Lithotomy

6. A laboring woman:
   A. Who is kept NPO will have reduced gastric acidity
   B. Needs routine IV hydration to reduce the risk of hypoglycemia in her newborn
   C. Should be encouraged to empty her bladder every 2 hours
   D. Must have routine IV hydration during the first 12 hours of labor

7. Pain experienced by the laboring woman can:
   A. Cause hyperventilation and subsequent increased blood flow to the uterus
   B. Trigger the release of epinephrine, which ultimately reduces blood flow to the placenta
   C. Reduce both her cardiac output and blood pressure
   D. Trigger the release of epinephrine, which ultimately causes fetal hypoglycemia

8. Slow chest breathing:
   A. Involves taking deep breaths in through the nose and exhaling out the mouth
   B. Is used in stage II of labor
   C. Should be done with the eyes closed to be effective
   D. Should only be done with a coach or support person present

9. Treatment for a postepidural spinal headache includes:
   A. Maintaining the patient in a semiupright position
   B. Using a blood patch to seal the puncture site
   C. Restricting fluid intake
   D. Withholding analgesia to prevent masking the symptoms

10. Effleurage is:
    A. Light abdominal massage recommended between contractions
    B. Gentle abdominal massage performed with the palm of the hand
    C. Firm abdominal massage performed with the fingertips
    D. Light abdominal massage recommended during contractions

LIPPINCOTT WILLIAMS & WILKINS
CONTINUING EDUCATION ENROLLMENT FORM

Intrapartum Management Modules: A Perinatal Education Program
4th Edition

Module 5—Caring for the Laboring Woman
Nursing CE contact hours: 5.0
Fee: $38.95 (For every four tests submitted, get the lowest priced test for free. Submit all tests for $299, a savings of more than 50%.)

A. Last Name _____ First Name _____ MI _____

Address _____

City _____ State _____ Zip _____

Telephone _____ Fax number _____

E-mail _____

☐ Please check here to have your certificate faxed

State of Licensure #1 _____ License #1 Number _____

☐ LPN   ☐ RN   ☐ CNM   ☐ CNS   ☐ NP   ☐ Other _____

State of Licensure #2 _____ License #2 Number _____

☐ LPN   ☐ RN   ☐ CNM   ☐ CNS   ☐ NP   ☐ Other _____

State of Licensure #3 _____ License #3 Number _____

☐ LPN   ☐ RN   ☐ CNM   ☐ CNS   ☐ NP   ☐ Other _____

☐ From time to time, we make our mailing list available to outside organizations to announce special offers. Please check here if you do not wish us to release your name and address.

B. Test answers: Please record your answers by filling in the appropriate boxes.

	a	b	c	d
1.	☐	☐	☐	☐
2.	☐	☐	☐	☐
3.	☐	☐	☐	☐
4.	☐	☐	☐	☐
5.	☐	☐	☐	☐
6.	☐	☐	☐	☐
7.	☐	☐	☐	☐
8.	☐	☐	☐	☐
9.	☐	☐	☐	☐
10.	☐	☐	☐	☐

C. Course Evaluation
1. Did this CE activity's learning objectives relate to its general purpose? ☐ Yes ☐ No
2. Was this format an effective way to present the material? ☐ Yes ☐ No
3. Was the content relevant to your nursing practice? ☐ Yes ☐ No
4. How long did it take you to complete this CE activity? _____ Hours _____ Minutes
5. Suggestion for future topics_____

■ ■ ■ ■

Continuing Education Posttests

INTRAPARTUM MANAGEMENT MODULES
MODULE 6
INTRAPARTUM FETAL MONITORING

General Purpose: To present registered professional nurses and other providers of women's health care with detailed guidelines for fetal monitoring.

Objectives
After reading this module and taking this test, you will be able to:
1. Compare and contrast the capabilities of and techniques and equipment involved with intermittent auscultation and electronic fetal monitoring
2. Discuss the physiologic basis for at least three parameters used to monitor fetal status
3. Plan interventions for the laboring woman based on interpretation of fetal monitoring parameters

Directions
To earn continuing education credit, follow these instructions:
1. Read Module 6.
2. Complete the following posttest. Each question has only one answer. Choose the one that is best in each case and darken the corresponding box on the Enrollment Form (Section B).
3. Complete Section A and record your answers to the Evaluation Questions (Section C) on the Enrollment Form.
4. The passing score for this CE activity posttest is 7 correct answers (70%).
5. Registration deadline is May 25, 2010. After this date, please contact Lippincott Williams & Wilkins Continuing Education Department at 800-787-8985 for course renewal information.
6. Send the completed Enrollment Form with the appropriate fee (U.S. checks, money order, or Visa, Mastercard, or American Express credit card) to:

Lippincott Williams & Wilkins
Continuing Education Department
333 Seventh Avenue, 19th Floor
New York, NY 10001

1. Using intermittent auscultation alone, an experienced clinician cannot necessarily:
   A. Determine baseline variations such as bradycardia
   B. Identify the baseline rhythm
   C. Approximate the baseline rate
   D. Distinguish the different kinds of decelerations accurately

2. Which of the following devices detects changes in the shape of the laboring woman's abdomen as a result of uterine contractions?
   A. An ultrasonic transducer
   B. A tocodynamometer
   C. A fetoscope
   D. An intrauterine pressure catheter

3. Essential to reading a fetal monitor strip is understanding that:
   A. The space between each light vertical line represents 10 seconds, and the space between each light horizontal line represents 10 beats per minute
   B. The space between each light vertical line represents 1 minute, and the space between each light horizontal line represents 30 beats per minute

C. The space between each light vertical line represents 10 seconds, and the space between each light horizontal line represents 30 beats per minute
D. The space between each light vertical line represents 1 minute, and the space between each light horizontal line represents 10 beats per minute

4. Blood flow to the placenta is completely blocked when uterine tone:
   A. Drops below 10 mmHg
   B. Drops below 15 mmHg
   C. Rises above 25 mmHg
   D. Rises above 40 mmHg

5. During a 10-minute period, a laboring woman has five contractions. The first two are 45 mmHg in intensity, the third is 50 mmHg, and the last two are 60 mmHg. Resting uterine tone between each contraction is 10 mmHg. Using the Montevideo units standard, what is the calculated MVS?
   A. 260
   B. 210
   C. 310
   D. There is insufficient information to determine the MVU

6. A drop in the pH of fetal blood is recognized by:
   A. Baroreceptors, which trigger a decrease in fetal heart rate
   B. Baroreceptors, which trigger an increase in fetal heart rate
   C. Chemoreceptors, which trigger an initial decrease in fetal heart rate
   D. Chemoreceptors, which trigger an initial increase in fetal heart rate

7. Which of the following interventions is recommended for absent variability?
   A. Positioning the patient on her back
   B. Discontinuing oxygen therapy
   C. Turning the patient to the side
   D. Avoiding any actions that might stimulate the fetus

8. A drop in fetal heart rate that typically lasts less than 2 minutes and is usually associated with umbilical cord compression is called:
   A. An early deceleration
   B. A late deceleration
   C. A variable deceleration
   D. A prolonged deceleration

9. The fetal heart rate pattern most likely to indicate fetal metabolic acidosis is:
   A. Absent variability
   B. Early decelerations
   C. Variable decelerations
   D. Accelerations

10. Select the appropriate umbilical artery cord gas interpretation based on the following values: pH, 7.08; P_{CO_2}, 54 mmHg; P_{O_2}, 15 mmHg; BE 13
    A. Mixed academia
    B. Respiratory acidemia
    C. Metabolic acidemia
    D. Normal values

LIPPINCOTT WILLIAMS & WILKINS
CONTINUING EDUCATION ENROLLMENT FORM

Intrapartum Management Modules: A Perinatal Education Program
4th Edition

Module 6—Intrapartum Fetal Monitoring
Nursing CE contact hours: 8.0
Fee: $56.95 (For every four tests submitted, get the lowest priced test for free. Submit all tests for $299, a savings of more than 50%.)

A. Last Name _____ First Name _____ MI _____

Address _____

City _____ State _____ Zip _____

Telephone _____ Fax number _____

E-mail _____

☐ Please check here to have your certificate faxed

State of Licensure #1 _____ License #1 Number _____

☐ LPN ☐ RN ☐ CNM ☐ CNS ☐ NP ☐ Other _____

State of Licensure #2 _____ License #2 Number _____

☐ LPN ☐ RN ☐ CNM ☐ CNS ☐ NP ☐ Other _____

State of Licensure #3 _____ License #3 Number _____

☐ LPN ☐ RN ☐ CNM ☐ CNS ☐ NP ☐ Other _____

☐ From time to time, we make our mailing list available to outside organizations to announce special offers. Please check here if you do not wish us to release your name and address.

B. Test answers: Please record your answers by filling in the appropriate boxes.

	a	b	c	d
1.	☐	☐	☐	☐
2.	☐	☐	☐	☐
3.	☐	☐	☐	☐
4.	☐	☐	☐	☐
5.	☐	☐	☐	☐
6.	☐	☐	☐	☐
7.	☐	☐	☐	☐
8.	☐	☐	☐	☐
9.	☐	☐	☐	☐
10.	☐	☐	☐	☐

C. Course Evaluation
1. Did this CE activity's learning objectives relate to its general purpose? ☐ Yes ☐ No
2. Was this format an effective way to present the material? ☐ Yes ☐ No
3. Was the content relevant to your nursing practice? ☐ Yes ☐ No
4. How long did it take you to complete this CE activity? _____ Hours _____ Minutes
5. Suggestion for future topics_____

■ ■ ■ ■

Continuing Education Posttests

INTRAPARTUM MANAGEMENT MODULES
MODULE 7
INDUCTION AND AUGMENTATION OF LABOR

General Purpose: To present registered professional nurses and other providers of women's health care with detailed guidelines for inducing and augmenting labor, including procedures for implementing various mechanical and pharmacologic interventions.

Objectives
After reading this module and taking this test, you will be able to:
1. Discuss the indications, contraindications, and precautions for implementing the various methods of labor induction and/or augmentation
2. Discuss at least two assessment parameters useful for monitoring pregnancy and labor progression
3. Plan interventions for the laboring woman undergoing labor induction and/or augmentation

Directions
To earn continuing education credit, follow these instructions:
1. Read Module 7.
2. Complete the following posttest. Each question has only one answer. Choose the one that is best in each case and darken the corresponding box on the Enrollment Form (Section B).
3. Complete Section A and record your answers to the Evaluation Questions (Section C) on the Enrollment Form.
4. The passing score for this CE activity posttest is 7 correct answers (70%).
5. Registration deadline is May 25, 2010. After this date, please contact Lippincott Williams & Wilkins Continuing Education Department at 800-787-8985 for course renewal information.
6. Send the completed Enrollment Form with the appropriate fee (U.S. checks, money order, or Visa, Mastercard, or American Express credit card) to:

Lippincott Williams & Wilkins
Continuing Education Department
333 Seventh Avenue, 19th Floor
New York, NY 10001

1. Of the following, which is an absolute contraindication for induction and augmentation of labor?
   A. Multiple gestation
   B. Hydramnios
   C. Breech presentation
   D. Total placenta previa

2. Oxytocin infusions should always be regulated using a
   A. Free-flow infusion set
   B. A saline lock
   C. An infusion pump
   D. A Y-connector at the distal port on the mainline

3. A Bishop's score includes evaluation of all of the following except:
   A. Station
   B. Cervical consistency
   C. Presentation
   D. Cervical effacement

4. Of the following, which is a contraindication for cervical ripening with prostaglandin E_2 vaginal inserts?
   A. Active genital herpes
   B. Ruptured membranes
   C. Vertex presentation
   D. Early decelerations in fetal heart rate

5. After endocervical instillation of prostaglandin E_2 gel, the patient should be positioned:
   A. On her side for 30 minutes
   B. On her back for 1 hour
   C. On her side for 1 to 2 hours
   D. Supine for 2 hours

6. If fetal bradycardia develops after prostaglandin E_2 is instilled, the patient should be placed:
   A. On her left side
   B. In a high-Fowler's position
   C. In semi-Fowler's position
   D. In Trendelenburg's position

7. Optimal safety for the mother and the fetus during misoprostol administration is most likely when:
   A. The woman is having 12 or more contractions per hour
   B. The Bishop's score is greater than 6
   C. The woman has had plenty of fluids by mouth in the previous 3 hours
   D. The fetus has had a reactive nonstress test before medication placement

8. During oxytocin administration:
   A. Flow rate should be adjusted according to unit/institutional guidelines
   B. Contractions should not exceed 60 to 70 mmHg in strength
   C. Contractions should not occur more frequently than six times in 10 minutes
   D. Contractions should not exceed 60 to 90 seconds in duration

9. A desirable fetal heart rate pattern during oxytocin administration includes:
   A. A fetal heart rate of 170 to 180 beats per minute
   B. A resting uterine tone of 15 to 25 mmHg
   C. Moderate variability in the fetal heart baseline
   D. Five contractions in 10 minutes

10. The recommended dose of misoprostol is
   A. 100 μg by mouth every 12 hours
   B. 25 μg in posterior fornix of vagina as the initial dose
   C. 50 μg by mouth every 6 hours
   D. 100 μg per vagina as needed to maintain contractions

LIPPINCOTT WILLIAMS & WILKINS
CONTINUING EDUCATION ENROLLMENT FORM

Intrapartum Management Modules: A Perinatal Education Program
4th Edition

Module 7—Induction and Augmentation of Labor

Nursing CE contact hours: 3.0

Fee: $27.95 (For every four tests submitted, get the lowest priced test for free. Submit all tests for $299, a savings of more than 50%.)

A. Last Name _____ First Name _____ MI _____

Address _____

City _____ State _____ Zip _____

Telephone _____ Fax number _____

E-mail _____

☐ Please check here to have your certificate faxed

State of Licensure #1 _____ License #1 Number _____

☐ LPN ☐ RN ☐ CNM ☐ CNS ☐ NP ☐ Other _____

State of Licensure #2 _____ License #2 Number _____

☐ LPN ☐ RN ☐ CNM ☐ CNS ☐ NP ☐ Other _____

State of Licensure #3 _____ License #3 Number _____

☐ LPN ☐ RN ☐ CNM ☐ CNS ☐ NP ☐ Other _____

☐ From time to time, we make our mailing list available to outside organizations to announce special offers. Please check here if you do not wish us to release your name and address.

B. **Test answers:** Please record your answers by filling in the appropriate boxes.

	a	b	c	d
1.	☐	☐	☐	☐
2.	☐	☐	☐	☐
3.	☐	☐	☐	☐
4.	☐	☐	☐	☐
5.	☐	☐	☐	☐
6.	☐	☐	☐	☐
7.	☐	☐	☐	☐
8.	☐	☐	☐	☐
9.	☐	☐	☐	☐
10.	☐	☐	☐	☐

C. Course Evaluation

1. Did this CE activity's learning objectives relate to its general purpose? ☐ Yes ☐ No
2. Was this format an effective way to present the material? ☐ Yes ☐ No
3. Was the content relevant to your nursing practice? ☐ Yes ☐ No
4. How long did it take you to complete this CE activity? _____ Hours _____ Minutes
5. Suggestion for future topics_____

Continuing Education Posttests

■ ■ ■ ■

INTRAPARTUM MANAGEMENT MODULES
MODULE 8
CARING FOR THE WOMAN AT RISK FOR PRETERM LABOR OR WITH PREMATURE RUPTURE OF MEMBRANES

General Purpose: To present registered professional nurses and other providers of women's health care with detailed guidelines for evaluating and managing preterm labor and premature rupture of membranes.

Objectives

After reading this module and taking this test, you will be able to:

1. Discuss the risk factors associated with preterm level and key assessment parameters
2. Outline the indications, contraindications, mechanisms of action, and side effects of various tocolytic agents
3. Plan interventions for the woman with premature rupture of membranes and/or undergoing preterm labor

Directions

To earn continuing education credit, follow these instructions:

1. Read Module 8.
2. Complete the following posttest. Each question has only one answer. Choose the one that is best in each case and darken the corresponding box on the Enrollment Form (Section B).
3. Complete Section A and record your answers to the Evaluation Questions (Section C) on the Enrollment Form.
4. The passing score for this CE activity posttest is 7 correct answers (70%).
5. Registration deadline is May 25, 2010. After this date, please contact Lippincott Williams & Wilkins Continuing Education Department at 800-787-8985 for course renewal information.
6. Send the completed Enrollment Form with the appropriate fee (U.S. checks, money order, or Visa, Mastercard, or American Express credit card) to:

Lippincott Williams & Wilkins
Continuing Education Department
333 Seventh Avenue, 19th Floor
New York, NY 10001

1. Which of the following is a key finding in preterm labor?
   A. Cervical effacement of at least 60%
   B. At least 16 weeks' gestation
   C. Cervical dilation of at least 2 cm
   D. Two or three contractions in 60 minutes

2. Which of the following factors is associated with an increased risk of preterm labor?
   A. Previous preterm delivery
   B. A lengthy interpregnancy interval
   C. Previous first trimester abortion
   D. A cervix that is 40 mm or longer

3. Which of the following biochemical markers of preterm labor can be detected in cervicovaginal secretions?
   A. Estriol
   B. Fetal fibronectin
   C. Alpha-fetoprotein
   D. Corticotropin-releasing hormone

4. At the onset of symptoms of preterm labor, it is recommended that the woman:
   A. Restrict fluids
   B. Lie on her back
   C. Resume her usual activities
   D. Empty her bladder

5. Common side effects of tocolytic therapy with β-adrenergic agonists include:
   A. Bradycardia
   B. Hypercalcemia
   C. Palpitations
   D. Diarrhea

6. Which of the following tocolytic agents works by reducing the production of prostaglandins?
   A. Calcium channel blockers
   B. Nonsteroidal anti-inflammatory drugs
   C. β-Adrenergic agonists
   D. Magnesium sulfate

7. Which of the following tocolytic agents requires the nurse to closely monitor maternal lungs sounds, reflexes, and urine output?
   A. Calcium channel blockers
   B. Nonsteroidal anti-inflammatory drugs
   C. β-Adrenergic agonists
   D. Magnesium sulfate

8. All of the following is true about 17-alpha-hydroxyprogesterone caproate administration in preterm labor, except:
   A. It can be given intramuscularly or as a vaginal suppository
   B. It is given each week from 15 to 20 weeks' gestation until 36 weeks' gestation
   C. It is recommended for women who have had a previous preterm birth
   D. It is a naturally occurring metabolite of progesterone

9. Most women with premature rupture of membranes:
   A. Go on to deliver at term
   B. Deliver within a week of membrane rupture
   C. Can postpone delivery for 2 to 3 weeks with tocolytic therapy
   D. Deliver within 24 hours of membrane rupture

10. Antenatal corticosteroid therapy:
    A. Is most effective within the first 24 hours of administration
    B. Should be repeated every 2 weeks if the patient remains undelivered
    C. Is especially effective before 24 weeks' gestation
    D. Reduces the risk of neonatal intraventricular hemorrhage

Intrapartum Management Modules: A Perinatal Education Program
4th Edition

Module 8—Caring for the Woman at Risk for Preterm Labor or With Premature Rupture of Membranes
Nursing CE contact hours: 4.0
Fee: $32.95 (For every four tests submitted, get the lowest priced test for free. Submit all tests for $299, a savings of more than 50%.)

A. Last Name _____ First Name _____ MI _____

Address _____

City _____ State _____ Zip _____

Telephone _____ Fax number _____

E-mail _____

☐ Please check here to have your certificate faxed

State of Licensure #1 _____ License #1 Number _____

☐ LPN   ☐ RN   ☐ CNM   ☐ CNS   ☐ NP   ☐ Other _____

State of Licensure #2 _____ License #2 Number _____

☐ LPN   ☐ RN   ☐ CNM   ☐ CNS   ☐ NP   ☐ Other _____

State of Licensure #3 _____ License #3 Number _____

☐ LPN   ☐ RN   ☐ CNM   ☐ CNS   ☐ NP   ☐ Other _____

☐ From time to time, we make our mailing list available to outside organizations to announce special offers. Please check here if you do not wish us to release your name and address.

B. Test answers: Please record your answers by filling in the appropriate boxes.

	a	b	c	d
1.	☐	☐	☐	☐
2.	☐	☐	☐	☐
3.	☐	☐	☐	☐
4.	☐	☐	☐	☐
5.	☐	☐	☐	☐
6.	☐	☐	☐	☐
7.	☐	☐	☐	☐
8.	☐	☐	☐	☐
9.	☐	☐	☐	☐
10.	☐	☐	☐	☐

C. Course Evaluation
1. Did this CE activity's learning objectives relate to its general purpose? ☐ Yes ☐ No
2. Was this format an effective way to present the material? ☐ Yes ☐ No
3. Was the content relevant to your nursing practice? ☐ Yes ☐ No
4. How long did it take you to complete this CE activity? _____ Hours _____ Minutes
5. Suggestion for future topics_____

■ ■ ■ ■

INTRAPARTUM MANAGEMENT MODULES
MODULE 9
CARING FOR THE LABORING WOMAN WITH HYPERTENSIVE DISORDERS COMPLICATING PREGNANCY

General Purpose: To present registered professional nurses and other providers of women's health care with comprehensive guidelines for understanding, evaluating, and managing the hypertensive disorders that complicate pregnancy.

Objectives

After reading this module and taking this test, you will be able to:
1. Discuss principles or factors helpful for understanding hypertension during pregnancy
2. List guidelines essential for evaluating hypertension during pregnancy
3. Describe interventions for the pregnant woman with a hypertensive disorder

Directions

To earn continuing education credit, follow these instructions:
1. Read Module 9.
2. Complete the following posttest. Each question has only one answer. Choose the one that is best in each case and darken the box on the Enrollment Form (Section B).
3. Complete Section A and record your answers to the Evaluation Questions (Section C) on the Enrollment Form.
4. The passing score for this CE activity posttest is 7 correct answers (70%).
5. Registration deadline is May 25, 2010. After this date, please contact Lippincott Williams & Wilkins Continuing Education Department at 800-787-8985 for course renewal information.
6. Send the completed Enrollment Form with the appropriate fee (U.S. checks, money order, or Visa, Mastercard, or American Express credit card) to:

Lippincott Williams & Wilkins
Continuing Education Department
333 Seventh Avenue, 19th Floor
New York, NY 10001

1. A woman whose blood pressure rises to 140/90 mmHg after 20 weeks' gestation with no protein detected in her urine and whose blood pressure returns to baseline by the time she is 12 weeks' postpartum would probably be diagnosed as having:
   A. Gestational hypertension
   B. Chronic hypertension
   C. Preeclampsia
   D. Eclampsia

2. Mild preeclampsia is characterized by:
   A. More than 500 mg of protein in a 24-hour urine sample
   B. Weight gain of more than 2 pounds per week during the third trimester
   C. Infrequent seizures
   D. Two rises in blood pressure to 160/110 mmHg or higher in a 4-hour period

3. Hemolysis, elevated liver enzymes, and low platelets (HELLP) syndrome is most common:
   A. In primigravid women
   B. In African-American women

C. Late in the first and early in the second trimester
D. With cesarean delivery

4. Women with preeclampsia have a shift in the usual balances of vasoactive substances, with especially high levels of:
   A. Prostacyclin
   B. Angiotensin II
   C. Thromboxane
   D. Endothelin

5. When evaluating a pregnant woman's blood pressure, it is important to use which of the following guidelines?
   A. An elevated blood pressure reading on two occasions at least a week apart confirms gestational hypertension.
   B. A blood pressure of 140/90 mmHg or higher constitutes an abnormally high blood pressure with diagnostic significance during pregnancy.
   C. Common preference is to use an electronic device to measure blood pressure because of its increased accuracy, even in various positions.
   D. An elevation of 30 mmHg systolic or 15 mmHg diastolic over baseline constitutes an abnormally high blood pressure with diagnostic significance during pregnancy.

6. When checking for proteinuria, a false-positive value is likely when:
   A. Urine specific gravity is 1.030 or higher
   B. Urine pH is 8.0 or higher
   C. Urine specific gravity is less than 1.010
   D. Diluted urine is used

7. Management of preeclampsia includes all of the following except:
   A. Bed rest
   B. Magnesium sulfate to prevent seizures
   C. Evaluation by a clinician as often as twice per week
   D. Sodium restriction

8. The optimal resting position for a woman with severe preeclampsia is:
   A. Semirecumbent
   B. High Fowler's
   C. Supine
   D. Lateral Trendelenburg

9. Which of the following represents an appropriate guideline for administering magnesium sulfate?
   A. Mixing the drug in isotonic saline solution
   B. Giving a loading dose of 1 to 2 g
   C. Infusing the loading dose over 30 minutes
   D. Giving the drug at the rate of 1 g/min to stop a seizure

10. The drug of choice for treating seriously elevated maternal blood pressure near term is:
    A. Labetalol
    B. Calcium gluconate
    C. Hydralazine
    D. Nifedipine

LIPPINCOTT WILLIAMS & WILKINS
CONTINUING EDUCATION ENROLLMENT FORM

Intrapartum Management Modules: A Perinatal Education Program
4th Edition

Module 9—Caring for the Laboring Woman With Hypertensive Disorders Complicating Pregnancy
Nursing CE contact hours: 6.0
Fee: $44.95 (For every four tests submitted, get the lowest priced test for free. Submit all tests for $299, a savings of more than 50%.)

A. Last Name _____ First Name _____ MI _____

Address _____

City _____ State _____ Zip _____

Telephone _____ Fax number _____

E-mail _____

☐ Please check here to have your certificate faxed

State of Licensure #1 _____ License #1 Number _____

☐ LPN   ☐ RN   ☐ CNM   ☐ CNS   ☐ NP   ☐ Other _____

State of Licensure #2 _____ License #2 Number _____

☐ LPN   ☐ RN   ☐ CNM   ☐ CNS   ☐ NP   ☐ Other _____

State of Licensure #3 _____ License #3 Number _____

☐ LPN   ☐ RN   ☐ CNM   ☐ CNS   ☐ NP   ☐ Other _____

☐ From time to time, we make our mailing list available to outside organizations to announce special offers. Please check here if you do not wish us to release your name and address.

B. Test answers: Please record your answers by filling in the appropriate boxes.

	a	b	c	d
1.	☐	☐	☐	☐
2.	☐	☐	☐	☐
3.	☐	☐	☐	☐
4.	☐	☐	☐	☐
5.	☐	☐	☐	☐
6.	☐	☐	☐	☐
7.	☐	☐	☐	☐
8.	☐	☐	☐	☐
9.	☐	☐	☐	☐
10.	☐	☐	☐	☐

C. Course Evaluation
1. Did this CE activity's learning objectives relate to its general purpose? ☐ Yes ☐ No
2. Was this format an effective way to present the material? ☐ Yes ☐ No
3. Was the content relevant to your nursing practice? ☐ Yes ☐ No
4. How long did it take you to complete this CE activity? _____ Hours _____ Minutes
5. Suggestion for future topics_____

Continuing Education Posttests

■ ■ ■ ■

INTRAPARTUM MANAGEMENT MODULES
MODULE 10
CARING FOR THE LABORING WOMAN WITH HIV INFECTION OR AIDS

General Purpose: To present registered professional nurses and other providers of women's health care with an overview of HIV infection, specific guidelines for testing and managing HIV infection and preventing perinatal transmission.

Objectives
After reading this module and taking this test, you will be able to:
1. Discuss factors helpful for understanding HIV infection
2. Outline the criteria for identifying HIV infection
3. Describe interventions for an HIV-infected mother and her infant

Directions
To earn continuing education credit, follow these instructions:
1. Read Module 10.
2. Complete the following posttest. Each question has only one answer. Choose the one that is best in each case and darken the corresponding box on the Enrollment Form (Section B).
3. Complete Section A and record your answers to the Evaluation Questions (Section C) on the Enrollment Form.
4. The passing score for this CE activity posttest is 7 correct answers (70%).
5. Registration deadline is May 25, 2010. After this date, please contact Lippincott Williams & Wilkins Continuing Education Department at 800-787-8985 for course renewal information.
6. Send the completed Enrollment Form with the appropriate fee (U.S. checks, money order, or Visa, Mastercard, or American Express credit card) to:

Lippincott Williams & Wilkins
Continuing Education Department
333 Seventh Avenue, 19th Floor
New York, NY 10001

1. Replication of HIV includes which of the following steps?
   A. Viral DNA is released from the host lymphocyte surface.
   B. Transcription of viral RNA generates multiple copies of viral DNA.
   C. The virus' RNA is converted to DNA via reverse transcription.
   D. Viral RNA is incorporated into host RNA.

2. False-positive enzyme immunosorbent assay (EIA) results are common in people who:
   A. Have hemophilia
   B. Are in the first trimester of pregnancy
   C. Have diabetes
   D. Have never been pregnant

3. An acceptable sequence of confirming HIV infection is:
   A. A positive Western blot confirmed with a reactive EIA
   B. Two reactive EIAs followed by an indeterminate Western blot followed by a positive immunofluorescent antibody test
   C. A positive single-use diagnostic system (SUDS)
   D. A reactive EIA followed by a positive SUDS

4. HIV is transmitted via:
   A. Vaginal secretions
   B. Amniotic fluid
   C. Urine
   D. Cerebrospinal fluid

5. To reduce the risk of vertical transmission of HIV, which of the following is advised?
   A. Giving eye prophylaxis immediately as the infant is delivered
   B. Performing an episiotomy to prevent unexpected blood flow from a perineal tear
   C. Conducting internal fetal monitoring throughout labor
   D. Bathing the infant with soap and water before blood sampling

6. An HIV-infected pregnant woman with a high viral load can reduce her risk of vertical transmission from 25% to 2% with:
   A. Zidovudine (ZDV) therapy
   B. ZDV therapy and vaginal delivery without forceps and without an episiotomy
   C. ZDV therapy and cesarean section as soon as labor begins
   D. ZDV therapy and cesarean section before labor and with amniotic membranes intact

7. All of the following vaccines are considered safe for an HIV-infected pregnant woman except:
   A. The hepatitis B series
   B. The pneumococcal vaccine
   C. Measles/mumps/rubella (MMR)
   D. *Haemophilus influenzae* type B (Hib)

8. Which of the following is recommended for infants of HIV-infected women?
   A. *Pneumocystis carinii* prophylaxis at birth and before initiation of ZDV therapy
   B. A baseline complete blood count with differential just after initiation of ZDV therapy
   C. *Pneumocystis carinii* prophylaxis at 12 weeks of age
   D. Hemoglobin measurements at the completion of ZDV therapy and again at 12 weeks of age

9. Which of the following is used to diagnose HIV infection in the infant of an HIV-infected mother?
   A. Western blot
   B. Serial EIAs
   C. DNA polymerase chain reaction
   D. Maternal HIV antibodies in the infant's blood

10. When caring for an HIV-infected woman during delivery and the postpartum period, you would:
    A. Promote maternal-infant contact as soon as possible after delivery
    B. Encourage the mother to breastfeed to foster maternal-infant bonding
    C. Discourage family participation in the birth to reduce the risk of opportunistic infection
    D. Plan your interventions carefully to minimize contact with the mother to reduce your risk of occupational exposure

LIPPINCOTT WILLIAMS & WILKINS
CONTINUING EDUCATION ENROLLMENT FORM

Intrapartum Management Modules: A Perinatal Education Program
4th Edition

Module 10—Caring for the Laboring Woman With HIV Infection or AIDS
Nursing CE contact hours: 5.0
Fee: $38.95 (For every four tests submitted, get the lowest priced test for free. Submit all tests for $299, a savings of more than 50%.)

A. Last Name _____ First Name _____ MI _____

Address _____

City _____ State _____ Zip _____

Telephone _____ Fax number _____

E-mail _____

☐ Please check here to have your certificate faxed

State of Licensure #1 _____ License #1 Number _____

☐ LPN   ☐ RN   ☐ CNM   ☐ CNS   ☐ NP   ☐ Other _____

State of Licensure #2 _____ License #2 Number _____

☐ LPN   ☐ RN   ☐ CNM   ☐ CNS   ☐ NP   ☐ Other _____

State of Licensure #3 _____ License #3 Number _____

☐ LPN   ☐ RN   ☐ CNM   ☐ CNS   ☐ NP   ☐ Other _____

☐ From time to time, we make our mailing list available to outside organizations to announce special offers. Please check here if you do not wish us to release your name and address.

B. Test answers: Please record your answers by filling in the appropriate boxes.

	a	b	c	d
1.	☐	☐	☐	☐
2.	☐	☐	☐	☐
3.	☐	☐	☐	☐
4.	☐	☐	☐	☐
5.	☐	☐	☐	☐
6.	☐	☐	☐	☐
7.	☐	☐	☐	☐
8.	☐	☐	☐	☐
9.	☐	☐	☐	☐
10.	☐	☐	☐	☐

C. Course Evaluation
1. Did this CE activity's learning objectives relate to its general purpose? ☐ Yes ☐ No
2. Was this format an effective way to present the material? ☐ Yes ☐ No
3. Was the content relevant to your nursing practice? ☐ Yes ☐ No
4. How long did it take you to complete this CE activity? _____ Hours _____ Minutes
5. Suggestion for future topics_____

■ ■ ■ ■

INTRAPARTUM MANAGEMENT MODULES
MODULE 11
HEPATITIS INFECTIONS

General Purpose: To present registered professional nurses and other providers of women's health care with a detailed overview of viral hepatitis and specific guidelines for testing, managing hepatitis infection, and preventing mother-to-baby transmission.

Objectives
After reading this module and taking this test, you will be able to:
1. Discuss factors helpful for understanding viral hepatitis and distinguishing the five types
2. Outline the criteria for identifying hepatitis infection status
3. Discuss interventions for a hepatitis-infected mother and her baby

Directions
To earn continuing education credit, follow these instructions:
1. Read Module 11.
2. Complete the following posttest. Each question has only one answer. Choose the one that is best in each case and darken the box on the Enrollment Form (Section B).
3. Complete Section A and record your answers to the Evaluation Questions (Section C) on the Enrollment Form.
4. The passing score for this CE activity posttest is 7 correct answers (70%).
5. Registration deadline is May 25, 2010. After this date, please contact Lippincott Williams & Wilkins Continuing Education Department at 800-787-8985 for course renewal information.
6. Send the completed Enrollment Form with the appropriate fee (U.S. checks, money order, or Visa, Mastercard, or American Express credit card) to:

Lippincott Williams & Wilkins
Continuing Education Department
333 Seventh Avenue, 19th Floor
New York, NY 10001

1. Which of the following is a true statement about the danger of hepatitis infection during pregnancy and postpartum?
   A. Hepatitis B cannot be transmitted via breast milk.
   B. Hepatitis A is usually much more severe in pregnant women than it is in other individuals.
   C. Maternal antibodies to the hepatitis C virus protect the infant from transmission.
   D. Neonatal mortality is greater with hepatitis E than with any other type of viral hepatitis.

2. Hepatitis B e antigen (HBeAg):
   A. Is found only when the hepatitis B core antigen (HBcAg) is also found
   B. Reflects a high level of hepatitis B infectivity
   C. Seems to be derived from the hepatitis B surface antigen (HBsAg)
   D. Can be detected only through liver biopsy

3. Immunity to hepatitis B is indicated by the presence of:
   A. The antibody to the hepatitis B surface antigen (anti-HBs)
   B. The antibody to the hepatitis B core antigen (anti-HBc)
   C. The antibody to the hepatitis B e antigen (anti-HBe)
   D. The hepatitis B surface antigen (HBsAg)

4. Hepatitis B carriers:
   A. Represent about 25% of adults who acquired acute hepatitis B infection
   B. Always have symptoms intermittently
   C. Show evidence of viral infection on liver biopsy
   D. Can clear HBsAg from their blood despite high levels of anti-HBs

5. The risk of vertical transmission of hepatitis B during pregnancy is greatest when the mother becomes infected:
   A. During the first trimester
   B. During the second trimester
   C. During the third trimester
   D. At any time during the pregnancy because no single trimester increases the infant's risk

6. Maternal hepatitis B infection during pregnancy:
   A. Often goes unrecognized
   B. Results in jaundice and liver tenderness in most women
   C. Usually requires hospitalization and careful dietary restrictions
   D. Causes symptoms within 2 to 3 weeks of exposure

7. Hepatitis B vaccination tends to be less effective in pregnant women who are:
   A. In the third trimester
   B. Smokers
   C. Undernourished
   D. Younger than the age of 18 years

8. The best choice for conferring immediate passive immunity to someone who has had a significant exposure to the hepatitis B virus is:
   A. Recombivax HB
   B. Engerix-B
   C. Hepatitis B immune globulin (HBIG)
   D. A plasma-derived hepatitis B vaccine

9. After a hepatitis B series, boosters are recommended:
   A. After 10 years in all individuals
   B. For immunosuppressed individuals with low antibody titers
   C. For those who have responded adequately to the primary course
   D. For anyone who has since contracted another sexually transmitted disease

10. An infant born to a woman whose hepatitis B status cannot be immediately identified must be:
    A. Given HBIG and hepatitis B vaccine within 24 hours of delivery
    B. Breastfed to receive protection from maternal antibodies
    C. Given HBIG immediately and the hepatitis B vaccine within the first 3 months of life
    D. Considered a carrier

LIPPINCOTT WILLIAMS & WILKINS
CONTINUING EDUCATION ENROLLMENT FORM

Intrapartum Management Modules: A Perinatal Education Program
4th Edition

Module 11—Hepatitis Infections
Nursing CE contact hours: 6.0
Fee: $44.95 (For every four tests submitted, get the lowest priced test for free. Submit all tests for $299, a savings of more than 50%.)

A. Last Name _____ First Name _____ MI _____

Address _____

City _____ State _____ Zip _____

Telephone _____ Fax number _____

E-mail _____

☐ Please check here to have your certificate faxed

State of Licensure #1 _____ License #1 Number _____

☐ LPN   ☐ RN   ☐ CNM   ☐ CNS   ☐ NP   ☐ Other _____

State of Licensure #2 _____ License #2 Number _____

☐ LPN   ☐ RN   ☐ CNM   ☐ CNS   ☐ NP   ☐ Other _____

State of Licensure #3 _____ License #3 Number _____

☐ LPN   ☐ RN   ☐ CNM   ☐ CNS   ☐ NP   ☐ Other _____

☐ From time to time, we make our mailing list available to outside organizations to announce special offers. Please check here if you do not wish us to release your name and address.

B. Test answers: Please record your answers by filling in the appropriate boxes.

	a	b	c	d
1.	☐	☐	☐	☐
2.	☐	☐	☐	☐
3.	☐	☐	☐	☐
4.	☐	☐	☐	☐
5.	☐	☐	☐	☐
6.	☐	☐	☐	☐
7.	☐	☐	☐	☐
8.	☐	☐	☐	☐
9.	☐	☐	☐	☐
10.	☐	☐	☐	☐

C. Course Evaluation
1. Did this CE activity's learning objectives relate to its general purpose? ☐ Yes ☐ No
2. Was this format an effective way to present the material? ☐ Yes ☐ No
3. Was the content relevant to your nursing practice? ☐ Yes ☐ No
4. How long did it take you to complete this CE activity? _____ Hours _____ Minutes
5. Suggestion for future topics_____

■ ■ ■ ■

INTRAPARTUM MANAGEMENT MODULES
MODULE 12
CARING FOR THE PREGNANT WOMAN WITH DIABETES

General Purpose: To provide registered professional nurses and other providers of women's health care with information on diabetes during pregnancy, including the physiology, implications, screening guidelines, and management of mother and baby.

Objectives
After reading this module and taking this test, you will be able to:
1. Discuss factors helpful for understanding diabetes during pregnancy
2. Outline the risks to mother and baby, as well as screening recommendations for diabetes during pregnancy
3. Discuss interventions for the pregnant woman with diabetes and her baby

Directions
To earn continuing education credit, follow these instructions:
1. Read Module 12.
2. Complete the following posttest. Each question has only one answer. Choose the one that is best in each case and darken the box on the Enrollment Form (Section B).
3. Complete Section A and record your answers to the Evaluation Questions (Section C) on the Enrollment Form.
4. The passing score for this CE activity posttest is 7 correct answers (70%).
5. Registration deadline is May 25, 2010. After this date, please contact Lippincott Williams & Wilkins Continuing Education Department at 800-787-8985 for course renewal information.
6. Send the completed Enrollment Form with the appropriate fee (U.S. checks, money order, or Visa, Mastercard, or American Express credit card) to:

Lippincott Williams & Wilkins
Continuing Education Department
333 Seventh Avenue, 19th Floor
New York, NY 10001

1. Gestational diabetes is a result of:
   A. Increased insulin secretion
   B. Overeating during pregnancy
   C. Increased insulin resistance
   D. Decreasing levels of human placental lactogen

2. Diabetic women who become pregnant are most likely to have an increased need for insulin:
   A. At the beginning of the first trimester
   B. At the end of the first trimester
   C. During the second and third trimesters
   D. In the postpartum period

3. Which of the following is a true statement about diabetic nephropathy during pregnancy?
   A. Nephropathy with hypertension can lead to macrosomia.
   B. The incidence of preeclampsia is increased if the woman has nephropathy.

C. Progression toward renal failure always accelerates with pregnancy.
D. Even without hypertension, nephropathy usually has a profound adverse effect on the fetus.

4. The most common cause of diabetic ketoacidosis in pregnancy is:
   A. Preeclampsia
   B. Infection
   C. Multiparity
   D. Polyhydramnios

5. Maternal hyperglycemia results in fetal:
   A. Distress
   B. Hypotension
   C. Hypoglycemia
   D. Hyperinsulinism

6. A neonate born to a diabetic mother is at risk for:
   A. Hypoglycemia, typically 6 to 12 hours after birth
   B. Hypoglycemia, typically 24 to 48 hours after birth
   C. Hyperglycemia, typically 6 to 12 hours after birth
   D. Hyperglycemia, typically 24 to 48 hours after birth

7. To control maternal blood glucose levels during delivery, which of the following is recommended?
   A. Increasing the woman's morning dose of insulin
   B. Infusing regular insulin to maintain a maternal glucose level at approximately 100 mg/dL
   C. Infusing only isotonic saline or lactated Ringer's throughout delivery
   D. Adding a long-acting insulin to the usual morning insulin regimen

8. When breastfeeding her infant, a mother with diabetes is likely to experience:
   A. A sudden steady increase in blood glucose over time
   B. An increased need for insulin
   C. Good glycemic control with oral hypoglycemic agents
   D. Episodes of hypoglycemia during a typical nursing session

9. Which of the following statements about screening for gestational diabetes is true?
   A. Screening is routinely recommended for all pregnant women at the initial visit.
   B. Screening with a 1-hour glucose challenge test is recommended between 24 and 28 weeks' gestation.
   C. Screening with a 3-hour glucose tolerance test is recommended between 18 and 28 weeks' gestation.
   D. Screening is routinely recommended for all underweight pregnant women older than the age of 30 years.

10. Infants of diabetic mothers are especially at risk for shoulder dystocia when:
    A. The first stage of labor is prolonged
    B. It is a preterm delivery
    C. The mother is a primigravida
    D. The baby is macrosomic

LIPPINCOTT WILLIAMS & WILKINS
CONTINUING EDUCATION ENROLLMENT FORM

Intrapartum Management Modules: A Perinatal Education Program
4th Edition

Module 12—Caring for the Pregnant Woman With Diabetes
Nursing CE contact hours: 4.0
Fee: $32.95 (For every four tests submitted, get the lowest priced test for free. Submit all tests for $299, a savings of more than 50%.)

A. Last Name _____ First Name _____ MI _____

Address _____

City _____ State _____ Zip _____

Telephone _____ Fax number _____

E-mail _____

☐ Please check here to have your certificate faxed

State of Licensure #1 _____ License #1 Number _____

☐ LPN   ☐ RN   ☐ CNM   ☐ CNS   ☐ NP   ☐ Other _____

State of Licensure #2 _____ License #2 Number _____

☐ LPN   ☐ RN   ☐ CNM   ☐ CNS   ☐ NP   ☐ Other _____

State of Licensure #3 _____ License #3 Number _____

☐ LPN   ☐ RN   ☐ CNM   ☐ CNS   ☐ NP   ☐ Other _____

☐ From time to time, we make our mailing list available to outside organizations to announce special offers. Please check here if you do not wish us to release your name and address.

B. Test answers: Please record your answers by filling in the appropriate boxes.

	a	b	c	d
1.	☐	☐	☐	☐
2.	☐	☐	☐	☐
3.	☐	☐	☐	☐
4.	☐	☐	☐	☐
5.	☐	☐	☐	☐
6.	☐	☐	☐	☐
7.	☐	☐	☐	☐
8.	☐	☐	☐	☐
9.	☐	☐	☐	☐
10.	☐	☐	☐	☐

C. Course Evaluation
1. Did this CE activity's learning objectives relate to its general purpose? ☐ Yes ☐ No
2. Was this format an effective way to present the material? ☐ Yes ☐ No
3. Was the content relevant to your nursing practice? ☐ Yes ☐ No
4. How long did it take you to complete this CE activity? _____ Hours _____ Minutes
5. Suggestion for future topics_____

Continuing Education Posttests

■ ■ ■ ■

INTRAPARTUM MANAGEMENT MODULES
MODULE 13
DELIVERY IN THE ABSENCE OF A PRIMARY CARE PROVIDER

General Purpose: To present registered professional nurses and other providers of women's health care with detailed guidelines for managing an unexpected delivery in the absence of a primary care provider.

Objectives

After reading this module and taking this test, you will be able to:

1. List the signs of imminent delivery and plan appropriate interventions for safe delivery
2. Describe the appropriate actions for handling at least two potential problems during delivery

Directions

To earn continuing education credit, follow these instructions:

1. Read Module 13.
2. Complete the following posttest. Each question has only one answer. Choose the one that is best in each case and darken the box on the Enrollment Form (Section B).
3. Complete Section A and record your answers to the Evaluation Questions (Section C) on the Enrollment Form.
4. The passing score for this CE activity posttest is 7 correct answers (70%).
5. Registration deadline is May 25, 2010. After this date, please contact Lippincott Williams & Wilkins Continuing Education Department at 800-787-8985 for course renewal information.
6. Send the completed Enrollment Form with the appropriate fee (U.S. checks, money order, or Visa, Mastercard, or American Express credit card) to:

Lippincott Williams & Wilkins
Continuing Education Department
333 Seventh Avenue, 19th Floor
New York, NY 10001

1. A sign of impending delivery is:
   A. Spontaneous amniotic membrane rupture
   B. Anal bulging
   C. Strong, regular contractions
   D. Panting respirations

2. You would instruct a woman about to deliver to "feather blow" to help:
   A. Increase intra-abdominal pressure
   B. Her control her urge to push
   C. Enhance her uterine contractions
   D. Improve her oxygenation

3. After the baby's head is delivered and before the shoulders are delivered, you would first:
   A. Suction the baby's oropharynx
   B. Stimulate respirations
   C. Suction the baby's nasopharynx
   D. Have the mother push

4. You would manage shoulder dystocia by:
   A. Placing the mother in an upright position
   B. Applying suprapubic pressure from the side opposite the fetal back
   C. Having two attendants pull back on the mother's legs to sharply flex her knees and hips
   D. Trying to manipulate the baby so that the shoulders are in an anteroposterior position

5. If you suspect a hematoma in the perineal area, you would:
   A. Apply firm pressure to the area
   B. Reduce the infusion rate to just enough to keep the vein "open"
   C. Massage the fundus
   D. Take and record the patient's blood pressure and pulse

6. For an unexpected delivery of an infant with a breech presentation, you would:
   A. Maintain a firm hold on the infant's abdomen until the head is delivered
   B. Use a towel to lift the body after the shoulders are delivered
   C. Keep the baby's head flexed using suprapubic pressure
   D. Lower the baby's body to deliver the shoulders

7. If the amniotic membranes do not rupture spontaneously, you would:
   A. Rupture them when the head crowns
   B. Attempt delivery with the membranes intact
   C. Rupture them as the head is delivered
   D. Rupture them before active labor begins

8. If the umbilical cord is tightly wrapped around the baby's neck, you would:
   A. Try to force a loop of cord down over the head
   B. Leave it alone until the baby is delivered and remove it then
   C. Clamp the cord and deliver the baby, then cut the cord
   D. Apply two clamps 1 inch apart, cut the cord between them, and loosen the cord

9. Between delivery of the anterior and the posterior shoulder, you would:
   A. Apply upward, outward traction to the head
   B. Apply upward, inward traction to the head
   C. Apply downward, outward traction to the head
   D. Apply downward, inward traction to the head

10. As you deliver the placenta, you would:
    A. Massage the fundus vigorously
    B. Exert gentle downward traction on the cord
    C. Tug firmly on the cord once you see a gush of blood
    D. Instruct the mother to avoid bearing down

LIPPINCOTT WILLIAMS & WILKINS
CONTINUING EDUCATION ENROLLMENT FORM

Intrapartum Management Modules: A Perinatal Education Program
4th Edition

Module 13—Delivery in the Absence of a Primary Care Provider
Nursing CE contact hours: 2.5
Fee: $24.95 (For every four tests submitted, get the lowest priced test for free. Submit all tests for $299, a savings of more than 50%.)

A. Last Name _____ First Name _____ MI _____

Address _____

City _____ State _____ Zip _____

Telephone _____ Fax number _____

E-mail _____

☐ Please check here to have your certificate faxed

State of Licensure #1 _____ License #1 Number _____

☐ LPN   ☐ RN   ☐ CNM   ☐ CNS   ☐ NP   ☐ Other _____

State of Licensure #2 _____ License #2 Number _____

☐ LPN   ☐ RN   ☐ CNM   ☐ CNS   ☐ NP   ☐ Other _____

State of Licensure #3 _____ License #3 Number _____

☐ LPN   ☐ RN   ☐ CNM   ☐ CNS   ☐ NP   ☐ Other _____

☐ From time to time, we make our mailing list available to outside organizations to announce special offers. Please check here if you do not wish us to release your name and address.

B. Test answers: Please record your answers by filling in the appropriate boxes.

	a	b	c	d
1.	☐	☐	☐	☐
2.	☐	☐	☐	☐
3.	☐	☐	☐	☐
4.	☐	☐	☐	☐
5.	☐	☐	☐	☐
6.	☐	☐	☐	☐
7.	☐	☐	☐	☐
8.	☐	☐	☐	☐
9.	☐	☐	☐	☐
10.	☐	☐	☐	☐

C. Course Evaluation

1. Did this CE activity's learning objectives relate to its general purpose? ☐ Yes ☐ No
2. Was this format an effective way to present the material? ☐ Yes ☐ No
3. Was the content relevant to your nursing practice? ☐ Yes ☐ No
4. How long did it take you to complete this CE activity? _____ Hours _____ Minutes
5. Suggestion for future topics_____

■ ■ ■ ■

Continuing Education Posttests

INTRAPARTUM MANAGEMENT MODULES
MODULE 14
ASSESSMENT OF THE NEWBORN AND NEWLY DELIVERED MOTHER

General Purpose: To present registered professional nurses and other providers of women's health care with detailed guidelines for assessing the mother and her baby immediately after delivery.

Objectives
After reading this module and taking this test, you will be able to:
1. Describe assessment parameters for the infant immediately after delivery and plan appropriate interventions
2. Describe assessment parameters for the mother immediately after delivery and plan appropriate interventions
3. Discuss key aspects of infant and mother care after delivery

Directions
To earn continuing education credit, follow these instructions:
1. Read Module 14.
2. Complete the following posttest. Each question has only one answer. Choose the one that is best in each case and darken the corresponding box on the Enrollment Form (Section B).
3. Complete Section A and record your answers to the Evaluation Questions (Section C) on the Enrollment Form.
4. The passing score for this CE activity posttest is 7 correct answers (70%).
5. Registration deadline is May 25, 2010. After this date, please contact Lippincott Williams & Wilkins Continuing Education Department at 800-787-8985 for course renewal information.
6. Send the completed Enrollment Form with the appropriate fee (U.S. checks, money order, or Visa, Mastercard, or American Express credit card) to:

Lippincott Williams & Wilkins
Continuing Education Department
333 Seventh Avenue, 19th Floor
New York, NY 10001

1. A recommended stimulus for evaluating a newborn's reflexes for Apgar scoring is:
   A. Tapping the sole of the infant's foot
   B. Slapping the infant on the buttocks
   C. Pricking the heel for a capillary blood specimen
   D. Taking a rectal temperature

2. The 1-minute Apgar score of an infant with a heart rate of 120 bpm, a sporadic respiratory effort, a grimace response to a catheter placed in the nares, some extremity flexion, and who is mostly pinkish with blue extremities is:
   A. 4
   B. 5
   C. 6
   D. 7

3. Some degree of resuscitation is usually indicated when an infant's Apgar score is below:
   A. 10
   B. 9
   C. 8
   D. 7

4. Cord compression just before delivery is most likely to cause which of the following in the infant?
   A. Respiratory acidosis
   B. Metabolic acidosis
   C. Respiratory alkalosis
   D. Mixed acidosis

5. The appropriate procedure for assessing the fundus after delivery includes:
   A. Cupping your hand and applying pressure just above the symphysis pubis
   B. Starting palpation at midline well above the umbilicus
   C. Calculating fundal height in fingerbreadths above or below the symphysis pubis
   D. Starting palpation at midline just below the umbilicus

6. Normal lochia immediately after delivery should be:
   A. Brown and scant
   B. Red and flowing lightly
   C. Red and flowing moderately
   D. Red and flowing heavily

7. When evaluating fundal height, it is helpful to understand that the fundus:
   A. Might be displaced to one side if the baby was unusually large
   B. Should be at the level of the umbilicus on the second postpartum day
   C. Should be at the level of the symphysis pubis about 5 days after delivery
   D. Might be higher than usual if the uterus contains multiple blood clots

8. Guidelines for assisting with breastfeeding include:
   A. Not initiating breastfeeding until several hours after delivery to be sure the infant is able to suck and to swallow water
   B. Positioning the mother so that she is semireclining
   C. Making sure the mother always begins with the same breast
   D. Encouraging the mother to breastfeed her infant as often as every 2 to 3 hours initially

9. Breastfeeding is contraindicated for women who:
   A. Are recovering from spinal anesthesia
   B. Have preeclampsia
   C. Are HIV positive
   D. Have a boggy uterus

10. When assisting parents whose infant has died, it is helpful to:
    A. Save any declined mementos of the infant in case the parents request them weeks or months later
    B. Dissuade them from holding the child's body for more than a few minutes
    C. Spend as little time as possible with the family, even if asked to stay, so that they can better share their grief with each other privately
    D. Repress one's own feelings about perinatal loss to better focus on the situation at hand

LIPPINCOTT WILLIAMS & WILKINS
CONTINUING EDUCATION ENROLLMENT FORM

Intrapartum Management Modules: A Perinatal Education Program
4th Edition

Module 14—Assessment of the Newborn and Newly Delivered Mother
Nursing CE contact hours: 4.0
Fee: $32.95 (For every four tests submitted, get the lowest priced test for free. Submit all tests for $299, a savings of more than 50%.)

A. Last Name _____ First Name _____ MI _____

   Address _____

   City _____ State _____ Zip _____

   Telephone _____ Fax number _____

   E-mail _____

   ☐ Please check here to have your certificate faxed

   State of Licensure #1 _____ License #1 Number _____

   ☐ LPN   ☐ RN   ☐ CNM   ☐ CNS   ☐ NP   ☐ Other _____

   State of Licensure #2 _____ License #2 Number _____

   ☐ LPN   ☐ RN   ☐ CNM   ☐ CNS   ☐ NP   ☐ Other _____

   State of Licensure #3 _____ License #3 Number _____

   ☐ LPN   ☐ RN   ☐ CNM   ☐ CNS   ☐ NP   ☐ Other _____

   ☐ From time to time, we make our mailing list available to outside organizations to announce special offers. Please check here if you
      do not wish us to release your name and address.

B. **Test answers:** Please record your answers by filling in the appropriate boxes.

	a	b	c	d
1.	☐	☐	☐	☐
2.	☐	☐	☐	☐
3.	☐	☐	☐	☐
4.	☐	☐	☐	☐
5.	☐	☐	☐	☐
6.	☐	☐	☐	☐
7.	☐	☐	☐	☐
8.	☐	☐	☐	☐
9.	☐	☐	☐	☐
10.	☐	☐	☐	☐

C. **Course Evaluation**
1. Did this CE activity's learning objectives relate to its general purpose? ☐ Yes ☐ No
2. Was this format an effective way to present the material? ☐ Yes ☐ No
3. Was the content relevant to your nursing practice? ☐ Yes ☐ No
4. How long did it take you to complete this CE activity? _____ Hours _____ Minutes
5. Suggestion for future topics_____

Continuing Education Posttests

■ ■ ■ ■

INTRAPARTUM MANAGEMENT MODULES
MODULE 15
LIABILITY ISSUES IN INTRAPARTUM NURSING

General Purpose: To present registered professional nurses and other providers of women's health care with an overview of liability issues as they apply to perinatal care.

Objectives

After reading this module and taking this test, you will be able to:
1. Discuss principles relating to the process of obtaining informed consent
2. Define the standards that apply to counseling a patient about the risks and outcomes of treatment
3. Outline legal requirements for medical documentation

Directions

To earn continuing education credit, follow these instructions:
1. Read Module 15.
2. Complete the following posttest. Each question has only one answer. Choose the one that is best in each case and darken the box on the Enrollment Form (Section B).
3. Complete Section A and record your answers to the Evaluation Questions (Section C) on the Enrollment Form.
4. The passing score for this CE activity posttest is 7 correct answers (70%).
5. Registration deadline is May 25, 2010. After this date, please contact Lippincott Williams & Wilkins Continuing Education Department at 800-787-8985 for course renewal information.
6. Send the completed Enrollment Form with the appropriate fee (U.S. checks, money order, or Visa, Mastercard, or American Express credit card) to:

Lippincott Williams & Wilkins
Continuing Education Department
333 Seventh Avenue, 19th Floor
New York, NY 10001

1. The essential components of informed consent are:
   A. Condition, information, and voluntariness
   B. Capacity, information, and permission
   C. Emancipation, information, and permission
   D. Capacity, information, and voluntariness

2. In most states, all of the following qualify a person for emancipated status EXCEPT:
   A. Getting married
   B. Becoming orphaned
   C. Becoming a parent
   D. Becoming financially independent

3. A patient's need for information about risks specifically related to that particular individual's lifestyle is considered the:
   A. Subjective patient standard
   B. Professional standard
   C. Objective patient standard
   D. Reasonable patient standard

4. A patient's need for information about risks and expected outcomes for that patient is considered the:
   A. Subjective patient standard
   B. Professional standard
   C. Objective patient standard
   D. Reasonable patient standard

5. The informed refusal is:
   A. A patient's decision not to receive treatment
   B. Information given to the patient about that patient's risk when declining to receive treatment or testing
   C. A health care provider's decision not to offer a patient a specific treatment or test
   D. A family's decision to override a patient's wish for a specific treatment

6. Which of the following is a true statement about informed consent?
   A. Written consent must be obtained for every patient contact.
   B. Consent is necessary only for major procedures, such as surgery.
   C. The components of informed consent must be integral to every patient contact.
   D. Written consent is especially necessary when the patient's health is rapidly deteriorating.

7. When an adult patient is comatose:
   A. Informed consent is not needed
   B. Family members may give consent
   C. A cohabitating significant other may give consent
   D. The patient's attorney may give consent

8. When a patient questions the advisability of having a surgical procedure done, the person responsible for answering the patient's questions is:
   A. The nurse
   B. The nurse practitioner
   C. The physician
   D. Any licensed health care professional

9. The correct procedure for correcting an error in a medical chart is:
   A. Erasing the error or obscuring it with liquid correction fluid, writing in the correct information over the error, and writing in the date and time and initialing it
   B. Drawing a line through the error, writing in the correct information just above the crossed-out information, and writing in the date and time and initialing it
   C. Erasing the error or obscuring it with liquid correction fluid, writing in the date and time and initialing it, and entering the new material as an addendum in the next available space
   D. Drawing a line through the error, writing in the date and time and initialing it, and entering the new material as an addendum in the next available space

10. Countersigning another person's charting means that you:
    A. Also provided the documented care to that patient
    B. Approved the care that person gave
    C. Are passing no judgment on that person's care or documentation but are just following your institution's policies
    D. Carry no legal responsibility for that person's actions

LIPPINCOTT WILLIAMS & WILKINS
CONTINUING EDUCATION ENROLLMENT FORM

Intrapartum Management Modules: A Perinatal Education Program
4th Edition

Module 15—Liability Issues in Intrapartum Nursing

Nursing CE contact hours: 3.5

Fee: $29.95 (For every four tests submitted, get the lowest priced test for free. Submit all tests for $299, a savings of more than 50%.)

A. Last Name _____ First Name _____ MI _____

Address _____

City _____ State _____ Zip _____

Telephone _____ Fax number _____

E-mail _____

☐ Please check here to have your certificate faxed

State of Licensure #1 _____ License #1 Number _____

☐ LPN   ☐ RN   ☐ CNM   ☐ CNS   ☐ NP   ☐ Other _____

State of Licensure #2 _____ License #2 Number _____

☐ LPN   ☐ RN   ☐ CNM   ☐ CNS   ☐ NP   ☐ Other _____

State of Licensure #3 _____ License #3 Number _____

☐ LPN   ☐ RN   ☐ CNM   ☐ CNS   ☐ NP   ☐ Other _____

☐ From time to time, we make our mailing list available to outside organizations to announce special offers. Please check here if you do not wish us to release your name and address.

B. Test answers: Please record your answers by filling in the appropriate boxes.

	a	b	c	d
1.	☐	☐	☐	☐
2.	☐	☐	☐	☐
3.	☐	☐	☐	☐
4.	☐	☐	☐	☐
5.	☐	☐	☐	☐
6.	☐	☐	☐	☐
7.	☐	☐	☐	☐
8.	☐	☐	☐	☐
9.	☐	☐	☐	☐
10.	☐	☐	☐	☐

C. Course Evaluation

1. Did this CE activity's learning objectives relate to its general purpose? ☐ Yes ☐ No
2. Was this format an effective way to present the material? ☐ Yes ☐ No
3. Was the content relevant to your nursing practice? ☐ Yes ☐ No
4. How long did it take you to complete this CE activity? _____ Hours _____ Minutes
5. Suggestion for future topics_____

Continuing Education Posttests

■ ■ ■ ■

INTRAPARTUM MANAGEMENT MODULES
MODULE 16
MATERNAL TRANSPORT

General Purpose: To present registered professional nurses and other providers of women's health care with detailed guidelines for maternal transport to a regional perinatal center.

Objectives

After reading this module and taking this test, you will be able to:

1. Outline the indications and contraindications for maternal transport to a regional center
2. Describe three interventions for the high-risk mother and her infant

Directions

To earn continuing education credit, follow these instructions:

1. Read Module 16.
2. Complete the following posttest. Each question has only one answer. Choose the one that is best in each case and darken the corresponding box on the Enrollment Form (Section B).
3. Complete Section A and record your answers to the Evaluation Questions (Section C) on the Enrollment Form.
4. The passing score for this CE activity posttest is 7 correct answers (70%).
5. Registration deadline is May 25, 2010. After this date, please contact Lippincott Williams & Wilkins Continuing Education Department at 800-787-8985 for course renewal information.
6. Send the completed Enrollment Form with the appropriate fee (U.S. checks, money order, or Visa, Mastercard, or American Express credit card) to:

Lippincott Williams & Wilkins
Continuing Education Department
333 Seventh Avenue, 19th Floor
New York, NY 10001

1. Transferring a mother pregnant with an infant who is likely to require intensive care after delivery to a Level III regional center is most optimal:
   A. When delivery is not expected for the next 24 hours
   B. When delivery is expected within the next 6 hours
   C. When delivery is not expected within the next 48 hours
   D. Immediately after a postdelivery stabilization period

2. Transferring a mother who is in early labor and is expected to deliver a compromised neonate is best when:
   A. Delivery is anticipated within 3 hours
   B. Transport time is estimated to be 4 hours or less
   C. The family can transport the mother in a private vehicle
   D. Transport time is estimated to be 2 hours or less

3. Transport to a regional center should be deferred for a mother who:
   A. Has reached term and is 3 cm dilated
   B. Has mild preeclampsia
   C. Is in preterm labor and is 6 cm dilated
   D. Has placenta previa but is not bleeding

4. Which of the following circumstances is least likely to require maternal transport to a regional center?
   A. Preterm labor at 35 weeks' gestation with a fetus likely to weigh more than 2,000 g
   B. Preterm labor at 34 weeks' gestation with a fetus likely to weigh between 1,500 and 2,000 g
   C. Preterm labor at 33 weeks' gestation in a mother with poorly controlled diabetes mellitus
   D. Ruptured amniotic membranes at 33 weeks' gestation

5. A cyanotic neonate is most likely to have a cardiac abnormality when he or she:
   A. Has only peripheral cyanosis
   B. Also has significant respiratory distress
   C. Is term and is experiencing little respiratory distress
   D. Experiences a rise in PO2 while on 100% oxygen

6. A consensus panel sponsored by the National Institutes of Health concluded that corticosteroid therapy:
   A. Decreased the incidence of respiratory distress syndrome (RDS) in infants born between 24 and 28 weeks' gestation
   B. Decreased the severity of RDS in infants born between 24 and 28 weeks' gestation
   C. Decreased both the severity and the incidence of RDS in infants born between 24 and 28 weeks' gestation
   D. Decreased the severity of RDS only in infants born after 29 weeks' gestation

7. Current recommendations for corticosteroid therapy include:
   A. Giving repeat courses of betamethasone or dexamethasone over the entire month before delivery is anticipated
   B. Giving four doses of betamethasone intramuscularly 24 hours apart within 7 days of the anticipated delivery
   C. Giving two doses of dexamethasone intramuscularly 24 hours apart within 14 days of the anticipated delivery
   D. Giving two doses of betamethasone intramuscularly 24 hours apart within 7 days of the anticipated delivery

8. The most appropriate way to transport most women expected to deliver a compromised neonate is by:
   A. Ambulance
   B. Helicopter
   C. Private vehicle
   D. Fixed-wing aircraft

9. When the infant is in the neonatal intensive care unit, it is appropriate to:
   A. Restrict parental visits until the infant is stable
   B. Stay with the parents throughout all visits
   C. Have the attending neonatologist make all decisions about the infant's care
   D. Make sure the parents participate, even if minimally, in the infant's care during visits

10. During maternal transport, the patient should be positioned:
    A. Supine
    B. In high semi-Fowler's
    C. In Trendelenburg
    D. In a lateral position

Intrapartum Management Modules: A Perinatal Education Program
4th Edition

Module 16—Maternal Transport
Nursing CE contact hours: 3.0
Fee: $27.95 (For every four tests submitted, get the lowest priced test for free. Submit all tests for $299, a savings of more than 50%.)

A. Last Name _____ First Name _____ MI _____

Address _____

City _____ State _____ Zip _____

Telephone _____ Fax number _____

E-mail _____

☐ Please check here to have your certificate faxed

State of Licensure #1 _____ License #1 Number _____

☐ LPN ☐ RN ☐ CNM ☐ CNS ☐ NP ☐ Other _____

State of Licensure #2 _____ License #2 Number _____

☐ LPN ☐ RN ☐ CNM ☐ CNS ☐ NP ☐ Other _____

State of Licensure #3 _____ License #3 Number _____

☐ LPN ☐ RN ☐ CNM ☐ CNS ☐ NP ☐ Other _____

☐ From time to time, we make our mailing list available to outside organizations to announce special offers. Please check here if you do not wish us to release your name and address.

B. Test answers: Please record your answers by filling in the appropriate boxes.

	a	b	c	d
1.	☐	☐	☐	☐
2.	☐	☐	☐	☐
3.	☐	☐	☐	☐
4.	☐	☐	☐	☐
5.	☐	☐	☐	☐
6.	☐	☐	☐	☐
7.	☐	☐	☐	☐
8.	☐	☐	☐	☐
9.	☐	☐	☐	☐
10.	☐	☐	☐	☐

C. Course Evaluation
1. Did this CE activity's learning objectives relate to its general purpose? ☐ Yes ☐ No
2. Was this format an effective way to present the material? ☐ Yes ☐ No
3. Was the content relevant to your nursing practice? ☐ Yes ☐ No
4. How long did it take you to complete this CE activity? _____ Hours _____ Minutes
5. Suggestion for future topics_____

Continuing Education Posttests

■ ■ ■ ■

INTRAPARTUM MANAGEMENT MODULES
MODULE 17
INTIMATE PARTNER VIOLENCE DURING PREGNANCY

General Purpose: To present registered professional nurses and other providers of women's health care with detailed guidelines for understanding, evaluating and managing intimate partner violence during pregnancy.

Objectives

After reading the module and taking this test, you will be able to:
1. Discuss factors helpful for identifying pregnant victims of abuse
2. Outline risks of violence to both mother and baby, as well as screening recommendations for abuse during pregnancy
3. Describe appropriate responses and interventions for the pregnant victim of abuse

Directions

To earn continuing education credit, follow these instructions:
1. Read Module 17.
2. Complete the following posttest. Each question has only one answer. Choose the one that is best in each case and darken the corresponding box on the Enrollment Form (Section B).
3. Complete Section A and record your answers to the Evaluation Questions (Section C) on the Enrollment Form.
4. The passing score for this CE activity posttest is 7 correct answers (70%).
5. Registration deadline is May 25, 2010. After this date, please contact Lippincott Williams & Wilkins Continuing Education Department at 800-787-8985 for course renewal information.
6. Send the completed Enrollment Form with the appropriate fee (U.S. checks, money order, or Visa, Mastercard, or American Express credit card) to:

Lippincott Williams & Wilkins
Continuing Education Department
333 Seventh Avenue, 19th Floor
New York, NY 10001

1. Abuse of a pregnant woman by a known perpetrator is known as:
   A. Intimate partner violence
   B. Child abuse
   C. Elder abuse
   D. Assault

2. Pushing, slapping, restraining, and refusals of access to care are examples of:
   A. Sexual violence
   B. Psychological abuse
   C. Physical violence
   D. Control

3. Violence against a pregnant woman can best be characterized by which of the following statements?
   A. Violence against a woman ceases when she becomes pregnant.
   B. Violence during pregnancy is overestimated.
   C. Violence frequently begins or increases during pregnancy.
   D. Violence during pregnancy is common enough to warrant general screening.

4. Current research has demonstrated a higher prevalence of violence during pregnancy in which of the following groups of women?
   A. African-American women
   B. Adolescents
   C. Unmarried women
   D. Less than 12 years of completed schooling

5. The phase of the "cycle of violence" that is characterized by a compliant victim and increasing threats of harm, humiliation, or intimidation is known as the:
   A. Acute violence phase
   B. Reconciliation phase
   C. Honeymoon phase
   D. Tension-building phase

6. Upon assessment, a physical indicator of violence might include:
   A. Evasiveness in answering questions
   B. Displaying irrational jealousy
   C. Injuries to centrally located areas of the body
   D. Flat affect

7. To fulfill the essential components of screening for IPV, the nurse must complete all of the following except:
   A. Observation and documentation of behaviors of the mother and partner
   B. Review of the mother's history, medical and obstetrical
   C. Complete physical examination
   D. Questioning of the mother about abuse with documentation of response

8. If the pregnant woman discloses abuse, the nurse should first:
   A. Acknowledge the abuse to validate her concerns
   B. Assist with development of a safety plan
   C. Contact a social worker immediately
   D. Disclose personal experiences with abuse

9. Which of the following statements about disclosure and mandatory reporting of IPV during pregnancy is true?
   A. Mandatory reporting of IPV increases the rate of disclosure.
   B. A victim may not disclose abuse if she knows it will be reported in fear of retaliation.
   C. Mandatory reporting of IPV exists in all states.
   D. A victim must disclose abuse under mandatory reporting statutes.

10. Complete nursing documentation of IVP during pregnancy would include which of the following?
    A. Chief complaint and body map
    B. Referrals given, a safety plan, and reports made
    C. Statements about ongoing abuse, even if the woman denies it.
    D. Relevant history, assessment/procedure/lab results, and interventions

LIPPINCOTT WILLIAMS & WILKINS
CONTINUING EDUCATION ENROLLMENT FORM

Intrapartum Management Modules: A Perinatal Education Program
4th Edition

Module 17—Intimate Partner Violence During Pregnancy
Nursing CE contact hours: 2.5
Fee: $24.95 (For every four tests submitted, get the lowest priced test for free. Submit all tests for $299, a savings of more than 50%.)

A. Last Name _____ First Name _____ MI _____

Address _____

City _____ State _____ Zip _____

Telephone _____ Fax number _____

E-mail _____

☐ Please check here to have your certificate faxed

State of Licensure #1 _____ License #1 Number _____

☐ LPN   ☐ RN   ☐ CNM   ☐ CNS   ☐ NP   ☐ Other _____

State of Licensure #2 _____ License #2 Number _____

☐ LPN   ☐ RN   ☐ CNM   ☐ CNS   ☐ NP   ☐ Other _____

State of Licensure #3 _____ License #3 Number _____

☐ LPN   ☐ RN   ☐ CNM   ☐ CNS   ☐ NP   ☐ Other _____

☐ From time to time, we make our mailing list available to outside organizations to announce special offers. Please check here if you do not wish us to release your name and address.

B. Test answers: Please record your answers by filling in the appropriate boxes.

	a	b	c	d
1.	☐	☐	☐	☐
2.	☐	☐	☐	☐
3.	☐	☐	☐	☐
4.	☐	☐	☐	☐
5.	☐	☐	☐	☐
6.	☐	☐	☐	☐
7.	☐	☐	☐	☐
8.	☐	☐	☐	☐
9.	☐	☐	☐	☐
10.	☐	☐	☐	☐

C. Course Evaluation
1. Did this CE activity's learning objectives relate to its general purpose? ☐ Yes ☐ No
2. Was this format an effective way to present the material? ☐ Yes ☐ No
3. Was the content relevant to your nursing practice? ☐ Yes ☐ No
4. How long did it take you to complete this CE activity? _____ Hours _____ Minutes
5. Suggestion for future topics_____

Continuing Education Posttests

■ ■ ■ ■

INTRAPARTUM MANAGEMENT MODULES
MODULE 18
INTRAPARTUM EMERGENCIES

General Purpose: To present registered professional nurses and other providers of women's health care with detailed guidelines for understanding, evaluating and managing selected intrapartum emergencies.

Objectives

After reading the module and taking this test, you will be able to:

1. Discuss emergent complications during the intrapartum period, including prolapsed cord, shoulder dystocia, AFE, uterine rupture, postpartum hemorrhage, and placental abruption
2. Outline risk factors for prolapsed cord, shoulder dystocia, AFE, uterine rupture, postpartum hemorrhage, and placental abruption
3. Describe appropriate nursing responses and interventions during selected intrapartum emergencies including prolapsed cord, shoulder dystocia, AFE, uterine rupture, postpartum hemorrhage, and placental abruption

Directions

To earn continuing education credit, follow these instructions:

1. Read Module 18.
2. Complete the following posttest. Each question has only one answer. Choose the one that is best in each case and darken the corresponding box on the Enrollment Form (Section B).
3. Complete Section A and record your answers to the Evaluation Questions (Section C) on the Enrollment Form.
4. The passing score for this CE activity posttest is 7 correct answers (70%).
5. Registration deadline is May 25, 2010. After this date, please contact Lippincott Williams & Wilkins Continuing Education Department at 800-787-8985 for course renewal information.
6. Send the completed Enrollment Form with the appropriate fee (U.S. checks, money order, or Visa, Mastercard, or American Express credit card) to:

Lippincott Williams & Wilkins
Continuing Education Department
333 Seventh Avenue, 19th Floor
New York, NY 10001

1. Upon doing a vaginal examination, you determine that there is a prolapsed umbilical cord. Your first action should be to:
   A. Give the mother oxygen
   B. Help the mother into a knee-chest position
   C. Notify the primary care provider
   D. Cover the cord with a sterile pad soaked with saline solution

2. When a prolapsed cord extends outside the mother's vagina, you should:
   A. Clamp the cord
   B. Reposition the cord
   C. Cover the cord with saline-soaked gauze
   D. Reinsert the cord

3. The first nursing response to a shoulder dystocia should be:
   A. Fundal pressure
   B. Empty the maternal bladder
   C. McRobert's maneuver with suprapubic pressure
   D. Alert anesthesia for operative delivery

4. The most common sign of an amniotic fluid embolism is:
   A. Headache
   B. Seizure
   C. Hypertension
   D. Cardiopulmonary collapse

5. The hallmark sign of placental abruption is:
   A. Painless, bright red vaginal bleeding
   B. Fetal tachycardia
   C. Rigid, board-like abdomen, vaginal bleeding
   D. Absence of uterine contractions

6. If symptoms of placental abruption are mild, the FHR tracing is reassuring, and the fetus is preterm, the most likely management course will be:
   A. Bed rest, corticosteroids, close fetal and maternal assessment
   B. Immediate cesarean delivery
   C. Administration of oxygen, anticipate central line placement
   D. Preparation for a vaginal delivery and a high-risk newborn

7. Uterine rupture is most commonly associated with:
   A. Trauma from a motor vehicle crash
   B. Vaginal birth after cesarean
   C. Shoulder dystocia
   D. Placenta previa

8. If the fetal monitor tracing demonstrates a non reassuring fetal heart rate pattern with a sudden change in uterine activity, the nurse may suspect:
   A. Uterine rupture
   B. Impending postpartum hemorrhage
   C. Placenta accreta
   D. Cord prolapse

9. You might anticipate a postpartum hemorrhage in which of the following laboring mothers?
   A. 28-year-old gravida 1, laboring for 18 hours
   B. 40-year-old gravida 6, vaginal delivery of twins, with a manual removal of the placenta
   C. 36-year-old gravida 2, 6-hour labor augmented with oxytocin
   D. 30-year-old gravida 3, vacuum-assisted vaginal delivery after 5-hour labor

10. If a mother is experiencing an immediate postpartum hemorrhage due to uterine atony, the nurse's first action should be:
    A. Placement of an IV catheter
    B. Uterine massage
    C. Administration of methergine
    D. Examination for lacerations

LIPPINCOTT WILLIAMS & WILKINS
CONTINUING EDUCATION ENROLLMENT FORM

Intrapartum Management Modules: A Perinatal Education Program
4th Edition

Module 18—Intrapartum Emergencies

Nursing CE contact hours: 3.0

Fee: $27.95 (For every four tests submitted, get the lowest priced test for free. Submit all tests for $299, a savings of more than 50%.)

A. Last Name _____ First Name _____ MI _____

Address _____

City _____ State _____ Zip _____

Telephone _____ Fax number _____

E-mail _____

☐ Please check here to have your certificate faxed

State of Licensure #1 _____ License #1 Number _____

☐ LPN   ☐ RN   ☐ CNM   ☐ CNS   ☐ NP   ☐ Other _____

State of Licensure #2 _____ License #2 Number _____

☐ LPN   ☐ RN   ☐ CNM   ☐ CNS   ☐ NP   ☐ Other _____

State of Licensure #3 _____ License #3 Number _____

☐ LPN   ☐ RN   ☐ CNM   ☐ CNS   ☐ NP   ☐ Other _____

☐ From time to time, we make our mailing list available to outside organizations to announce special offers. Please check here if you do not wish us to release your name and address.

B. Test answers: Please record your answers by filling in the appropriate boxes.

	a	b	c	d
1.	☐	☐	☐	☐
2.	☐	☐	☐	☐
3.	☐	☐	☐	☐
4.	☐	☐	☐	☐
5.	☐	☐	☐	☐
6.	☐	☐	☐	☐
7.	☐	☐	☐	☐
8.	☐	☐	☐	☐
9.	☐	☐	☐	☐
10.	☐	☐	☐	☐

C. Course Evaluation

1. Did this CE activity's learning objectives relate to its general purpose? ☐ Yes ☐ No
2. Was this format an effective way to present the material? ☐ Yes ☐ No
3. Was the content relevant to your nursing practice? ☐ Yes ☐ No
4. How long did it take you to complete this CE activity? _____ Hours _____ Minutes
5. Suggestion for future topics_____

■ ■ ■ ■

INTRAPARTUM MANAGEMENT MODULES
MODULE 19
CARING FOR THE WOMAN UNDERGOING
AN INSTRUMENTED OR OPERATIVE DELIVERY

General Purpose: To present registered professional nurses and other providers of women's health care with detailed guidelines and information for understanding, evaluating and managing women undergoing an instrumented or operative delivery.

Objectives
After reading the module and taking this test, you will be able to:
1. Discuss nursing implications for assisted birth.
2. Outline indications for cesarean birth.
3. Describe appropriate nursing actions in caring for women experiencing forceps assisted, vacuum assisted, or cesarean delivery.

Directions
To earn continuing education credit, follow these instructions:
1. Read Module 19.
2. Complete the following posttest. Each question has only one answer. Choose the one that is best in each case and darken the corresponding box on the Enrollment Form (Section B).
3. Complete Section A and record your answers to the Evaluation Questions (Section C) on the Enrollment Form.
4. The passing score for this CE activity posttest is 7 correct answers (70%).
5. Registration deadline is May 25, 2010. After this date, please contact Lippincott Williams & Wilkins Continuing Education Department at 800-787-8985 for course renewal information.
6. Send the completed Enrollment Form with the appropriate fee (U.S. checks, money order, or Visa, Mastercard, or American Express credit card) to:

Lippincott Williams & Wilkins
Continuing Education Department
333 Seventh Avenue, 19th Floor
New York, NY 10001

1. A vacuum-assisted birth is contraindicated in:
   A. A face or breech presentation
   B. Severe maternal or fetal compromise requiring rapid delivery
   C. Evidence of CPD
   D. All of the above

2. Shoulder dystocia is encountered more frequently with:
   A. Fetal malpresentation
   B. A vacuum-assisted birth
   C. A forceps-assisted birth
   D. A preterm birth

3. The nurse's role in a vacuum assisted birth is:
   A. Education and support
   B. To apply the vacuum
   C. The nurse does not have a role in a vacuum-assisted birth

4. A nursing consideration during an operative vaginal birth would be to:
   A. Place the mother in the lithotomy position
   B. Empty the mother's bladder
   C. Remind the mother to push with uterine contractions
   D. Ensure adequate pain relief for the mother
   E. All of the above

5. After a vacuum-assisted birth, a normal finding that the nurse may anticipate to find in the neonate is:
   A. Retinal hemorrhaging
   B. Cephalohematoma
   C. Caput succedaneum
   D. Blistering

6. Forceps are preferred over the use of a vacuum in which of the following situations?
   A. Delivering a preterm fetus
   B. Assisting the delivery of the fetal head in a breech delivery
   C. Delivering a fetus with cord prolapse in the second stage of labor
   D. All of the above

7. High forceps applications are used when:
   A. The leading part of the fetal head is at $+2$ station
   B. The fetal head is engaged but above $+2$ station
   C. The fetal head is visible at the vaginal introitus without separating the labia
   D. High forceps applications are no longer a part of current obstetric practice

8. Maternal medical indications for a cesarean birth include:
   A. Depression
   B. History of previous back surgery
   C. Hypertensive disorders
   D. Fear of vaginal birth

9. Maternal risks of cesarean birth include:
   A. Infection
   B. Hemorrhage
   C. Wound complications
   D. Increased costs
   E. All of the above

10. When a patient is being considered for a VBAC, which of the following are important considerations?
   A. Knowledge of prior uterine incisions
   B. Birth setting
   C. The patient's anticipated family size
   D. All of the above

LIPPINCOTT WILLIAMS & WILKINS
CONTINUING EDUCATION ENROLLMENT FORM

Intrapartum Management Modules: A Perinatal Education Program
4th Edition

Module 19—Caring for the Woman Undergoing an Instrumented or Operative Delivery
Nursing CE contact hours: 3.0
Fee: $27.95 (For every four tests submitted, get the lowest priced test for free. Submit all tests for $299, a savings of more than 50%.)

A. Last Name _____ First Name _____ MI _____

Address _____

City _____ State _____ Zip _____

Telephone _____ Fax number _____

E-mail _____

☐ Please check here to have your certificate faxed

State of Licensure #1 _____ License #1 Number _____

☐ LPN ☐ RN ☐ CNM ☐ CNS ☐ NP ☐ Other _____

State of Licensure #2 _____ License #2 Number _____

☐ LPN ☐ RN ☐ CNM ☐ CNS ☐ NP ☐ Other _____

State of Licensure #3 _____ License #3 Number _____

☐ LPN ☐ RN ☐ CNM ☐ CNS ☐ NP ☐ Other _____

☐ From time to time, we make our mailing list available to outside organizations to announce special offers. Please check here if you do not wish us to release your name and address.

B. Test answers: Please record your answers by filling in the appropriate boxes.

	a	b	c	d
1.	☐	☐	☐	☐
2.	☐	☐	☐	☐
3.	☐	☐	☐	☐
4.	☐	☐	☐	☐
5.	☐	☐	☐	☐
6.	☐	☐	☐	☐
7.	☐	☐	☐	☐
8.	☐	☐	☐	☐
9.	☐	☐	☐	☐
10.	☐	☐	☐	☐

C. Course Evaluation
1. Did this CE activity's learning objectives relate to its general purpose? ☐ Yes ☐ No
2. Was this format an effective way to present the material? ☐ Yes ☐ No
3. Was the content relevant to your nursing practice? ☐ Yes ☐ No
4. How long did it take you to complete this CE activity? _____ Hours _____ Minutes
5. Suggestion for future topics_____

■ ■ ■ ■